D1708170

Handbook of
Behavior Modification
with the
Mentally Retarded

SECOND EDITION

APPLIED CLINICAL PSYCHOLOGY

Series Editors:
Alan S. Bellack, *Medical College of Pennsylvania at EPPI, Philadelphia, Pennsylvania,*
and Michel Hersen, *University of Pittsburgh, Pittsburgh, Pennsylvania*

Current Volumes in this Series

THE AIDS HEALTH CRISIS
Psychological and Social Interventions
  Jeffrey A. Kelly and Janet S. St. Lawrence

BEHAVIORAL CONSULTATION AND THERAPY
  John R. Bergan and Thomas R. Kratochwill

BEHAVIORAL CONSULTATION IN APPLIED SETTINGS
An Individual Guide
  Thomas R. Kratochwill and John R. Bergan

HANDBOOK OF BEHAVIOR MODIFICATION WITH THE MENTALLY RETARDED
Second Edition
  Edited by Johnny L. Matson

HANDBOOK OF THE BRIEF PSYCHOTHERAPIES
  Edited by Richard A. Wells and Vincent J. Giannetti

HANDBOOK OF CLINICAL BEHAVIORAL PEDIATRICS
  Edited by Alan M. Gross and Ronald S. Drabman

HANDBOOK OF SEXUAL ASSAULT
Issues, Theories, and Treatment of the Offender
  Edited by W. L. Marshall, D. R. Laws, and H. E. Barbaree

HANDBOOK OF TREATMENT APPROACHES IN CHILDHOOD
PSYCHOPATHOLOGY
  Edited by Johnny L. Matson

PSYCHOLOGY
A Behavioral Overview
  Alan Poling, Henry Schlinger, Stephen Starin, and Elbert Blakely

A Continuation Order Plan is available for this series. A continuation order will bring delivery of each new volume immediately upon publication. Volumes are billed only upon actual shipment. For further information please contact the publisher.

Handbook of
Behavior Modification
with the
Mentally Retarded

SECOND EDITION

Edited by

Johnny L. Matson

Louisiana State University
Baton Rouge, Louisiana

Plenum Press · New York and London

Library of Congress Cataloging-in-Publication Data

Handbook of behavior modification with the mentally retarded / edited
by Johnny L. Matson. -- 2nd ed.
      p.   cm. -- (Applied clinical psychology)
   Includes bibliographical references.
   ISBN 0-306-43309-5
   1. Mentally handicapped--Rehabilitation. 2. Mentally handicapped
children--Rehabilitation. 3. Behavior modification.   I. Matson,
Johnny L. II. Series.
   [DNLM: 1. Behavior Therapy. 2. Mental Retardation-
-rehabilitation.   WM 308 H236]
RC570.2.H36 1990
616.85'8806--dc20
DNLM/DLC
for Library of Congress   89-23235
                                                              CIP

© 1990 Plenum Press, New York
A Division of Plenum Publishing Corporation
233 Spring Street, New York, N.Y. 10013

Printed in the United States of America

Contributors

MARTIN AGRAN, Department of Special Education, Utah State University, Logan, Utah 84322

BETSEY A. BENSON, Department of Psychology, University of Illinois at Chicago, Chicago, Illinois 60680

DIANE M. BROWDER, Department of Counseling Psychology, School Psychology, and Special Education, Lehigh University, Bethlehem, Pennsylvania 18015

JOSEPH A. BUCKHALT, Department of Counseling and Counseling Psychology, Auburn University, Auburn, Alabama 36849

VINCENT A. CAMPBELL, Department of Mental Health and Mental Retardation, 135 South Union Street, Montgomery, Alabama 36130

ENNIO CIPANI, Department of Special Education, University of the Pacific, Stockton, California 95211

CHRISTINE L. COLE, School Psychology Program, Lehigh University, Bethlehem, Pennsylvania 18015

JEFFREY S. DANFORTH, Department of Psychiatry, University of Massachusetts Medical School, 55 Lake Avenue North, Worcester, Massachusetts 01655

RONALD S. DRABMAN, Department of Psychiatry and Human Behavior, University of Mississippi Medical Center, 2500 North State Street, Jackson, Mississippi 39216

WILLIAM I. GARDNER, Behavioral Research Unit, Waisman Center on Mental Retardation and Human Development, University of Wisconsin, Madison, Wisconsin 53706

CAROLYN W. GREEN, Department of Psychology, Western Carolina Center, Enola Road, Morganton, North Carolina 28655

DONALD A. HANTULA, Department of Psychology, University of Notre Dame, Notre Dame, Indiana 46556

DINAH S. HENSARLING, Department of Psychology, Louisiana State University, Baton Rouge, Louisiana 70803

JAMES V. HUSCH, Department of Special Education, University of Colorado at Colorado Springs, Colorado Springs, Colorado 80933

RAMASAMY MANIKAM, Department of Psychology, Louisiana State University, Baton Rouge, Louisiana 70803

ALLEN G. MARCHETTI, Georgia Retardation Center, 4770 Peachtree Road N.E., Atlanta, Georgia 30338

JAMES E. MARTIN, Department of Special Education, University of Colorado at Colorado Springs, Colorado Springs, Colorado 80933

MARY MATESE, Department of Psychology, Louisiana State University, Baton Rouge, Louisiana 70803

JOHN R. McCARTNEY, Alabama Department of Mental Health and Mental Retardation, Applied Research Bureau, University of Alabama, Tuscaloosa, Alabama 35486

JAMES F. McCOY, Department of Psychology, Auburn University, Auburn, Alabama 36849

BARBARA EVANS McKINNEY, Shapiro Developmental Center, 100 East Jeffery Street, Kankakee, Illinois 60901

DENNIS E. MITHAUG, Department of Special Education, University of Colorado at Colorado Springs, Colorado Springs, Colorado 80933

JAMES A. MULICK, The Nisonger Center, Ohio State University, Columbus, Ohio 43201

JAMES T. NAPOLITAN, Ray Graham Association for the Handicapped, 420 West Madison Street, Elmhurst, Illinois 60126

DENNIS H. REID, Department of Psychology, Western Carolina Center, Enola Road, Morganton, North Carolina 28655

STEVEN REISS, Department of Psychology, University of Illinois at Chicago, Chicago, Illinois 60680

JOHANNES ROJAHN, The Nisonger Center, Ohio State University, Columbus, Ohio 43201

CAROLYN S. SCHROEDER, Department of Pediatrics, University of North Carolina, Chapel Hill, North Carolina 27514

STEPHEN R. SCHROEDER, The Nisonger Center, Ohio State University, Columbus, Ohio 43201

EDWARD S. SHAPIRO, Department of Counseling Psychology, School Psychology, and Special Education, Lehigh University, Bethlehem, Pennsylvania 18015

LORI A. SISSON, Western Psychiatric Institute and Clinic, University of Pittsburgh School of Medicine, Pittsburgh, Pennsylvania 15238

BRENDA H. SPENCE, Department of Psychology, University of Notre Dame, Notre Dame, Indiana 46556

MARIE E. TARAS, Department of Psychology, Louisiana State University, Baton Rouge, Louisiana 70803

RON VAN HOUTEN, Department of Psychology, Mount Saint Vincent University, Halifax, Nova Scotia B3M 2J6, Canada

PAUL WEISBERG, Department of Psychology, University of Alabama, Tuscaloosa, Alabama 35487

THOMAS L. WHITMAN, Department of Psychology, University of Notre Dame, Notre Dame, Indiana 46556

Preface to the Second Edition

The development of behavior modification principles and procedures and the ensuing research have had a dramatic impact on services for mentally retarded persons. This book is the second edition of a volume that is designed to update readers on some of these many developments. Although many of the chapter titles and authors from the first edition remain unchanged, we have added additional chapters to reflect new areas of research. The book is thus a critical review of this literature and, as such, provides essential and important notions about what we know and what can be done to expand our current knowledge. The authors of the chapters are all recognized experts who have been active in publishing in the research areas they critique. As a result, they have a good understanding of what are the major issues in the field. And because they are also active in service provision to persons with identified handicaps, their material will be especially useful to practitioners and, it is hoped, to those professionals who are working in the field in establishing data-based treatments.

One important change in the field has concerned the terminology used to describe handicapped persons. We are aware that persons with mental retardation are no longer referred to as "the mentally retarded," and although no disrespect is intended, for the sake of continuity the original title has been retained on the advice of the publisher.

It is hoped that this book will reflect the growing and quite exciting body of behavioral research for persons with handicaps. The book is therefore dedicated to all those we hope to assist in leading happier and more productive lives.

Finally, I would like to thank my wife Deann and my children Meggan and Michael for all their support, and Vetta M. Johnson for her fine secretarial assistance and good humor.

JOHNNY L. MATSON

Preface to the First Edition

The emphasis on habilitation of the mentally retarded in the last few years had led to a substantial increase in the amount of research devoted to training adaptive skills and reducing inappropriate behavior in this population. Behavior modification procedures have been the primary basis for these attempts to improve the independence and quality of life of the mentally retarded. These procedures have been successful in achieving behavioral changes when applied appropriately for a broad range of skills, including such diverse behaviors as toilet training and interpersonal behavior.

As in many other areas of scientific endeavor, there has been an information explosion in this field, making it difficult for the practitioner to stay abreast of the literature. The goal of this volume is to provide reviews of the major topics addressed in behavior modification research with the mentally retarded to date. Chapters are based on specific types of behavior that have been treated. They are presented in a roughly developmental sequence to give a more systematic presentation.

Chapter authors have considerable clinical and research experience with the mentally retarded. As a result, they are fully cognizant of the problems facing the practitioner in this area. We feel that the analysis of what treatments work best under different conditions is aptly made by the various authors. Also, and perhaps more important, they have pointed out the limitations of the procedures currently available. Certainly behavior modification is not a panacea for the habilitation of the mentally retarded. However, these methods have proven utility. Thus, it is hoped that this book will be of value to those who are currently involved in research, treatment, and administration at some level of applied work.

No attempt is made to resolve broad general issues regarding the degree of trainability of the severely retarded, the viability of the concept of normalization, or our interpretation of it. These concepts are certainly important and impact strongly on the behavior modification treatments that are used. It is our position that these and related questions are subject to empirical and legal resolutions that fall outside the purview of a discussion of behavior modification technology. Rather, it is our hope that the reader will benefit from the technical information presented in this volume with respect to the current state of behavior modification procedures for treating the mentally retarded.

JOHNNY L. MATSON
JOHN R. McCARTNEY

Contents

PART II.   ASSESSMENT AND TREATMENT

PART III.   TREATING DISRUPTIVE BEHAVIOR

8

WILLIAM I. GARDNER AND CHRISTINE L. COLE

PART IV.   TREATING SELF-HELP PROBLEMS

9

JOHN R. MCCARTNEY

10

MARIE E. TARAS AND MARY MATESE

PART V.   TREATING SOCIAL AND EMOTIONAL PROBLEMS

14

Emotional Problems I: Anxiety Disorders and Depression 391

BETSEY A. BENSON

15

Emotional Problems II: Autism 421

RON VAN HOUTEN

PART VI. ACADEMIC AND MANAGEMENT ISSUES

16

Language Acquisition 445

JAMES F. McCOY AND JOSEPH A. BUCKHALT

17

Academic Training 467

PAUL WEISBERG

18

Sexual Behavior 503

RAMASAMY MANIKAM AND DINAH S. HENSARLING

Introduction

JOHNNY L. MATSON

HISTORY

The field of mental retardation has been a central area for research and clinical practice for behavior modifiers and therapists. Much of the early application of learning principles has focused on this population, and much of what we know and do springs from the research with this group. Such procedures as the token economy, overcorrection, a good deal of the self-control and regulation literature, and many of the early differential reinforcement of other behavior (DRO) studies are among those that have emerged from this research. It should also be noted that behavior modification therapy has become the dominant mode of treatment for mentally retarded persons. As recently as the early 1960s, people who evinced mental retardation were all too often considered untreatable. The state of affairs then is a far cry from current research and practice, which is highly optimistic with respect to these handicapped persons. We now know that, with the proper training, these individuals have the potential to learn not only how to dress themselves but also to achieve toileting, dining, computer computation, shopping, vocational, and pedestrian skills, plus a host of other equally important behaviors that will allow them to live in a more normalized environment.

Until recently, another major concern of some persons with mental retardation, which was largely ignored, was emotional problems. In fact, many mental health professionals held the concept that these persons could not have emotional problems because of their lack of "proper ego strength" resulting from their intellectual deficiencies. Research has shown this to be a false assumption. Concurrent with this trend, however, was the excessive almost indiscriminate use of major tranquilizers (e.g., Haldol, Mellaril, Thorazine) with mentally retarded persons. In a survey that was conducted in 1969, for example, it was found that over half of the institutionalized persons in the United States who were categorized as mentally retarded were receiving these drugs at the time of their review. Various serious side effects, such as tardive dyskinesia (permanent neurological damage), may result from these medications and were among the reasons for this grave concern.

Once again, behavior therapists have had a major and positive impact with respect to this medication issue, and, as a result, numerous effective

1

treatments have been developed that are behavioral in nature. Similarly, a number of assessment methods that were developed are of particular note, because they assist in delineating more clearly who is and who is not a candidate for psychotropic drugs. The trends that have emerged include the identification of persons who might benefit from psychotropic drugs, the decreasing use of drugs by combining or using behavior modification alone and by maximizing effective treatments for persons with mental retardation and mental health problems (also referred to as "dual diagnosis"), and the development of specialized programs to treat these persons.

PHILOSOPHY

Perhaps more so than with any other population, professionals and the parents of persons with mental retardation have also indulged in the development of philosophical camps that have markedly affected the type of treatment procedures they consider acceptable for mentally retarded persons. Thus, it is common to see state legislatures and major national organizations involved in determining what is and what is not acceptable treatment based on their philosophy. For example, a heated debate has emerged over the use of aversive (punishment) methods. Similarly, a more radical camp has espoused the notion that no behavioral or other data-based methods of treatment should be available. These persons view normalization not only as a goal but also as a treatment; that is, not only should the issue be to ensure that people are trained to live in the most normal fashion possible, but the method of doing this should be to treat the person normally. Of course, considerable debate also has arisen as to what factors constitute being "normal."

RECENT DEVELOPMENTS

Although much has changed in the mental retardation field, many of the issues noted in this book, such as dual diagnosis and the philosophy of treatment, are basically new categories since the appearance of the first volume of the *Handbook of Behavior Modification with the Mentally Retarded*. Similarly, because research has been increasing at an amazingly fast pace, there is much to report on these various developments. In particular, several topics have appeared and have become substantial additions to the existing behavioral methods of treatment and assessment for developmentally disabled persons. One such issue is the increased attention to behaviorally based assessments. The emphasis is on better determining the effective antecedents and consequences of various target behaviors that the clinician would like to increase or decrease. Thus, the development of the scatter plot, which is another way of determining patterns of behavior displayed by a client, has gained some popularity. Using a grid with behaviors listed on one axis and with time on the other, the object is to determine if appropriate or inappropriate behaviors are occurring at set points. When that is the case, environmental arrangements can be altered, thus ensuring that the person with whom the client is always coming into contact is not present or the particular demand situation that results in aggression may be avoided or at least that the behavior may be anticipated more accurately.

Self-control strategies are other areas receiving a good deal of attention. Methods that allow clients to learn how to self-record their own target behaviors, to be more aware of times when they are becoming upset, and to develop strategies to delay such urges as hitting themselves by learning self-restraint (e.g., by sitting on their hands, clasping their hands, or holding their hands behind their back) are typical procedures that are taught. Often, the emphasis is to make handicapped persons more aware of their environment or surroundings and how best to control and monitor them.

The major developments in behavior modification approaches for mentally retarded persons might best be described as *refinement*. For example, most often efforts are being made to find more socially acceptable treatments where effective but less socially acceptable alternatives are currently being used. Similarly, the extension of effective treatments to other target behaviors, populations, and environments continues to be a high priority. Along these same lines, such issues as the generalization and maintenance of various target behaviors are of considerable importance, because we now know that they do not typically carry over to different settings, persons, or activities and do not typically continue to be displayed after treatment has been concluded, unless some type of planning and some variation of a successful treatment is put into place. Although little has been done, research is now emerging to determine the best method of making such alterations. In the future, this should be and most likely will develop into an important area of research. It is ironic, however, that although many criticize others for not doing such research, the critics themselves rarely do it for the simple reason that it is difficult to conduct research of the type that is proposed (e.g., socially valid generalization and maintenance oriented). Maintenance and generalization research is very labor intensive, and it is often difficult to get permission to do research in more applied settings, particularly in schools. Thus, even though it is important to encourage professionals to conduct research of this type, it is also vital to acknowledge that such research is often quite difficult to perform and that developments in this area, because of logistical concerns, are likely to be much slower than in other areas.

THE PRESENT TEXT

The second edition of this volume is composed of 18 chapters reflecting the primary areas where research in behavior modification has been conducted. It is always difficult to provide chapters of roughly equal length when the amount of published research for each of the topics is not equal or, in some cases, is not even remotely close. In this regard, our best effort was to provide example studies in some areas in which an exhaustive review would have been a book in and of itself, with, for example, self-help and self-injury being two such topics. In the first edition, this was not necessary, but the information explosion of current research will, in time, make the approach of an illustrative rather than an exhaustive review far more essential. Other topics, such as sex education for mentally handicapped individuals, have actually had little empirical research, but they are of sufficient importance that it would be unwise to leave them out of any book on applied topics.

This Handbook is divided into six sections. An attempt was made to place the topics into the most logical groupings possible, although, in reality, an even distribution of material that has been written in journals does not fit this objective as well as one might hope. In Part I, General Issues, the first chapter provides an overview of the handicapped behavior modification literature and a brief discussion of the various trends and topics. Chapter 2 treats service models. In my view, this chapter is of considerable importance because behavioral technology is not implemented in a vacuum but rather the type of treatment system that is developed has a major impact on the effectiveness, generalization, and maintenance of positive outcomes. Only recently have professionals begun to take this issue as seriously as it should be taken. Chapter 3 is related to another important issue that must be addressed if effective treatments are to be employed; that is, useful staff training programs. The effectiveness of any treatment is only as good as the weakest staff member implementing it. Unfortunately, few researchers in the behavior modification arena have looked into what is the best way to train staff to do a good job and how can efficient staff performance be maintained. These first three chapters then provide a basis from which to judge behavioral programs and from which professionals can establish and evaluate effective programs.

In Part II, Assessment and Treatment, the emphasis is on describing the basics of behavior modification technology in their present forms as they apply to the most up-to-date approaches. Many new developments exist and are briefly presented.

The three chapters in Part III pertain to the treatment of disruptive behavior, and are likely to be of considerable interest to any reader. The topics of self-injury, stereotypy, and aggression and related conduct disorder are the most discussed behavior disorders in the mental retardation system. For obvious reasons, persons with these problems seem to get all the attention. For self-injury and stereotypy, the best description of the treatments currently being employed might be entitled "more of the same" but with a more refined slant. On the other hand, aggression and conduct disorder have been the focus of some of the most innovative research in recent years. Much of the self-control and social learning procedures developed for mentally retarded persons are with this particular group. This situation may also be the case because self-injury and stereotypy, in their most severe forms, tend to be associated with the most severely mentally retarded persons, many of whom have various physical handicaps, including being nonambulatory. The reverse holds true with aggression, with the most extreme cases observed in persons with greater intellectual skills but still in the mentally retarded range. Additionally, aggressive persons also tend to have good ambulatory skills and coordination. Thus, it seems only reasonable that treatment procedures that require greater intellectual abilities are confined more likely to methods of self-control, cognitive behavior therapy, and social learning. Thus, researchers working with self-injury and stereotypy are not necessarily less creative. What must be understood by the reader is that the considerable disparity in intellectual and physical skills of the client dictates, to a great degree, the type of treatment method that is likely to be feasible and effective.

In Part IV, the chapters that deal with treating self-help problems have become the core area for special education and psychology as applied to mentally retarded persons. Toilet training, the first topic of these chapters, is in a sense the building block for all community living programs and for life in less restrictive settings. Few community programs will accept a person without toileting skill, and little additional more complex community skills are likely to occur or be targeted for training for such a person. Toilet training of handicapped individuals has been a real success story for mental retardation professionals and has as long a tradition in the habituation area as any other treatment research. Dressing, grooming, and many other self-help skills are also reviewed. However, given the expansion of research in the self-help area, it is difficult to cover all that has been written. Thus, only selected examples are included in the present review. The final chapter in this section pertains to community living skills, an area, which I predict, will see the greatest advances in the next five years. People are interested in this topic, and, for the most part the mentally handicapped persons, too, are more interested and motivated in learning than in many of the compliance problems that are being researched (e.g., with regard to self-injury and aggression). Further, the persons who are being trained are, in the main, the less severely mentally retarded individuals, given that the vast majority of mentally retarded persons are mildly mentally retarded and the fact that the most severely impaired multiply handicapped persons are likely the last to be researched and to receive the benefits of such training. These are the areas that best exemplify the notion that mentally retarded persons do have great potential.

Part V deals with social and emotional problems. Although this topic has existed for a good deal of time, research and clinical practice in this area have flourished only recently. A considerable amount of behavioral research has emerged in an area that was previously dominated by drug therapy. However, drugs do not teach new behaviors, and it is these new adaptive responses that have become the hallmark of modern treatment planning for mentally retarded persons. Of the four chapters that are included in this section, the first begins with a discussion of social skills. Researchers now know that social behavior is a major factor in the etiology of most forms of emotional disturbance, and that nowhere is this factor more pronounced than among mentally retarded persons, in whom social excesses and deficiencies are a defining aspect of their condition. Naturally, this issue leads to the next chapter on vocational skills, given the finding that social skills are also the primary reason why persons with mental retardation fail in competitive employment. Further, vocational training has traditionally been seen as an important adjunct in the training of mentally ill persons. Thus, Chapter 13,

"Consumer-Centered Transition and Supported Employment" seems to be a natural fit with the other topics presented in this section. Chapters 14 and 15 cover some of the major emotional problem areas, and it is in these two chapters perhaps more than in any other that it is difficult to provide a balanced discussion of the various emotional problems of mentally retarded persons as these problems occur in frequency and severity. Researchers, for whatever reason, have been interested in a few infrequently occurring conditions. Thus, self-abuse has received one hundred times more attention from researchers than depression. Therefore, if we could place one item on the wish list for researchers, it would be to have them study a much broader range of emotional problems of mentally retarded persons, particularly such high-incidence conditions as depression and anxiety disorders. The amount of attention that these topics have received is actually quite embarrassing.

Part VI, the final group of chapters in the book, covers topics that are likely to be of interest to teachers and psychologists who are working in the classroom setting. The first of these topics, which is probably the most controversial for professionals and parents alike, is sex education. It is my view that some happy medium should be possible between the various factions that have such strong opinions about this topic. Furthermore, if parents and professionals are serious about normalizing handicapped persons to the fullest extent possible, sex education can no longer be ignored. The advent of AIDS and other serious health risks associated with unrestrained and uneducated sexual conduct may result in the handicapped person's health being put at grave risk. Much work is needed to reconcile such issues.

The other chapters in this section are less controversial but are no less important. An entire chapter is devoted to language development, given the frequency with which persons with mental retardation are likely to experience such problems, and another chapter is provided on the best ways to teach the more typical academic materials. Given the difficulty in teaching mentally retarded persons relative to the general population, this is an issue deserving serious attention by the reader.

CONCLUSIONS

It is my hope that the present volume will be instructive to the reader. It is a book that has been prepared by many noted contributers, who are expert in the areas that they discuss. Most certainly, this volume will not be the last word on any topic; however, it should provide the interested reader with a good overview, in one source, of what is happening in the area of developmental disabilities. After reading the book, I hope that you will feel as I do that quite a lot is new and exciting, and that the future is promising not only for developmentally disabled persons but also for the professionals who hope to teach them how to make their lives better and more fulfilled.

I

General Issues

Current Issues in Behavior Modification with Mentally Retarded Persons

Thomas L. Whitman, Donald A. Hantula, and Brenda H. Spence

The treatment and education of mentally retarded individuals has changed considerably over the years, alternating between compassionate concern and neglect and ridicule (Gearhart & Litton, 1975). Although residential institutions for mentally retarded persons in the United States were initially conceived for the purpose of treatment and education, a custodial-care orientation emerged early in the twentieth century, and, as a consequence, treatment and educational programs virtually disappeared. It was not until the 1950s that a growing concern for mentally retarded persons led to social change. In 1952, the National Association for Retarded Children (NARC, now called the Association for Retarded Citizens) was formed through the efforts of parents of mentally retarded children. Subsequently, the NARC and its state and local member units catalyzed community agencies into developing services for mentally retarded persons and provided, when necessary, direct services. Concurrent with this type of development, public enlightenment and awareness about mental retardation increased. The 1960s and 1970s were times of moral indignation, during which man's inhumanity to man was exposed in such books as *Christmas in Purgatory* (Blatt & Kaplan, 1966). During the Kennedy and Johnson administrations, a national effort began to address the needs of mentally retarded persons and the problems associated with mental retardation. As a consequence of these social and political concerns, an educational movement occurred, as movements to normalize, educate, and treat, and secure civil rights for mentally retarded persons gained impetus.

Concomitant with these changes in societal attitudes, new programs for mentally retarded persons were established, and active treatment and educa-

Thomas L. Whitman, Donald A. Hantula, and Brenda H. Spence • Department of Psychology, University of Notre Dame, Notre Dame, Indiana 46556.

tion programs were introduced into institutional environments. Many mentally retarded persons who historically would have been placed in institutions now remained at home, participating in a variety of newly developed community-based programs. Community educational and recreational services for moderately and mildly handicapped individuals were developed or extended. Perhaps the major catalyst of change during the 1960s occurred as a consequence of the behavior modification movement.

When behavioral educators first entered institutions for mentally retarded persons in the 1960s, they were confronted with a major challenge. At that time, institutional programming was almost entirely directed toward giving basic physical care to the residents and providing general types of stimulation programs. Systematic training programs were nonexistent because of the prevailing belief about the uneducability of this population, the inadequate numbers of staff, and the ignorance concerning what the nature of such programs should be. Within the past three decades, through the efforts of behavior modifiers, a technology has been developed that has influenced the training programs of nearly all agencies serving mentally retarded persons (Whitman, Scibak, & Reid, 1983). In this chapter, traditional and behavioral conceptualizations concerning the definition, assessment, and treatment of retardation will be compared, an overview of research evaluating behavior modification programs for retarded persons will be presented, future directions that behavioral research should take will be explored, and general issues relating to the development of behavior programs will be discussed.

TRADITIONAL VERSUS BEHAVIORAL CONCEPTUALIZATIONS OF MENTAL RETARDATION

Definition

Historically, there has been considerable agreement about what retardation is. Early definitions put forth by Tredgold (1937), Doll (1941), and Kanner (1957) focused on retarded individuals' inability to adapt adequately to their surrounding environment because of their "mental deficiency." The development of the intelligence test led to definitions of retardation emphasizing intellectual rather than adaptive behavior problems (Terman & Merrill, 1973; Wechsler, 1955). A relatively recent and widely accepted definition of retardation that combines basic features of previous definitions was put forth by the American Association on Mental Deficiency (AAMD) in 1973. This definition states that "mental retardation refers to significantly subaverage general intellectual functioning existing concurrently with deficits in adaptive behavior and manifested during the development period" (Grossman, 1973). According to this definition, individuals are defined as mentally retarded only if they manifest both intellectual and behavioral deficiencies. Moreover, individuals are described as "intellectually deficient" only if they are significantly subaverage in this regard, which means operationally that their performance is more than two standard deviations below the mean of the intelligence test employed. As a result of defining retardation in this fashion, the size of the population of people who are labeled as mentally retarded has diminished. Individuals who are intellectually subaverage but whose adaptive-behavior skills are adequate, individuals who are deficient in adaptive behavior but intellectually who are not subaverage, and individuals who are of borderline intelligence are no longer labeled mentally retarded.

From a more behavioral perspective, Whitman *et al.* (1983) defined a *retarded person* as an individual who has one or more response deficiencies that, at least in part, are produced and/or maintained by the environment. This definition, although similar to that of the American Association on Mental Deficiency presented earlier, is also different in a number of important ways. First, this definition makes no reference to the existence of an intellectual deficiency. It does not attempt to interconnect existing response deficiencies with any specific hypothetical cause or internal deficit. However, it does not specifically deny that such deficits may be present. Second, this definition emphasizes that the response deficiencies are partially a function of the external surroundings in which the individual has been reared, thereby suggesting that such deficiencies can be prevented or ameliorated through systematic arrangement of environmental contingencies.

In contrast to previous definitions of mental retardation, Whitman *et al.* (1983) pointed out that their definition stresses implicitly the following: (1) the uniqueness of the individual labeled retarded and more specifically the fact that retarded individuals differ considerably from each other in the number, type, and extent of their response deficiencies; and (2) the existence of a continuum of retardation ranging from individuals, commonly referred to as "profoundly retarded," who have numerous extensive response deficiencies, to individuals who are deficient only in certain academic, social, or vocational situations. This definition does not exclude from the category of retardation individuals who are intellectually normal and whose deficiency is restricted to one response category; for example, a child who has reading problems or a child who has a problem interacting with other children. The intent of this definition was not to broaden the concept of retardation *per se* but rather to suggest that all individuals lie on a behavioral continuum, and that they are all more or less retarded and all more or less normal. Consequently, individuals are not placed into absolute categories of either retardation or nonretardation.

Classification

Associated with most definitions of mental retardation is a classification system. In general, classification systems assign mental retarded individuals to various categories on the basis of IQ, adaptive behavior, and/or etiology. Although a number of systems for classifying the mentally retarded are available, the schemata employed are not mutually exclusive. Schools in the United States have traditionally used a classification scheme in which low IQ children are defined as "educable mentally retarded" (EMR) or "trainable mentally retarded" (TMR). This system not only labels children but also places them into classes with certain assumptions concerning what they should be learning and what they are capable of learning.

Another classification system that has been commonly employed emphasizes the adaptive behavior and behavioral deficiencies in the retarded individual (cf. Meyers, Nihira, & Zetlin, 1979). It is different from the preceding classification scheme in that it does not seek or use IQ information. Rather, it involves a detailed cataloging of what a retarded individual can and cannot do. Although there is variation between specific adaptive-behavior scales, behaviors in the sensorimotor, communication and language, self-help, socialization, academic, and vocational areas are generally assessed. In addition, maladaptive behavior of various types, for example, stereotypy and self-injurious behavior, can be evaluated. A classification schema, based on both IQ and adaptive behavior, is presented in a 1973 manual published by the American Association on Mental Deficiency. In this system, mentally retarded individuals are classified according to the severity of their symptoms into four categories of retardation: mild, moderate, severe, and profound (Grossman, 1973).

In contrast, another classification system that has been employed categorizes mentally retarded individuals on the basis of etiology or purported etiology. Such categories include disorders that are associated with discrete genetic problems, chromosomal abnormalities, disease, injury, ingestion of toxic agents, and malnutrition. The major advantage of this type of schema is that it may have direct implications for the scientific study, treatment, and prevention of mental retardation.

In contrast to these four classification systems, formal placement of individuals into broad categories does not occur within a behavioral model. The uniqueness of the individual who is labeled "retarded" is emphasized. Classifications, such as severe or moderate retardation, though they simplify communication, convey little information concerning the persons described, implying simply that they are behaviorally deficient in several ways. In general, it is felt that classification labels at this level of abstraction have little scientific or educational value (Whitman et al., 1983). Although labeling allows for gross categorization, this process is dangerous as Bellack and Hersen (1977) point out, because it facilitates a generalized response on the part of a clinical community and the public at large toward the person labeled and reduces the likelihood of accurate perception and discrimination. Instead of a formal classification system, behavior modifiers prefer a listing of the adaptive behaviors and response deficiencies of the individual; that is, a behavioral profile. This type of schema is both descriptive of how the person is presently behaving and also prescriptive in the sense that it suggests objectives for training programs.

Assessment and Treatment

As suggested in the previous section, there is a close association between the assessment and classification process. Ideally, there should also be a close interrelationship between assessment and treatment. The purpose of assessment is to learn why a person is retarded, how this retardation manifests itself, and how it can be treated. If, through assessment, it can be discovered why a person is retarded, this often has immediate treatment implications. Assessment occurring early in the life of the child who is at risk for retardation may assist in the prevention of later retardation. In contrast, assessment, which occurs after an individual is already labeled retarded, aids more habilitative than preventive treatment.

Unfortunately, the dynamic relationship that should exist between assessment and treatment, through an understanding of the factors that produce retardation and prevent normal development, is often not achieved in reality. Frequently, the specific condition that causes and maintains retarded behavior is unknown. Perhaps for this reason, nonbehavioral assessment programs have relied on the use of descriptive classification systems, which place individuals in specific categories based on the presence of common symptom or behavior patterns. Assumptions about underlying defects as well as decisions concerning curability and educability are made based on the configuration of these symptoms. Evaluation before treatment is stressed, with less emphasis placed on evaluation during or after treatment. Central to the use of the nonbehavioral assessment approach and its conception of the nature of retardation is the notion of intellectual deficit. Despite the success the intelligence tests have had in predicting who will do well and who will have problems in regular academic classroom situations, these tests have had little specific value for educational planning or for predicting how a person functions outside a classroom.

Because of their limited utility for treatment planning, the exclusive use of intellectual assessments has been discouraged, and more complex, multidimensional assessment systems that emphasize the evaluation of adaptive behavior have been developed. The inclusion of adaptive behavior as well as intellectual criteria in the AAMD definition of mental retardation (Grossman, 1973, 1977) reflects the professional concern about the adequacy of traditional conceptualization and classification systems. The interest in adaptive behavior also precipitated the development of a variety of instruments. A number of these instruments, such as the Adaptive Behavior Scales (Nihira, Foster, Shellhaas, & Leland, 1974), the Balthazar Scales of Adaptive Behavior (Balthazar, 1971, 1973), and the Progress Assessment Chart of Social and Personal Development (Gunzburg, 1976), were designed to determine an individual's level of independence and ability to cope with the environment.

Although adaptive-behavior assessments and the behavior assessments employed by behavior modifiers focus on the evaluation of behavior, their methods of assessment differ greatly. Typically, when adaptive-behavior scales are used, they are filled out by or with the informational input of persons who are presumed to be well acquainted with the individual being rated. Direct observation is sometimes employed, but more often the information about the skills and deficits of mentally retarded persons is both retrospective and subjective. This is in distinct contrast to the measurement approach used in direct behavior-assessment programs.

When behavior modification assessment procedures are employed, response definitions are developed and emphasis is placed on establishing the reliability of the rating procedures. Behavior is evaluated, not only directly, but repeatedly; not only before, but also during and after treatment; not in one setting, but in many settings. The rationale behind the use of such repeated observations lies in the fact that single observations of an individual's behavior do not present a complete picture of the way the person acts. Behavior is observed in more than one setting in order to determine how the person generally acts and whether his or her behaviors are situation specific. The purposes of this type of behavioral evaluation are to assess the extent to which a particular target behavior occurs before treatment, to determine which stimulus events appear to be controlling behavior, and to evaluate through the use of appropriate experimental designs whether behavior changes are a function of the treatment employed.

In a provocative study by Millham, Chilcutt, and Atkinson (1978), one retrospective observational instrument, the Adaptive Behavior Scale, was compared with a direct behavior-assessment procedure. Both instruments were used to evaluate the behavior of mentally retarded individuals in a community residential setting. The investigation revealed a number of differences between the two techniques in the rated levels of adaptive behavior. In general, the retarded individuals were seen as more behaviorally proficient when the Adaptive Behavior Scales were used. The results indicated that generalizations should not be made from one of these assessment procedures to the other. The authors suggested that retrospective observations of retarded persons' behaviors obtained from parents, peers, or counselors may reveal more about the observer than the individual who is observed. If one accepts the premise that direct observation procedures are more accurate, this raises serious questions about the validity of retrospective assessment procedures. Future research needs to examine further the relationship between retrospective and direct behavior-assessment procedures, the accuracy of each of these instruments, and how they might be used in conjunction. It may be that, for certain behaviors, the more time-efficient retrospective procedures will provide an acceptable substitute for direct behavior assessment.

Medical and Behavioral Approaches to Retardation

Mental retardation has often been characterized as a medical syndrome; that is, it has been asserted that the causes are organic in nature and that treatment must address itself to an underlying pathology. The more proximal causes of retardation are assumed to be neurological in nature: the brain either fails to develop properly or undergoes deterioration. The more distal causes of retardation and these brain problems are stated to range from genetic deficiencies that are present at conception to disease and other traumatic processes that occur before, during, and after birth (Robinson & Robinson, 1976). At the present time, there is a consensus that conceptualizations deriving from the medical model are most applicable to the severely and profoundly mentally retarded persons.

Advocates of the medical model believe that by using knowledge of underlying biological causes, it may be possible to prevent future cases of retardation and to prevent further deterioration of individuals who are already retarded. Examples of such prevention strategies include (1) counseling of couples who are at risk of having genetically defective children; (2) programs directed at reducing conception rates of females who are at high risk of having retarded children, such as teenagers and older women; (3) the abortion of high-risk pregnancies with risk assessed through such diagnostic techniques as amniocentesis; (4) improved health services for high-risk mothers during pregnancy; (5) dietary interventions with children who have certain genetic disorders, such as phenylketonuria and galactosemia; and (6) surgical treatment of such disorders as hydrocephalus. The contribution of the medical model to the treatment of retardation once it has already occurred is not clear. Cure in the medical sense of reversal of retardation symptoms is not presently thought possible because of irreversible neurological deterioration.

In general, it is difficult to evaluate the impact of medically based prevention programs. It has been suggested on the one hand that the incidence of severe and profound mental retardation may be on the decline because of such programs and on the other that this incidence may be increasing because of increased survival rates of profoundly handicapped newborns (cf. Wolfensberger, 1969). Perhaps one of the most negative features associated with the medical model relates to the issue of the "educable" level of severely and profoundly mentally retarded individuals. Historically, physicians have often thought of retardation of this type to be medically incurable. Institutionalization has frequently been recommended, not as a treatment but as an alternative that would free the family from the burdensome responsibility of providing basic care to their child. Unfortunately, the notion of medical incurability has become associated with negative educational prognostic statements concerning the retarded individuals' ability to learn.

In striking contrast to this viewpoint is that taken by practitioners of behavior modification. Within the behavioral model, predictions about an individual's ability to learn are based on a person's performance in a specific learning situation rather than on knowledge of his or her biological condition. Assertions concerning whether a person will learn in a certain situation are related to whether he or she has learned in similar situations previously. However, the fact that an individual has not learned in a specific situation does not mean that he or she could not learn if the situation were slightly altered. Behavior modifiers contend that whether a retarded person can or cannot learn a particular skill is an empirical question that can be answered only by providing a maximal learning environment (Gardner, 1971). When a retarded person fails to perform adequately in a specific learning situation, it is often suggested that an ineffective teaching strategy may have been employed rather than asserting categorically that the person is incapable of learning.

When developing behaviorally oriented educational programs for mentally retarded individuals, behavior modifiers must identify through systematic observation specific environmental circumstances preventing the development of adaptive behaviors. Additionally, they must consider general hypotheses about environmental conditions that are associated with retardation from learning-based theories of behavior development. Bijou (1966) and Gardner (1971) discussed at length factors that might account for the behavior deficits of mentally retarded individuals. These factors include inadequate reinforcement for appropriate behavior, limitations in the stimulus environment, a history of aversive experiences, and reinforcement of inappropriate behavior. In general, the assumption that appropriate behaviors are absent from the repertoires of mentally retarded persons because of environmental circumstances, such as those just described, implies that learning might occur if these circumstances were systematically changed.

In summary, the medical and behavioral models generate quite different conceptualizations concerning the nature, prevention, and treatment of mental retardation. Although these two conceptualizations are divergent, they can be viewed as complementing one another. As our understanding of the biological and environmental mechanisms that control behavior develops, it is likely that an integrated biobehavioral model of severe and profound mental retardation will evolve. At present, however, it is fair to state that use of the medical model has not yet led to a "cure" for most types of severe and profound retardation and that such cures are not likely to occur in the near future. Although the behavioral model has not and is not likely to lead to a cure either, there are both theoretical reasons and substantial evidence to suggest that the severely and profoundly mentally retarded as well as the mildly and moderately mentally retarded can be habilitated and taught skills that will allow them to adapt more effectively to their social environment and live in a more "normalized" fashion.

The Educability of Mentally Retarded Persons

Since the nineteenth century, there has been considerable refinement in our knowledge of and conceptualizations about the nature of mental retardation and its treatment. However, the basic issue concerning the extent to which this condition, particularly in its more severe form, is modifiable remains largely unresolved. It is obvious that society and, particularly, the parents, professionals, and paraprofessionals who interact on a daily basis with mentally retarded individuals are often pessimistic concerning the potential in these persons for achievement. Moreover, it is clear that society's expectations also differ depending on the extent of the retarded individual's behavioral and intellectual deficiency (Gottlieb, 1977).

Whitman et al. (1983) pointed out that the negative view of society concerning the educability of severely and profoundly mentally retarded persons appears to be based on several assumptions:

> First, it is assumed that persons with lower IQs, as measured by an intelligence test, have less potential for achievement. Second, it is asserted that there is a direct relationship between the degree of present behavioral deficiency manifested by an individual and his or her potential for future behavioral development. Specifically,

it is believed that persons who are more behaviorally deficient have less potential for behavioral development. Third, it is believed that persons who demonstrate significant learning when placed in educational programs have greater potential than those who learn only a little or do not learn at all. A corollary to this assumption is that an individual who shows minimal or no progress after being in an education program for a "reasonable" amount of time, is probably not capable of learning. Although numerous counterarguments can be brought to bear concerning the validity of these assumptions, they, nevertheless, often influence decisions concerning the type and extent of educational services offered to the retarded. (p. 400)

Despite the many published reports that suggest that behavior modification programs can be employed successfully in teaching mentally retarded persons, there is disagreement about whether this technology can be employed successfully in educating those individuals who are most deficient in adaptive skills, that is, those who are severely and profoundly mentally retarded. However, the fundamental question concerning the educability of these persons is not whether they are educable but to what extent they are educable. Most scientists and practitioners now recognize that the answer to this question, for any specific individual, cannot be arrived at on an *a priori* basis, but must be based on careful evaluation of the individual's response to the educational programming he or she receives. In this regard, it should be recognized that even when a person fails to learn under a particular teaching regimen, it cannot be concluded that he or she is not capable of learning in other situations when other approaches are employed. Ultimately, as Whitman *et al.* (1983) have pointed out, the issue concerning the educability of mentally retarded persons is really a practical rather than a theoretical one. The decision about whether to educate this population relates less to the issues concerning the educational potential of this population and more to society's value system concerning the importance of such educational programs and how much time and resources society is willing to devote to the development of these programs. Whereas during the first half of this century there was considerable emphasis on custodial care and eugenics programs for mentally retarded persons (Sarason & Doris, 1969), currently there is a commitment to recognize the rights of these persons and provide them with the best possible treatment and education. The extent to which society continues this commitment to mentally retarded individuals in the future will be, at least in part, a function of the success of behavior modification programs that are developed.

BEHAVIOR MODIFICATION RESEARCH WITH MENTALLY RETARDED PERSONS

In order to examine more recent trends in behavior modification programs conducted with mentally retarded individuals, a literature review was carried out. This review complements that completed by Whitman and Scibak (1981), which appeared in the first edition of this book. In the 1981 review by Whitman and Scibak, eight journals were surveyed in order to examine be-

*Behavior Modification Research with Mentally Retarded Individuals
Published in Various Journals from 1979 to 1987*

Journal	Number of studies
American Journal of Mental Deficiency	124
Analysis and Intervention in Developmental Disabilities	40
Applied Research in Mental Retardation	63
Behavior Modification	32
Behaviour Research and Therapy	17
Journal of Applied Behavior Analysis	161
Journal of Autism and Developmental Disabilities	26
Journal of Behavior Therapy and Experimental Psychiatry	58
Total	521

havior modification research conducted from 1962 to 1979 with severely and profoundly mentally retarded individuals. In this earlier review, 280 studies were surveyed. For the current review, behavior modification research conducted from 1979 to 1987 with mentally retarded individuals, regardless of level of retardation, was examined. The journals surveyed were: *American Journal of Mental Deficiency, Analysis and Intervention in Developmental Disabilities, Applied Research in Mental Retardation, Behavior Modification, Behaviour Research and Therapy, Journal of Applied Behavior Analysis, Journal of Autism and Developmental Disabilities*, and the *Journal of Behavior Therapy and Experimental Psychiatry*. In reviewing each study, the following information was recorded for descriptive purposes: journal name, subject age and level of retardation, target behaviors addressed, training procedures employed, who applied the training procedures, the setting in which the procedures were applied, whether maintenance and generalization were assessed, and whether a group or single subject design was employed. Table 1 shows for each journal the number of articles devoted to behavior modification research with mentally retarded persons.

A total of 521 relevant studies were published in the aforementioned journals during the 8-year period. Three hundred ninety-nine of these studies evaluated behavior modification programs for mentally retarded individuals. Fifty-four studies evaluated behavior management procedures for training institutional staff (19 studies), parents (16 studies), siblings (2 studies), peers (15 studies), and teachers (2 studies) to work with mentally retarded individuals. An additional 68 studies dealt with assessment issues, such as research evaluating the reliability and validity of new or existing behavioral scales.

Analysis of the 399 studies devoted to evaluating behavioral programs for mentally retarded persons revealed that a large number, 238 (60%), of the behavior modification studies were conducted with severely and profoundly mentally retarded individuals. This number of studies is quite similar to the number reported in the Whitman and Scibak survey (1981) for an earlier but a

TABLE 2
General Target Behaviors Addressed in
Behavior Modification Research
with Mentally Retarded Individuals

Target behaviors	Number of studies[a]
Language	56
Discrimination	24
Social skills	41
Self-help/daily living	39
Academic/cognitive	38
Vocational	29
Physical/motor skills	16
Leisure/play	17
Computer use	2
Coping/fear	2

[a]Studies add to more than 399 because some studies addressed more than one target behavior.

comparable time frame (1971–1979). One hundred eighty-seven studies (47%) evaluated behavioral programs with mildly and moderately mentally retarded individuals, and 60 (16%) dealt with mentally retarded autistic individuals. When the age of the target population in these studies was examined, 221 (55%) were found to have been conducted with children, 112 (28%) with adolescents, and 152 (38%) with adults. Four studies were found that evaluated programs serving mentally retarded individuals over age 65. Of these four programs, only two were specifically designed to serve the needs of elderly mentally retarded individuals. (Percentages add to more than 100% because subjects within a study often varied in level of retardation and age.)

Further analysis of the survey data showed that 189 (47%) of the studies focused on decreasing maladaptive behavior, whereas 264 (66%) focused on increasing adaptive behavior. The adaptive behaviors most frequently addressed were in language, discrimination learning, and in academic, social, self-help, and vocational areas. Of the studies devoted to decreasing maladaptive responses, 142 (75%) were conducted with severely and profoundly retarded subjects, with 66% of these studies directed at reducing self-injurious behavior. Table 2 presents a more complete breakdown of the adaptive target goals addressed in these studies.

Procedurally, a wide array of techniques for changing behavior have been evaluated. Nearly all of the studies reviewed have employed some sort of positive reinforcement procedure. Table 3 shows other techniques that have been used. Among the more frequently utilized techniques were self-management, modeling, and behavioral rehearsal. Punishment procedures were employed in 76 of the studies, almost always in conjunction with a positive reinforcement technique. The aversive stimuli utilized in the punishment programs were diverse, changing considerably over the last decade. For example, such aversive agents as restraint, shock, slaps, and lemon juice have

TABLE 3
*Behavior Modification Procedures Employed in Research
with Mentally Retarded Individuals*

Procedures	Number of studies
Punishment	76
Self-management	44
Environmental change	15
Stimulus control	20
Adaptive devices, computer aids	17
Increased stimulation, enriched environment	8
Picture prompts	9
Modeling, behavior rehearsal	43
Drugs	16
Drugs and behavior modification	6
Satiation	7
Incidental learning	5
Videotape with feedback	2

been employed less frequently in recent years, whereas verbal reprimands, facial screening, and brief response interruption are more often used.

Table 4 shows the agents who have administered the behavioral procedures and the settings in which the training programs have been conducted. The majority of the studies occurred in naturalistic settings, that is, in a setting where the targeted individual normally spent part or most of his or her day. The therapist–trainer agent was often not specified. When this infor-

TABLE 4
*Therapists Applying Procedures and Settings
in Which Behavior Modification Research
with Mentally Retarded Individuals
Has Been Conducted*

Therapists		Settings[a]	
Unspecified	122	Institution	159
Author	68	Classroom	152
Institutional staff	39	Outpatient clinic	21
Teacher	54	Vocational	30
Therapists	42	Hospital	17
Parent	14	Community	19
Undergraduates	13	Home	24
Graduate students	14	Group home	21
Volunteer	3	Day program	10
Other	30	Unspecified	11

[a]Studies add to more than 399 because training took place in more than one setting or because settings were double classified (i.e., institution and classroom).

mation is not provided, it is, of course, impossible to make any valid inferences about who might be able to apply effectively the evaluated change procedure. When the therapist was specified, the person administering the behavioral program was typically not an individual in daily contact with the client. In only about 25% of the studies were institutional staff, classroom teachers, or parents explicitly designated as the change agent.

Since the inception of behavior modification research programs with mentally retarded individuals, the measurement procedures that were employed have been improving. In contrast to the Whitman and Scibak (1981) survey, in which it was found that only 50% of the studies assessed the reliability of their measurement procedures, nearly all of the studies in the current survey have conducted some type of reliability check. Brief descriptive information concerning the observers and the manner in which they were trained was typically provided. Reported reliability coefficients were generally above .90. Although a few studies use more sophisticated on-line recording procedures, most studies continue to rely on paper-and-pencil counts.

From a design perspective, there also appears to be an improvement in the quality of research published since 1978 (see Whitman & Scibak, 1981). In the present survey, 48 studies employed a group design, while the remainder utilized some type of single subject design. The majority of the studies employed experimental designs allowing the functional relationship between treatment procedures and target behaviors to be assessed. The majority of the studies also examined maintenance of program effects from one week to several months after training. A subanalysis of studies conducted in 1986 indicated that over 70% of the studies evaluated for maintenance and/or generalization of program effects. However, as in the earlier Whitman and Scibak (1981) survey, the current review indicated that treatment applications were seldom monitored to see if they were correctly implemented. Consequently, it should be noted that failure to monitor technique implementation reduces the confidence which may be placed in statements asserting a functional relationship between an intervention and behavior change.

In summary, the present survey indicates that a large number of studies have been conducted evaluating the efficacy of behavioral techniques with mentally retarded individuals. An extensive technology for teaching a variety of adaptive behaviors and for suppressing numerous deviant responses has been developed. In general, the methodological quality of these studies is good and getting better. However, a great deal more research remains to be conducted. Although numerous techniques have been evaluated and their effectiveness established across subjects within a study, systematic attempts to assess a technique's general effectiveness across different types of client and therapist populations and across different types of settings have been infrequent. Moreover, although research indicates that existing techniques can produce dramatic positive short-term changes in behavior in a treatment situation, the programming and evaluation of long-term and generalized changes needs to be addressed more extensively. Research in a number of important areas remains undeveloped. Some directions that future research might take are discussed in the next section.

Future Research Directions

Behavioral Pharmacology

Although drugs cannot create behavior (Peffer-Smith, Smith, & Byrd, 1983), pharmacological interventions can be employed effectively to increase desirable behavior rates as well as to decrease the occurrence of undesirable behaviors. Because drugs exert their influence at a great temporal distance, in contrast to physical restraints, their use is often viewed in a positive fashion by the casual observer. However, pharmacotherapy is not without its problems. Drugs are chemical agents that affect the entire biochemical as well as the behavioral complex of the individual. Major tranquilizers, which inhibit aggressive behaviors, as well as other psychotropic drugs may also interfere with the acquisition and maintenance of adaptive behaviors (Burgio, Page, & Capriotti, 1985; Marholin, Touchette, & Stewart, 1979; Wysoki, Fuqua, Davis, & Breuning, 1981). Furthermore, long-term use of major tranquilizers may cause a variety of physiological side effects, such as tardive dyskinesia and other parkinsonian-like syndromes (Gualtieri & Hawk, 1980).

Since the advent of the behavior modification movement, researchers have been interested in the behavioral effects of pharmacological programs, the utility of combined behavioral and pharmacological programs, as well as the relative efficacy of the two approaches. In addition, because drugs may not only affect targeted behaviors but also modify many other behaviors, clinical research has investigated the effects drugs exert on the diminution of nontargeted inappropriate behaviors, as well as on the acquisition and maintenance of nontargeted adaptive and prosocial behaviors (Schroeder, Gualtieri, & Van Bourgondien, 1986).

Although pharmacological approaches may be effective, other research indicates that contingency management procedures may work as well as or better than pharmacological programs in reducing the frequency of inappropriate or maladaptive behaviors (Burgio et al., 1985; Durand, 1982; Luiselli, 1986; Rapport, Murphy, & Bailey, 1982; Shafto & Sulzbacher, 1977; Singh & Winton, 1984). Evidence from behavioral pharmacological research also suggests that once sufficient stimulus control over behavior is obtained, the need for the use of drugs is reduced (Laties, Wood, & Cooper, 1981). Given the efficacy of nondrug behavioral treatments and the fact that therapeutic drug usage may expose an individual to a host of undesirable and sometimes permanent side effects, it is often advised that pharmacological agents be employed only as a last resort, and then only as a temporary means to gain environmental control over the behavior. Nevertheless, because pharmacological interventions can potentially serve a vital function in the habilitation of mentally retarded persons, it is imperative that their effects be thoroughly investigated in a methodologically rigorous fashion. A number of reviews suggest that a considerable amount of published clinical behavioral pharmacological research is methodologically unsound, although the quality of this research is improving (Aman, 1983; Marholin & Phillips, 1976; Wysoki & Fuqua, 1982).

Based on existing statistics, it appears that the majority of mentally retarded persons receive one or more behaviorally active drugs, including stimulants, anticonvulsants, antidepressants, major tranquilizers, and anxiolytics (see Breuning & Poling, 1982, for a review). A recent survey of mentally retarded persons revealed that 48% were being given medication for behavioral control (Martin & Agran, 1985). The rate of drug administration is perhaps highest for institutionalized retarded populations. For example, Craig and Behar (1980) reported that 86% of their institutionalized sample were receiving medications.

Despite the powerful effects drugs exert on behavior, applied researchers evaluating behavioral techniques often ignore the potentially important interactions between behavioral and pharmacological interventions. Drugs may act as reinforcers, punishers, discriminative stimuli, and establishing operations. Drug effects on behavior are determined not only by the nature of the drug *per se* but also are dependent upon the baseline rate of the behavior undergoing treatment (Dews, 1958), as well as on the contingencies under which the behavior is maintained (Barrett & Katz, 1981). Behavior modification researchers who ignore these relationships may well report results that are experimentally confounded. Most researchers evaluating behavior modification programs do not report whether the subjects in their study were receiving drug therapy or if pharmacological interventions were attempted prior to a behavioral intervention (Poling, Grosset, Karas, & Breuning, 1985). When therapeutic drug interventions are described, precise information about the characteristics of the program is typically lacking. Based on standard practices and recommendations of pharmacological researchers (Poling, Picker, & Hall-Johnson, 1983), the following points need to be reported if a clear picture of drug-behavior interactions is to emerge in the applied literature: (1) the type of drug administered, (2) the amount administered, (3) the route of administration, (4) the time of drug administration relative to the time the behavior was measured, (5) the chronicity of drug exposure, (6) the relevant organismic variables, and (7) the previous and concomitant drug use by the subjects.

More specifically, the type of drug administered should be expressed by its chemical name and trade name (e.g., thioridazine [Mellaril]) to permit precise identification of the pharmacological agent. The amount of drug administered should be expressed in milligrams of drug per kilogram of body weight or blood serum level, given that drug effects are partially a function of the recipient's body weight. Because drug effects may vary with the route of administration that is due to differential rates of absorption, the route of administration should be delineated. The most common methods of administration employed with mentally retarded persons are oral and by injection. Drugs may be injected under the skin, in a muscle, in a vein, or into a body cavity.

Since drugs vary in the latency and duration of their effects, it is also critical that administration schedules be reported. For example, some widely used major tranquilizers produce immediately after administration such effects as drowsiness and sedation, which dissipate within approximately an hour's time. The evaluation of behavioral interventions can yield widely discrepant results depending upon the temporal interface of the intervention and medication schedules. Information concerning the period over which a drug has been given (chronicity of exposure) is also important, given that tolerance may develop, thereby changing the drug's impact on behavior as well as its mode of interaction with other drugs. Finally, organismic variables, such as existing infirmities, illnesses or handicaps, and previous or concurrent experience with other drugs, need to be specified given their potential impact on current pharmacological and behavior programs. Different drugs administered concurrently can interact in a variety of ways with each other and with the general physiological status of the individual, as well as with behavioral interventions, thereby confounding attempts at systematic evaluation.

In summary, future research needs to address the interactions between pharmacological and behavioral interventions. Those situations under which pharmacological, behavioral, or combined intervention are most desirable need to be identified. Research needs to address the issue of behavioral covariation, more specifically to evaluate nontargeted behaviors that might be affected by pharmacotherapy in addition to those which the drug was intended to change. Special attention needs to be directed toward the effects drugs have on the acquisition and maintenance of adaptive behaviors. As this research is published, it is imperative that comprehensive and precise information about the structure of the drug programs be reported.

Technology and Behavioral Control

The task of the behavior modification specialist is to maximize the mentally retarded person's adaptive repertoires. Traditionally, behavior modifiers have relied upon contingency management procedures to shape and maintain desired behavior changes. Although very effective in many cases, it is unlikely, because of the physical handicaps associated with some types of retardation, that direct changes in behavior can always be effected through such an intervention strategy. Moreover, this type of intervention is sometimes extremely labor intensive and difficult to implement. To address these problems, Lindsley (1964) proposed the use of prosthetic or "artificial" devices to extend and maximize the behavioral repertoires of mentally retarded individuals. Prosthetic instruments, such as voice synthesizers, communication boards, and special cueing devices, can help a wide variety of individuals compensate for behavioral deficiencies (Mulick, Scott, Gaines, & Campbell, 1983). These devices not only provide special assistance to persons who have seemingly irreversible adaptive-behavior deficiencies (particularly those whose disabilities have a biological basis), but also aid their caregivers.

Culturally, there has been a tendency to reduce human labor by mechanizing jobs as much as possible. Even though "mechanization" does not replace human activity, it has made living easier. In contrast, in the area of behavior modification, mechanization has been slow in arriving, with only occasional studies in the literature describing adaptive devices for mentally retarded persons. There is evidence, however, that behavior analysts are recognizing the potential of new and existing technologies as clinical tools. For example, Ball, McCrady, and Teixeira (1978) employed a mercury switch and electronic timer to cue staff to deliver reinforcement for client standing and to implement a DRO (differential reinforcement of other behavior) schedule for maladaptive behavior. Lebouf and Boeverts (1981) used a similar device to cue staff to punish rectal digging, as did Macurik (1979) to control slouching. A response amplification device involving microswitches was used by Wacker, Berg, Wiggins, Muldoon, and Cavanaugh (1985) to evaluate reinforcer preferences. Other electromechanical equipment, which has been developed in earlier years, includes devices to signal inappropriate urination or defecation and to treat nocturnal enuresis (Foxx & Azrin, 1973). Browning (1983) and Smith, McConnell, Walter, and Miller (1985) described other devices to assist in stimulus control and prompting at temporal and spatial distances. A variety of equipment has also been developed to assist mentally retarded individuals more directly. For example, McClure, Moss, McPeters, and Kirkpatrick (1986) used a switch-operated vibratory stimulus to decrease hand-mouthing in a profoundly retarded boy, and Smith, Olson, Berger, and McConnell (1981) used an auditory response amplification device to improve the verbal behavior of an autistic child.

Although behavioral educators have not emphasized the development of prosthetic aids and environments, the integration of prosthetics and behavior management seems to have much to offer severely and profoundly handicapped individuals. The behavioral programmer could teach mentally retarded persons how to use prosthetic devices or how to interact with prosthetically arranged environments. For example, more emphasis might be placed on using reinforcement procedures in teaching retarded persons to use elevators, wheelchairs, and canes, and to wear and use other prosthetic devices, such as artificial limbs, hearing aids, and eyeglasses.

At present, the outlook for the development and utilization of a prosthetic technology is bright. The rapidly expanding availability of microcomputers and general electrical-mechanical equipment may signal the dawning of a new age in the development of behavioral prosthetics with mentally retarded individuals (Coker, 1984; Pfadt & Tryon, 1983). Electromechanical devices are relatively inexpensive, easily constructed and maintained, and may be adapted to a wide variety of client needs (Mulick et al., 1983). Although these devices are very useful in many situations, there are problems and limitations associated with their usage. For example, electromechanical devices are difficult to employ when complex or multiresponse operants are targeted or when the input to such devices is not a simple on–off or limited linear input. However, when interfaced with a microcomputer, electromechanical devices allow minute responses, such as wrist turns or head nods, to control significant environmental events. In many respects, the microcomputer could become a universal behavioral prosthetic, allowing the retarded person continuous access to previously inaccessible environments.

The microcomputer can also serve functions besides that of a behavioral prosthetic; for example, it can be employed as an individualized tutor. Much of the training and education performed with mentally retarded persons is highly individualized. The advent of computer-assisted instruction (CAI) provides a means for delivering individualized instruction, without focusing all of the teacher's time on one student. Applications of CAI with mentally retarded persons can be used to teach academic skills, such as reading and mathematics, or to teach more basic discrimination and conceptual skills (see Ager, 1985; Conners, Caruso, & Detterman, 1986; and Tighe & Groeneweg, 1985, for reviews, and Lally, 1981, 1982, for CAI applications on minicomputers). Although existing CAI systems cannot always be employed with mentally retarded individuals, they can be adapted and modified to meet the specific physical and behavioral needs of retarded individuals, by providing, for example, alternative input devices (other than the usual keyboard) and/or software (see Wood, 1986, for a review).

The potential for implementation of this technology has not even been approached, with the technological advancements occurring much more quickly than behavioral researchers can adapt them for use with mentally retarded persons. Special attention should be addressed to the development of microcomputer-controlled "performance assistants," which would allow the mentally retarded individual to function independently in the environment.

Of course, microcomputer systems may also be employed as data collection and information storage devices. Adaptation of existing microcomputer technologies permits the collection of multiple-response data *in vivo* or from a videotape. Microcomputers can be used to store and retrieve client records in the form of a database, and many commercial software packages are available for database development (for reviews of clinical applications, see Romanczyk, 1986).

In summary, with the increasing sophistication, low cost, and wide availability of electronic equipment and microcomputers, it is becoming more commonplace to employ this new technology with mentally retarded persons. However, behavioral researchers need to become more broadly aware of the potential of this technology and to evaluate its utility with mentally retarded clients. With effort, behavior modifiers may be able to realize in the near future Lindsley's (1964) call for the development of truly adaptive behavioral prosthetics.

Staff Training and Management

The practice of behavior modification involves changing a client's behavior by manipulating critical aspects of the environment. In the case of mentally retarded persons, the environment most frequently altered is social in nature. For example, in institutions and group homes, direct care staff spend the largest amount of time with the clients (Iwata, Bailey, Brown, Foshee, & Alpern, 1976). Although direct care staff have a profound influence on the client's behavior, the influence that they exert is often less than satisfactory

(Burg, Reid, & Lattimore, 1979; Reid & Whitman, 1983; Repp, Barton, & Brulle, 1981). As a consequence, their behavior constitutes a critical social environment that must be programmed to manage the client's behavior (Faw, Reid, Schepis, Fitzgerald, & Welty, 1981; Iwata et al., 1976). In developing programs for staff training and management, behavior modifiers have emphasized the employment of the same sorts of generic techniques utilized in programs for mentally retarded persons. Although these programs have been successful in the short-term, evidence of long-term maintenance of targeted staff behaviors is relatively meager (Reid & Whitman, 1983).

Given this maintenance problem, it is surprising that staff management researchers do not show more cognizance of work conducted in closely related areas, such as human resource management. A large body of research, examining procedures for maximizing human performance in the work setting, reflects a burgeoning organizational behavior management (OBM) movement. See Prue, Frederiksen, and Bacon (1978), and Rapp, Carstensen, and Prue (1983) for annotated bibliographies; Frederiksen (1982), and O'Brien, Dickinson, and Rosow (1982) for examples and reviews of research; and Hall (1982), Luthans and Kreitner (1975), and Scott and Podsakoff (1985) for overviews of the OBM area. The *Journal of Organizational Behavior Management* also provides intriguing perspectives on staff training and how behavior analysis can be a powerful tool for staff management. To illustrate the potential relevance of this literature for staff management research and programs in the mental retardation area, a brief review of some basic conceptualizations put forth by OBM investigators will be presented and their implications explored.

Within the OBM area, the supervisor–worker relationship is analogous to the supervisor–staff relationship in facilities serving mentally retarded persons. The supervisor–worker component is examined as part of a complex system of interlocking and interdependent parts (Krapfl & Gasparotto, 1982). An adaptation of the "behavior management triangle" (Luthans & Kreitner, 1975) illustrates the nature of this system. In this conceptualization, organizations are seen to be dependent upon the occurrence of organizationally important *outcomes* (such as increased profits), which are products of employee *accomplishments* (such as sales), which, in turn, are related to employee *behaviors* (such as calling on clients). A close parallel exists in institutions for the mentally retarded. The *outcome* might be an increased overall rate and frequency of adaptive behaviors by clients; the *accomplishments*, the establishment of specific client repertoires, such as handwashing; and the *behaviors* necessary for these accomplishments to occur, a number of direct care responses, such a staff prompting and reinforcement. The ultimate success or failure of a management program is viewed as resting with those who control the supervisor's environment, specifically with higher level supervisors and a broad supervision chain (see Page, Iwata, & Reid, 1982). Proceeding down from the top of the organizational chart, higher level supervisor behavior is a major determinant of lower level supervisor behavior, which, in turn, controls worker (line-staff) behavior. Organizational behavior managers recognize that this "top down" chain of behavior management is a major determinant of whether or not positive changes in worker behavior are ultimately maintained (see Crowell & Anderson, 1982, for further discussion). In distinct contrast, staff management researchers in the area of mental retardation have typically focused their programs more narrowly and exclusively on the behavior of staff who are low in the supervisory chain (see Reid & Whitman, 1983).

Another potentially important contribution of the OBM literature to the development of staff training and management programs for mentally retarded clients lies in the area of leadership development. In a successful behavioral intervention, a supervisor must be able to monitor a subordinate's behavior directly, evoke and shape the desired employee behaviors, provide appropriate discriminative stimuli, reinforce desired behaviors, inhibit or extinguish undesired behaviors, and develop these same abilities in their subordinates. Collectively, this response class has been referred to in the OBM literature as leadership (Scott & Podsakoff, 1982). Leadership is an operant that may be measured and managed (Komaki, 1986; Komaki, Zlotnick, & Jensen, 1986; Scott & Podsakoff, 1982, 1985). Perhaps the most important characteristic of effective leaders is that they become a potent source of social reinforcement for staff.

Although the general importance of social reinforcement has been acknowledged in the staff management of mentally retarded persons, little attention has been given to how one establishes social reinforcement capabilities in supervisors. This issue of the development social reinforcers is of particular significance in institutions for mentally retarded persons. In these institutions, direct care staff often have low pay, low prestige, and aversive working conditions. Tangible reinforcers cannot be readily manipulated because of union regulations and lack of material resources. When tangible reinforcers cannot be employed, social reinforcement becomes a prime intervention technique. Social reinforcers are particularly useful because they can be dispensed immediately and in a wide variety of forms, are hard to satiate, difficult to legislate against, and tend to be self-replenishing and, most importantly, can insure program maintenance. In general, the more a supervisor becomes a dispenser of social reinforcement, the more potent such reinforcers become as the supervisor acquires greater conditioned reinforcing properties. Social reinforcement has the added benefit of making the workplace a more positive context. It has been suggested that staff behavior is often governed by avoidance contingencies (Skinner, 1953, 1986). The imposition of a regular social reinforcement schedule by supervisors is likely to reduce their use of aversive contingencies and thereby evoke more prosocial behaviors as well as reduce interpersonal conflict and aggressive verbal behavior in those they supervise (Emurian, Emurian, & Brady, 1985).

Despite the importance of social reinforcement to the success of a staff management program, little attention has been given to how this should be accomplished procedurally. Although social reinforcement can be a powerful means of controlling behavior, the specific conditions that lead a supervisor to acquire social reinforcement capabilities have not been fully articulated. Future research needs to examine the condition under which supervisors become potent social reinforcers, and the types of social reinforcement that are most effective. As this research is conducted, the effects of such social reinforcement manipulations need to be broadly assessed; for example, in terms of their impact on staff absenteeism, behavior generalization and maintenance, and employee acceptance of behavior modification programs.

Programs for Aging Mentally Retarded Individuals

Although evidence suggests that mentally retarded individuals are living longer (Lubin & Kiely, 1985), research directed at developing and evaluating behavior modification programs for this elderly population has been sparse (Foxx, McMorrow, Bittle, & Ness, 1986; Kleitsch, Whitman, & Santos, 1983; Schleien, Weyman, & Kiernan, 1981). The reason for this lack of research is unclear. It appears that applied researchers do not view elderly mentally retarded individuals as distinct from younger mentally retarded individuals and assume that the needs of older retarded individuals can be met through the same types of programs developed for younger populations. Available research suggests, however, that the needs of the aging mentally retarded individuals may be different from those of younger mentally retarded individuals, as well as from aging individuals of normal intellectual capacity (Heller, 1985; Puccio, Janicki, Otis, & Rettig, 1983).

Although it is generally accepted that mentally retarded individuals differ from nonretarded individuals in their development during childhood, it now appears that they may also differ in their development during later adulthood. Whereas normal older individuals remain relatively intact, both physically and cognitively, well into their 70s, there is evidence to suggest that mentally retarded individuals may begin to deteriorate earlier (Eyman & Widaman, 1987; Puccio et al., 1983). For example, the gradual loss of cognitive abilities associated with Alzheimer's disease occurs earlier for Down syndrome individuals who survive into their 40s and 50s than for non-Down syndrome Alzheimer patients (Wisniewski & Merz, 1985). Eyman and Widaman (1987) also found a pattern of cognitive decline, as early as age 30, in institutionalized moderately mentally retarded individuals. Moreover, there is evidence that the percentage of elderly severely and profoundly mentally retarded individuals is considerably lower than in the normal population (Janicki & MacEachron, 1984). Because longevity is associated with cognitive decline, with the "terminal drop" perhaps beginning approximately five years before death (Reigel & Reigel, 1972), it is logical to assume that a loss of cognitive and behavioral skills occurs earlier in retarded than nonretarded individuals. In summary, there is reason to believe that the development of mentally retarded individuals as a group may follow a somewhat different trajectory across the life span, with slower development in childhood and a lower ultimate peak of performance and an earlier onset of decline than for the normal population. Such a developmental curve may resemble the one depicted in Figure 1.

Although much is known about development in nonretarded elderly individuals (Baltes & Schaie, 1976; Denney, 1984; Horn & Donaldson, 1976; Salthouse & Somberg, 1982), relatively little specific data are available con-

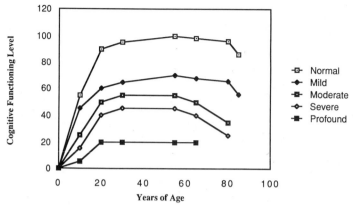

FIGURE 1. Hypothetical curves describing the functioning levels of normal and of mildly, moderately, severely, and profoundly retarded persons over their life spans.

cerning the cognitive and behavioral development of mentally retarded individuals in their later years (Eyman & Widaman, 1987). Before relevant treatment programs can be developed for aging mentally retarded individuals, more information is required concerning their specific and unique behavioral needs. Based on available data, it appears that program development is needed in a number of areas (Catapano, Levy, & Levy, 1985; Heller, 1985; Janicki & MacEachron, 1984). For example, special behavioral programs are needed to assist aging mentally retarded individuals in preparing for and dealing with age-related physical changes. Because mentally retarded individuals are usually unable to read and frequently are unaware of the educational information provided by television and other sources, they are likely to be ignorant of normal aging processes. Programs are needed to teach them how to recognize the signs of aging, and to identify these signs in themselves, as well as how to cope with and adapt to the aging process. Moreover, programs are needed to teach new behaviors, such as being responsible for taking medication, using community medical facilities, and using such prosthetic devices as a cane or walker—behaviors that will allow aging mentally retarded individuals to live more independently as long as possible.

Programs are also needed to help mentally retarded individuals adapt to new living arrangements. Older mentally retarded individuals, dependent upon elderly parents, may suddenly be placed in nursing homes when a parent becomes ill or dies. Elderly group home residents who are unable to participate in existing day programs may also be relocated. Such relocations in the nonretarded elderly are often associated with increases in stress, illness, and higher mortality rates (Heller, 1985). Transition for retarded individuals might be eased by appropriate behavioral training programs that allow for a gradual transition into a new setting. In addition, cognitive-behavioral programming may assist retarded individuals in coping with personal loss, particularly loss due to the death of relatives and friends. Programs that prepare them in advance for the death of a loved one would be particularly helpful. Such deaths are less likely to be accepted by retarded individuals who do not have spouses or children to provide them with active support.

Finally, programs teaching caregivers how to implement the above programs and how to cope with the unique problems of the aging retarded individuals are needed. Emphasis in such programs must be directed at maintaining existing client skills. The challenge behavior modifiers must confront is to recognize when existing behavioral interventions are adequate with this population, and when such programs need to be revised and tailored to the developmental needs of the aging retarded individuals. However, to insure proper program selection, behavioral practitioners must first conduct a thorough and systematic needs assessment.

Family Interventions

Currently, most mentally retarded children are reared in a family environment. In sharp contrast to societal practices followed several decades ago, even children who are severely retarded are cared for more often at home than in an institution (Vitello & Soskin, 1985). As home-care programs have become more common, there has been a growing recognition by professionals that certain parenting practices may be less than ideal, inhibiting development in the children and producing tension among family members. Thus, it is not surprising that in order to train children with mental retardation, behavioral programmers have focused increasingly on working with families and especially parents. More generally, it has been argued that training programs for parents should be an essential component of all child education programs. Graziano (1977) has pointed out that parents are the natural choice to be primary mental health agents because they have the most frequent contact with their children, they have the most significant impact on their children's development, and because they have moral, ethical, and legal responsibilities for their children. Graziano emphasized that it is not the task of the therapist to assume the burden for treatment, but rather, through training programs, to assist parents in fulfilling their educational responsibilities to their children.

In an attempt to identify variables that impede development in children, several researchers have described an interactive-deficiency model of parenting. Research suggests that deficiencies in parent–child interactions not only contribute to developmental delay but also provide the natural focus for intervention programs (Allen, Affleck, McQuenney, & McGrade, 1982). Past research has demonstrated that parents can be taught to use behavioral techniques to address these deficiencies and facilitate the progress of developmentally delayed children (Cowart, Iwata, & Poynter, 1984; Harris, Wolchik, & Milch, 1983). Research also suggests that parental training is superior to direct child intervention (see Kaiser & Fox, 1986).

Although numerous behaviorally oriented training programs for parents have been shown to be effective in working with mentally retarded children, little attention has been given to evaluating the utility of such programs when administered with infants. This is surprising given that during the past two decades it has become increasingly evident that early intervention constitutes an effective approach to working with a wide range of clients (Field, Widmayer, Stringer, & Ignatoff, 1980; Moran & Whitman, 1985). Intervening early in the life of the child, while parents are just developing a parenting style, not only assists in the habilitative process but also has the added potential advantage of preventing further retardation in that child.

Implicit in past behavioral training research programs involving parents of retarded children is a narrow conceptualization of the parenting unit. Most parent training research has involved only the mother. Parke (1986) has argued that conceptualizations of the child's environment must be expanded to include also the father–child unit and the mother–father–child relationships. Inclusion of the father in parent training programs makes sense from a variety of perspectives. Lamb (1976, 1977) points out that fathers as well as mothers have significant impact on child development, although the type of influence each parent exerts may differ. Although empirical studies of early education programs for young delayed children have not examined the impact of fathers on development (Wiegerink, Hocutt, Posante-Loro, & Bristol, 1980), it has been observed that fathers of mentally retarded children show more signs of stress, are less effective copers, and are less involved with their handicapped child than mothers (Bristol & Gallagher, 1986; Cummings, 1976; Gallagher, Scharfman, & Bristol, 1984). Results by Stoneman and Brody (1982) indicate that despite the fact that a developmentally delayed child puts increased demands on the family, fathers of these children do not help mothers any more than comparable fathers of nonhandicapped children. They observed that fathers of handicapped children are only half as likely as mothers to assume a teaching role with their children. In combination, these studies suggest that inclusion of fathers of mentally retarded children in parenting training programs may have positive effects on their children's development and on paternal and maternal well-being.

A broader family system's conceptualization also suggests that inclusion of nonhandicapped siblings in intervention programs may be advisable. Farber (1975) contends that families of severely retarded children are better able to cope when siblings are able to assume helping roles in the family. In support of this contention, a variety of studies indicate the positive effects of sibling interaction on child development (see Brody & Stoneman, 1986, for a review). In a more general vein, the influence of social support systems, extrafamilial as well as intrafamilial, on family stability needs to be examined. Research suggests that the presence of a mentally retarded child in a family may not only increase stress but also lead to family schism (Reed & Reed, 1965). Bristol (1979) found that one variable that differentiated high-stress from low-stress mothers of autistic children was the adequacy of the informal social supports provided them by the nuclear family, extended family, friends, neighbors, and parents of other developmentally delayed children. Data from Wahler's (1980) study indicate that a mother's successful implementation of a behavioral intervention program is directly related to the availability of social supports.

In summary, past research and theory indicate that behavior modifiers could benefit considerably by taking a broader life-span and family systems perspective as they structure home intervention programs for retarded children. More attention needs to be given to the development of early behavioral intervention programs when the handicapped individual first shows signs of delay. More emphasis also needs to be placed on structuring training programs that include the fathers and siblings of retarded family members, as well as the mothers. In evaluating various types of family intervention programs, broader based measurement systems are needed to evaluate the comparative effects of these programs on the development, maintenance, and generalization of the handicapped child's adaptive behavior across different settings. It seems likely that inclusion of multiple family members in a training program should facilitate more enduring and generalized behavioral changes. From a social validity perspective, evaluations of family intervention programs should include measurements of the impact of these programs on the perceived level of stress and feelings of well-being of various family members, and their perception of the retarded family member. A family system's perspective suggests that in addition to the direct and indirect effects of the program on each family member, the status of various family relationships, such as the marital relationship and the nonhandicapped sibling–parent relationships, should be assessed. An ideal intervention program should not only facilitate the development of the handicapped family member but also reduce family stress and strengthen family relationships.

Interventions with Mentally Retarded Parents

It has been estimated that about 50% of mentally retarded individuals marry (Bass, 1973). Although accurate data concerning the number of children reared by mentally retarded parents are not available, there has been considerable discussion about the adequacy of caregiving provided by these parents (Greenspan & Budd, 1986). On the one hand, it has been suggested, that the children of mentally retarded parents are not well cared for and are at great risk for mental retardation (Schilling, Shinke, Blythe, & Barth, 1982). In fact, in many states, the child is routinely removed from the custody of parents who are labeled mentally retarded (Hertz, 1979). On the other hand, it has been pointed out that mentally retarded parents are not a homogeneous group and that many function within or close to normal limits (Mira & Roddy, 1980). Because few studies have examined the parenting styles of mentally retarded individuals and the long range impact of these styles on child development, empirical data are needed to document if and to what extent problems occur. There is, however, general agreement that, as a group, mentally retarded parents are in need of and can benefit from interventions directed at developing their parenting skills (Greenspan & Budd, 1986). It is questionable whether programs for other parent populations can be utilized with mentally retarded parents without being modified. The challenge to behavioral educators is to evaluate the utility of training programs empirically validated with other types of parents and as necessary to develop innovative training programs for retarded parents and their children. For further general background information on mentally retarded parents and general approaches to developing creative training environments, the reader is referred to a chapter by Greenspan and Budd (1986).

Self-Regulation

Implicit in most characterizations of mentally retarded individuals is a picture of a person who displays not only specific adaptive behavior deficiencies, but who also has more general self-regulatory problems. These problems of self-regulation are manifested in a variety of ways: such as by failing to act in an appropriate manner when such action is within the individual's response capabilities; by engaging in behaviors that are generally adaptive but at the wrong time or wrong place; by depending on others to direct their action; and by not transferring learned action patterns to new situations. As a consequence of these types of self-regulatory problems, society has often placed mentally retarded individuals in protective environments.

Because of the mentally retarded individual's dependency on others, it is not surprising that behavior modifiers have turned their attention to the development of technologies that teach self-control and self-management skills. Through such technologies, retarded individuals have been taught to define problem situations, to provide verbal cues to themselves, to monitor and evaluate their behavior, and to use reinforcement procedures to motivate their own behavior (Whitman, Burgio, & Johnston, 1984). In order for a self-management program to be judged successful, individuals trained must be able to change their own behavior by altering either the external and/or their own internal (covert) environment (Thoresen & Mahoney, 1974). Although self-regulatory behavior is taught initially within a context of external control, the goal of self-management programs is to shift control of the behavior of individuals from external social agents to the individuals themselves.

The advantages of teaching mentally retarded individuals to manage their behavior have been discussed at length by others (O'Leary & Dubey, 1979; Rosenbaum & Drabman, 1979). First, independent behavior is evaluated positively by our society. Second, the need for supervision is minimized when an individual exerts self-control. In this regard, reduction of supervision is important because continuous monitoring is time-consuming, often impossible, and ties up valuable human resources that could be used in other ways. Third, self-management skills allow a person to generalize behavior to situations in which training has not been explicitly given.

Past reviews of research directed at developing self-management skills in mentally retarded individuals suggest that such skills can be taught and when utilized result in more appropriate academic, job-related, and community-living behaviors (Shapiro, 1981, 1986; Whitman, 1987; Whitman et al., 1984). Shapiro (1986) concluded that while it is unlikely that mentally retarded individuals will acquire self-control skills without instruction, these persons are quite capable of learning these skills with a minimum of effort. However, the aforementioned reviews emphasize that more attention needs to be given by researchers to assessing the characteristics of those individuals who benefit most from self-management training and to examining how these type of training can be structured to serve a broader number of individuals.

For example, Whitman (1987), in discussing one type of self-management program, self-instruction, has suggested that its utility may vary depending on the language skills of the individual. He argues that self-instruction will benefit most persons who have difficulty processing and utilizing information given through an external instructional format. He suggests that self-instruction has special utility for retarded individuals because of their receptive language deficiencies, which make it difficult for them to understand the spoken word and their expressive language problems, which prevent them from dynamically using words to cue their behavior. Future research needs to examine the relative utility of external and self-instructional formats as well as to examine whether and how the specific linguistic characteristic of retarded individuals determines the amount of benefit they derive from these programs. Research to date, while not definitive, suggests that self-instruction may be more effective than external instruction when teaching mentally retarded individuals (Keogh, Whitman, & Maxwell, 1987; Whitman, Spence, & Maxwell, 1987).

As indicated earlier, one major reason for teaching mentally retarded individuals to self-regulate is that it enables them to control their behavior in situations beyond those in which training occurred. To facilitate generalization, it may be easier to program an individual's verbal behavior than the external environment. Systematic situation analyses, however, must be conducted before such verbal training strategies can be developed. Insofar as environments have common stimulus components and require similar behaviors, it is reasonable to expect that verbally mediated generalization can be produced. Retarded individuals must be taught the dynamic relationship between their verbal behaviors, situational characteristics, and the generalization process. Ultimately, to show extensive generalization, trainees must be taught not only specific verbal strategies, but also be taught to perform situational analyses themselves and to develop their own strategies. This type of research is likely to be demanding from both an assessment and a training perspective. Because generalized self-control is perhaps the ultimate sign of an individual's ability to adapt to the environment, the benefits of this type of research and training program are considerable.

Applications of Basic Research to Clinical Practice

Because the conceptual and methodological roots of behavior modification lie in the experimental analysis of behavior and its accompanying philosophy of science, that is, radical behaviorism (Branch, 1987; Skinner, 1953, 1978), it would seem that practitioners and researchers working in the area of behavior modification should be conversant with and draw upon this basic literature as a resource and database. In reality, the influence of basic research on applied work is minimal (Poling, Picker, Grosset, Hall-Johnson, & Holbrook, 1981). Baer (1981) suggested that because behavior modification has sufficiently advanced and has its own unique set of questions and concerns, it does not need to depend on basic research to develop. However, other investigators have indicated that the widening gulf between basic and applied research may lead to the stagnation of research and practice in behavior modification (Birnbrauer, 1981; Deitz, 1978; Hayes, Rincover, & Solnick, 1980; Michael, 1980; Pierce & Epling, 1980).

Epling and Pierce (1986) have suggested that basic and applied researchers have much to learn from one another. They point out that the areas of experimental and applied behavior analysis share not only the same intellectual heritage, aims, scope and metatheoretical stance, but also that these two areas are often addressing the same problems. On the one hand, applied research can generate new and socially important experimental questions for basic researchers to examine. On the other hand, basic research assists applied researchers by developing innovative treatment methods, methods which might not be otherwise developed given the ethical and practical constraints of clinical research. Applied researchers can also derive from the basic literature new methods for evaluating programs (Epling & Pierce, 1986). Thus, in this section, several recent trends in basic research that might provide assistance to those involved in developing behavior modification programs for retarded persons will be discussed.

One potentially productive interface between basic and applied research is in the area of verbal behavior (Skinner, 1957), a response domain in which the mentally retarded have extensive deficiencies. Research on language acquisition by chimpanzees has already yielded a sophisticated and potentially effective technology for teaching communication skills to mentally retarded individuals through the use of computer-controlled language boards (Romski, White, Millen, & Rumbaugh, 1984; Rumbaugh, 1977). In addition, procedures used for teaching language (Savage-Rumbaugh, 1984) and counting skills (Rumbaugh, Savage-Rumbaugh, & Hegel, 1987) to chimpanzees may prove useful to the behavior modification practitioner. Other basic research has indicated that when verbal behavior is acquired, mands (e.g., requesting) and tacts (e.g., labeling) are initially functionally separate repertoires (Lamarre & Holland, 1985), as are speaker and listener repertoires (Guess, 1969; Guess & Baer, 1973; Silverman, Anderson, Marshall, & Baer, 1986). This research suggests that teaching tacts before mands mimics the "natural" sequence of language development and that verbal operants must be taught explicitly, not relied upon to emerge as a result of "learning words."

In still other basic research, the conditional relations between words and phrases have been studied (Chase, Johnson, & Sulzer-Azaroff, 1985), and successful teaching strategies based on this work have been developed (Braam & Poling, 1983). The importance of conditional relations between stimuli in the development of reading has been particularly emphasized (Lee, 1981; Lee & Pegler, 1982; Sidman, 1977). Research into the training and formation of stimulus classes has shown that when certain sets of stimulus equivalences are taught, untaught equivalences will emerge (Devaney, Hayes, & Nelson, 1986; Dube, McIlvane, Mackay, & Stoddard, 1987; Lazar, Davis-Lang, & Sanchez, 1984; Sidman, Kirk, & Wilson-Morris, 1985; Sidman, Rauzin, Lazar, Cunningham, Tailby, & Carrigan, 1982; Sidman & Tailby, 1982). For example, MacKay and Sidman's (1984) research indicates that if a retarded child is taught to point to a picture of a cat and to the word "cat" upon hearing the spoken word "cat," the child will subsequently point to the picture of a cat upon seeing the word "cat," and vice-versa, without any explicit training. Apparently, the latter two stimulus relations emerge "spontaneously" as a result of training. It is reasonable to assume that programs designed to capitalize on the emergence of these untaught conditional relations could improve the efficiency and scope of programs in language training for the retarded. For a review of this research, the reader is referred to Fields, Verhave, and Fath (1984), Sidman (1986, and a special issue of *Analysis and Intervention in Developmental Disabilities* (Stoddard, 1986).

Once receptive language skills are taught, behavior can come under the control of verbal contingencies. Research into rule-governed behavior has shown that teaching linguistic rules facilitates learning (Vaughan, 1985) and that rules may alter the way in which people interact with the prevailing contingencies and their subsequent behavior (Bentall & Lowe, 1987; Bentall, Lowe, & Beasty, 1985; Buskist & Miller, 1982; Hayes, Brownstein, Zettle, Rosenfarb, & Korn, 1986; Lowe, Beasty, & Bentall, 1983; Matthews, Catania, & Shimoff, 1985; Shimoff, Catania, & Matthews, 1981). Rule-governed behavior (Skinner, 1969), that is, behavior which is controlled by words which describe contingencies, need not, however, come into direct contact with actual environmental contingencies to be maintained (see Baron & Galizio, 1983, for a review). Indeed, one characteristic of rule-governed behavior is its relative insensitivity to prevailing environmental contingencies (Catania, Matthews, & Shimoff, 1982). The efficiency of using instructional control, directions, commands, and verbal prompts rather than direct contingencies is considerable, because rule-governed behavior allows for the bridging of spatio/temporal gaps and produces behavioral changes more quickly than contingency management programs. Moreover, because rule-governed behavior can be regulated by the person, as well as others, it provides the basis for self-control training. For example, using a rule-governed behavior paradigm, Woods and Lowe (1985) taught mentally retarded adults to self-regulate inappropriate social behavior.

Another important area of basic research that could have substantial impact on applied work with retarded individuals has to do with the scheduling of behavior-consequence relationships (Ferster & Skinner, 1957; see Zeiler, 1977, for a review). It is clear that temporal relations between events in the environment and behavior can exert a profound influence on behavior, and that reinforcement schedules are fundamental determinants of behavior (Dews, 1958; Morse & Kelleher, 1970). Although practitioners in the area of mental retardation show familiarity with some schedules, such as DRO (Poling & Ryan, 1982), there are many other schedules which they might employ. Schedules may be formulated mathematically to allow for more precise prediction and control of behavior. One long-studied mathematical formulation is the matching law (deVilliers, 1977; Herrnstein, 1970). The matching law describes the allocation of two or more concurrent operants under different schedules of reinforcement and holds that the relative amount of time or number of responses allocated to a particular schedule is a function of that schedule's relative density of reinforcement. The matching law can be applied to determine the relative value of reinforcing events by analyzing the temporal distribution of behavior between two or more alternatives. Indirect manipulation of a behavior may be accomplished by changing the reinforcement density available to other concurrently available behaviors (see McDowell, 1982; Myerson & Hale, 1984; and Pierce & Epling, 1983, for further discussions of applications of the matching law).

Manipulation of the temporal relations between the opportunities to engage in behaviors in accordance with the response deprivation hypothesis (Allison, Miller, & Wozny, 1979; Hanson & Timberlake, 1983; Konarski, 1987; Podsakoff, 1982; Timberlake, 1984a,b; Timberlake & Allison, 1974) provides a particularly powerful method for controlling behavior in an applied setting (Holburn & Dougher, 1986; Konarski, Crowell, & Duggan, 1985; Konarski, Crowell, Johnson, & Whitman, 1982; Konarski, Johnson, Crowell, & Whitman, 1980, 1981). Expanding upon Premack's (1965) observation that the opportunity to engage in high-probability behaviors will reinforce the occurrence of low-probability behaviors, the response deprivation hypothesis states that under certain conditions any response can serve as a reinforcer or punisher for another response. Reinforcement is conceptualized not as a discrete event, but as an opportunity to engage in behavior which was previously suppressed. The significance of the response deprivation hypothesis for applied work is that it expands considerably the types and number of reinforcers and punishers available to trainers and provides a precise method for their selection. It has particular importance for behavioral interventions with mentally retarded persons because of the problems of locating effective reinforcers for certain retarded individuals, particularly the severely and profoundly handicapped.

In addition to the research reviewed, there are numerous other basic research programs that might make a substantial contribution to research and practice in mental retardation, such as research on stereotyped behaviors in animals (Anderson, Crowell, Hantula, Siroky, & Brown, 1989; Iversen, Ragnasdottir, & Randrup, 1984; Peffer-Smith et al., 1983; Zentall & Zentall, 1983), trust and cooperation (Hake & Schmid, 1981; Schmid & Hake, 1983; Schmitt, 1984), and the experimental analysis of human operant behavior (Buskist et al., 1987; Lowe, 1979, 1983; see also Buskist & Miller, 1982, for a bibliography). To the extent that applied behavior analysts can become intelligent consumers of this research and basic researchers can clearly communicate the applied implications of their work, it seems obvious that new and effective intervention programs for mentally retarded individuals are likely to emerge.

CRITICAL ISSUES IN BEHAVIORAL PROGRAMMING

More research must be conducted before it can be concluded that generally effective techniques exist for modifying the behavior of mentally retarded persons. Although research examining the efficacy of behavioral techniques in numerous behavioral domains is available, data concerning the efficacy of technologies in other areas are just beginning to emerge. It can also be argued persuasively that research alone does not generate a better technology and that other factors must be taken into account as complex and critical decisions concerning program objectives and educational procedures are made. The bases on which these decisions are made often involve a multitude of *a priori* as well as empirical considerations.

Although a behavioral model can be extremely useful in defining the various behavioral deficiencies of mentally retarded individuals, this model does not specify in an *a priori* fashion criteria for determining which behavioral goals should be addressed first and in what sequence specific behavior-change programs should occur. In other words, a behavioral model does not provide information about whether a specific program being considered for a retarded individual is the most educationally appropriate. White and Haring (1978) have pointed out that "it is important to know exactly what we want our pupils to accomplish, for without specific goals and objectives, education may amount to little more than a series of loosely related intrusions upon their lives." Ultimately, decisions concerning goal selection and achievement relate to the value structure of society and the demands society places on its members. Despite the existence of general societal guidelines, practitioners are often forced to make decisions on a somewhat arbitrary basis because of the absence of any absolute and specific criteria for selecting goals and evaluating behavior changes.

To assist in making program decisions, educators who are involved in developing programs often either explicitly or implicitly employ a normal developmental model. This model suggests that the skills taught to a mentally retarded child and the order in which the skills are taught should be dictated by how a normal child's behavior develops (Haring & Bricker, 1976). In sharp contrast to this development perspective is a position taken by Switzky, Rotatori, Miller, and Freagon (1979), who suggest that educators should take a remedial approach to strengthening skills regardless of hypothesized developmental sequences. They emphasize that human beings are plastic and that rigid or invariant developmental sequences of behavior probably do not exist (cf. Bower, 1976). Whichever perspective one might adopt, the point that should be emphasized is that such conceptualizations have been adopted but not empirically examined by educators. At present, a scientifically valid instructional model for the retarded individual does not exist.

Although conceptualizations such as those provided by the developmental model can specify what objectives should be pursued in an educational program and serve as a standard of reference against which to evaluate behavior change, they do not stipulate the type of environment in which treatment should take place. Behavior modifiers espouse the position that treatment should take place in the setting that best assists behavioral growth. Within the behavioral model, a training environment that produces more rapid and generalized changes is typically considered superior to one that effects change more slowly. Although learning rate and generalization considerations should ideally dictate where educational programs take place, in reality a variety of practical and legal concerns also influence this choice. For example, although education for mentally retarded persons should often involve one-on-one instruction, the nature of the curricula, the lack of personnel, and the limited physical facilities often demand that children be grouped. White and Haring (1978) pointed out that in regular educational programs, children are generally assigned to classes on the basis of age, with only minimal attention given to skill level.

From a legal perspective, Public Law 94-142 states that handicapped children, including those in institutions, should, whenever possible, be educated with children who are not handicapped. Moreover, it stipulates that separate schooling or removal of handicapped children should occur only when the severity of the handicap is such that education in regular classrooms with the use of supplementary aids and services cannot be easily achieved. When removal does occur for these reasons, this law indicates that there must be a continuum of alternative placements available including special classrooms, special schools, home instruction and instruction in hospitals and institutions. Kenowitz, Zweibel, and Edgar (1978) pointed out that decisions concerning what constitutes the least restrictive educational setting should take into account the physical setting in which education takes place, the nature of the educational program, and the child's opportunity to interact with the nonhandicapped.

The formulation of PL 94-142 and its emphasis on program delivery in the least restrictive setting was undoubtedly influenced by the promulgation of the normalization principle in this country (Nirje, 1969; Wolfensberger, 1972). In discussing the implication of this principle, Wolfensberger (1972) suggested that, in human services, both the means of establishing or maintaining personal behaviors as well as the nature of the personal behaviors towards which these services are directed should be as culturally normative as possible. However, it has been persuasively argued that just because a procedure is normative, it is not necessarily as effective as or more effective than specialized procedures (National Association for Retarded Children, 1972). In fact, Throne (1975) indicated that using normative rather than specialized procedures for educating retarded children is inadvisable because the nature of retardation dictates that extraordinary means be employed. In this regard, Mesibov (1976) suggested that because the normalization model is concerned with service systems rather than individuals, it fails to recognize the basic differences between retarded persons and nonretarded persons and the diverse needs of retarded individuals. If the normalization principle is taken literally, any new approach to education might be excluded because it varies from the procedures ordinarily employed. Insofar as behavior modification represents a radical departure from traditional educational procedures, a literal interpretation of the normalization principle would exclude it from at least primary consideration when educational procedures are chosen.

The foregoing discussion points out that there is by no means uniform agreement concerning what goals should be pursued in educational programs with mentally retarded individuals, what techniques should be employed in these programs, and where programs should take place. Ultimately, there is even a question about what constitutes a successful program outcome. Whether one adopts a developmental model, follows the normalization principle, or assumes a pragmatic stance in planning and implementing behavior modification programs, it is imperative that the recipients of these educational programs, along with their advocates, their parents, the educators implementing the programs, and the larger societal structure that supports and monitors these programs be satisfied with them. It is hoped that future program development and society's evaluation of these programs will be based on the finding of scientifically acceptable research.

REFERENCES

Ager, A. (1985). The role of microcomputers in teaching mentally retarded individuals. In J. M. Berg (Ed.), *Science and service in mental retardation* (pp. 224–231). New York: Methuen.

Allen, D. A., Affleck, G., McQuenney, M., & McGrade, B. J. (1982). Validation of the parent behavior progression in an early intervention program. *Mental Retardation, 20,* 159–163.

Allison, Jr., Miller, M., & Wozny, M. (1979). Conservation in behavior. *Journal of Experimental Psychology: General, 108,* 4–34.

Aman, M. (1983). Psychoactive drugs in mental retardation. In J. L. Matson & F. Andrasik (Eds.) *Treatment issues and innovations in mental retardation* (pp. 455–513). New York: Plenum Press.

Anderson, D. C., Crowell, C. R., Hantula, D. A., Siroky, L., & Brown, J. S. (1989). Spontaneous alleyway "pacing" behavior in the rat (*Rattus Norvegicus*): I. Effects of food and water privation, distribution of runaway access time, variations in reward conditions and relationships with other spontaneous behaviors. Manuscript submitted for publication.

Baer, D. M. (1981). A flight of behavior analysis. *Behavior Analyst, 4,* 85–91.

Ball, T. S., McCrady, R. E., & Teixeira, J. (1978). Automated monitoring and cuing for positive reinforcement and differential reinforcement of other behavior. *Journal of Behavior Therapy and Experimental Psychiatry, 9,* 33–37.

Baltes, P. B., & Schaie, K. W. (1976). On the plasticity of intelligence in adulthood and old age: Where Horn and Donaldson fail. *American Psychologist, 36,* 720–724.

Balthazar, E. E. (1971). *Balthazar Scales of Adaptive Behavior: I. Scales for functional independence.* Champaign, IL: Research Press.

Balthazar, E. E. (1973). *Balthazar Scales of Adaptive Behavior: II. Scales of social adaptation.* Palo Alto, CA: Consulting Psychologists Press.

Baron, A., & Galizio, M. (1983). Instructional control of human operant behavior. *Psychological Record, 33,* 495–520.

Barrett, J. E., & Katz, J. L. (1981). Drug effects on behavior maintained by different events. In T. Thompson, P. B. Dews, & W. A. McKim (Eds.), *Advances in behavioral pharmacology* (Vol. 3, pp. 119–168). New York: Academic Press.

Bass, M. S. (1973). Marriage and parenthood. In M. S. Bass (Ed.), *Sexual rights and responsibilities of the mentally retarded.* Santa Barbara: Channel Lithographs.

Bellack, A., & Hersen, M. (1977). *Behavior modification: An introductory textbook.* Baltimore, Williams & Wilkins.

Bentall, R. P., & Lowe, C. F. (1987). The role of verbal behavior in human learning: III. Instructional effects in children. *Journal of the Experimental Analysis of Behavior, 47,* 177–190.

Bentall, R. P., Lowe, C. F., & Beasty, A. (1985). The role of verbal behavior in human learning: II. Developmental differences. *Journal of the Experimental Analysis of Behavior, 43,* 165–181.

Bijou, S. W. (1966). A functional analysis of retarded development. In N. Ellis (Ed.), *International review of research in mental retardation* (Vol. 1, pp. 1–20). New York: Academic Press.

Birnbrauer, J. S. (1981). External validity and experimental investigation of individual behavior. *Analysis and Intervention in Developmental Disabilities, 1,* 117–123.

Blatt, B., & Kaplan, F. (1966). *Christmas in purgatory.* Boston: Allyn & Bacon.

Bower, T. (1976). Repetitive processes in child development. *Scientific American, 234,* 38–47.

Braam, S. J., & Poling, A. (1983). Development of intraverbal behavior in mentally retarded individuals through transfer of stimulus control procedures: Classification of verbal responses. *Applied Research in Mental Retardation, 4,* 279–302.

Branch, M. N. (1987). Behavior analysis: A conceptual and empirical base for behavior therapy. *Behavior Therapist, 4,* 79–84.

Breuning, S. E., & Poling, A. D. (Eds.). (1982). *Drugs and mental retardation.* Springfield, IL: Charles C Thomas.

Bristol, M. M. (1979). *Maternal coping with autistic children: The effect of child characteristics and interpersonal support.* Unpublished doctoral dissertation, University of North Carolina at Chapel Hill.

Bristol, M. M., & Gallagher. (1986). Research on fathers of young handicapped children. In J. J. Gallagher & P. M. Vietze (Eds.), *Families of handicapped persons* (pp. 81–100). Baltimore: Brookes.

Brody, G. H., & Stoneman, Z. (1986). Contextual issues in the study of sibling socialization. In J. J. Gallagher & P. M. Vietze (Eds.), *Families of handicapped persons* (pp. 197–217). Baltimore: Brookes.

Browning, E. R. (1983). A memory pacer for improving stimulus generalization. *Journal of Autism and Developmental Disabilities, 13,* 427–432.

Burg, M. M., Reid, D. H., & Lattimore, J. (1979). Use of a self-recording and supervision program to change institutional staff behavior. *Journal of Applied Behavior Analysis, 12,* 363–375.

Burgio, L. D., Page, T. J., & Capriotti, R. M. (1985). Clinical behavioral pharmacology: Methods for evaluating medications and contingency management. *Journal of Applied Behavior Analysis, 18,* 45–59.

Buskist, W., Deitz, S. M., Etzel, B., Galizio, M., Brownstein, A., Shull, R. L., & Michael, J. (1987). The experimental analysis of human behavior: History, current status and future directions. *Psychological Record, 37,* 3–42.

Buskist, W. F., & Miller, H. L. (1982). A study of human operant behavior, 1958–1981: A topical bibliography. *Psychological Record, 32,* 249–268.

Catania, A. C., Matthews, B. A., & Shimoff, E. (1982). Instructed versus shaped human verbal behavior: Interactions with nonverbal responding. *Journal of the Experimental Analysis of Behavior, 38,* 233–248.

Catapano, P. M., Levy, J. M., & Levy, P. H. (1985). Day activity and vocational program services. In M. P. Janicki & H. M. Wisniewski (Eds.), *Aging and the developmental disabilities* (pp. 305–316). Baltimore: Brookes.

Chase, P. N., Johnson, K. R., & Sulzer-Azaroff, B. (1985). Verbal relations within instruction: Are there subclasses of the intraverbal? *Journal of the Experimental Analysis of Behavior, 43,* 301–313.

Coker, W. B. (1984). Homemade switches and toy adaptation for early training with nonspeaking persons. *Language, Speech, and Hearing Services in the Schools, 15,* 32–36.

Conners, F. A., Caruso, D. R., & Detterman, D. K. (1986). Computer-assisted instruction for the mentally retarded. In N. R. Ellis & N. W. Bray (Eds.) *International review of research in mental retardation* (Vol. 14, pp. 105–129). Orlando, Fl: Academic Press.

Cowart, J. D., Iwata, B. A., & Poynter, H. (1984). Generalization and maintenance in training parents of the mentally retarded. *Applied Research in Mental Retardation, 5,* 233–244.

Craig, T. J., & Behar, R. C. (1980). Trends in the prescription of psychotropic drugs (1970–1977) in a state hospital. *Comprehensive Psychiatry, 21,* 336–345.

Crowell, C. R., & Anderson, D. C. (1982). Systematic behavior management: General program considerations. *Journal of Organizational Behavior Management, 4,* 129–163.

Cummings, S. T. (1976). The impact of the handicapped child on the father: A study of fathers of mentally retarded and chronically ill children. *American Journal of Orthopsychiatry, 36,* 246–255.

Deitz, S. M. (1978). Current status of applied behavior analysis: Science versus technology. *American Psychologist, 33,* 805–814.

Denney, N. W. (1984). A model of cognitive development across the life-span. *Developmental Review, 4,* 171–191.

Devaney, J. M., Hayes, S. C., & Nelson, R. O. (1986). Equivalence class formation in language-able and language-disabled children. *Journal of the Experimental Analysis of Behavior, 46,* 243–257.

deVilliers, P. (1977). Choice in concurrent schedules and a quantitative formulation of the law of effect. In W. K. Honing & J. E. R. Staddon (Eds.), *Handbook of operant behavior* (pp. 233–287). Englewood Cliffs, NJ: Prentice-Hall.

Dews, P. B. (1958). Studies on behavior: IV. Stimulant actions of methamphetamine. *Journal of Pharmacology and Experimental Therapeutics, 122,* 137–147.

Doll, E. A. (1941). The essentials of an inclusive concept of mental deficiency. *American Journal of Mental Deficiency, 465,* 214–219.

Dube, W. V., McIlvane, W. J., Mackay, H. A., Stoddard, L. J. (1987). Stimulus class membership established via stimulus-reinforcer relations. *Journal of the Experimental Analysis of Behavior, 47,* 159–175.

Durand, V. M. (1982). A behavioral/pharmacological intervention for the treatment of severe self-injurious behavior. *Journal of Autism and Developmental Disabilities, 12,* 243–251.

Emurian, H. H., Emurian, C. S., & Brady, J. V. (1985). Positive and negative reinforcement effects in a three-person microsociety. *Journal of the Experimental Analysis of Behavior, 44,* 157–174.

Epling, W. F., & Pierce, W. D. (1986). The basic importance of applied behavior analysis. *Behavior Analyst, 9,* 89–99.

Eyman, R. K., & Widaman, K. F. (1987). Life-span development of institutionalized and community-based mentally retarded persons revisited. *American Journal of Mental Deficiency, 91,* 559–569.

Farber, B. (1975). Family adaptations to severely mentally retarded children. In M. J. Begab & S. A. Richardson (Eds.), *The mentally retarded and society: A social science perspective* (pp. 247–266). Baltimore: University Park Press.

Faw, G. D., Reid, D. H., Schepis, M. M., Fitzgerald, J., & Welty, P. A. (1981). Involving institutional staff in the development and maintenance of sign language skills with profoundly retarded persons. *Journal of Applied Behavior Analysis, 14,* 411–423.

Ferster, C. B., & Skinner, B. F. (1957). *Schedules of reinforcement.* NY: Appleton-Century-Crofts.

Field, T. M., Widmayer, S. M., Stringer, S., & Ignatoff, E. (1980). Teenage, lower-class, black mothers and their pre-term infants: An intervention and developmental follow-up. *Child Development, 51,* 426–436.

Fields, L., Verhave, T., & Fath, S. (1984). Stimulus equivalence and transitive associations: A methodological analysis. *Journal of the Experimental Analysis of Behavior, 42,* 143–157.

Foxx, R. M., & Azrin, N. H. (1973). *Toilet training the retarded: A rapid program for day and nighttime independent toileting.* Champaign, IL: Research Press.

Foxx, R. M., McMorrow, M. J., Bittle, R. G., & Ness, J. (1986). An analysis of social skills generalization in two settings. *Journal of Applied Behavior Analysis, 19,* 299–306.

Frederiksen, L. W. (Eds.). (1982). *Handbook of organizational behavior management.* New York: Wiley.

Gallagher, J. J., Scharfman, W., & Bristol, M. M. (1984). The division of responsibilities in families with preschool handicapped and nonhandicapped children. *Journal of the Division of Early Childhood, 8,* 3–11.

Gardner, W. (1971). *Behavior modification in mental retardation.* Chicago: Aldine-Atherton.

Gearhart, B., & Litton, F. (1975). *The trainable retarded.* St. Louis: Mosby.

Gottlieb, J. (1977). Attitudes toward mainstreaming retarded children and some possible effects on educational practices. In P. Mittler (Ed.), *Research to practice in mental retardation* (Vol. 1, pp. 269–293). Baltimore: University Park Press.

Graziano, A. M. (1977). Parents as behavior therapists. In M. Hersen, R. M. Eisler, & P. M. Miller (Eds.), *Progress in behavior modification* (Vol. 14, pp. 251–298). New York: Academic Press.

Greenspan, S., & Budd, K. S. (1986). Research on mentally retarded parents. In J. J. Gallagher & P. M. Vietze (Eds.), *Families of handicapped persons* (pp. 115–128). Baltimore: Brookes.

Grossman, H. (1973). *Manual on terminology and classification in mental retardation* (1973 revision). Washington, DC: American Association on Mental Deficiency.

Grossman, H. (1977). *Manual on terminology and classification in mental retardation* (rev. ed.). Washington, DC: American Association on Mental Deficiency.

Gualtieri, C. T., & Hawk, B. (1980). Tardive dyskinesia and other drug-induced movement disorders among handicapped children and youth. *Applied Research in Mental Retardation, 1,* 55–69.

Guess, D. (1969). A functional analysis of receptive language and productive speech: Acquisition of the plural morpheme. *Journal of Applied Behavior Analysis, 2,* 55–64.

Guess, D., & Baer, D. (1973). An analysis of individual differences in generalization between receptive and productive language in retarded children. *Journal of Applied Behavior Analysis, 6,* 311–329.

Gunzburg, H. C. (1976). *Progress assessment chart of social and personal development* (4th ed.). Stratford-Avon, England: SEFA.

Hake, D. F., & Schmid, T. L. (1981). Acquisition and maintenance of trusting behavior. *Journal of the Experimental Analysis of Behavior, 35,* 109–124.

Hall, B. L. (Ed.). (1982). *OBM in multiple business environments.* New York: Haworth Press.

Hanson, S. J., & Timberlake, W. (1983). Regulation during challenge: A general model of learned performance under schedule constraint. *Psychological Review, 90,* 261–282.

Haring, N., & Bricker, D. (1976). *Overview of comprehensive services for the severely/profoundly handicapped.* New York: Grune & Stratton.

Harris, S. L., Wolchik, S. A., & Milch, R. E. (1983). Changing the speech of autistic children and their parents. *Child and Family Behavior Therapy, 4,* 151–173.

Hayes, S. C., Rincover, A., & Solnick, J. V. (1980). The technical drift of applied behavior analysis. *Journal of Applied Behavior Analysis, 13,* 275–286.

Hayes, S. C., Brownstein, R. J., Zettle, R. D., Rosenfarb, I., & Korn, Z. (1986). Rule-governed behavior and sensitivity to changing consequences of responding. *Journal of the Experimental Analysis of Behavior, 45,* 237–256.

Heller, T. (1985). Residential relocation and reactions of elderly mentally retarded persons. In M. P. Janicki & H. M. Wisniewski (Eds.), *Aging and the developmental disabilities* (pp. 367–378). Baltimore: Brookes.

Herrnstein, R. J. (1970). On the law of effect. *Journal of the Experimental Analysis of Behavior, 13,* 243–266.

Hertz, R. A. (1979). Retarded persons in neglect proceedings: Erroneous assumptions of parental inadequacy. *Stanford Law Review, 31,* 785–805.

Holburn, C. S., & Dougher, M. J. (1986). Effects of response satiation procedures in the treatment of aerophagia. *American Journal of Mental Deficiency, 91,* 72–77.

Horn, J., & Donaldson, G. (1976). On the myth of intellectual decline in adulthood. *American Psychologist, 31,* 701–719.

Iversen, I. H., Ragnasdottir, G. A., & Randrup, K. I. (1984). Operant conditioning of autogrooming in vervet monkeys (*Cercopithecus aethiops*). *Journal of the Experimental Analysis of Behavior, 42,* 171–189.

Iwata, B. A., Bailey, J. S., Brown, K. M., Foshee, T. J., & Alpern, M. (1976). A performance based lottery to improve residential care and training by institutional staff. *Journal of Applied Behavior Analysis, 9,* 417–431.

Janicki, M. P., & MacEachron, A. E. (1984). Residential, health, and social service needs of elderly developmentally disabled persons. *Gerontologist, 24,* 128–137.

Kaiser, A. P., & Fox, J. J. (1986). Behavioral parent training research: Contributions to an ecological analysis of families of handicapped children. In J. J. Gallagher & P. M. Vietze (Eds.), *Families of handicapped persons* (pp. 219–236). Baltimore: Brookes.

Kanner, L. (1957). *Child psychiatry* (3rd ed.). Springfield, IL: Charles C Thomas.

Kenowitz, L., Zweibel, S., & Edgar, E. (1978). Determining the least restrictive opportunity for the severely and profoundly handicapped. In N. Haring & D. Bricker (Eds.), *Teaching the severely handicapped* (Vol. 3, pp. 54–79). Columbus, OH: Special Press.

Keogh, D., Whitman, T. L., & Maxwell, S. E. (1989). Self-instruction versus external instruction: Individual differences and training effectiveness. *Cognitive Therapy and Research, 12,* 591–610.

Kleitsch, E. C., Whitman, T. L., & Santos, J. (1983). Increasing verbal interaction among elderly socially isolated mentally retarded adults: A group language training procedure. *Journal of Applied Behavior Analysis, 16,* 217–233.

Komaki, J. L. (1986). Toward effective supervision: An operant analysis and comparison of managers at work. *Journal of Applied Psychology, 71,* 270–279.

Komaki, J. L., Zlotnick, S., & Jensen, M. (1986). Development of an operant-based taxonomy and observational index of supervisory behavior. *Journal of Applied Psychology, 71,* 260–269.

Konarski, E. A. (1987). Effects of response deprivation on the instrumental performance of mentally retarded persons. *American Journal of Mental Deficiency, 91,* 537–542.

Konarski, E. A., Johnson, M. R., Crowell, C. R., & Whitman, T. L. (1980). Response deprivation and reinforcement in applied settings. A preliminary analysis. *Journal of Applied Behavior Analysis, 13,* 595–609.

Konarski, E. A., Johnson, M. R., Crowell, C. R., & Whitman, T. L. (1981). An alternative approach to reinforcement for applied researchers: Response deprivation. *Behavior Therapy, 12,* 653–666.

Konarski, E. A., Crowell, C. R., Johnson, M. R., & Whitman, T. L. (1982). Response deprivation, reinforcement, and instrumental academic performance in an EMR classroom. *Behavior Therapy, 13,* 94–102.

Konarski, E. A., Crowell, C. R., & Duggan, L. M. (1985). The use of response deprivation to increase the academic performance of EMR students. *Applied Research in Mental Retardation, 6,* 15–31.

Krapfl, J. E., & Gasparotto, G. (1982). Behavioral systems analysis. In L. W. Frederiksen (Ed.), *Handbook of organizational behavior management.* New York: Wiley.

Lally, M. (1981). Computer-assisted teaching of sight-word recognition for mentally retarded school children. *American Journal of Mental Deficiency, 85,* 383–388.

Lally, M. (1982). Computer-assisted handwriting instruction and visual/kinaesthetic feedback processes. *Applied Research in Mental Retardation, 3,* 397–405.

Lamarre, J., & Holland, J. G. (1985). The functional independence of mands and tacts. *Journal of the Experimental Analysis of Behavior, 43,* 5–19.

Lamb, M. E. (1976). Effects of stress and cohort on mother- and father-infant interaction. *Development Psychology, 12,* 435–443.

Lamb, M. E. (1977). Father-infant and mother-infant interaction in the first year of life. *Child Development, 48,* 167–181.

Laties, V. G., Wood, R. W., & Cooper, R. D. (1981). Stimulus control and the effect of drugs. *Psychopharmacology, 75,* 277–282.

Lazar, R. M., Davis-Lang, D., & Sanchez, L. (1984). The formation of stimulus equivalences in children. *Journal of the Experimental Analysis of Behavior, 41,* 251–266.

Lebouf, A., & Boeverts, M. (1981). Automatic detection and modification of aberrant behaviors: Two case studies. *Journal of Behavior Therapy and Experimental Psychiatry, 12,* 153–157.

Lee, V. L. (1981). Prepositional phrases spoken and heard. *Journal of the Experimental Analysis of Behavior, 35,* 227–242.

Lee, V. L., & Pegler, A. M. (1982). Effects on spelling of teaching children to read. *Journal of the Experimental Analysis of Behavior, 37,* 311–322.

Lindsley, O. R. (1964). Direct measurement and prosthesis of retarded behavior. *Journal of Education, 147,* 62–81.

Lowe, C. F. (1979). Determinants of human operant behavior. In M. D. Zeiler & P. Harzem (Eds.), *Advances in the analysis of behavior: Reinforcement and the organization of behavior* (pp. 159–192). New York: Wiley.

Lowe, C. F. (1983). Radical behaviourism and human psychology. In G. C. L. Davey (Ed.), *Animal models of human behavior* (pp. 71–93). New York: Wiley.

Lowe, C. F., Beasty, A., & Bentall, R. P. (1983). The role of verbal behavior in human learning: Infant performance on fixed-interval schedules. *Journal of the Experimental Analysis of Behavior, 39,* 157–164.

Lubin, R. A., & Kiely, M. (1985). Epidemiology of aging in development disabilities. In M. P.

Janicki & H. M. Wisniewski (Eds.), *Aging and the development disabilities* (pp. 95–113). Baltimore: Brookes.

Luiselli, J. K. (1986). Behavior analysis of pharmacological and contingency management interventions for self-injury. *Journal of Behavior Therapy and Experimental Psychiatry, 17,* 275–284.

Luthans, F., & Kreitner, R. (1975). *Organizational behavior modification.* Glenview, IL: Scott, Foresman.

Mackay, H. A., & Sidman, M. (1984). Teaching new behavior via equivalence relations. In P. H. Brooks, R. Sperber, & C. McCauley (Eds.), *Learning and cognition in the mentally retarded* (pp. 493–513). Hillsdale, NJ: Lawrence Erlbaum.

Marholin, D., & Phillips, D. (1976). Methodological issues in psychopharmacological research. *American Journal of Orthopsychiatry, 46,* 477–495.

Marholin, D., Touchette, P. E., & Stewart, R. M. (1979). Withdrawal of chronic chlorpromazine medication: An experimental analysis. *Journal of Applied Behavior Analysis, 12,* 159–171.

Martin, J. E., & Agran, M. (1985). Psychotropic and anticonvulsant drug use by mentally retarded adults across community, residential, and vocational placements. *Applied Research in Mental Retardation, 6,* 33–49.

Matthews, B. A., Catania, A. C., & Shimoff, E. (1985). Effects of uninstructed verbal behavior on nonverbal responding: Contingency descriptions versus performance descriptions. *Journal of the Experimental Analysis of Behavior, 43,* 155–164.

McClure, J. T., Moss, R. A., McPeters, J. W., & Kirkpatrick, M. A. (1986). Reduction of hand-mouthing by a boy with profound mental retardation. *Mental Retardation, 24,* 219–222.

McDowell, J. J. (1982). The importance of Herrnstein's mathematical statement of the law of effect for behavior therapy. *American Psychologist, 37,* 771–779.

Macurik, K. M. (1979). An operant device to reinforce correct head position. *Journal of Behavior Therapy and Experimental Psychiatry, 10,* 237–239.

Mesibov, G. (1976). Alternative to the principle of normalization. *Mental Retardation, 14,* 30–32.

Meyers, C. E., Nihira, K., & Zetlin, A. (1979). The measurement of adaptive behavior. In N. Ellis (Ed.), *Handbook of mental deficiency, psychological theory and research* (pp. 431–482). Hillsdale, NJ: Lawrence Erlbaum.

Michael, J. (1980). Flight from behavior analysis. *Behavior Analyst, 3,* 1–24.

Millham, M., Chilcutt, J., & Atkinson, B. (1978). Comparability of naturalistic and controlled observation assessment of adaptive behavior. *American Journal of Mental Deficiency, 83,* 52–59.

Mira, M., & Roddy, J. (1980). *Parenting competencies of retarded persons: A critical review.* Unpublished manuscript. (Available from Children's Rehabilitation Unit, University of Kansas Medical Center, Kansas City, KS 66103)

Moran, D., & Whitman, T. (1985). The multiple effects of a play-oriented, parent-training program for mothers of developmentally delayed children. *Analysis and Intervention in Developmental Disabilities, 5,* 73–96.

Morse, W. H., & Kelleher, R. T. (1970). Schedules as fundamental determinants of behavior. In W. N. Schoenfeld (Ed.), *The theory of reinforcement schedules* (pp. 139–186). Englewood Cliffs, NJ: Prentice-Hall.

Mulick, J. A., Scott, F. D., Gaines, R. F., & Campbell, B. M. (1983). Devices and instrumentation for skill development and behavior change. In J. L. Matson & F. Andrasik (Eds.), *Treatment issues and innovations in mental retardation* (pp. 515–580). New York: Plenum Press.

Myerson, J., & Hale, S. (1984). Practical implications of the matching law. *Journal of Applied Behavior Analysis, 17,* 367–380.

National Association for Retarded Children (NARC) (1972). Comparability of naturalistic and controlled observation assessment of adaptive behavior. *American Journal of Mental Deficiency, 83,* 52–59.

Nihira, K., Foster, R., Shellhaas, M., & Leland, H. (1974). *AAMD Adaptive Behavior Scale.* Washington, DC: American Association on Mental Deficiency.

Nirje, B. (1969). The normalization principle and its human management implications. In R. Krigel & W. Wolfensberger (Eds.), *Changing patterns in residential services for the mentally retarded* (pp. 179–196). Washington, DC: U.S. Government Printing Office.

O'Brien, R. M., Dickinson, A. M., & Rosow, M. P. (Eds.). (1982). *Industrial behavior modification.* New York: Pergamon Press.

O'Leary, S. D., & Dubey, D. R. (1979). Applications of self-control procedures by children: A review. *Journal of Applied Behavior Analysis, 12,* 449–466.

Page, T. J., Iwata, B. A., & Reid, D. H. (1982). Pyramidal training: A large-scale application with institutional staff. *Journal of Applied Behavior Analysis, 15,* 335–351.

Parke, R. D. (1986). Fathers, families, and support systems: Their role in the development of at-risk and retarded infants and children. In J. J. Gallagher & P. M. Vietze (Eds.), *Families of handicapped persons* (pp. 101–113). Baltimore: Brookes.

Peffer-Smith, P. G., Smith, E. O., & Byrd, L. D., (1983). Effects of d-amphetamine and posturing in stumptailed macaques. *Journal of the Experimental Analysis of Behavior, 40,* 313–320.

Pfadt, A., & Tryon, W. W. (1983). Issues in the selection and use of mechanical transducers to directly measure motor activity in clinical settings. *Applied Research in Mental Retardation, 4,* 251–270.

Pierce, W. D., & Epling, W. F. (1980). What happened to analysis in applied behavior analysis? *Behavior Analyst, 3,* 1–9.

Pierce, W. D., & Epling, W. F. (1983). Choice, matching and human behavior: A review of the literature. *Behavior Analyst, 6,* 57–76.

Podsakoff, P. M. (1982). Effects of schedule changes on human performance: An empirical test of predictions of the law of effect, the probability differential model, and the response deprivation approach. *Organizational Behavior and Human Performance, 29,* 322–351.

Poling, A., & Ryan, C. (1982). Differential reinforcement of other behavior schedules: Therapeutic applications. *Behavior Modification, 6,* 3–21.

Poling, A., Picker, M., Grossett, D., Hall-Johnston, E., & Holbrook, M. (1981). The schism between experimental and applied behavior analysis: Is it real and who cares? *Behavior Analyst, 4,* 93–102.

Poling, A., Picker, M., & Hall-Johnson, E. (1983). Human behavioral pharmacology. *Psychological Record, 33,* 457–472.

Poling, A., Grosset, D., Karas, C. A., & Breuning, S. E. (1985). Medication regimen: A subject characteristic rarely reported in behavior modification studies. *Applied Research in Mental Retardation, 6,* 71–77.

Premack, D. (1965). Reinforcement theory. In D. Levine (Ed.), *Nebraska symposium on motivation* (pp. 123–180). Lincoln: University of Nebraska Press.

Prue, D. M., Frederiksen, L. W., & Bacon, A. (1978). Organizational behavior management: An annotated bibliography. *Journal of Organizational Behavior Management, 1,* 216–257.

Puccio, P., Janicki, M., Otis, J., & Rettig, J. (1983). Report of the committee on aging and developmental disabled. Albany: Office of Mental Retardation and Developmental Disabilities.

Rapp, S. R., Carstensen, L. L., & Prue, D. M. (1983). Organizational behavior management 1978–1982: An annotated bibliography. *Journal of Organizational Behavior Management, 5,* 5–50.

Rapport, M. D., Murphy, H. A., & Bailey, J. S. (1982). Ritalin vs. response cost in the control of hyperactive children: A within-subject comparison. *Journal of Applied Behavior Analysis, 15,* 205–216.

Reed, E. W., & Reed, S. C. (1965). *Mental retardation: A family study.* Philadelphia: W. B. Saunders.

Reid, D. H., & Whitman, T. L. (1983). Behavioral staff management in institutions: A critical review of effectiveness and acceptability. *Analysis and Intervention in Developmental Disabilities, 3,* 131–149.

Reigel, K. F., & Reigel, R. M. (1972). Development drop and death. *Developmental Psychology, 6,* 306–319.

Repp, A. C., Barton, L. E., & Brulle, A. R. (1981). Correspondence between effectiveness and staff use of instructions for severely retarded persons. *Applied Research in Mental Retardation, 2,* 237–245.

Robinson, N., & Robinson, H. (1976). *The mentally retarded child: A psychological approach.* New York: McGraw-Hill.

Romanczyk, R. G. (1986). *Clinical utilization of microcomputer technology.* New York: Pergamon Press.

Romski, M. A., White, R. A., Millen, C. E., & Rumbaugh, D. M. (1984). Effects of computer-keyboard teaching on the symbolic communication of severely retarded persons: Five case studies. *Psychological Record, 34,* 39–54.

Rosenbaum, M. S., & Drabman, R. S. (1979). Self-control training in the classroom: A review and critique. *Journal of Applied Behavior Analysis, 12,* 467–485.

Rumbaugh, D. M. (Ed.). (1977). *Language learning by a chimpanzee: The Lana project.* New York: Academic Press.

Rumbaugh, D. M., Savage-Rumbaugh, E. S., & Hegel, M. T. (1987). Summation in the chimpanzee (*Pan troglodytes*). *Journal of Experimental Psychology: Animal Behavior Processes, 13,* 107–115.

Salthouse, T. A., & Somberg, B. L. (1982). Isolating the age deficit in speeded performance. *Journal of Gerontology, 37,* 59–63.

Sarason, S., & Doris, J. (1969). *Psychological problems in mental deficiency.* New York: Harper & Row.

Savage-Rumbaugh, E. S. (1984). Verbal behavior at a procedural level in the chimpanzee. *Journal of the Experimental Analysis of Behavior, 41,* 223–250.

Schilling, R. F., Schinke, S. P., Blythe, B. J., & Barth, R. P. (1982). Child maltreatment and mentally retarded parents: Is there a relationship? *Mental Retardation, 20,* 201–209.

Schleien, S. J., Weyman, P., Kiernan, J. (1981). Teaching leisure skills to severely handicapped adults: An age-appropriate dart game. *Journal of Applied Behavior Analysis, 14,* 513–519.

Schmid, T. L., & Hake, D. F. (1983). Fast acquisition of cooperation and trust: A two-stage view of trusting behavior. *Journal of the Experimental Analysis of Behavior, 40,* 179–190.

Schmitt, D. R. (1984). Interpersonal relations: Cooperation and competition. *Journal of the Experimental Analysis of Behavior, 42,* 377–383.

Schroeder, S. R., Gualtieri, C. T., & Van Bourgondien, M. E. (1986). Autism. In M. Hersen (Ed.), *Pharmacological and behavioral treatment: An integrative approach* (pp. 89–107). New York: Wiley.

Scott, W. E., & Podsakoff, P. M. (1982). Leadership, supervision, and behavior control: Perspectives from an experimental analysis. In L. W. Frederiksen (Ed.), *Handbook of organizational behavior management* (pp. 39–70). New York: Wiley.

Scott, W. E., & Podsakoff, P. M. (1985). *Behavioral principles in the practice of management.* New York: Wiley.

Shafto, F., & Sulzbacher, S. (1977). Comparing treatment tactics with a hyperactive preschool child: Stimulant medication and programmed teacher intervention. *Journal of Applied Behavior Analysis, 10,* 13–20.

Shapiro, E. S. (1981). Self-control procedures with the mentally retarded student. In M. Hersen, R. M. Eisler, & P. M. Miller (Eds.), *Progress in behavior modification* (Vol. 12, pp. 265–297). New York: Academic Press.

Shapiro, E. S. (1986). Behavior modification: Self-control and cognitive procedures. In R. P. Barrett (Ed.), *Severe behavior disorders in the mentally retarded* (pp. 61–97). New York: Plenum Press.

Shimoff, E., Catania, A. C., & Matthews, B. A. (1981). Uninstructed human responding: Sensitivity of low-rate performance to schedule contingencies. *Journal of the Experimental Analysis of Behavior, 36,* 207–220.

Sidman, M. (1977). Teaching some basic prerequisites for reading. In P. Mittler (Ed.), *Research and practice in mental retardation: Vol. 2. Education and training* (pp. 353–360). Baltimore: University Park Press.

Sidman, M. (1986). Functional analysis of emergent verbal classes. In T. Thompson & M. D. Zeiler (Eds.), *Analysis and integration of behavioral units* (pp. 223–245). Hillsdale NJ: Lawrence Erlbaum.

Sidman, M., & Tailby, W. (1982). Conditional discrimination vs. matching-to-sample: An expansion of the testing paradigm. *Journal of the Experimental Analysis of Behavior, 37,* 5–24.

Sidman, M., Rauzin, R., Lazar, R., Cunningham, S., Tailby, W., & Carrigan, P. (1982). A search for symmetry in the conditional discriminations of Rhesus monkeys, baboons, and children. *Journal of the Experimental Analysis of Behavior, 37,* 23–44.

Sidman, M., Kirk, B., & Willson-Morris, M. (1985). Six-member stimulus classes generated by conditional-discrimination procedures. *Journal of the Experimental Analysis of Behavior, 43,* 21–42.

Silverman, K., Anderson, S. R., Marshall, A. M., & Baer, D. M. (1986). Establishing and generalizing audience control of new language repertoires. *Analysis and Intervention in Developmental Disabilities, 6,* 21–40.

Singh, N. N., & Winton, A. S. W. (1984). Behavioral monitoring of pharmacological interventions for self-injury. *Applied Research in Mental Retardation, 5,* 161–170.

Skinner, B. F. (1953). *Science and human behavior.* New York: Macmillan.

Skinner, B. F. (1957). *Verbal behavior.* Englewood Cliffs, NJ: Prentice-Hall.

Skinner, B. F. (1969). *Contingencies of reinforcement: A theoretical analysis.* Englewood Cliffs, NJ: Prentice-Hall.

Skinner, B. F. (1978). *About behaviorism.* New York: Knopf.

Skinner, B. F. (1986). What's wrong with daily life in the western world? *American Psychologist, 41,* 568–574.

Smith, D. E. P., Olson, M., Berger, F., & McConnell, J. V. (1981). The effects of improved auditory feedback on the verbalizations of an autistic child. *Journal of Autism and Developmental Disabilities, 11,* 449–454.

Smith, D. E. P., McConnell, J. V., Walter, T. L., & Miller, S. D. (1985). Effects of using an auditory trainer on the attentional, language, and social behaviors of autistic children. *Journal of Autism and Developmental Disabilities, 15,* 285–302.

Stoddard, L. T. (Ed.). (1986). Special issue: Stimulus control research and developmental disabilities. *Analysis and Intervention in Developmental Disabilities, 6,* 155–178.

Stoneman, Z., & Brody, G. H. (August, 1982). *Observational research on retarded children, their parents, and their siblings.* Paper presented at the National Institute of Child Development Lake Wilderness Conference, University of Washington, Seattle, WA.

Switzky, H., Rotatori, A., Miller, T., & Freagon, S. (1979). The developmental model and its implications for assessment and instruction for the severely/profoundly retarded. *Mental Retardation, 13,* 23–25.

Terman, L. M., & Merrill, M. A. (1973). *The Stanford-Binet intelligence scale* (3rd rev.). Boston: Houghton Mifflin.

Thoresen, C. E., & Mahoney, N. J. (1974). *Behavioral self-control.* New York: Holt, Rinehart & Winston.

Throne, J. (1975). Normalization through the normalization principle: Right ends, wrong means. *Mental Retardation, 13,* 23–25.

Tighe, R. J., & Groeneweg, G. (1985). A comparison of input and output alternatives with a computer-assisted basic concept program. In J. M. Berg (Ed.), *Science and service in mental retardation* (pp. 232–239). New York: Methuen.

Timberlake, W. (1984a). Behavior regulation and learned performance: Some misapprehensions and disagreements. *Journal of the Experimental Analysis of Behavior, 41,* 355–375.

Timberlake, W. (1984b). Further thoughts on behavior regulation. *Journal of the Experimental Analysis of Behavior, 41,* 383–386.

Timberlake, W., & Allison, J. (1974). Response deprivation: An empirical approach to instrumental performance. *Psychological Review, 81,* 146–164.

Tredgold, A. F., (1937). *A textbook of mental deficiency* (6th ed.). Baltimore: William Wood.

Vaughan, M. E. (1985). Repeated acquisition in the analysis of rule-governed behavior. *Journal of the Experimental Analysis of Behavior, 44,* 175–184.

Vitello, S. J., & Soskin, R. M. (1985). *Mental retardation: Its social and legal context.* Englewood Cliffs, NJ: Prentice-Hall.

Wacker, D. P., Berg, W. K., Wiggins, B., Muldoon, M., & Cavanaugh, J. (1985). Evaluation of reinforcer preferences for profoundly handicapped students. *Journal of Applied Behavior Analysis, 18,* 173–178.

Wahler, R. G. (1980). The insular mother: Her problems in parent-child treatment. *Journal of Applied Behavior Analysis, 13,* 207–219.

Wechsler, D. (1955). *Wechsler adult intelligence scale, manual.* New York: Psychological Corporation.

White, O., & Haring, N. (1978). Evaluating educational programs serving the severely and profoundly handicapped. In N. Haring & P. Bricker (Eds.), *Teaching the severely handicapped* (Vol. 3). Columbus, OH: Special Press.

Whitman, T., Burgio, L., & Johnston, M. B. (1984). Cognitive behavior therapy with the mentally retarded. In A. Myers & E. Craighead (Eds.), *Cognitive behavior therapy with children* (pp. 193–227). New York: Plenum Press.

Whitman, T. L. (1987). Self-instruction and mental retardation: Theoretical, research and educational perspectives. *American Journal of Mental Deficiency, 92,* 213–223.

Whitman, T. L., & Scibak, J. W. (1981). Behavior modification with the mentally retarded: Treatment and research perspectives. In J. Matson & J. McCartney (Eds.), *Handbook of behavior modification with the mentally retarded* (pp. 1–35). New York: Plenum Press.

Whitman, T. L., Scibak, J., & Reid, D. (1983). *Behavior modification with the mentally retarded: Treatment and research perspectives.* New York: Academic Press.

Whitman, T. L., Spence, B. H., & Maxwell, S. E. (1987). A comparison of external and self-instructional teaching formats with mentally retarded adults in a vocational training setting. *Research in Developmental Disabilities, 8,* 371–388.

Wiegerink, R., Hocutt, A., Posante-Loro, R., & Bristol, M. (1980). Parent involvement in early education programs for handicapped children. *New Directions for Exceptional Children, 1,* 67–85.

Wisniewski, H. M., & Merz, G. S. (1985). Aging, Alzheimers's disease, and developmental disabilities. In M. P. Janicki & H. M. Wisniewski (Eds.), *Aging and the developmental disabilities* (pp. 177–184). Baltimore: Brookes.

Wolfensberger, W. (1969). Twenty predictions about the future of residential services in mental retardation. *Mental Retardation, 7,* 51–54.

Wolfensberger, W. (1972). *Principle of normalization in human services.* Toronto: National Institute on Mental Retardation.

Wood, D. L. (1986). Designing microcomputer programs of disabled students. *Computers in Education, 10,* 35–42.

Woods, P. A., & Lowe, C. F. (1985). Verbal regulation of inappropriate social behavior with mentally handicapped adults. In J. M. Berg (Ed.), *Science and service in mental retardation* (pp. 353–362). New York: Methuen.

Wysoki, T., & Fuqua, R. W. (1982). Methodological issues in the evaluation of drug effects. In S. E. Breuning & A. D. Poling (Eds.), *Drugs and mental retardation* (pp. 138–167). Springfield, IL: Charles C Thomas.

Wysoki, T., Fuqua, W., Davis, V. J., & Breuning, S. E. (1981). Effects of thioridazine (Mellaril) on titrating matching to sample performance of mentally retarded adults. *American Journal of Mental Deficiency, 85,* 539–547.

Zeiler, M. (1977). Schedules of reinforcement: The controlling variables. In W. K. Honig & J. E. R. Staddon (Eds.), *Handbook of operant behavior* (pp. 201–232). Englewood Cliffs, NJ: Prentice-Hall.

Zentall, S. S., & Zentall, T. R. (1983). Optimal stimulation: A model of disordered activity and performance in normal and deviant children. *Psychological Bulletin, 94,* 446–471.

2

Three New Mental Retardation Service Models

Implications for Behavior Modification

STEVEN REISS, BARBARA EVANS MCKINNEY, AND
JAMES T. NAPOLITAN

THREE NEW SERVICE MODELS FOR MENTALLY RETARDED PEOPLE

Every year new service models are demonstrated by energetic professionals who are seeking better ways to serve mentally retarded people (e.g., Menolascino & Stark, 1984). The new models are constantly challenging behavior modifiers to broaden their horizons or risk the possibility of becoming outdated (Reiss, 1987). In this chapter, we will consider three new models for serving people with mental retardation and discuss some of the ways in which behavior modifiers might relate to these models. The models are outpatient mental health services, inpatient mental health services, and foster care. Two of the models, outpatient and inpatient mental health services, relate to the critical need for services to people who are *dually diagnosed* (i.e., mentally retarded and emotionally disturbed). The third model, foster care for persons with mental retardation, provides a desirable alternative to residential placement in state institutions and other restrictive environments. Although the three models discussed here are from Illinois, similar programs have been created in many places across the United States. Thus, the models are relevant to important national trends in the field of developmental disabilities. Because two thirds of this chapter is concerned with behavior modification and service models for the dually diagnosed, our discussion begins with a consideration of general information on the importance of increasing the supply of mental health services for mentally retarded people.

STEVEN REISS • Department of Psychology, University of Illinois at Chicago, Chicago, Illinois 60680.   BARBARA EVANS MCKINNEY • Shapiro Developmental Center, 100 East Jeffery Street, Kankakee, Illinois 60901.   JAMES T. NAPOLITAN • Ray Graham Association for the Handicapped, 420 West Madison Street, Elmhurst, Illinois 60126.

MENTAL HEALTH NEEDS OF MENTALLY RETARDED PEOPLE

Historically, behavior modifiers working with mentally retarded people have concentrated their efforts on the treatment of severe behavior disorders. As important as this contribution has been, the treatment of severe behavior disorders represents only a small part of the total mental health needs of mentally retarded people. For every mentally retarded person who needs treatment for a severe behavior disorder, there are 10 who need training in social skills, and 2 who need treatment for depression. Although severe behavior disorders are important problems that should be treated, there is no justification for concentrating on the treatment of these problems to the point that other, more prevalent disorders are virtually ignored. Yet this is what happened during much of the period from 1960 to 1985.

There is a need to broaden the behavioral approach to include the treatment of the full range of mental health problems. The development of behavioral programs for social skills training was a major step in this direction. We need to continue these efforts and to develop treatments for other underserved mental health problems, such as depression (Kazdin, Matson, & Senatore, 1983; Sovner & Hurley, 1983), anxiety disorders (Matson, 1981; McNally & Ascher, 1985), and personality disorders (Eaton & Menolascino, 1982; Zigler, 1971). We believe that the behavioral approach should be adapted to address the full range of mental health problems with mentally retarded people.

Prevalence

The importance of developing behavioral treatments for persons with dual diagnosis is suggested by a number of prevalence studies (Lund, 1985; Philips, 1967; Philips & Williams, 1975; Reiss, 1982). There are numerous findings that the prevalence of emotional disorders is much higher among mentally retarded than among nonretarded people (Dewan, 1948; Rutter, Tizard, Yule, Graham, & Whitemore, 1976; Weaver, 1946). Jacobson's (1982) survey of mentally retarded people in New York State found that about 1 in every 6 mildly mentally retarded adults had a mental illness. Other surveys reported even higher estimates, with some studies suggesting that as many as one third of all mentally retarded persons may need mental health services (Matson & Barrett, 1982).

Steven Reiss recently completed a survey of a fairly random sample of 205 mentally retarded adolescents and adults from 17 community-based day programs in the Chicago metropolitan area. The sample included 94, 73, and 35 people with, respectively, mild, moderate, and severe mental retardation (the level of mental retardation was unknown for 3 subjects). The age range was from 18 to 79; there were 82 women and 123 men. The ethnic background comprised 126 whites, 53 blacks, 15 Hispanics, and 10 "others."

In the first part of the study, the Reiss Screen for Maladaptive Behavior was completed by caretakers who knew the subjects well. The Reiss Screen has scales for conduct disorder, schizophrenia, paranoia, depression (behavioral symptoms), depression (physical symptoms), dependent personality disorder, and avoidant disorder. A scale for autism was added after the prevalence study was completed. The test also screens for seven significant psychological problems, including drug abuse, euphoria (mood disorder), hyperactivity, self-injury, sexual problem, suicidal problem, and stealing. The caretaker rates the extent to which each of 38 psychopathological symptoms is "no problem," "a problem," or a "major problem" in the life of the subject who is being rated. The operational definitions of the rating scale provide instructions for rating the frequency, intensity, and consequences of the behavior problem.

The results of the survey indicated that as many as 45% of the sample needed help with social adjustment. Anxiety was rated as a problem for 37.5% of the sample; withdrawal for 22.4%; and excessive attention-seeking for 39.5%. Much less common were such problems as self-abusive behavior, which was rated as a problem for 4.4% of the sample, and alcoholism/drug abuse, which was rated as a problem for only 2.5%. Of course, these figures include only those mentally retarded people who needed a mental health service at the time that the survey was conducted; the percentage of mentally retarded people who might need a mental health service at some point in their lives should be much higher than these numbers.

The results of the Chicago survey suggest that poor social skills is the foremost mental health problem among mentally retarded people. For every individual in the survey who suffered from self-abusive behavior, there were approximately 10 people who needed social skills training. Because behavior modification techniques can be especially helpful in teaching social skills to mentally retarded people (e.g., Matson, Kazdin, & Esveldt-Dawson, 1981), the results of the Chicago survey point to the relevance of behavior modification to the dual diagnosis movement.

Reasons for Inadequate Services

Although mental health problems are common among mentally retarded people, these people are not receiving the mental health services they need (Reiss, 1982, 1985; Szymanski & Tanguay, 1980). Part of the problem is that there is a tendency for professionals to assume that everything a mentally retarded person does is a result of that person's mental retardation. At the University of Illinois in Chicago, Steven Reiss, Joseph Szyszko, and Grant Levitan studied this tendency to overlook the mental health needs of mentally retarded people (Goldsmith & Schloss, 1984; Levitan & Reiss, 1983; Reiss, Levitan, & Szyszko, 1982; Reiss & Szyszko, 1983). In one of the studies, two groups of psychologists were asked to diagnose a person who was afraid to ride a bus. One group was given information suggesting that the person has normal intelligence, and the other group was given information suggesting that the person is mentally retarded. The study found that some psychologists diagnosed fear and recommended appropriate treatment when the patient has normal intelligence but not when the patient has mental retardation. This tendency for the presence of mental retardation to decrease the diagnostic significance of signs of emotional problems has been called "diagnostic overshadowing" (Reiss *et al.*, 1982).

Another problem is that people with both mental retardation and emotional disorder fall through a gap in the service delivery systems between agencies serving mentally retarded people and those serving mentally ill people (Reiss, 1982). The dually diagnosed are sometimes referred back and forth between mental retardation and mental health agencies so that nobody provides the mental health and the developmental disability services that are needed. Moreover, some dually diagnosed people have combinations of handicaps requiring special services that are not available from either mental retardation or mental health agencies (Reiss, 1985). In order to meet the mental health needs of mentally retarded people, we will need special programs serving the dually diagnosed and much greater cooperation between mental retardation and mental health agencies.

OUTPATIENT MENTAL HEALTH CLINIC

The greatest need for mental health services for mentally retarded people is for outpatient services that promote adjustment to community-based facilities (Reiss & Trenn, 1984). The community mental health centers in the United States should be opened to persons with mental retardation. As things stand now, some community mental health centers serve mentally retarded people, but many do not. Consequently, many mentally retarded people living in community-based facilities or with their families have no place to turn to for needed services.

In 1980, Steven Reiss and Joseph Szyszko set up a developmental disabilities mental health clinic: the Institute for the Study of Developmental Disabilities (ISDD) Mental Health Clinic. The ISDD clinic, which is located on the Chicago campus of the University of Illinois, serves all age groups of mildly, moderately, and severely mentally retarded people on a first-come, first-served basis. The clinic, which provides only mental health services for mentally retarded people, has no services to diagnose mental retardation, test intelligence, or operate programs of early intervention. Because all the referrals to the clinic are for mentally retarded people needing a mental health service, the referrals represent a previously unmet consumer demand for services.

Total Consumer Demand for Services

The ISDD clinic demonstrated a high level of consumer demand for mental health services for mentally retarded people (Reiss & Trenn, 1984). From 1981 through 1984, the clinic served approximately 70 clients per week and about 125 new clients per year. Most of the clients were seen on an individual basis. Some dually diagnosed people were refused services because the clinic already was operating at maximum capacity at the time that services were requested. The frequent periods during which new clients could not be accepted probably discouraged some referrals, reducing the level of consumer demand that could be demonstrated. Nevertheless, the strong level of consumer demand for services experienced at the ISDD demonstrated the need for more outpatient mental health services for mentally retarded people, especially in metropolitan areas.

Referral Sources

During the first 27 months that clients were accepted for services, the clinic received 274 referrals. A total of 181 referrals, or 66.1% of the sample, came from 36 community agencies, such as community-based residential programs and sheltered workshops. The remaining referrals came from 9 state facilities, 6 private hospitals, 8 schools, and other sources including the client's family. All the clients were referred by a third party so that no person with mental retardation referred himself or herself. These data suggest that the ISDD clinic functioned primarily as a support service to help mentally retarded people adjust to community-based facilities.

To a large degree, the demand for more mental health services for mentally retarded people is related to the movement for community-based care. As much as one third or more of the mentally retarded people placed in community-based facilities need mental health services, especially social skills training. Moreover, operators of large state facilities have discovered that some mentally retarded people cannot be placed in community agencies because they also have emotional disorders. In one way or another, dual diagnosis is a major obstacle to the integration of many mentally retarded people into the community.

Client Age

Although client age at time of referral ranged from 5 to 59, approximately two thirds of the clients were adolescents or young adults between the ages of 15 and 29. This finding suggests that unmet consumer demand for mental health services for mentally retarded people was greatest for adolescents and young adults. Because this is the age at which people normally establish their independence from their parents, mentally retarded people often cannot do this well. This is also the age at which mildly retarded people lose the public schools as a major social support system. The stress of trying to become independent, plus the perception of being different from other people, might contribute to the development of emotional problems.

Psychopathology

Although clients were referred for the full range of emotional problems, the problems seen most frequently were conduct disorder, depression, avoidant disorder, and dependent personality disorder. These problems accounted for about 80% of the referrals to the ISDD clinic (Benson, 1985; Reiss, 1982; Reiss & Trenn, 1984).

The results of the ISDD clinic studies supported the previous findings that mentally retarded people are vulnerable to affective disorders (Matson, 1982; Reid, 1972; Sovner & Hurley, 1983). As late as 1984, many authorities in the field of mental retardation questioned whether or not depression is an important mental health problem among mentally retarded people. Prior to the early 1980s, for example, there were no published behavioral studies on the treatment of depression. Yet depression accounted for as many as 20% of the referrals to the ISDD clinic. In the ISDD client sample, depression was more commonly seen in women than in men and among mildly retarded people than among severely retarded people (Benson & Reiss, 1985; Reiss & Trenn, 1984).

Another important finding was that personality disorders and avoidant behavior accounted for a significant portion of the demand for services. The most commonly seen symptoms included avoidant behavior, excessive inter-personal anxiety, excessive attention-seeking, anger-management problems, and a wide range of social skill deficiencies. Over the course of many years, researchers consistently reported that there is a high prevalence of person-ality problems among persons with mental retardation (e.g., Eaton & Men-olascino, 1982). The results of the ISDD clinic added to these findings by demonstrating that caretakers will refer large numbers of people with person-ality problems to mental health clinics.

The large number of referrals for conduct problems was expected. If there is one subgroup of dually diagnosed people who have long been recognized as needing mental health services, it would be mentally retarded people with conduct problems such as aggression. In the ISDD clinic sample, more males than females were referred for conduct disorder.

The ISDD results are interesting partially because certain types of prob-lems did not lead to as many referrals as was initially expected. There were a surprisingly small number of referrals for phobias. Although a few clients were referred because they drank too much alcohol, there were no referrals for other types of drug abuse. Only a few clients were referred for sex prob-lems. These and other infrequently seen problems accounted for less than one fifth of the referrals to the ISDD clinic.

Therapy

The ISDD clinic is a demonstration program with the goal of stimulating greater professional and research interest in the mental health aspects of mental retardation. The administrators of the program have interpreted this goal to mean that the program should welcome qualified practitioners from all legitimate schools of therapy. Accordingly, the ISDD clinic has offered a wide range of therapies, including psychotherapy, chemotherapy, behavior thera-py, cognitive therapy, pretherapy, and art therapy. This philosophy has served the ISDD clinic well; clinicians representing a wide range of theoretical orientations have been able to work together at the ISDD clinic in an atmosphere of mutual respect.

The behaviorally oriented psychologists at the ISDD clinic have been engaged in a variety of activities in addition to the treatment of severe behavior problems. Perhaps the best known of these activities is Betsey Benson's cognitive-behavioral program for the treatment of anger-management problems (Benson, 1986). This 12-week, structured program is based on the cognitive-behavioral techniques pioneered by Novaco (1975). The therapists use reinforcement principles, relaxation training, modeling, and behavioral rehearsal to teach mentally retarded people to identify the situations that make them angry, to identify appropriate and inappropriate responses to anger, and to learn how to respond to anger in appropriate ways. The weekly training sessions are provided in a small-group format. Because the clients are mentally handicapped, the training proceeds at a slow pace with a fair amount of practice and rehearsal.

Benson's treatment program is extremely popular with mentally retarded clients at the ISDD, and there is also some preliminary evidence that it has positive benefits (Benson, Rice, & Miranti, 1986). If future studies support the positive results from the initial study, the Benson program would provide an attractive therapy for the management of anger problems in mildly and some moderately retarded people.

Another application of behavior therapy to the problems of dual diagnosis was demonstrated at the ISDD clinic by Denise Valenti-Hein and Kim Mueser (Mueser, Valenti-Hein, & Yarnold, 1987). These investigators addressed the problem of romantic loneliness among young adults with mental retardation. They developed a dating-skills training program that is based largely on such learning principles as reinforcement and modeling. An initial evaluation of this program, which is administered in a small-group format, suggested some positive outcomes (Mueser *et al.*, 1987). It is anticipated that Valenti-Hein's doctoral dissertation will provide a more detailed evaluation of the effects of the program.

Conclusion

Outpatient community mental health clinics are needed to help persons with mental retardation adjust to community-based facilities. Outpatient clinics can reach significant numbers of people in a cost-effective manner. The outpatient model is best suited for urban and suburban areas, where there is a sufficiently large population base to support an outpatient mental health service for persons with mental retardation. Outpatients clinics serve mentally retarded people who suffer from a wide range of mental health problems, including depression, anger-management, social skill deficiencies, and personality disorder.

There is a need to increase the relevance of behavior modification to the outpatient mental health service model, including the need to develop more programs for teaching social skills to mentally retarded people. For example, many mentally retarded people can benefit from training in dating and other interpersonal skills. There also is a need to develop cognitive-behavioral therapy programs for use with mentally retarded persons (Reiss, 1982).

STATE-OPERATED INPATIENT PROGRAMS

Behavior modifiers also need to expand their activities for dually diagnosed people who live in state institutions. This means more treatment for people who suffer from such problems as hallucinations, inappropriate affect, sexual misconduct, and bizarre behavior rituals. Although behavior modifiers provide some services for inpatients with these conditions, they are not providing as much service as is needed, especially with regard to affective disorders.

Although relatively few dually diagnosed people need institutional care, the problem requires much more attention than the prevalence numbers would suggest. The cost of providing appropriate care can be considerable, and sometimes there is genuine concern that an individual's behavior problems cannot be managed effectively. Dually diagnosed people with severe behavior problems sometimes are referred from one state-operated institution to another because of the burdens of managing their behavior.

Placement in Mental Health versus Developmental Center

Residential placement is often a controversial issue in state systems that serve people with dual diagnosis. Some people feel that dually diagnosed people should be placed in institutions for the developmentally disabled, whereas others feel that they should be placed in institutions for the mentally ill or in special units for the dually diagnosed. The problem is that many dually diagnosed people do not fit well into any of these programs (Reiss, 1985). On the one hand, many dually diagnosed people do not belong in the state-operated mental health hospitals because they are unlikely to profit from the traditional verbal therapies that are commonly used in these facilities. On the other hand, many dually diagnosed people do not belong in state-operated facilities for the mentally retarded because their mental retardation is often too mild to justify placement in an institution for mentally retarded persons.

Sometimes dually diagnosed people are the victims of mistrust between the mental health and the mental retardation service systems. For example, Reiss (1985) reported the case of a dually diagnosed person who was caught between mental health administrators who recommended the person be placed in a developmental disabilities center and mental retardation administrators who recommended a mental health facility. The mental health administrators argued that the person should be placed in a developmental center because the behavioral problems appeared to be a result of emotional immaturity, which they thought was a sign of mental retardation. These administrators knew that the individual did not fit any of the existing mental health programs, so they assumed that the needed services were provided by the mental retardation system. The mental retardation administrators argued that the person should be placed in a mental health facility because the behavioral problems appeared to be an expression of mental illness. These administrators knew that the individual did not fit any of the existing programs in the developmental centers. Furthermore, they strongly suspected that the mental health administrators were not telling the truth when they claimed that they did not have an appropriate placement for the person. Thus, each side knew that the person did not fit its service programs and concluded that the appropriate placement must therefore be with the other side. An outside consultant had to be called in to convince both sides that this particular person had such a unique combination of handicaps that she did not fit any of the existing service programs offered by the state.

Because some dually diagnosed people do not fit well into existing inpatient programs, many states have created special inpatient units for dually diagnosed persons. Some states house these units with the Mental Retardation Division, whereas others house them with the Mental Health Division. Regardless of where the units are housed, a common problem is that they tend to be dead-end placements in which patients stay for very long periods of time. The mere fact that a person has been placed in an inpatient unit for the dually diagnosed sometimes tags that person as a "problem." This attitude can make it difficult to place the person in a less restrictive program even when treatment has been successful and behavioral improvement has occurred.

There is very little research on the question of whether it is best to place dually diagnosed people in mental health versus developmental centers. Different policies seem to have evolved in different states, with no one policy being obviously superior to any other. It is clear, however, that the dually diagnosed are an extremely heterogeneous group of people with diverse treatment needs. The needs of one dually diagnosed person can be very different from the needs of another. For this reason, we favor an approach that evaluates each individual according to his or her needs and finds the needed services from whatever service system is most appropriate for that individual. Thus, some dually diagnosed people might be served best by the mental health system, others by the mental retardation system, and still others by combinations of programs from various systems.

Illinois System

In this chapter, we will consider the inpatient services for dually diagnosed people that are provided by the state of Illinois. These services have been influenced significantly by a consent decree entered in October, 1985 to settle the *Nathan v. Levitt* lawsuit. This consent decree protects the right of dually diagnosed individuals to habilitation as well as treatment. Under the terms of the decree, mentally retarded people may receive services in mental health centers if they have mental health needs and a documented psychiatric diagnosis. Such persons must be evaluated and treated according to both the mental illness and the developmental disabilities codes of the Illinois Department of Mental Health and Developmental Disabilities. They must receive a habilitation plan as well as a treatment plan, and a "Qualified Mental Retardation Professional" must be assigned to each individual case. The facility director is required to certify that these services are being provided and that each individual is appropriately placed. If the individual or guardian disagrees with the facility director, he or she has the right to request a utilization review hearing. If psychiatric symptoms remit, or if subsequent evaluation finds that the service recipient no longer has a condition warranting treatment in a mental health setting, discharge or transfer must occur within 30 days of the facility director's decertification.

These rules apply only to dually diagnosed people with mild or moderate mental retardation. Persons with profound or severe mental retardation are not permitted treatment in a mental health setting even if they have a psychosis. When persons with severe or profound mental retardation present at a mental health center, they may be admitted for a period of up to 72 hours for the purpose of evaluation and/or transfer. By the end of the 72-hour period, however, the person must be discharged or transfered to a developmental center.

In order to insure that the Illinois Department of Mental Health and Developmental Disabilities complies with the terms of the *Nathan v. Levitt* consent decree, the court ordered that compliance be monitored by Protection and Advocacy, Inc., which is a federally-funded program providing advocacy for persons with developmental disabilities. The Protection and Advocacy officers report to the court the status of mental health facility compliance with the consent decree.

Figure 1 outlines the network of inpatient services for dually diagnosed people that were available in Illinois at the time of this writing (summer, 1987). Mentally retarded recipients with a psychiatric disorder or behavioral episode usually enter the system through MI (mentally ill) admissions and are placed initially on an acute care unit. Some may be discharged after a brief period of stabilization; however, those who stay must be evaluated within 14 days. Under the consent order and mental health code, the evaluation must include psychological, developmental/social, educational, medical, neurological, and psychiatric examinations as well as any other examination that is recommended by the multidisciplinary team. The team may recommend discharge, continuation of treatment, initiation of habilitation of the acute care unit for the mentally ill, transfer to a unit for the dually diagnosed, or transfer to a developmental disability facility.

Illinois Inpatient Units for Dually Diagnosed

By the summer of 1987, Illinois was operating for dually diagnosed people three units that had a total of 141 beds. Two of the units, Units 1 and 2,

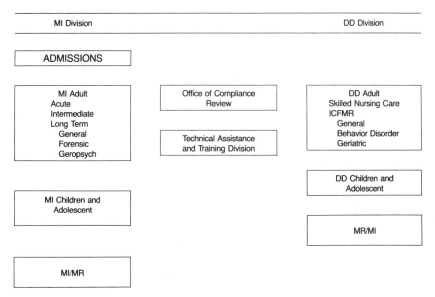

FIGURE 1. Illinois Department of Mental Health and Developmental Disabilities residential service options for the dually diagnosed. Key: MI = mental illness; MR = mental retardation; DD = developmental disability; Geropsych = gerontology/psychiatric; ICFMR = intermediate care facility/mental retardation.

were located at different mental health centers. Approximately 70% of the population served in these units had mild mental retardation; the remaining 30% of the population had moderate mental retardation. Approximately one half of the dually diagnosed people served by these units suffered from schizophrenia; many of the other dually diagnosed people suffered from personality disorder and impulse control disorder. The most commonly practiced treatments were behavior modification, chemotherapy, psychotherapy, and special focus groups for substance abuse and family issues.

Unit 3, the third Illinois unit for dually diagnosed people, is located at a developmental center, and serves 55 people who have a primary diagnosis of mental retardation. Approximately 40% of the people residing in Unit 3 also have a diagnosis of schizophrenia; other residents have such diagnoses as personality disorder or "psychosis." Although the mental health services for the dually diagnosed provided by Unit 3 are similar to those provided by Units 1 and 2, the training and habilitation services for mental retardation are more comprehensive. The primary treatment objective is to prepare persons with developmental disabilities for reintegration with the general population.

A fourth unit for dually diagnosed people has been proposed. This unit would serve people on a short-term, "flow-through" basis with the staff of the unit evaluating clients and recommending appropriate services and placements. Not all dually diagnosed individuals would be evaluated by this unit. It would be reserved for those who meet one of the following criteria: (1) people who have been difficult to evaluate in mental health facilities; (2)

people who need short-term behavior management to make a successful adjustment to community placement; (3) people transferring from mental health
to a developmental disabilities setting who require a period of adjustment to a
more structured environment; (4) people with complex problems who need
extended observation by a specialized team of professionals in order to identify treatment and habilitation needs; and (5) people from general developmental disabilities units who are acutely psychotic and need short-term stabilization in a developmental disabilities setting.

The Illinois Department of Mental Health and Developmental Disabilities
assigned internal responsibility for monitoring dually diagnosed people to a
Technical Assistance and Training Division. When a person suspected of
being dually diagnosed presents at a mental health center for an intake interview, the Technical Assistance and Training Team is notified within 24 hours.
The team then monitors the progress of the case until discharge, transfer to a
general developmental disabilities unit, or until a determination is made that
the individual is not mentally retarded. The division also provides assistance
and training in the diagnosis, evaluation, habilitation, and placement of persons suspected of dual diagnosis.

Inpatient Population Characteristics

During a recent 18-month period, the Illinois Department of Mental
Health and Developmental Disabilities served 763 people with dual diagnosis
in either its mental health programs or its special units for the dually diagnosed (see Tables 1 and 2). This number does not include the dually diag-

TABLE 1

Illinois State Discharges of Persons with Dual Diagnosis
during 18-Month Period

Receiving facility	Number of cases
Home	235
Intermediate care facility/DD	75
Intermediate care facility/MI	40
Group home	21
Jail	18
Community living facility	16
Community residential alternative	16
Sheltered care	11
Hospital	9
Skilled nursing	6
Out-of-state	4
Child care institution	3
Supported living arrangement	3
Independent living	2
Psychiatric hospital	2
Miscellaneous	6

TABLE 2
Illinois State Transfers of Persons with Dual
Diagnosis during 18-Month Period

Receiving facility	Number
Home	235
Community	230
State-operated DD facility	150
State-operated MI facility	54
State dual diagnosis unit	10

nosed people who are served within the general population of the developmentally disabled at state-operated centers for persons with mental retardation. Of the 763 people, 98 are recidivists with one or more readmissions to the same or to another state-operated facility. The total number of persons reported to the court each month, combined for 13 mental health and 1 dual diagnosis unit on the campus of a developmental disability center, averaged 286. Approximately 70% of the 763-person sample was served by one of the six facilities in the Chicago metropolitan area, with the remaining 30% served by one of the seven downstate facilities. The number of individuals admitted each month averaged 41 with recidivists included and 26.6 with recidivists excluded.

The age range for the 763 people was from 5 to 72 years, with the majority being young to middle-aged adults. Approximately 72% of the sample was mildly retarded, 24% was moderately retarded, and 3% was severely or profoundly retarded. Schizophrenia was diagnosed for more than one-third of the sample. In order of prevalence, the other common diagnoses were personality disorder, organic brain syndrome, atypical psychosis, impulse control disorder, adjustment disorder, substance abuse, conduct disorder, and affective disorder.

These statistics indicate that the population of dually diagnosed people served by inpatient facilities in Illinois was heterogeneous. The dually diagnosed people showed a very wide range of intelligence, personality characteristics, emotional functioning, and cultural background.

Transfers and Discharges

During the 18-month period of the study, 465 dually diagnosed persons were discharged from state-operated mental health facilities in Illinois. This number represents 235 people who were discharged to their families and 230 who were discharged to publicly funded residential facilities in the community. The discharges to community facilities included 75 placements at Intermediate Care Facilities for the Developmentally Disabled (ICF/DD) and 40 placements at Intermediate Care Facilities for the Mentally Ill (ICF/MI). Approximately 75% of the placements were made to developmental disabilities agencies, with the remainder made to mental health programs.

Although many of the dually diagnosed people had the skills to function at an adequate level of adaptive behavior, only two persons were discharged to independent living. This finding is consistent with the view that dual diagnosis often results in placement in a more restrictive residential setting than would have been necessary, based on the handicaps caused by the mental retardation. The cost of not treating dual diagnosis is considerable because untreated cases often require placement in a restrictive residential setting.

Our 18-month survey of Illinois inpatient services also found 214 instances in which a dually diagnosed person was transferred from one state-operated facility to another. There were 150 instances in which a dually diagnosed person had been transferred to a state-operated developmental disabilities facility; 61 of these transfers were mandated by *Nathan v. Levitt* because the individual was either severely or profoundly retarded. The other transfers were caused by findings that the most prominent need was for habilitation or skill development or by findings that there was minimal need for mental health services. Transfers of dually diagnosed persons to state-operated mental health centers were less frequent, accounting for only 24% of all transfers of dually diagnosed people. Some transfers to mental health facilities were made to return the person to the state-operated facility nearest to his or her family, whereas other transfers occurred because of a need for increased security in the case of persons who were considered to be a danger to themselves or to others. In a few instances, a transfer was made because of a finding that an individual at a mental retardation/mental illness unit was primarily mentally ill, at least from the viewpoint of current treatment needs.

Individualizing Placement Services

As noted previously, our experience in Illinois suggests that the dually diagnosed population is so diverse that no one housing plan is appropriate for the entire population. Instead, the best plan provides a wide range of residential options and an evaluation process to determine which option is best for each individual. Although units for the dually diagnosed have a place in the system, not all dually diagnosed people should be placed in such units, because many of them can be served in community settings if appropriate mental health services are provided to support the placement. Moreover, some dually diagnosed persons might best be served in developmental centers, whereas others might best be served in mental health facilities. Which setting is best may depend on the needs of the particular individual who is being placed.

The successful placement of dually diagnosed people requires a comprehensive evaluation of each individual, because a psychiatric diagnosis and the level of mental retardation are insufficient to determine proper placement. Other factors that should be taken into account include the degree to which the individual perceives himself or herself as mentally retarded, the individual's response to structured environments, and the vulnerability of the individual to manipulation or physical threat.

Comment on Behavior Modification

In Illinois, behavior modification is probably used more often in inpatient units for dually diagnosed people than in outpatient clinics for the dually diagnosed. Nevertheless, we still need to broaden the behavioral approaches used with inpatient populations. For example, behavior modifiers working in inpatient units do not seem to be treating depression as often as they should. There is evidence that some inpatients suffer from affective disorders and that these treatment needs are often overlooked (Sovner & Hurley, 1983).

FOSTER CARE

The third new service model is the placement of mentally retarded people in foster care homes. Foster care is important because it provides an alternative to the placement of mentally retarded people in restrictive environments, including state institutions. Moreover, behavior modification is relevant to foster care because behavior specialists are needed to assist foster parents in developing habilitation plans and in treating problem behaviors. Foster care is one of the ways in which behavior modifiers are supporting the community-integration movement. In this chapter, we will consider the foster care program of the Ray Graham Association for the Handicapped, which is located in the suburban Chicago area. This program, which began in 1977, consists of a social worker, three behavior specialists, and a psychologist, and was the first of its type in Illinois.

Parent Training

The Ray Graham program prepares people for foster parenthood by teaching them about developmental disabilities. All parents approved for the foster care program attend a four-session training course that is taught by a psychologist. The purpose of the training is to teach the parents the following details:

1. The concepts of mental retardation and developmental disabilities and how people are identified as having these conditions; the history of care of persons with mental retardation; the principles of reinforcement, extinction, and punishment
2. Specific behavior modification training techniques, including prompting, fading, modeling, and forward and backward chaining
3. Defining and observing behavior, data recording, and problem behavior management

4. The general conduct expected of a foster parent at home and in the community; preparation of the home; program record keeping; dealing with public agencies and schools

The fourth training class is usually taught with the assistance of veteran foster parents who can describe day-to-day experiences in foster care, including common problems and how they managed to cope with them.

After training is completed, placement is planned as soon as a child is available who meets the desires of the foster parent. The child visits the foster family three or four times prior to placement. If everything goes well, the child is then placed with the foster family.

The Training Home Concept

Once placement has occurred, parents are given the option of providing the child with concentrated training in the development of new skills and the remediation of problem behavior. The parents who accept this option are paid for 60 hours per month of special training in addition to the usual payments for the child's room and board. A distinction is drawn between these training homes, or Special Home Placements, and regular foster placements, or Maintenance Homes. Foster parents of the latter do not carry the expected extra training responsibilities and do not earn the extra pay. Virtually all of the foster parents in the Ray Graham program have opted for the special training responsibilities.

Intensive Behavioral Services

In contrast to the standard foster care approach in which families see a caseworker intermittently, the Ray Graham foster care program assigns a behavior specialist to each family. This person makes biweekly home visits and more frequent telephone contacts. Working with the foster parents, the behavior specialist does a behavioral assessment and generates an annual habilitation plan that includes a detailed list of behavioral objectives for the coming year. Specific behavioral training programs are developed, written, and explained to the parents. Progress is reviewed on each visit, and a formal written review of all objectives occurs every 6 months. In a number of instances, foster parents implemented sophisticated behavioral programs for problems, such as noncompliance, aggression, and self-injurious behavior.

The behavior specialist has many duties in addition to the development and implementation of the habilitation plan, including participation in all school, workshop, and public agency reviews of the developmentally disabled child. Also included are traditional casework duties, such as obtaining social security insurance funding, public aid, and food stamps. The behavior specialist also arranges for a limited amount of respite resources at the rate of

3.5 hours per child per week. Each behavior specialist has a caseload of about 15 to 20 clients at any one time.

Results and Discussion

A total of 80 placements have been made since the program began. At the time this chapter was written, 52 mentally retarded people were still in the foster care program and 28 had left the program. The primary reasons for leaving the program included a return to the natural parents, the presence of problem behavior that made the foster placement unsuccessful, and the occurrence of medical conditions or death.

Table 3 shows some of the characteristics of the people who were served by the foster care program, with little more than one half being severely or profoundly retarded and approximately 35% being multiply handicapped. These figures suggest that, compared with other foster care programs for the persons with developmental disabilities (Bruininks, Hill, & Thorsheim, 1982; Freeman, 1978), the Ray Graham program was more oriented toward serving persons with severe handicaps.

As shown in Table 3, the largest single referral source was the child's natural home. For most of these children, foster care provided an alternative to institutional placement. The program also received many referrals from private nursing homes and intermediate care facilities. Only 10 children came from prior placements in a state-operated institution.

TABLE 3
Handicapping Characteristics of Persons with Dual Diagnosis in the Ray Graham Foster Care Program

Characteristic	Number of clients
A. Mental retardation	
No mental retardation	1
Borderline impairment	8
Mild retardation	9
Moderate retardation	20
Severe retardation	42
B. Other handicaps	
Physical	13
Visual	7
Seizure	6
Hearing	4
C. Prior placement	
Natural home	33
Private institution	44
Other foster program	8

We analyzed the discharge data for the 28 children and adults who have left the program. On average, these people were in the program for 2.5 years. No data were available regarding the quality of the placement after discharge or the degree to which the individual made a successful adjustment.

Conclusions

The Ray Graham foster care program not only provided a relatively stable placement for most of the children and adults in the program, but also provided a nonrestrictive residential alternative to placement in state institutions and other special facilities for mentally retarded people. Behavior specialists played an important role in helping foster parents care for mentally retarded people.

GENERAL CONCLUSION

Three new service models in developmental disabilities were considered. Each of these models provides new opportunities and challenges for behavior modifiers. The dual diagnosis models provide opportunities to use the behavioral approach to address a broad range of emotional and social problems, such as depression, anxiety, personality disorder, and social skills deficiencies. The foster care model provides opportunities to use established behavioral techniques in new situations, such as foster care. Whether the behavior modifier is asked to develop new techniques or to use established techniques in new situations, the need is to adapt the behavioral approach to the changing priorities in the field. The greater the degree to which behavior modification is made relevant to dual diagnosis, and the greater the degree to which behavioral techniques assist the community-integration movement, the more relevant will be the future of behavior modification.

REFERENCES

Benson, B. A. (1985). Behavior disorders and mental retardation associations with age, sex, and levels of functioning in an outpatient clinic sample. *Applied Research in Mental Retardation, 6,* 79–85.

Benson, B. A. (1986). Anger management training. *Psychiatric Aspects of Mental Retardation, 5,* 51–56.

Benson, B. A., & Reiss, R. (1985). A factor analysis of emotional disorders in mentally retarded people. *Australia and New Zealand Journal of Developmental Disabilities, 10,* 135–139.

Benson, B. A., Rice, C. J., & Miranti, S. V. (1986). Effects of anger management training with mentally retarded adults in group treatment. *Journal of Consulting and Clinical Psychology, 54,* 728–729.

Bruininks, R. H., Hill, B. K., & Thorsheim, M. J. (1982). Deinstitutionalization and foster care for mentally retarded people. *Health and Social Work, 7,* 198–205.

Dewan, J. G. (1948). Intelligence and emotional stability. *American Journal of Psychiatry, 104,* 548–554.

Eaton, L. F., & Menolascino, F. J. (1982). Psychiatric disorders in the mentally retarded: Types, problems, and challenges. *American Journal of Psychiatry, 139*, 1297–1303.

Freeman, H. (1978). Foster homes for retarded children. *Child Welfare, 57*, 113–121.

Goldsmith, L., & Schloss, P. J. (1984). Diagnostic overshadowing among learning-disabled and hearing-impaired learners with an apparent secondary diagnosis of behavior disorders. *International Journal of Partial Hospitalization, 2*, 209–217.

Jacobson, J. W. (1982). Problem behavior and psychiatric impairment in a developmentally disabled population: I. Behavior frequency. *Applied Research in Mental Retardation, 3*, 121–139.

Kazdin, A. E., Matson, J. L., & Senatore, V. (1983). Assessment of depression in mentally retarded adults. *American Journal of Psychiatry, 140*, 1040–1043.

Levitan, G. W., & Reiss, S. (1983). Generality of diagnostic overshadowing across disciplines. *Applied Research in Mental Retardation, 4*, 59–69.

Lund, J. (1985). The prevalence of psychiatric morbidity in mentally retarded adults. *Acta Psychiatrica Scandinavica, 72*, 563–570.

Matson, J. L. (1981). A controlled outcome study of phobias in mentally retarded adults. *Behaviour Research and Therapy, 19*, 101–107.

Matson, J. L. (1982). The treatment of behavioral characteristics of depression in the mentally retarded. *Behavior Therapy, 13*, 209–218.

Matson, J. L., & Barrett, R. P. (1982). *Psychopathology in the mentally retarded.* New York: Grune & Stratton.

Matson, J. L., Kazdin, A. E., & Esveldt-Dawson, K. (1981). Training interpersonal skills among mentally retarded and socially dysfunctional children. *Behaviour Research and Therapy, 18*, 419–427.

McNally, R. J., & Ascher, L. M. (1985). Anxiety disorders in mentally retarded people. In L. Michelson & L. M. Ascher (Eds.), *Cognitive-behavioral assessment and treatment of anxiety disorders.* New York: Guilford Press.

Menolascino, F. J., & Stark, J. A. (1984). *Handbook of mental illness in the mentally retarded.* New York: Plenum Press.

Mueser, K. T., Valenti-Hein, D., & Yarnold, P. R. (1987). Dating-skills groups for the developmentally disabled. *Behavior Modification, 11*, 200–227.

Novaco, R. W. (1975). *Anger control: The development and evaluation of an experimental treatment.* Lexington, MA: Lexington Books.

Philips, I. (1967). Psychopathology and mental retardation. *American Journal of Psychiatry, 124*, 29–35.

Philips, I., & Williams, N. (1975). Psychopathology and mental retardation: A study of 100 mentally retarded children: I. Psychopathology. *American Journal of Psychiatry, 132*, 1265–1271.

Reid, A. H. (1972). Psychoses in adult mental defectives: I. Manic depressive psychosis. *British Journal of Psychiatry, 120*, 205–212.

Reiss, S. (1982). Psychopathology and mental retardation: Survey of a developmental disabilities mental health program. *Mental Retardation, 20*, 128–132.

Reiss, S. (1985). The mentally retarded, emotionally disturbed adult. In M. Sigman (Ed.), *Children with dual diagnosis: Mental retardation and mental illness* (pp. 171–192). New York: Grune & Stratton.

Reiss, S. (1987). Overview of symposium on dual diagnosis. *Mental Retardation, 25*, 323–324.

Reiss, S., & Szyszko, J. (1983). Diagnostic overshadowing and professional experience with mentally retarded persons. *American Journal of Mental Deficiency, 87*, 396–402.

Reiss, S., & Trenn, E. (1984). Consumer demand for outpatient mental health services for mentally retarded people. *Mental Retardation, 22*, 112–115.

Reiss, S., Levitan, G. W., & Szyszko, J. (1982). Emotional disturbance and mental retardation: Diagnostic overshadowing. *American Journal of Mental Deficiency, 86*, 567–574.

Rutter, M., Tizard, J., Yule, W., Graham, P., & Whitemore, K. (1976). Research report: Isle of Wight studies, 1964–74. *Psychological Medicine, 6*, 313–332.

Sovner, R., & Hurley, A. (1983). Do the mentally retarded suffer from affective illness? *Archives of General Psychiatry, 40*, 61–67.

Szymanski, L. S., & Tanguay, P. E. (1980). *Emotional disorders of mentally retarded persons.* Baltimore: University Park Press.

Valenti-Hein, D. (1989). An evaluation of treatment approaches for romantic loneliness of mentally retarded adults. Doctoral dissertation, University of Illinois at Chicago.

Weaver, T. R. (1946). The incident of maladjustment among mental defectives in military environment. *American Journal of Mental Deficiency, 51,* 238–315.

Zigler, E. (1971). The retarded child as a whole person. In H. E. Adams & W. K. Boardman (Eds.), *Advances in experimental clinical psychology* (Vol. 1). New York: Pergamon.

3

Staff Training

DENNIS H. REID AND CAROLYN W. GREEN

One of the most critical determinants of the effectiveness of human service systems for persons who are mentally retarded is the proficiency with which staff members, who work in those systems, fulfill their job roles. In essence, if service programs are to meet effectively the needs of mentally retarded clients, then human service staff must perform in a competent and efficient manner. Without proficient staff performance, human service programs, at best, are ineffective and, at worst, detrimental to client welfare.

If human service staff are to perform their job roles proficiently, then they must, of course, be *able* to do their jobs; that is, they must possess the work skills that are required to assist their mentally retarded clients. In most human service settings, in order to ensure that staff do indeed have the necessary work skills, staff training programs are usually needed.

The need for staff training programs in settings serving mentally retarded persons has been well recognized (Bensberg & Barnett, 1966; Gardner, 1973). Although a variety of reasons have been discussed why staff training programs are frequently needed, two reasons appear most critical. First, most persons who are hired for a human service job to work with the mentally retarded—and particularly into paraprofessional positions in residential settings—have had no formal preparation for the job in terms of relevant education and training experiences (cf. Burch, Reiss, & Bailey, 1987; Zlomke & Benjamin, 1983). Consequently, without some type of orientation or training program, such individuals realistically cannot be expected to have the necessary work skills that are required for a specific job. The second critical reason for staff training is that the skills required by staff members are frequently changing because the technology of providing various types of human services is consistently changing. In particular, in habilitative and educational settings, the technology for teaching new skills to mentally retarded clients and for reducing maladaptive behaviors is continuously being expanded and refined. Unless they are trained in the appropriate habilitative and educational techniques, human service staff cannot be expected to have the skills to apply this new technology.

DENNIS H. REID AND CAROLYN W. GREEN • Department of Psychology, Western Carolina Center, Enola Road, Morganton, North Carolina 28655.

The importance of, and need for, staff training is particularly germane in regard to the use of behavior modification with mentally retarded persons. Training human service staff in the use of behavior modification procedures for working with mentally retarded clients has received widespread acceptance (Frazier, 1972; Gardner, 1973). Furthermore, behavioral procedures represent an important means of training the numerous work skills that staff members need in order to perform various job roles that do not involve behavior modification (Ford, 1983; Reid, Schepis, & Fitzgerald, 1984).

Largely because of the recognized importance of staff training, there has been a rather considerable amount of applied research pertaining to behavior modification and staff training in human service settings for the mentally retarded. Thus, our purpose in this chapter is to review the work that has been conducted, as well as what we have learned as a result of the existing research.

FOCUS OF CHAPTER

Like the basic content of this volume, the orientation of this chapter is behavioral in nature. Specifically, we will address staff training in regard to research that (1) demonstrated and/or evaluated the use of behavior modification procedures to teach various types of job-related skills to human service staff working with mentally retarded persons; (2) demonstrated and/or evaluated methods of training staff to apply behavior modification procedures with their mentally retarded clients; and (3) addressed staff training issues that used applied behavioral research designs to conduct the respective investigations (see Baer, Wolf, & Risley, 1968; Kazdin, 1982; for elaboration on applied behavioral research, see Reid, 1987, Chapter 5).

No attempt will be made within this chapter to review and discuss *all* areas of behavior modification and staff training research with mentally retarded persons. Rather, the focus will be on staff training programs and research in residential settings, with particular emphasis on institutional environments. The rationale for focusing on staff training in residential facilities is severalfold. First, the bulk of the staff training research in settings serving mentally retarded persons has occurred in residential locations. Second, discussions of the (relatively little) research on staff training in mental retardation service settings other than residential environments, such as schools, has been discussed elsewhere (e.g., Reid, McCarn, & Green, 1989). Third, most of our experience in conducting and investigating staff training programs has been in residential settings.

Another focus of the chapter that warrants mentioning is the emphasis on staff training *per se*. There has been considerable discussion regarding the differences, as well as the similarities in certain contexts, between staff *training* and staff *management* (Reid & Whitman, 1983). For our purposes here, staff training is used to refer to the process of teaching new skills to staff members; that is, training them to perform duties which previously they did not know how to do. In contrast, staff management refers to changing and maintaining staff's application of skills that they already have in their performance repertoire. In this case, the focus is on assisting staff in doing what they already know how to do but, for whatever reason, are not doing appropriately.

Based on the description just provided, staff training represents a somewhat different set of issues than staff management. However, as discussed repeatedly elsewhere (see Miller & Lewin, 1980; Reid & Whitman, 1983; Whitman, Scibak, & Reid, 1983, Chapter 11, for reviews), the two sets of issues are clearly related. Essentially, the relationship between staff training and staff management, in regard to improving staff performance where such performance is less than optimal, can be categorized into three types of situations. In the first situation, staff performance can be improved by teaching new skills to staff through a staff training endeavor (Burch et al., 1987; Page et al., 1981). In the second situation, new skills via staff training are needed to improve performance along with a staff management program (e.g., Greene, Willis, Levy, & Bailey, 1978). In the third situation, improved staff performance can result from the application of a staff management program without teaching any new skills via a staff training process (Burg, Reid, & Lattimore, 1979). Considering all three situations, staff training endeavors should be considered as a step that is *frequently needed* for improving staff performance but *not necessarily sufficient* in this regard (Reid & Whitman, 1983). This relationship between staff training and management will be discussed intermittently across different contexts throughout the text. Because staff training is so frequently needed as one step in improving staff performance, or in some cases as an entire process in and of itself, our focus will be on those programs and investigations that are explicitly concerned with teaching staff new work skills.

FORMAT OF THE CHAPTER

This chapter consists of four main sections. In the first section, the use of behavior modification *procedures* to teach relevant job skills to human service staff working with the mentally retarded will be discussed in light of the applied research that has occurred in this area. The second section will address the *types of skills* that have been taught to staff personnel via the behavioral training processes discussed in the first section. The third section will discuss the *adequacy of the research* that addressed the topics investigated in the first two sections in order to determine, in essence, the degree of definitiveness with which conclusions about training processes and outcomes can be made. Finally, based on the information provided, as well as what was not provided, in the research summarized in the first three sections, areas warranting attention for *future research* will be highlighted in the fourth section.

PROCEDURES USED TO TRAIN NEW SKILLS TO STAFF

A variety of procedures have been evaluated in behavior modification research on the training of staff members in relevant work skills. However, the efficacy of any one of the various procedures rarely has been evaluated. Rather, in most cases, two or more procedures have been used as part of a staff training package so that the effectiveness of the procedures as a group can be determined but not the effectiveness of any individual component procedure within the package. Nevertheless, in order to understand the use of these types of *multifaceted* training procedures, the specific procedural components must be clearly delineated. This section describes the basic training procedures that have been used to date in the behavior modification research on staff training.

Verbal Instruction

Probably the most common component of staff training programs is verbal (spoken) instruction—a trainer providing information to staff by word of mouth. Essentially, every staff training program entails some type of verbally provided information. For example, the instruction may be brief and describe only the basic performance skills that a trainer wants a staff member to learn how to perform (cf. Lattimore, Stephens, Favell, & Risley, 1984). Alternatively, verbally presented information can be quite elaborate and can discuss, in addition to the explicit performance skills expected, the rationale for the training program, the importance of the targeted behaviors, and other related information (Reid *et al.*, 1985). Verbal instruction can be provided either individually to staff persons or to a group through a lecture or seminar format (Fitzgerald *et al.*, 1984).

As a means of teaching skills to staff, verbal instruction often has the advantage of requiring minimal preparation on the part of the trainer relative to other training procedures to be discussed. Also, verbal instruction can have the advantage of allowing for a two-way interaction between the trainer and staff trainees so that the latter can have the opportunity to ask questions and seek appropriate clarification. On the other hand, effective verbal instruction requires that the trainer be able to articulate clearly the relevant aspects about the skills that are targeted to be taught to the staff. Additionally, verbal instruction typically provides only as much exposure to the content of the training as the trainer provides while talking to staff; staff members often do not have the opportunity to review the information at their convenience or at the respective times when the information may be particularly needed during routine work performance. Furthermore, verbal instruction seems to be effective for teaching verbal skills to staff but not for teaching actual performance skills (Gardner, 1972); verbal instruction teaches staff what to say more effectively about a job than how actually to perform the job.

Written Instruction

As a means of staff training, written instruction refers to the presentation of information in writing regarding new job skills that staff must learn to perform. Like verbal or vocal instruction, written instruction can take many forms, including the use of published papers that describe performance techniques and various types of background material (Page *et al.*, 1981), self-instructional manuals (Fitzgerald *et al.*, 1984), and performance checklists that essentially list only concise descriptions of performance skills (Lattimore *et al.*, 1984). Written instruction has also been used in the form of pictures of various job-related duties (Fielding, Errickson, & Bettin, 1971; Stoddard, McIlvane, McDonagh, & Kledaras, 1986), as well as in combined form involving pictures with accompanying written descriptions (Fitzgerald *et al.*, 1984).

Perhaps the most important advantage of written instruction as a means of staff training is that the written material can provide a permanent representation regarding desired performance areas of staff. Once staff members receive the written material, they can refer repeatedly to the text information for assistance in knowing what duties are expected regarding a given job. Also, whereas the specific content of verbal instruction may vary depending on the consistency of a trainer's presentation across training sessions, written instruction provides a consistent source of information. On the negative side, appropriate written material must of course be available for the trainer's use. In many cases, commercially available and/or published material is often too general or irrelevant, in terms of the exact skills which are expected of a staff member in a given job situation, to be of much use to a trainer. Consequently, a trainer must be able to write about performance areas of staff in a clear and accurate manner, or at least have ready access to someone who can transcribe the information proficiently. Written instruction also requires a certain degree of reading comprehension skills of staff members—skills that are not always sufficiently adequate among some paraprofessional staff persons (Stoddard *et al.*, 1986).

Performance Demonstration

A type of staff training procedure that is becoming more common in the applied research literature is performance demonstration. This approach involves physically demonstrating for staff members the new skills that are targeted for them to learn. A relatively frequent application of performance demonstration is the *modeling* of job skill usage by someone who engages in the designated performance behavior while staff members observe (Gladstone & Spencer, 1977). Modeling may be conducted by the job supervisor of staff (Ivancic, Reid, Iwata, Faw, & Page, 1981), a specialty or professional staff member (Fitzgerald *et al.*, 1984; Mansdorf & Burstein, 1986), or a staff peer or colleague who is already skilled in the performance area of concern (van den Pol, Reid, & Fuqua, 1983). Another type of performance demonstration is the use of films or videotapes (Kissel, Whitman, & Reid, 1983) that present individuals performing designated staff skills.

Performance demonstration can be particularly helpful in that often the demonstration provides more relevant information regarding exactly what is expected of staff than verbal and written instructions. Considered in a more figurative vein, performance demonstration is useful in accordance with the adage that "a picture is worth a thousand words." Also, performance demonstration does not require a certain level of reading skills among staff trainees as do various types of written instructions. In addition, modeling of new staff skills can be a relatively well-received or popular method of staff training among trainees when the job demonstrations are conducted by a staff supervisor (see Whitman *et al.*, 1983, Chapter 11, for elaboration).

The advantages of performance demonstration as just described notwithstanding, one of the disadvantages of this approach to staff training is that such materials as films and videotapes are not always readily available for trainers. Similarly, considerable time and money are often required to prepare effective demonstrations, and appropriate equipment must be accessible. However, the rather rapid development, in recent years, in the use of videocassettes and videocassette recorders is helping to overcome this disadvantage at least partially. Another disadvantage of performance demonstration using modeling is that the trainers *may not be able* to demonstrate proficiently certain types of skills for staff members. This problem is likely to occur when trainers attempt to teach staff new skills, developed through research, that are highly specialized in nature, such as new methods of overcoming the feeding disabilities of multiply physically impaired clients or new behavior reduction strategies to remediate client maladaptive behaviors.

Performance Practice

Performance practice refers to the desired performance activity staff trainees engage in as part of a staff training program. Frequently, staff members are asked to try to practice a given skill after they have received verbal or written instruction or after having viewed a demonstration of the target performance (Faw, Reid, Schepis, Fitzgerald, & Welty, 1981). A related type of performance practice is role playing. Role playing requires that a staff person briefly assume the (simulated) job of someone else and attempt to perform the necessary skills that comprise that particular job (Gardner, 1972). A modified type of practice has also been used in which trainees are required to describe, either verbally or through written exercises, critical components of a job task that is to be learned (Stoddard *et al.*, 1986).

An important advantage of performance practice is that it represents probably the best way for a trainer to know for sure that a staff member can perform a new work skill. No matter what a staff member may say or write about his or her knowledge of a performance skill, a trainer should not be totally convinced that a staff member can indeed perform the skill unless the trainer actually sees the skill demonstrated. Another advantage of performance practice is that the procedure does not require a certain level of reading proficiency among staff trainees.

A disadvantage of performance practice is that typically a staff trainer can work with only one trainee at a time. Consequently, relative to the training procedures noted previously that can be implemented by one trainer with a group of trainees simultaneously, performance practice can be a rather time-consuming process when a number of staff members must be trained individually. Another disadvantage of this training strategy is that some staff members are uncomfortable when they attempt to demonstrate for a trainer a skill with which they do not yet feel proficient; hence, they may not be very willing to accept the performance demonstration approach.

Feedback

As applied research on staff training procedures has developed and expanded, performance feedback appears to have become the most widely accepted component of training programs among professional staff trainers. Most likely, this popularity is due to the frequently documented effectiveness of feedback procedures for changing staff performance (Reid & Whitman, 1983). As reflected in Table 1, there are a variety of formats for presenting performance feedback, and the various formats have been included in a number of investigations on staff training programs. Usually, the common procedure across the different formats is that the trainer provides descriptive and/or evaluative information regarding the proficiency of a staff trainee's performance to the trainee. Because feedback procedures have been investigated and discussed so frequently, elaboration on how feedback can be provided will not be presented here, and the interested reader is referred to the other sources cited in Table 1.

The relative advantages and disadvantages of performance feedback vary across the type of format used to provide the feedback. Verbal feedback presented individually to staff persons has an advantage similar to verbal instruction in that it can provide a two-way interaction between trainer and trainee. However, effective presentation of verbal feedback typically requires a certain degree of interpersonal skill on the part of staff trainers, which not all staff trainers necessarily possess. Also, individual verbal feedback must, of course, be presented to one staff person at a time, which can be a time-

TABLE 1
Formats Used for Presenting Feedback in Staff Training Investigations

Format	Reference
Verbal (vocal) feedback	Fabry & Reid, 1978; Gardner, 1972
Videotaped performance feedback	Kissel, Whitman, & Reid, 1983
Self-recorded feedback	Korabek, Reid, & Ivancic, 1981
Publicly posted feedback on client responsiveness to staff activities	Ivancic, Reid, Iwata, Faw, & Page, 1981
Publicly posted feedback on staff performance	Ivancic, Reid, Iwata, Faw, & Page, 1981
Privately written feedback	Fitzgerald et al., 1984

consuming process. Verbal feedback presented either publicly or in a group format shares the same advantages and disadvantages as individual verbal feedback, with the exception that it is typically more time efficient in that it is provided simultaneously to a group of staff trainees. However, the latter feedback procedure can have the additional disadvantage of being poorly received by staff trainees because some staff members do not like to have their performance discussed publicly, especially if the feedback is negative.

Privately written feedback may overcome the disadvantage that is sometimes associated with private (or individual) verbal feedback in that interpersonal skills in terms of face-to-face interactions on the part of the trainer are not as important. However, privately written feedback does require a certain level of writing proficiency by a trainer as well as reading skills by the trainee. Although it can be more time efficient, publicly posted feedback is similar to privately written feedback because of its focus on a group of staff trainees. However, publicly displayed feedback is also similar to public verbal feedback in that a number of staff may not be very receptive to that approach. Actually, this type of feedback can be more negatively received than public verbal feedback because it is more permanent (i.e., the feedback remains displayed for staff members to review). Indications of negative staff reaction to publicly posted feedback have been reported a number of times (see Reid & Whitman, 1983, for discussion), although such a reaction does not always occur (Greene *et al.*, 1978).

JOB SKILLS TARGETED IN BEHAVIORAL STAFF TRAINING

Although the types of skills targeted in staff training research have varied across different investigations, the skills generally fall into one of two groups. The first, and clearly the larger group, is behavior modification skills. The second group consists of work-related skills that do not involve the explicit use of behavior modification techniques.

Behavior Modification Skills

The general effectiveness of behavior modification as a means of teaching useful skills to mentally retarded persons and of reducing maladaptive behaviors has been demonstrated many times over (e.g., see *Journal of Applied Behavior Analysis*, Volumes 1–20). Once the effectiveness of this approach to habilitation and education became recognized in the 1970s, applied researchers began to address the issue of how to disseminate the developing behavioral technology. Rather quickly, it became apparent that if many mentally retarded persons were to benefit significantly from the application of behavior modification procedures, then their routine trainers and caregivers (e.g., institutional direct care staff) would need to be trained in behavior modification skills. Subsequently, a number of investigations were conducted to demonstrate methods of training behavior modification skills to mental retardation staff.

Multiskill Training Programs

One approach to teaching behavior modification skills that was especially common among the initial staff training investigations (see Gardner, 1973, for a review) was to focus on a broad range of behavior modification principles and procedures (see also Zlomke & Benjamin, 1983). Such an approach often targeted a number of principles of learning as well as various procedural applications, including data collecting, reinforcing, shaping, and modeling strategies for decelerating behavior and obtaining stimulus control (Gardner, 1973).

The major advantage in training staff to use a wide variety of behavior modification procedures is that conceivably they can acquire a robust set of skills useful across a variety of client habilitative situations. However, because of the number and variety of skills that are targeted in these types of training programs, a rather substantial amount of time is often required to conduct the training—sometimes several hundred hours (Gardner, 1973). Staff training programs that require large amounts of trainer time are often quite expensive. Similarly, requiring staff members to be away from their daily work site for extended periods of time in order to attend staff training programs can be problematic in terms of ensuring that routine work responsibilities are fulfilled during these absences.

Because of the large amount of information that the multiskill training programs attempt to teach, as well as the large amount of time required for training, these programs often rely on a considerable amount of verbal instruction as a teaching strategy. Verbal instruction requires less time than the demonstration-oriented and practice procedures noted earlier and can easily be conducted in a group format. However, as noted earlier, although verbal instruction is generally appropriate for teaching such things as an understanding of the principles of learning (i.e., verbal skills), it typically is not very useful for teaching how to apply the information (performance skills).

Procedurally Specific Training Programs

Generally, the more recent staff training investigations have focused on teaching one or a small set of behavior modification skills in contrast to a broad range of skills. By focusing on a small set of behavioral skills, less time is required for training staff, and more demonstration and practice-type training procedures can usually be incorporated into the training program. This type of approach can be particularly helpful if the targeted skills can be applied across a variety of client habilitation situations. For the most part, staff training research that has attempted to teach a small number of skills has focused on behavior modification procedures that can be used to accelerate the development of mentally retarded clients' adaptive behavior. These types of procedures include, for example, staff's skilled use of verbal instruction and physical guidance (Fabry & Reid, 1978; Kissel et al., 1983), backward chaining teaching strategies (Watson & Uzzell, 1980), and reinforcement procedures (Adams, Tallon, & Rimell, 1980; Parsonson, Baer, & Baer, 1974). A smaller number of investigations have focused on training staff in methods of decelerating maladaptive client behavior, such as through the proficient use of time-out procedures (Katz & Lutzker, 1980).

As indicated previously, an advantage of staff training programs that focus on a circumscribed, yet nevertheless important, set of behavior modification skills is that the programs are less time-consuming to implement than multiskill training programs. Consequently, it is easier to use demonstration- and practice-oriented training procedures in these types of training programs. Again, training procedures that involve demonstrations and trainee practice are generally more effective for training staff in how to perform necessary skills than are verbal and written instructional formats. Of course, staff training programs that focus on a small number of skills are limited in terms of the amount of new information or skills the staff trainees acquire as a result of participating in the training program.

Job-Related Skills Other Than Behavior Modification

As mentioned, the first behavior modification investigations involving staff performance focused on training staff members in the proficient application of behavior modification techniques with their mentally retarded clients. Generally, as the research in this area progressed, there was an increasing reliance within the staff training programs on the use of *behavioral* training strategies with staff trainees (e.g., trainee practice, performance feedback) to teach behavior modification skills and a decreasing emphasis on more traditional teaching formats (e.g., large group lectures). Because of the effectiveness of the behavioral training strategies in the earlier investigations that focused on teaching behavior modification skills to staff, these training strategies were extended to staff training programs that focused on job-related skills other than behavior modification applications with mentally retarded clients. In this regard, because of the varied, multiskill nature of the jobs of direct service providers, there are numerous skills that are needed by mental retardation staff that warrant the development of effective staff training programs.

With few exceptions (Ford, 1983), each of the investigations on the use of behavioral training procedures to teach various (nonbehavior modification) job skills to staff has focused on a relatively specific or circumscribed skill area. Table 2 shows the types of skills that are targeted in this area of research. As indicated in the table, a rather wide variety of service-related job responsibilities have been addressed in the staff training research.

CRITIQUE OF STAFF MANAGEMENT RESEARCH

As suggested in the preceding sections, a relatively large number of investigations to date have been conducted in the area of staff training and behavior modification. To illustrate, some 32 applied behavioral research studies involving the teaching of new job skills in institutional settings have

TABLE 2
*Examples of (Nonbehavior Modification) Job Skills Taught to
Mental Retardation Staff through Applied Behavioral Investigations*

Type of job skill	Reference
Writing client program objectives	Page *et al.*, 1981
Supervisory skills	Clark *et al.*, 1985
Fire safety procedures	van den Pol, Reid, & Fuqua, 1983
Physical therapy treatment procedures	Lattimore, Stephens, Favell, & Risley, 1984
Performing personal care for dependent clients	Ford, 1983
General information about mental retardation	Zlomke & Benjamin, 1983
Lifting and transferring nonambulatory clients	Stoddard, McIlvane, McDonagh, & Kledaras, 1986
Responding to client seizures	van den Pol, Reid, & Fuqua, 1983

been noted so far in this chapter. Such a body of research has resulted in a considerable amount of information in regard to training staff to provide therapeutic services to mentally retarded clients. However, the mere existence of a body of research does not necessarily guarantee that useful information has been obtained from each of these investigations. Rather, assurances are needed that given studies were conducted with an acceptable degree of scientific rigor such that definitive, or even near-definitive, conclusions can be drawn from the research (Whitman *et al.*, 1983, Chapter 3). Attention is warranted to determine if the results of the research actually represent an outcome that is truly significant or meaningful from a clinical perspective (Wolf, 1978) and not just an academic exercise; the outcome should be something that truly enhances staff work performance and, subsequently, service provision to clients.

Because of the importance of the scientific rigor and clinical utility of respective investigations in terms of the ability to draw informative conclusions from a body of research, these aspects of the research on staff training and behavior modification will be discussed in this section. Specifically, this area of research will be critiqued and summarized in regard to criteria for conducting experimentally sound and clinically useful applied behavioral research. Evaluative criteria to be used in this regard have been described in depth elsewhere (e.g., Baer *et al.*, 1968; Wolf, 1978) and have been used specifically with applied behavioral research on staff performance (Reid & Whitman, 1983; Whitman *et al.*, 1983, Chapter 11). Because of space limitations, no attempt will be made to summarize the research adequacy of each of the reported studies. Rather, *general* areas of concern that tend to exist throughout significant components of the staff training research will be discussed.

A primary reason for attempting to summarize the adequacy of the staff training research is to highlight areas that may be addressed in future research endeavors in order to continuously upgrade the sophistication of the research so that more useful information on staff training will be forthcoming. Consequently, this critique will focus on problematic areas that currently exist with the staff training research. However, the emphasis on areas of concern should not devalue the important advances that have resulted from applied research on staff training and behavior modification. This research has addressed numerous important areas of staff performance and has consistently demonstrated means of teaching staff new and relevant job skills. Thus, if applied research in this area continues, and attempts are made to improve the adequacy of the research in certain areas, our ability to assist human service staff to perform their jobs with proficiency will continue to be substantially enhanced.

Analyses of Components in Packaged Training Programs

As noted previously, with few exceptions (e.g., Gardner, 1972) investigations on approaches to staff training have evaluated multifaceted *packages* of procedures. Component analyses of the effectiveness of the respective component procedures that constitute the packages generally have been lacking. Consequently, it is possible that some of the components that comprise typical training programs are not needed (i.e., certain components may add little or nothing to the overall effectiveness of a training program). Research is warranted to evaluate the contribution of the component parts of effective training packages. Such research could be particularly useful if procedural components were identified within respective staff training programs that require a substantial amount of time to implement yet add little in the way of overall effectiveness. If identified, these types of procedures could then be eliminated from training programs with a subsequent reduction in the time requirements for conducting the programs. As discussed earlier, time efficiency is an important feature of staff training programs in terms of the cost of a trainer's time and the reduction in work performance while trainees are drawn away from routine work duties for training purposes.

Demonstrating Experimental Control of Training Programs

An essential feature in any behavior change investigation is the demonstration of experimental control of the intervention; specifically, demonstrating it is the intervention (the staff training program) that is responsible for the change in behavior of the participants (the newly acquired job skills of the staff trainees). Demonstrations of experimental or functional control require the use of an appropriate research design (Baer *et al.*, 1968; Barlow & Hersen, 1984; Kazdin, 1982). For the most part, investigations on staff training and behavior modification have employed adequate research designs, with improvement in this regard occurring in more recent investigations in the 1980s. However, there are some recent investigations that seriously lacked appropriate experimental controls. Several investigations used between-group-comparison designs to compare different training procedures without any preintervention measures to establish the equivalence of groups prior to training or to determine pretraining levels of staff skills (Ford, 1983; Katz & Lutzker, 1980). Other investigations evaluated respective training programs using pre- versus postintervention measures without any control group measures (Stoddard *et al.*, 1986; Zlomke & Benjamin, 1983).

These examples are cited not because they are representative of the general body of research on staff training and behavior modification—again, fortunately, most recent research has used adequate experimental designs— but because they are somewhat discouraging in that they represent regression in the state-of-the-art research in the staff training area. In essence, without adequate experimental control, no conclusions—and basically no validly useful information—can stem from an investigation. Such investigations may be useful in the initial stages of development of a given area of research (Bailey, 1987) but are generally not warranted once an area has progressed beyond a few studies. Consequently, investigations lacking in experimental control in the staff training area are really not beneficial at this point. However, in defense of some of the research in this area, it should also be noted that conducting research on staff performance can be a considerably more difficult research task than other areas of applied research in behavior modification and mental retardation (see Reid, 1987, for elaboration). Generally, good staff research requires that an applied researcher have access to authoritative and/or supervisory control over a component of an agency's staff population; such control is often difficult to obtain for professional researchers, such as investigators who operate out of a university setting. Additionally, effective access to a setting for successfully conducting research on staff performance usually necessitates a rather intimate knowledge of the inner workings of a given agency's organizational structure (Liberman, 1983). Staff training researchers who do not work routinely within a setting in which they conduct their research often do not possess such information.

Analyses of Duration of Training Effects

As the application of behavior modification procedures in human service settings became widespread in the 1970s and early to mid 1980s, and applied research with behavioral procedures in general began to proliferate, there was increasing concern with regard to the durability of treatment effects. Applied researchers began to realize that, to be useful, a treatment procedure (e.g., a staff training program) not only had to be effective in terms of initially *changing* behavior (such as teaching new skills), it also had to *maintain* the change in behavior. Consequently, more concern is currently directed in the general applied behavioral research literature to collecting follow-up data to demonstrate the durability of initial changes following a given behavior modification intervention. The trend of increasing attention given to maintenance of behavior change is also reflected in the research on staff performance (Reid & Whitman, 1983). However, numerous investigations on staff training continue to be reported without any systematic evaluation of the durability of the initial skills in which staff members were trained (e.g., Adams *et al.*, 1980; Ford, 1983; Katz & Lutzker, 1980). To maximize the amount of useful information that can result from an investigation on staff training, it would be helpful for future research endeavors to include follow-up data.

A major issue that arises when considering the durability of behavior changes resulting from a staff training program is the supervision or management of staff performance during the routine job situation following the staff training endeavor. As noted in the introductory comments to this chapter, staff training programs are often necessary for improving staff performance but are rarely sufficient. Actually, many applied behavioral researchers have become astutely aware of the need to effectively supervise staff performance in the daily job setting following a training program in order to ensure that the skills acquired by staff members during training are consistently applied (e.g., Greene *et al.*, 1978; Montegar, Reid, Madsen, & Ewell, 1977; Quilitch, 1975). Hence, some of the criticism of staff training research for not including follow-up measures is not entirely representative in that a number of recent studies focused on staff *management* instead of staff training *per se* but nevertheless included a staff training component and did provide systematic follow-up measures (e.g., Dyer, Schwartz, & Luce, 1984; Kissel *et al.*, 1983; Parsons, Schepis, Reid, McCarn, & Green, 1987; Reid *et al.*, 1985).

Analyses of Impact of Staff Training on Client Welfare

A well-recognized critical measure of the value of a training program which attempts to teach staff members skills that have a direct impact on their mentally retarded clients is the demonstration that client welfare actually is enhanced (Greene *et al.*, 1978; Reid & Whitman, 1983, Whitman *et al.*, 1983, Chapter 11). Investigators ought to demonstrate that not only do staff members acquire the skills addressed in a training program, but also that they acquire these skills sufficiently thoroughly to bring about desired changes in client welfare (e.g., improved client adaptive behavior). A number of investigations have subsequently included systematic measures of changes in client welfare as a function of a staff training program (e.g., Fabry & Reid, 1978; Kissel *et al.*, 1983) although, unfortunately, a rather large number of studies have not included such measures (e.g., Adams *et al.*, 1980; Ford, 1983; Katz & Lutzker, 1980). Of course, there are a variety of important staff skills that would not be expected to result in a relatively quick or direct change in client behavior (see Table 2) so that measures of client welfare then are not a crucial issue.

Analyses of the Acceptability or Nonacceptability of Staff Training Programs

A final concern with existing research on staff training and behavior modification is the demonstration of the degree of trainer and trainee acceptance of respective staff training programs (Kazdin, 1980). With very few exceptions (e.g., Fitzgerald *et al.*, 1984), research on staff training has not addressed the issue of program acceptability. The lack of research attention directed to this area is problematic because of the importance of staff acceptance or nonacceptance of behavior change programs as noted earlier, and especially because there have been several indications that behavioral training procedures have not been very well received by staff trainees (see Ford, 1983, and Gardner, 1973, for discussion). On the more positive side, however, where staff acceptability has been addressed with some behavioral staff *management* procedures that are similar to a number of staff training approaches, results have been more encouraging in terms of staff acceptance of the procedures (see Reid & Whitman, 1983, for a review).

FUTURE RESEARCH NEEDS

In the introductory comments to this chapter, we stressed the continuing need for staff training programs in mental retardation settings. When considering the lack of formal preparation of many persons who are hired by agencies serving the mentally retarded, along with the continuously changing processes involved in service provision that frequently require new skills of staff, staff training programs will continue to be needed on both a preservice basis for newly employed staff and an inservice basis for experienced staff. Consequently, continued research is warranted in order to develop and improve programs for effectively and efficiently training staff to perform with proficiency all aspects of their service jobs. This section summarizes our views regarding those staff training areas most in need of applied research.

Improving the Adequacy of Staff Training Research Methodology

Prior to discussing specific areas in need of research, the general approach to staff training research warrants mention. As indicated in the preceding section, there are a number of problems with investigations in the staff training area, ranging from the lack of a valid experimental design to inattention to the durability of the effects of respective staff training programs. Also methodological problems are likely due, at least in part, to the difficulty many researchers have in obtaining sufficient control over staff resources in mental retardation settings to conduct sound research on staff training issues. Nevertheless, if applied research is going to have a significant and beneficial impact on the improvement of staff training programs, then investigators must find a way to ensure that their research is experimentally sound and clinically thorough.

Targeting Additional Skill Areas

Although the skill areas addressed by staff training research have been expanded considerably since the initial behavior modification research with staff in the early 1970s (see Table 2 for examples), there are still a number of important skill areas that have not been addressed in the staff training research, or have been addressed only minimally. In particular, very little applied behavioral research to date (Clark *et al.*, 1985; Page, Iwata, & Reid, 1982) has focused on training effective management skills to staff supervisors. Ineffective supervisory practices have traditionally been somewhat common in many facilities serving mentally retarded persons (Mayhew, Enyart, & Cone, 1979). Hence, effective procedures for training proficient supervisory skills would be a valuable contribution to the mental retardation service delivery system.

Another skill area that has been addressed only minimally in the staff training research is teaching staff to proficiently apply behavioral decelerative procedures for treating client maladaptive behavior problems (Katz & Lutzker, 1980). Appropriate use of such decelerative techniques as, for example, time out and restraint procedures by mental retardation staff warrants serious attention because these techniques are frequently recommended as part of client habilitation plans. Thus, if staff are not trained appropriately and do not conduct decelerative procedures competently, not only will habilitation efforts be stymied, but there can also be rather deleterious effects on client welfare (cf. Reid & Schepis, 1986).

At this time, an area of staff training that is growing rapidly is teaching staff members the use of personal computers as part of their job routine (Smith & Wells, 1983). Computerization is steadily impacting many areas of service delivery for mentally retarded persons, including habilitative programming with clients. In some ways, the introduction of personal computers has progressed at a faster rate than our ability to teach staff how to use them in a maximally advantageous manner. Currently, many mental retardation staff members seem to be somewhat intimidated by the computerization movement. Hence, good staff training programs need to be developed that are effective *and* are well received by staff trainees so that the programs assist staff members in being more comfortable with various computerized systems.

Similar to the need for research on training a wider variety of skills is the need for additional investigations on training a wider variety of personnel in mental retardation agencies. With few exceptions (e.g., Fitzgerald *et al.*, 1984; Page *et al.*, 1981), the institutional staff training research has involved direct care personnel almost exclusively. Assisting other types of staff, such as specialty habilitative and support personnel, in developing improved job skills warrants research attention. One relatively specific need in this regard is training specialty staff (e.g., speech pathologists) to work with severely and profoundly handicapped clients—clients who are steadily becoming the primary population that resides in institutional settings relative to less seriously handicapped persons. In many cases, specialty personnel who assume jobs in institutions have no real preparation for applying their therapeutic skills with very low functioning populations and are in need of effective training in this area. In this regard, conducting training programs for professional specialists may represent somewhat of a different task in terms of which training procedures are most efficient and effective relative to implementing training programs with paraprofessional staff who have considerably less educational background (Page *et al.*, 1981). Whether or not there are such differences, and the resulting impact on respective types of training procedures that are most useful, warrants the attention of investigators.

Developing New and Refined Training Procedures

If applied behavioral research is to continue to find means of better preparing mental retardation staff members for their important job roles, then research on better methods or procedures for training staff is needed. In this respect, three criteria seem particularly relevant in terms of ensuring that new or revised training procedures do indeed represent improvements in staff training technology. First, and most apparent, is that new training processes must be *effective* in terms of teaching relevant work skills. Second, new approaches to training staff would be most helpful if they are more *efficient* regarding the amount of time required of staff trainers to teach skills to trainees. Third, and related to the second characteristic, is that newly developed training procedures should be *acceptable* to mental retardation staff; hence, for maximum utility, trainers and trainees should enjoy or, at the very least, not dislike the training programs in which they participate.

One approach to staff training that would be useful to investigate and that has been only minimally researched to date is self-management strategies (Kissel *et al.*, 1983). Self-management procedures in which staff members are instructed in means of changing and maintaining their own skills have been effective in several management programs (Burg *et al.*, 1979; Burgio, Whitman, & Reid, 1983) in institutional settings. Self-management procedures, such as performance goal setting and self-recording, also seem to be quite well received by staff (e.g., Burgio *et al.*, 1983). Additionally, these types of approaches can be relatively efficient in that they reduce the amount of trainer time and involvement in the training process (Kissel *et al.*, 1983).

Another rather novel approach to staff training that can reduce the participative requirements of trainers is peer training (van den Pol *et al.*, 1983). Actually, new (and, to a lesser degree, experienced) staff members probably learn a considerable amount of job skills from their staff peers on an informal basis during the routine course of their work. Formal peer training strategies could capitalize on such procedures and ensure that *what* is learned by new staff members from their peers is well organized and in accordance with supervisory expectations.

Finally, continued research on assisting supervisors in teaching staff important work skills during the day-to-day job routine in contrast to a geographically and temporally removed training program would be beneficial (Favell, Favell, Riddle, & Risley, 1984). Such *in situ* approaches to training have the advantage of not necessitating the removal of staff from their ongoing work responsibilities for training purposes. Also, on-site training strategies can alleviate concerns over whether the skills learned in a training program *carry over* to the daily work routine because, in these types of programs, the skills are taught as part of the ongoing work situation and carry over is not an issue.

Summary

Many advances have been made through research in staff training and behavior modification since behavioral procedures began to be applied significantly within mental retardation agencies in the early 1970s. We now have a rather broad repertoire of staff training procedures with which to establish staff training programs with relatively good documentation that the procedures are truly effective. Nevertheless, we still have significant gaps in our knowledge regarding how best to train staff members and how to ensure that what we do know about training is actually applied in typical service agencies. It is hoped that this chapter will help set the occasion for continued applied research in this important area and, subsequently, lead to better services for mentally retarded persons.

Acknowledgments. Appreciation is expressed to Carole McNew for her patient and competent assistance in preparing this chapter and to Marsha Parsons for her comments on an earlier draft.

References

Adams, G. L., Tallon, R. J., & Rimell, P. (1980). A comparison of lecture versus role-playing in the training of the use of positive reinforcement. *Journal of Organizational Behavior Management, 2,* 205–212.

Baer, D. M., Wolf, M. M., & Risley, T. R. (1968). Some current dimensions of applied behavior analysis. *Journal of Applied Behavior Analysis, 1,* 91–97.

Bailey, J. S. (1987). The editor's page. *Journal of Applied Behavior Analysis, 20,* 3–6.

Barlow, D. H., & Hersen, M. (1984). *Single case experimental designs: Strategies for studying behavior change* (2nd ed.). New York: Pergamon Press.

Bensberg, G. J., & Barnett, C. D. (1966). *Attendant training in southern residential facilities for the mentally retarded.* Atlanta: Southern Regional Education Board.

Burch, M. R., Reiss, M. L., & Bailey, J. S. (1987). A competency-based "hands-on" training package for direct care staff. *Journal of the Association for Persons with Severe Handicaps, 12,* 67–71.

Burg, M. M., Reid, D. H., & Lattimore, J. (1979). Use of a self-recording and supervision program to change institutional staff behavior. *Journal of Applied Behavior Analysis, 12,* 363–375.

Burgio, L. D., Whitman, T. L., & Reid, D. H. (1983). A participative management approach for improving direct-care staff performance in an institutional setting. *Journal of Applied Behavior Analysis, 16,* 37–53.

Clark, H. B., Wood, R., Kuehnel, T., Flanagan, S., Mosk, M., & Northrup, J. T. (1985). Preliminary validation and training of supervisory interactional skills. *Journal of Organizational Behavior Management, 7,* 95–115.

Dyer, K., Schwartz, I. S., & Luce, S. C. (1984). A supervision program for increasing functional activities for severely handicapped students in a residential setting. *Journal of Applied Behavior Analysis, 17,* 249–259.

Fabry, P. L., & Reid, D. H. (1978). Teaching foster grandparents to train severely handicapped persons. *Journal of Applied Behavior Analysis, 11,* 111–123.

Favell, J. E., Favell, J. E., Riddle, J. I., & Risley, T. R. (1984). Promoting change in mental retardation facilities: Getting services from the paper to the people. In W. P. Christian, G. T. Hannah, & T. J. Glahn (Eds.), *Programming effective human services: Strategies for institutional change and client transition* (pp. 15–37). New York: Plenum Press.

Faw, G. D., Reid, D. H., Schepis, M. M., Fitzgerald, J. R., & Welty, P. A. (1981). Involving institutional staff in the development and maintenance of sign language skills with profoundly retarded persons. *Journal of Applied Behavior Analysis, 14,* 411–423.

Fielding, L. T., Errickson, E., & Bettin, B. (1971). Modification of staff behavior: A brief note. *Behavior Therapy, 2,* 550–553.

Fitzgerald, J. R., Reid, D. H., Schepis, M. M., Faw, G. D., Welty, P. A., & Pyfer, L. M. (1984). A rapid training procedure for teaching manual sign language skills to multidisciplinary institutional staff. *Applied Research in Mental Retardation, 5,* 451–469.

Ford, J. E. (1983). Application of a personalized system of instruction to a large, personnel training program. *Journal of Organizational Behavior Management, 5,* 57–65.

Frazier, T. W. (1972). Training institutional staff in behavior modification principles and techniques. In R. D. Ruben, H. Fensterheim, J. D. Henderson, & L. P. Ullman (Eds.), *Advances in behavior therapy: Proceedings of the fourth conference of the Association for Advancement of Behavior Therapy* (pp. 171–178). New York: Academic Press.

Gardner, J. M. (1972). Teaching behavior modification to nonprofessionals. *Journal of Applied Behavior Analysis, 5,* 517–521.

Gardner, J. M. (1973). Training the trainers. A review of research on teaching behavior modification. In R. D. Rubin, J. P. Brady, & J. D. Henderson (Eds.), *Advances in behavior therapy* (Vol. 4, pp. 145–158). New York: Academic Press.

Gladstone, B. W., & Spencer, C. J. (1977). The effects of modelling on the contingent praise of mental retardation counsellors. *Journal of Applied Behavior Analysis, 10,* 75–84.

Greene, B. F., Willis, B. S., Levy, R., & Bailey, J. S. (1978). Measuring client gains from staff implemented programs. *Journal of Applied Behavior Analysis, 11,* 395–412.

Ivancic, M. T., Reid, D. H., Iwata, B. A., Faw, G. D., & Page, T. J. (1981). Evaluating a supervision program for developing and maintaining therapeutic staff-resident interactions during institutional care routines. *Journal of Applied Behavior Analysis, 14,* 95–107.

Katz, R. C., & Lutzker, J. R. (1980). A comparison of three methods for training timeout. *Behavior Research of Severe Developmental Disabilities, 1,* 123–130.

Kazdin, A. E. (1980). Acceptability of alternative treatments for deviant child behavior. *Journal of Applied Behavior Analysis, 13,* 259–273.

Kazdin, A. E. (1982). *Single-case research designs: Methods for clinical and applied settings.* New York: Oxford University Press.

Kissel, R. C., Whitman, T. L., & Reid, D. H. (1983). An institutional staff training and self-management program for developing multiple self-care skills in severely/profoundly retarded individuals. *Journal of Applied Behavior Analysis, 16,* 395–415.

Korabek, C. A., Reid, D. H., & Ivancic, M. T. (1981). Improving needed food intake of profoundly handicapped children through effective supervision of institutional staff performance. *Applied Research in Mental Retardation, 2,* 69–88.

Lattimore, J., Stephens, T. E., Favell, J. E., & Risley, T. R. (1984). Increasing direct care staff compliance to individualized physical therapy body positioning prescriptions: Prescriptive checklists. *Mental Retardation, 22,* 79–84.

Liberman, R. (1983). Guest editor's preface. *Analysis and Intervention in Developmental Disabilities, 3,* iii–iv.

Mayhew, G. L., Enyart, P., & Cone, J. D. (1979). Approaches to employee management: Policies and preferences. *Journal of Organizational Behavior Management, 2,* 103–111.

Mansdorf, I. J., & Burstein, Y. (1986). Case manager: A clinical tool for training residential treatment staff. *Behavioral Residential Treatment, 1,* 155–167.

Miller, R., & Lewin, L. M. (1980). Training and management of the psychiatric aide: A critical review. *Journal of Organizational Behavior Management, 2,* 295–315.

Montegar, C. A., Reid, D. H., Madsen, C. H., & Ewell, M. D., (1977). Increasing institutional staff-to-resident interactions through inservice training and supervisor approval. *Behavior Therapy, 8,* 533–540.

Page, T. J., Christian, J. G., Iwata, B. A., Reid, D. H., Crow, R. E., & Dorsey, M. F. (1981). Evaluating and training interdisciplinary teams in writing IPP goals and objectives. *Mental Retardation, 19,* 25–27.

Page, T. J., Iwata, B. A., & Reid, D. H. (1982). Pyramidal training: A large-scale application with institutional staff. *Journal of Applied Behavior Analysis, 15,* 335–351.

Parsons, M. B., Schepis, M. M., Reid, D. H., McCarn, J. E., & Green, C. W. (1987). Expanding the impact of behavioral staff management: A large-scale, long-term application in schools serving severely handicapped students. *Journal of Applied Behavior Analysis, 20,* 139–150.

Parsonson, B. S., Baer, A. M., & Baer, D. M. (1974). The application of generalized correct social contingencies: An evaluation of a training program. *Journal of Applied Behavior Analysis, 7,* 427–437.

Quilitch, H. R. (1975). A comparison of three staff-management procedures. *Journal of Applied Behavior Analysis, 8,* 59–66.

Reid, D. H. (1987). *Developing a research program in human service agencies: A practitioner's guidebook.* Springfield, IL: Charles C Thomas.

Reid, D. H., & Schepis, M. M. (1986). Direct care staff training. In R. P. Barrett (Ed.), *Severe behavior disorders in the mentally retarded* (pp. 297–322). New York: Plenum Press.

Reid, D. H., & Whitman, T. L. (1983). Behavioral staff management in institutions: A critical review of effectiveness and acceptability. *Analysis and Intervention in Developmental Disabilities, 3,* 131–149.

Reid, D. H., Schepis, M. M., & Fitzgerald, J. R. (1984). Innovations in organizational behavior management in institutions for the developmentally disabled. In S. E. Breuning, J. L. Matson & R. P. Barrett (Eds.), *Advances in mental retardation and developmental disabilities* (Vol. 2, pp. 181–204). Greenwich, CT: JAI Press.

Reid, D. H., Parsons, M. B., McCarn, J. E., Green, C. W., Phillips, J. F., & Schepis, M. M. (1985). Providing a more appropriate education for severely handicapped persons: Increasing and validating functional classroom tasks. *Journal of Applied Behavior Analysis, 18,* 289–301.

Reid, D. H., McCarn, J. E., & Green, C. W. (1988). Staff training and management in school programs for severely developmentally disabled students. In M. D. Powers (Ed.), *Severe developmental disabilities: Expanded systems of interactions* (pp. 199–215). Baltimore: Brookes.

Smith, D. W., & Wells, M. E. (1983). Use of a microcomputer to assist staff in documenting resident progress. *Mental Retardation, 21,* 111–115.

Stoddard, L. T., McIlvane, W. J., McDonagh, E. C., & Kledaras, J. B. (1986). The use of picture programs in teaching direct care staff. *Applied Research in Mental Retardation, 7,* 349–358.

van den Pol, R. A., Reid, D. H., & Fuqua, R. W. (1983). Peer training of safety-related skills to institutional staff: Benefits for trainers and trainees. *Journal of Applied Behavior Analysis, 16,* 139–156.

Watson, L. S., Jr., & Uzzell, R. (1980). A program for teaching behavior modification skills to institutional staff. *Applied Research in Mental Retardation, 1,* 41–53.

Whitman, T. L., Scibak, J. W., & Reid, D. H. (1983). *Behavior modification with the severely and profoundly retarded: Research and application.* New York: Academic Press.

Wolf, M. M. (1978). Social validity: The case for subjective measurement or how applied behavior analysis is finding its heart. *Journal of Applied Behavior Analysis, 11,* 203–214.

Zlomke, L. C., & Benjamin, V. A., Jr. (1983). Staff in-service: Measuring effectiveness through client behavior change. *Education and Training of the Mentally Retarded, 18,* 125–130.

II

Assessment and Treatment

4

Behavioral Assessment

EDWARD S. SHAPIRO AND DIANE M. BROWDER

INTRODUCTION

Interest in behavioral assessment has increased tremendously over the past 10 years. Prior to 1976, no major textbooks and only a few articles had been written expressly devoted to the topic of behavioral assessment (e.g., Bijou & Grimm, 1972; Kanfer & Saslow, 1969). Beginning in 1977, there was a virtual explosion of literature on behavioral assessment. No less than 10 textbooks (e.g., Ciminero, Calhoun, & Adams, 1977; Cone & Hawkins, 1977; Haynes, 1978; Hersen & Bellack, 1976) and two journals (*Behavioral Assessment* and the *Journal of Behavioral Assessment*) appeared devoted solely to the topic of behavioral assessment. Expansion of this literature has continued to include books related to behavioral assessment with specific populations (Powers & Handleman, 1984), ages (Barlow, 1981; Mash & Terdal, 1981) and for school-related settings (Shapiro, 1987; Shapiro & Kratochwill, 1988). Additionally, the methodology of behavioral assessment, which was originally developed to evaluate nonacademic problems of children, has been equally developed for assessing academically related school problems (Deno, 1985; Shapiro & Lentz, 1985, 1986).

As applied to persons with mental retardation, behavioral assessment methodology has shared equally in the expansion of the literature over the past decade. Actually, there has been a long standing use of behavioral assessment strategies in evaluating the problems of people with mild/moderate mental retardation (Shapiro & Barrett, 1983). Extensions and adaptations of behavioral assessment techniques have also been made to the evaluation of persons with severe handicaps (Browder, 1987; Snell, 1987). Clearly, behavioral assessment plays an important and critical role in the evaluation process. The methodology has gained increased acceptance as a useful, relevant, and valuable technique in attaining a better understanding of the types of problems of persons with mental retardation as well as providing a more empirical strategy for determining potential interventions and ongoing evaluation for referred problems.

EDWARD S. SHAPIRO AND DIANE M. BROWDER • Department of Counseling Psychology, School Psychology, and Special Education, Lehigh University, Bethlehem, Pennsylvania 18015.

Despite the very positive role that behavioral assessment can play in evaluation of persons with mental retardation, there are distinct differences in the assumptions that underlie traditional and behavioral assessment. These conceptual differences result in very differing methods for conducting assessments and provide answers to very different sets of questions. For example, although traditional assessment may be able to provide answers to questions of classification, these measures are inadequate to make specific recommendations for remediation. Additionally, traditional measures may not be very effective at pinpointing areas of difficulty and in need of further programming. Obviously, one must clearly understand the conceptual distinctions that underlie behavioral and traditional assessment.

In addition to differences between traditional and behavioral assessment, all methods of behavioral assessment may not be equally applicable across all levels of persons with mental retardation. In particular, assessment of persons with more severe handicaps may require the use of more indirect methods of assessment, such as interviewing or informant reports, as preliminary steps to the use of direct observation techniques.

The purpose of this chapter is to examine how behavioral assessment is applied to persons with mental retardation. Following a brief discussion of the conceptual differences between traditional and behavioral assessment, the various methods of behavioral assessment will be described. Applications of these procedures to persons with more mild/moderate levels of mental retardation will be presented. How these same principles and procedures are applied to persons with severe handicaps will then be discussed.

TRADITIONAL AND BEHAVIORAL ASSESSMENT: CONCEPTUAL DIFFERENCES

Hartmann, Roper, and Bradford (1979) provided an excellent discussion of the key differences between traditional and behavioral assessment (see Table 1). The most crucial differences can be found in the underlying assumptions that are employed in the assessment process. Whereas traditional assessment views persons as possessing a set of enduring traits or characteristics that need to be understood to better predict human behavior, behavioral assessment starts by assuming that human behavior can only be understood and predicted by careful evaluation of the environmental events that surround behavior. As such, behavioral assessment assumes situational specificity where traditional assessment assumes that behavior is cross-situational. An important implication of this distinction is that assuming behavior to be cross-situational allows one to make substantial inferences from observations conducted under one set of conditions to other conditions in which the person has not been directly observed. In behavioral assessment, such inferences are minimized, and predictions of responses under unobserved conditions are withheld until the person is actually seen in those conditions.

TABLE 1
Differences between Behavioral and Traditional Approaches to Assessment

	Behavioral	Traditional
I. Assumptions		
1. Conception of personality	Personality constructs mainly employed to summarize specific behavior patterns, if at all	Personality as a reflection of enduring underlying states or traits
2. Causes of behavior	Maintaining conditions sought in current environment	Intrapsychic or within the individual
II. Implications		
1. Role of behavior	Important as a sample of person's repertoire in specific situation	Behavior assumes importance only insofar as it indexes underlying causes
2. Role of history	Relatively unimportant, except, for example, to provide a retrospective baseline	Crucial in that present conditions seen as a product of the past
3. Consistency of behavior	Behavior thought to be specific to the situation	Behavior expected to be consistent across time and settings
III. Uses of data	To describe target behaviors and maintaining conditions	To describe personality functioning and etiology
	To select the appropriate treatment	To diagnose or classify
	To evaluate and revise treatment	To make prognosis; to predict
IV. Other characteristics		
1. Level of inferences	Low	Medium to high
2. Comparisons	More emphasis on intra-individual or idiographic	More emphasis on interindividual or nomothetic
3. Methods of assessment	More emphasis on direct methods (e.g., obsevations of behavior in natural environment)	More emphasis on indirect methods (e.g., interviews and self-report)
4. Timing of assessment	More ongoing; prior, during, and after treatment	Pre- and perhaps posttreatment, or strictly to diagnose
5. Scope of assessment	Specific measures and of more variables (e.g., of target behaviors in various situations, of side effects, context, strengths as well as deficiencies)	More global measures (e.g., of cure, or improvement) but only of the individual

Note. From "Some Relationships between Behavioral and Traditional Assessment," by D. P. Hartmann, B. L. Roper, and D. C. Bradford, 1979, *Journal of Behavioral Assessment, 1,* p. 4. Copyright 1979 by Plenum Press. Reprinted by permission.

Another important assumption that differentiates traditional and behavioral assessment are the specific causes of behavior. Traditional assessment assumes that observable behavior is primarily a function of intrapsychic causes. People behave the way they do as a result of the conditions of their past, their feelings at the time, and their unconscious motives. As a result, the observable behavior provides only a "window" to possible underlying psychological constructs that are the root causes of the behavior one sees. In contrast, because behavioral assessment views observable behavior as related to the conditions existing in the environment, no inferential leaps are made to root causes. The person's past is seen as important only in that it offers information about reinforcement history, and the observable behavior becomes *the* important data for assessment rather than a surface indication of some more deeply rooted problem.

Typically, traditional assessment is used for purposes of personality description and diagnosis. Indeed, behavioral assessment is not often an effective means of classification. However, behavioral assessment is more likely to offer assistance in describing target behaviors, selecting appropriate treatment, and evaluating ongoing treatment plans. Given that the overall purpose of assessment should be to identify problem areas and develop remediation plans, behavioral assessment may offer answers to a much broader range of questions than more traditional measures.

One of the most frequently cited conceptual models for behavioral assessment is the Behavioral Assessment Grid (BAG) (Cone, 1978). The model places behavioral assessment within three dimensions: contents, methods, and universes of generalization. Contents of behavioral assessment are commonly viewed as the three modalities of behavioral assessment (Nelson & Hayes, 1979) and include cognitive, physiological, and motor assessment. Motor contents include those activities that result in observable movement without instrumentation and would include such behaviors as walking, running, talking, hitting, or moving arms. Physiological contents are evident in activities that are typically measurable through instrumentation, such as muscle activity, respiration, heart rate, and so forth. Cognitive contents are more difficult to define but are considered to represent the internal thought process of the person and other similar private events. Obviously, direct access to these private events is impossible and can only be deciphered by examining the referent of cognitive activity, verbal and written reports.

Methods of assessment are ordered by Cone (1978) along the dimension of direct to indirectness of assessment. The degree to which an assessment method is considered direct is determined by the extent to which the method measures the behavior of interest as it naturally occurs in the environment. As one moves toward the indirect pole of the continuum, one gets further away from assessing behavior as it actually occurs and increases the inferences needed to describe behavior in the natural setting. Cone (1978) placed direct observation that occurs under naturalistic and analogue (simulation of the natural environment) conditions within the direct dimension. Additionally, self-observation is viewed as a direct method of assessment. Rat-

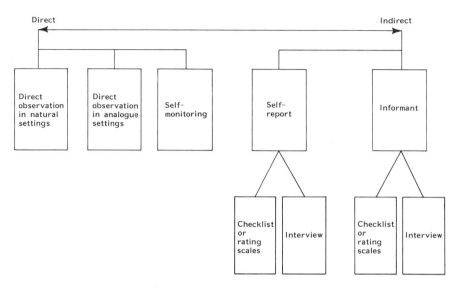

FIGURE 1. Continuum of behavioral assessment methods.

ings by others, self-report, and interview methods are placed within the indirect method. Figure 1 displays a somewhat modified version of the method dimension of Cone (1978). As evident from this figure, direct methods of assessment are viewed the same as Cone (1978), but interviews and rating scales are seen as subtypes of self-report and informant-report measures.

Finally, the third dimension of the BAG represents how behavioral assessment data can be used. Originally, Cone (1977) conceptualized behavioral assessment using generalizability theory described by Cronbach, Gleser, Nanda, and Rajaratnam (1972). Data derived from behavioral assessment measures are viewed as providing generalizability across scorers, items, time, settings, methods, and dimensions. Cone (1981) reconceptualized this dimension of the BAG as reflecting the accuracy of behavioral assessment rather than generalizability.

Although there is some disagreement regarding the conceptual relationship of generalizability to the evaluation of behavioral assessment methods (see Nelson, Hay, & Hay, 1977, and Hayes & Nelson, 1986, for extended discussions of this point), there is widespread acceptance of the methodological distinctions between direct and indirect assessment methods and the triple-response modality approach to behavioral assessment.

Another key area of difference between behavioral and traditional assessment is the accepted measures for evaluation. The psychometric properties that determine how one regards the value of traditional assessment measures are well known and would include test–retest reliability, internal consistency, concurrent validity, predictive validity, factorial validity, and normative sampling. These are metrics that have been well established through the years and are the standards against which traditional measurement devices will be judged. It is less clear what should be the comparable metrics for evaluating behavioral assessment measures. Although some researchers have argued that the psychometric properties applicable for traditional assessment are equally applicable for behavioral assessment (e.g., Hartmann *et al.*, 1979), others have argued that the underlying assumptions of behavioral assessment call for a different set of measurement procedures for evaluation. Specifically, Nelson and Hayes (1979), Hayes and Nelson (1986), and Nelson (1983) have suggested using measures that reflect accuracy of measurement (interobserver agreement) and treatment utility (Hayes, Nelson, & Jarrett, 1986, 1987) as being more consistent with behavioral assessment methodology. The key argument used by Nelson and Hayes (1987) is that traditional assessment treats subject variance as error, whereas the whole purpose of behavioral assessment is to explain this type of variance. Thus, psychometric properties, such as test–retest reliability or concurrent validity, consider good measures those that result in minimal between- or within-subject variance. On the other hand, behavioral assessment measures that show such variance are not discarded as "bad measures" if they are accurately showing the variability of the behavior. Indeed, the primary purpose of behavioral assessment is to investigate the reasons for subject variance, not dismiss it as error.

CONCLUSIONS AND SUMMARY

The conceptual differences between behavioral and traditional assessment will lead to very different methodologies of evaluation. Because traditional assessment measures assume the presence of internal, stable characteristics, the results of measurement procedures are used to infer traits and attributes that describe the structure of the person. Thus, results of performance on a measure assumed to assess "intelligence" is taken to reflect the construct of cognitive ability. Further, these measures are viewed as predictive of future behavior, because behavior is assumed to be consistent across time, place, and persons. Results of personality measures, such as projective tests, are assumed to represent stable traits and are used to describe persons as "aggressive," "dependent," "narcissistic," or with some other characteristic. Measurement procedures that do not show stability over time or place will be discarded as poor measures.

In contrast, behavioral assessment offers data on the function of behavior rather than its structure. An individual's performance observed during the assessment is not assumed to represent characteristics that are cross-situational or temporally stable. Only after behavior is found consistent across time or situations is any inference of temporal stability or cross-situationality made (Strosahl & Linehan, 1986). Additionally, measures that show variability across time are not discarded if they are demonstrated to be reflecting accurately the variability of the person's behavior.

These differing conceptual foundations of behavior result in very different interpretations of the same methods for assessing behavior. Although at times traditional assessment measures can be considered valuable in the behavioral assessment process (e.g., Nelson, 1980; Prout & Ferber, 1988), the interpretation of the measures from a behavioral assessment perspective is quite different. Likewise, many individuals conducting traditional assessments use many of the procedures (e.g., interviews, direct observation) employed in behavioral assessment. Again, the crucial difference is in how the data from the methods are interpreted. Using behavioral assessment to assess individuals with mental retardation is no different than using it with nonhandicapped persons. The only differences may be in the degree to which certain methods may be employed, particularly those indirect methods involving verbal and written self-reports. In the next section, the various methods of behavioral assessment will be described with special attention to applications of these methods for individuals with mild to moderate levels of mental retardation. Because of the large amount of material describing behavioral assessment methods in detail, only a brief discussion of these procedures will be provided. Readers who are interested in more extensive discussion of behavioral assessment methods in general should consult any of the excellent texts written on this topic (e.g., Barlow, 1981; Haynes, 1978; Hersen & Bellack, 1987; Mash & Terdal, 1981; Shapiro, 1987; Shapiro & Kratochwill, 1988).

METHODS OF BEHAVIORAL ASSESSMENT: APPLICATIONS FOR PERSONS WITH MILD TO MODERATE MENTAL RETARDATION

Direct Assessment Methods

Perhaps the hallmark of behavioral assessment has been the extensive development of a systematic methodology for collecting data through direct observation of behavior. Procedures for collecting these data usually employ four possible types of data: event recording, duration recording, time sampling, or permanent products.

Event Recording

This type of data requires the recording of individual instances of behavior. Typically, the observer records the number of times a specified behavior occurs within a particular time interval. The data are then reported as rate (frequency per unit of time) and represent the actual rate at which the behavior occurs. Event recording requires behavior to have a discrete beginning and end point. Hand raising and calling out are examples of behaviors that have inherently defined starting and finishing points. Interactions with others, rocking, and doing seatwork are somewhat ambiguous as to when they start and finish. Although these behaviors can be operationally defined to have such beginning and end points, other methods of recording these behaviors (e.g., time sampling) may be more appropriate. Recording events is straightforward and can require the use of paper-and-pencil or mechanical devices, such as golf-counters, beads, grocery store counters, and so forth.

Event recording is very useful for low or moderate frequency behaviors. Likewise, behaviors that occur in response bursts may also lend themselves to this type of recording. For example, aggressive behavior may include hitting, kicking, swearing, and throwing objects. Rather than record the individual frequencies of each behavior, one may more realistically treat the entire out-burst as a single incident, ending after a defined period of nonaggressive behavior.

Duration Recording

When a behavior persists for a sustained period of time, a recording of the duration may be appropriate. This recording is simply a measure of the amount of time from onset to termination of the behavioral response. Each episode is recorded separately, and a mean duration per episode is deter-mined. For example, if one is observing an individual who is engaged in high rates of stereotyped rocking, the duration of each episode of behavior may be useful. In particular, reductions in the frequency of behavior may not always coincide with reductions in duration. Thus, data taken by a mother during a child's trantrum may show no reduction in the *number* of tantrums but may display significant reductions of duration.

Recording duration is somewhat cumbersome. Usually, it requires the use of a stopwatch or some other timing device. This is difficult with behav-iors that occur at moderate or high rates. At low rates, however, duration may be a very valuable asset to the behavioral assessment process.

Time Sampling

Behaviors that do not have discrete beginnings and endings create prob-lems when one is trying to use event or duration recording. Additionally, it is not always possible to have persons who can engage in direct observation throughout the entire time period a behavior is likely to occur. An alternative method for these situations is to employ a time-sampling procedure. The purpose of time sampling is not to produce a detailed account of how often the behavior *actually* occurred, but instead to provide a best *estimate* of the behavior by collecting data only during a portion of the time the behavior actually occurred.

Time sampling is done by dividing the observation period into smaller units of time or intervals. These intervals can be of any duration but are typically 10, 15, or 30 seconds. Observations are conducted by using either whole interval, partial interval, or momentary data collection procedures. For whole interval recording, the targeted behavior would have to be present for the entire observed interval for the behavior to be recorded as present. Simi-larly, for partial interval sampling, the behavior is recorded as present if it occurs for any portion of the interval. Momentary time sampling records the presence or absence of the behavior only at the exact instant the interval begins. Because time sampling only estimates the actual rate of behavioral occurrence, the type of time sampling used may introduce specific biases into the data that are obtained.

Studies examining the relationships between whole interval, partial interval, and momentary time sampling have consistently demonstrated that whole interval sampling tends to overestimate performance whereas partial interval sampling underestimates performance (Powell, Martindale, Kulp, Martindale, & Bauman, 1977; Powell & Rockinson, 1978). Lentz (1982), comparing partial and momentary time sampling in recording mother–child interaction, found that the degree of error introduced by momentary time sampling was substantially less than partial interval recording.

Which type of time sampling should be chosen is best based on the type of behavior being observed. For example, Ollendick, Shapiro, and Barrett (1982) used a whole interval time-sampling procedure in recording the play behavior of severely, multihandicapped children. Use of whole interval was logical because playing is a behavior that must be sustained across time. Likewise, Shapiro, Barrett, and Ollendick (1980) used a partial interval recording system to record the stereotyped hand flapping of a girl with severe mental retardation. This system was used because the behavior was a high-frequency response that did not require any sustained time period. In this study, a momentary time-sampling technique would have been equally as logical.

Permanent Products

Certain behavioral responses result in permanent products. For example, in schools, children often complete worksheets that can be scored as permanent products. In teaching cooking to persons with mental retardation, the resulting food products can be used as permanent products—at least until they are eaten! An advantage of these measures is their simplicity and unobtrusive nature. Data using permanent products can easily be collected without the target subject's knowledge. However, the measure does require some inference from the data to the behavior. Because the behavior obtained from permanent products may not be observed directly, the resulting data are assumed to represent the actual behavioral response. For example, if the resulting food products are used to determine whether an individual being taught cooking skills has reached mastery, an appetizing food product may not necessarily mean that the *target individual* is responsible for the improved food. Further investigation may reveal that the individual had substantial assistance from other clients or staff to produce the improved tasting food. Clearly, the use of these types of data must be supported by additional data collection methods.

Direct Observation in the Natural Environment: Applications

The most direct form of behavioral assessment would be the observation of behavior as it actually occurs within the natural setting. This methodology of behavioral assessment has been broadly applied to persons of all levels of mental retardation. It is nearly impossible to open issues of the *American Journal of Mental Deficiency, Mental Retardation, Journal of Applied Behavior Analysis, Behavior Modification,* or *Research in Developmental Disabilities* without finding an article that uses this method. Given the large array of potential studies that illustrate this method, two examples are presented of studies that assessed persons with mild to moderate mental retardation.

Burgio, Whitman, and Johnson (1980) examined the effects of a self-instruction training program to increase attending behavior in children with mild mental retardation. Their assessment procedures incorporated direct observation in the natural environment and permanent product data. After defining self-instruction statements and in-seat/off-task behavior, Burgio and co-workers observed five students (ages 9–14) four days a week who were working on math, printing, and phonics tasks. An event-recording procedure was employed to record each instance of a self-instruction statement that students made while in the classroom. In-seat/off-task behavior was recorded using a 10-second partial interval recording system. Additionally, the number of problems completed on the arithmetic task and the number of letters printed on the printing task were tallied and divided by the number of problems assigned or letters possible. This provided a percentage correct score for each measure. The writing task was evaluated by using a transparent overlay to measure deviation of writing samples that were more than 2 millimeters from the standard.

This study is a good illustration of how observational data collected within the natural environment can be easily collected and supplemented by permanent products. Collecting data on the number of self-instructions actually employed by students in the classroom offered evidence to the experimenters that their training program could account for the observed impact. Data obtained on off-task behavior substantiated the experimenters' goals to increase attending behavior. Finally, the data on correct academic responding provided empirical evidence of the value of the training program on desired school-related behavior.

Shapiro *et al.* (1980) conducted a study employing both event recording and time sampling in measuring stereotypical behavior of three children with mental retardation. For two of the subjects who engaged in stereotypical mouthing, the number of face- or mouth-pats were counted during a 15-minute work session in a classroom. Number of face-/mouth-pats per minute served as the dependent measure in the study. A third child exhibited mouthing behavior that was continuous, which would make use of an event-recording procedure inappropriate. For this child, a 10-second, whole interval time-sampling procedure was employed. Additionally, the amount of time spent appropriately engaged with the assigned classroom tasks was obtained using once again a 10-second, whole interval recording procedure. Finally, for the first two children, a duration measure of the time spent engaged appropriately with the assigned tasks was obtained by starting and stopping a stopwatch each time the child began to use the materials. Cumulative total duration of appropriate behavior then served as the dependent measure.

This study helps to illustrate how several different types of direct observation measures can be employed simultaneously. Of critical importance is to note how the nature of the frequency and topography of the behavior being observed resulted in the differential selection of various direct observation measurement procedures.

Direct Observation in an Analogue Setting

Although observing behavior under its naturally occurring conditions offers probably the most accurate depiction of the behavior, it is not always possible either to observe or teach a new behavior in such settings. As an alternative to assessing behavior within the natural setting, an attempt is made to create a setting that simulates and approximates the natural conditions under which the behavior is likely to occur. A particular area in which this has been true is in the assessment and training of social skills.

A very common method for the assessment of social skills has been the use of role-play tests. One of the first of these measures was the Behavioral Assertiveness Test for Children (Bornstein, Bellack, & Hersen, 1977), which was developed based on the work of Eisler, Hersen, Miller, and Blanchard (1975) for adults. After specific scenes were developed, which reflected appropriate social skills among elementary aged children, instructions were given to children to pretend that these scenes were actually happening to them and to respond as they would in those situations. The child's response to each scene was scored on a number of predetermined variables, such as duration of reply, smiles, frequency of eye contact, and so forth.

Senatore, Matson, and Kazdin (1982) reported a similar strategy for assessing social skills across a wide range of persons with mental retardation. Four scenes were developed for each of three areas of social skills identified as problems for the individuals in their study: making positive statements, acknowledging others, and complaining. Assessment occurred during a weekly group meeting held in an outpatient hospital setting. Responses to each scene presented in the assessment were scored by independent raters on a 1 to 5 scale, depending on how many socially appropriate words were used by the subjects.

The most significant problem with this type of measure is that any change in behavior noted on this measure may have little or no relationship to changes in more natural settings. Recognizing this, Senatore *et al.* (1982) also assessed clients during an individual interview session, asking a standard set of questions and scoring responses the same as during the role-play test. Additionally, subjects were assessed during a party held at the end of the study for all clients. Six standard questions were asked by individuals who were unknown to the subjects during the natural conditions of the party. The subjects' responses were scored on a three-point scale, ranging from socially inappropriate responses to appropriate responses of two words or more.

Foxx, McMorrow, and Schloss (1983) used a similar procedure to assess and train social skills using a game format. After identifying the series of social skills to be trained, the subjects were taught a board game in which each of these social skills were assessed and taught. Criteria for correct responses were established, and each individual's response to the social skills situation card during the game was evaluated by an independent rater and scored as correct or incorrect. Recognizing the limitations of these data for any generalization to more natural conditions, Foxx, McMorrow, Bittle, and Ness (1983) replicated the previous study but assessed client behavior immediately prior to, during, and after playing the game. This assessment took place while clients were asked to "sit and talk" in the lounge for 10 minutes before and after the game was played. The interactions of clients were audiotaped and scored to provide the generalization data.

Using direct observation within analogue settings offers the opportunity to assess behavior that may be of low frequency within more natural settings. Additionally, if behavior occurs at times when it would be difficult to have observers present (e.g., at the bus stop or in the bathroom), using a simulated situation allows one to create opportunities for the behavior to occur. Unfortunately, the artificial nature of these settings may result in responses that are quite different than those seen under more natural conditions. Indeed, almost all studies that have examined the relationship of role-play assessment to more naturalistic evaluation have found significant but low to moderate correlations between the two types of measures (e.g., Matson *et al.*, 1980; Van Hasselt, Hersen, & Bellack, 1981; Williamson, Moody, Granberry, Lethermon, & Blouin, 1983). When using these types of analogue measures, it is very important to be cautious in drawing any inferences from the behavior observed under the analogue and the natural conditions. Still, direct observation of analogue conditions does provide some access and approximation of behavior that may not be easily obtained in other ways.

Self-Monitoring

Although direct observation is commonly conducted by having independent observers collect the data, it is also possible to have the individuals who are the targets of the data collection monitor their own behavior. Self-monitoring incorporates two components. First, the individual must self-observe that the behavior under question has actually occurred. Once the behavior is acknowledged, it is recorded by using some form of recording device. Although self-observation or self-recording can occur independently, they are usually combined into self-monitoring.

An extensive literature exists which discusses the theoretical and practical applications of self-monitoring (e.g., Browder & Shapiro, 1985; Ciminero, Nelson, & Lipinski, 1977; Haynes, 1978; Mace & Kratochwill, 1985; McFall, 1977; Nelson, 1977; Shapiro, 1984). This literature was concerned primarily with two issues—reactivity and accuracy. Simply engaging in the act of self-monitoring may cause behavior to change in the desired direction.

Much of the literature surrounding self-monitoring has examined the potential variables that may predict reactivity. Related to reactivity is the relationship between the accuracy of self-monitoring and behavior change. Studies have demonstrated that accuracy of self-monitoring may not be a prerequisite for reactive behavior change (Ciminero *et al.*, 1977; Haynes, 1978; Nelson, 1977).

Substantial applications of self-monitoring have been made to persons with mental retardation at all levels. Ackerman and Shapiro (1984) examined the effect of self-monitoring on the work productivity of five adults with moderate to mild mental retardation. Clients were trained to push a standard grocery store counter after completing each package they were assigned to assemble. Data obtained during a training session and a generalization session, which immediately followed training, showed that the self-monitoring procedure alone substantially improved the clients' performance. When self-monitoring was absent, however, clients reverted to former, slower rates of production. In this case, self-monitoring resulted in significant reactivity.

Using a similar task and population, Shapiro and Ackerman (1983) also demonstrated, in a series of studies, the unpredictability of reactivity in self-monitoring. In these studies, few improvements in productivity levels occurred after self-monitoring was employed. Results of these studies suggest that although self-monitoring may be a useful tool for both the assessment and intervention process with mentally retarded clients, effects may be idiosyncratic across individuals. Such idiosyncratic effects have been found in other investigations with children with mental retardation (Shapiro, Browder, & D'Huyvetters, 1984; Shapiro & Klein, 1980; Shapiro, McGonigle, & Ollendick, 1980).

Despite the somewhat mixed effects of studies on self-monitoring with persons with mental retardation, there has been a substantial increase in the number of studies that have shown how self-monitoring and other self-management strategies can be easily applied to improving the skills of persons with mental retardation (Martin, Burger, Elias-Burger, & Mithaug, 1988). Further, this technology has been widely applied in teaching community-living skills as well as school-related academic behavior for children (Agran & Martin, 1987). Clearly, self-monitoring can and should play a significant role in the assessment process for persons with mental retardation.

It is important to remember, however, that the possibility of reactivity of behavior may create problems if self-monitoring alone is used as a form of assessment. Although self-monitoring is a form of direct rather than indirect assessment, given that one is collecting data on the behavior of interest within the natural setting where it occurs, the data obtained through self-monitoring may not be an accurate baseline measure. Instead, the data may be a function of any possible reactive effects of the data collection process itself. Often, it is important that data be collected using an independent observer prior to beginning the self-monitoring process. This procedure would offer evidence whether the data collected under self-monitoring conditions represented reactive or nonreactive effects.

Indirect Methods of Assessment

At this point in the continuum of behavior assessment methods, one crosses the line between direct and indirect assessment. All of the three methods discussed previously—direct observation in natural settings, direct observation in analogue settings, and self-monitoring—still involved close relationships between the behavior actually occurring and its observation. Methods considered as indirect (e.g., self-report and informant report) involve collection of data that are obtained at a time other than when the behavior actually occurs. In one set of methods, the data are reported by the persons themselves and in the other by a significant other.

Self-Report

Self-reported data can be collected through either verbal or written modalities. A written self-report usually takes the form of having the person complete rating scales/checklists. These scales can be divided as assessing either global or specific categories of behavior. Global behavior rating scales and checklists provide respondents with a large array of questions about many different types of behavior problems. Often, these types of measures may be particularly useful as screening measures prior to conducting interview or having persons complete checklists/rating scales on a specific subarea noted on the global scale. A large number of these scales have appeared in the literature. Walls, Werner, Bacon, and Zane (1977) and Haynes and Wilson (1979) have provided some of the most extensive listings of these measures along with Hoge (1983), which provides an excellent review of many of the scales. Edelbrock (1988) and Witt, Cavell, Heffer, Carey, and Martens (1988) have also provided excellent reviews and discussions of many checklists/ rating scales that pertain to children.

Although the number of written self-report instruments that are used in behavioral assessment is very large, applications of this method of assessment to individuals with mental retardation is quite rare. Obviously, the cognitive levels of persons with mental retardation may make the data obtained on a paper-and-pencil rating scale quite suspect if completed independently by the client. Not only may individuals be unable to read the scales accurately, but they also may not have a clear idea regarding scaling processes and may not understand the differences between points that anchor the scale.

One alternative to using independently completed self-report instruments is to employ an interview format using a standardized protocol. Applications of structured interviewing formats have been made to persons with mental retardation. Heal and Chadsey-Rusch (1985) reported the development of the Lifestyle Satisfaction Scale (LSS) to assess individuals' satisfaction with their residence, community settings, and associated services. Each item on the scale required a yes or no answer and was read directly to clients with mental retardation. The subscales of the measure showed test—retest reliability ranging from .44 to .83, and internal-consistency correlations between .64

and .85. Other studies have also interviewed individuals with mental retardation regarding their views about their current living arrangements (e.g.,
Schalock, Harper, & Carver, 1981); however, few studies have derived a
systematic measure to assess client responses. Sigelman, Budd, Spanhel, and
Schoenrock (1981) noted that the use of yes–no and either–or questions,
when interviewing individuals with mental retardation, tend to produce substantially less response bias than more typical interviewing or rating scale
formats.

   Although the verbal reports of individuals with mental retardation are
important sources of data and obviously can be collected using systematic,
empirically validated procedures, several limitations of this method of data
collection must be recognized. It is not unusual to find that individuals are
selective about their recall of past events (Linehan, 1977). Further, even when
the interview is highly structured, agreements between interviewers regarding the identification of specific behavior problems have not been demonstrated (Gresham, 1984; Hay, Hay, Angle, & Nelson, 1979). When interviewing or using checklists/rating scales with persons with mental retardation, the
difficulties typically encountered with other persons are compounded. Often,
persons with mental retardation will acquiesce to questions and provide a
clear response bias when completing surveys and other self-report measures
(e.g., Sigelman *et al.* 1981). Despite these problems, however, it remains very
important that the opinions of persons with mental retardation continue to be
solicited directly when conducting a behavioral assessment. Continued
efforts, similar to those of Heal and Chadsey-Rusch (1985), are needed.

Informant Reports

   As with self-reports, informant reports involve data that are collected
either through written (paper-and-pencil) or verbal (interview) formats. There
is a large number of these measures, particularly checklists/rating scales, and
interested readers are referred to the listings of measures that are offered by
Walls *et al.* (1977), Haynes and Wilson (1979), and Hoge (1983).

   Unlike available self-report measures, a large number of informant report
instruments are available in application for persons with mental retardation.
Clearly, the range of these measures is far beyond the cope of this chapter,
but they include primarily scales designed to assess adaptive behavior (e.g.,
Meyers, Nihira, & Zetlin, 1979).

   Two adaptive behavior rating scales that have received significant and
positive receptions in the literature are the Vineland Adaptive Behavior Scales
(VABS) (Sparrow, Balla, & Cicchetti, 1984, 1985) and the American Association on Mental Deficiency (AAMD) Adaptive Behavior Scales (ABS). The
VABS is a complete revision of the Vineland Social Maturity Scale, first published in 1953 (Doll, 1953). Actually, the only remaining element of the original scale is the use of a semistructured interview in completing the scale.
Included in the VABS are three versions: the Interview Edition, Survey Form;
Interview Edition, Expanded Form; and the Classroom Edition. Each version

divided behavior into four domains: communication, daily living skills, socialization, and motor skills. Maladaptive behavior is also assessed on the survey and expanded editions.

Psychometrically, the VABS appears to have acceptable reliability for most domains. Unfortunately, a lower than anticipated interrater reliability may cast some doubt on its value. However, the scale appears to be most well suited for initial screening and assessment. Although global scores in each domain may suggest areas in need of further investigation and assessment, the scale does not appear to be useful for the development of interventions directly from the administration of the measure. Like most informant report measures, the scale requires verification of results through more direct measures of behavior.

Both the ABS (Nihira, Foster, Shellhaas, & Leland, 1969) and the ABS-Public School Version (ABS-PV) (Lambert, Windmiller, & Cole, 1981) assess behavior across 10 domains related to self-care and community living. An additional 14 domains for assessing maladaptive behavior are also included. The ABS is completed as a paper-and-pencil informant report, although an interview format can be employed. Although norms are provided for the scale, they represent populations of institutionalized persons. Given the emphasis on deinstitutionalization and the increasing number of persons with mental retardation living in the community, these norms may be quite problematic. However, norms for the ABS-PV do appear to be excellent and very representative of children attending public school settings who are mentally retarded. Like the VABS, the ABS and the ABS-PV offer good screening and background information but little in the way of detail regarding planning for intervention.

Despite the popularity of these scales in the assessment of persons with moderate/mild levels of mental retardation, adaptive behavior scales are more problematic when assessing individuals with more severe handicaps. These problems are addressed in more detail in the next section.

Applications of Behavioral Assessment to Individuals with Severe Retardation

Although the principles of behavioral assessment are applicable to individuals with severe and profound mental retardation, the way in which these methods are adapted will differ for several reasons. The first is the nature of the curriculum to which assessment will be linked. Persons with severe handicaps require direct instruction in the skills of daily living. With such instruction and ongoing support, persons with severe handicaps can live in the community (Conroy & Bradley, 1985) and hold paid, competitive jobs (Wehman, Hill, Wood, & Parent, 1987). Although a few life skills curricula have been developed in recent years (e.g., McGregor, Janssen, Larsen, & Tillery, 1986), most resources for instructors still emphasize the need to generate individualized curricula (e.g., Gaylord-Ross & Holvoet, 1985; Snell, 1987). Thus, curriculum-based assessment for persons with severe handicaps requires an initial step of curriculum development that is not typical of academic planning for persons with milder handicaps.

The curriculum development that must precede educational assessment for individuals with severe handicaps is further complicated by the fact that life skills do not have an established sequence for instruction. Without an easy-to-hard sequence to guide a point at which to begin and end assessment, the evaluator is faced with a nearly infinite number of skills that could be addressed. Thus, it is necessary to identify which of a vast number of potential skills should be selected for assessment. Once assessment has been conducted, further prioritization will be needed to set habilitation and educational goals. Delineating the curriculum that will form the basis for assessment requires a particular application of behavioral assessment known as the "ecological inventory" (Brown et al., 1979). A second reason behavioral assessment for individuals with severe handicaps requires special adaptations is related to curriculum delineation. Given the sparcity of published curricula in the area of life skills, it is understandable that few published tests exist for the assessment of these skills. Adaptive behavior scales have always provided a broad screening of skills related to daily living. However, assessment for habilitative planning requires consideration of more specific skills than these scales provide. Consideration must also be given to simpler skills. For example, individuals whose mental retardation is profound may be unable to perform any of the responses listed on an adaptive behavior scale but may have acquired simpler or alternative responses that enable them to participate in activities of daily living. Given the absence of published instruments, assessment of individuals with severe handicaps requires skill in utilizing several principles of behavioral assessment to create assessment tools. A third reason adaptations of behavioral assessment are required is because special consideration must be given to problem behaviors when an individual has few responses to influence others. Evans and Meyer (1985) have reviewed research on procedures to manage problem behaviors and advocate an alternative educative procedure. When an individual is highly dependent on others for supervision and most aspects of personal care, and has limited social and communication skills, behaviors that are obnoxious or annoying to others may actually be the only means that individual has to negotiate rest, social attention, or other needs. Thus, assessment of problem behaviors cannot be separated from skill assessment. Rather, the *function* of problem behaviors must be carefully considered to identify more adaptive responses to communicate personal needs or desires. With these special considerations, the principles of behavioral assessment can be utilized for educational planning for people with severe handicaps. Similar advantages exist in applying these principles to this population and to people with milder handicaps. That is, behavioral assessment provides information directly relevant to educational planning with consideration given to the environments in which the individual will function.

Indirect Assessment

In conducting assessment of individuals with severe handicaps, the evaluator will typically utilize more indirect methods of assessment to delineate the relevant curricula and specific skills to be considered in direct assessment. These procedures provide information on what skills are most critical to a person's current and future environments, identify a person's current repertoire of behavior (adaptive and maladaptive), and provide clues to the functions of any maladaptive behaviors. The various methods of indirect assessment have applications for each of these assessment purposes.

Curriculum Delineation

The methods of assessment to identify a life skills curriculum have been referred to collectively as "ecological inventories" (Brown *et al.*, 1979; Snell, 1982) and most typically include interviews or checklist assessments completed by informant report. The tradition of ecological inventories has its roots in social validation as described by Kazdin (1977) and by Wolf (1978). These researchers advocated that the selection of target responses to be modified must be socially valid and congruent with existing social standards as reflected in the judgment of experts or observations of "normative" behaviors. To identify the specific skills to be assessed, the evaluator may consult the "experts" in the person's life domains. For example, parents or other caregivers are the natural experts for the domestic skills a person needs to be more independent in personal care and to participate in such family responsibilities as housekeeping. Caregivers also can provide information on skills needed outside the home (e.g., for restaurants, physicians' offices, shopping malls). An example of a parental interview format to be used for curriculum delineation in preparation for assessment is shown in Figure 2. An alternative method to obtain this information would be to present a checklist of potential skills to be assessed for the parent to select and prioritize.

Besides parents, potential employers are experts in the skills that will be most critical for future employment. Interviews of potential employers and observations of co-workers in the environment are techniques recommended for assessment in preparation for supported employment training for people with severe handicaps (cf. Moon, Goodall, Barcus, & Brooke, 1985; Rusch, Chadsey-Rusch, & Lagomarcino, 1987).

Research on the design and utilization of ecological inventories has been limited. The research that does exist contains inventories of a wide sample of people to suggest skills that are valued by a broad range of experts. For example, Rusch, Schutz, and Agran (1982) summarized a list of competitive employment survival skills obtained from a checklist survey of employers in the state of Illinois. Aveno (1987) conducted a national survey of group homes to identify necessary skills. A unique feature of Aveno's research is that she validated the checklist survey with direct observations of clients in a small subsample of the homes.

In some research, the skill validation process has been reported but has

Individual's name: Sarah   Source: Mrs. Jones

Date: August 1, 1988   Place: Jones' residence

Age: 19

1.   What are Sarah's current family activities?

      — Informal socializing; Sarah eats separately; does not go out with
        family except to grandparents
      — Older sister sometimes plays music for Sarah

2.   What are some typical or frequent family activities/outings?

      —Grocery store; shopping at mall; annual vacation to beam (Sarah
        stays in respite), watching TV, cooking together

3.   What skills and preferences does Sarah have that might be en-
      hanced to increase her participation?

      —Likes to eat; can turn on the television

4.   What problems occur when Sarah participates at home or goes
      with the family?

      —Not toilet trained; loud screaming in public settings

5.   What skills do you hope to see Sarah acquire (your priorities)?

      —Some leisure skills for home; improved social behavior in public;
        job training; improved eating so can join family meals

6.   Evaluator's summary:

      —Assessment is needed of Sarah's leisure skills (e.g., games,
        crafts, sports); skills to use facilities (e.g., to make a
        purchase); eating skills; and job interests/skills.

FIGURE 2. Example of an ecological inventory conducted as an interview with the caregivers.

not been the major focus of the study (e.g., Cuvo, Jacobi, & Sipko, 1981;
Voeltz, Wuerch, & Bockhaut, 1982). Although some of the inventory procedures that have been described in the literature, such as that of Moon *et al.*
(1985) are explicit in nature, research is needed to demonstrate agreement
between experts. In the case of interviews with parents, it may be useful to
demonstrate consistency of responding through a repeated assessment across
a brief time period.

Adaptive Behavior Scales and Other Skill Screening

    Concurrent with curriculum delineation, the evaluator needs information
on the individual's adaptive and maladaptive behavior. One type of indirect
assessment that can be useful in initial skill screening is the adaptive behavior

scale. Some adaptive behavior scales utilize a checklist format that can be completed by the caregiver or a teacher (e.g., the Camelot Behavioral Checklist [Foster, 1974], the Comprehensive Test of Adaptive Behavior, and the Pyramid Scales). Others have an interview format to be administered by the professional with parents or other individuals familiar with the individual (e.g., the Woodcock–Johnson Scales of Independent Behavior [Bruininks, Woodcock, Weatherman, & Hill, 1984], the AAMD Adaptive Behavior Scales, and the Vineland Adaptive Behavior Scale). Some of the scales include assessment of problem behavior as well as daily living skills (e.g., the AAMD Adaptive Behavior Scale, the Woodcock–Johnson Scales of Independent Behavior, and the ABS).

For some individuals with very limited skills in daily living, adaptive behavior scales may yield little to no information. In such instances, the evaluator may need to develop a skills checklist with more specific responses to be considered or may have to use an interview format to identify any adaptive responses observed by caregivers in each of the students' environments. Browder (1987) provided examples of both checklists and interview formats to obtain information on students with very limited skills.

Research on agreement between informants for indirect assessment of adaptive behavior, though limited, has been reported for some scales (McLoughlin & Lewis, 1986). Information on agreement between these indirect measures and direct observations of behavior are rarely reported. A notable exception is the data Cone (1984) provided on agreement between both teachers and parents as informants with direct observations of children's behaviors. Checklists developed for an individual will have unknown reliability unless the evaluator utilizes and compares multiple sources of information (e.g., parents and teacher).

Indirect Assessment of Problem Behavior

As mentioned earlier, problem behaviors of an individual with few adaptive behaviors signal the need for skill development. These annoying or destructive behaviors may be the only responses in the individual's repertoire that effectively terminate an undesirable activity, secure attention, or meet other needs of the individual in a given situation. Although direct assessment of the problem behavior will be important to evaluate the effectiveness of treatment, and may be useful in some cases to validate the function of the problem behavior, indirect assessment will often provide the clues for treatment.

The two questions that this indirect assessment can answer are: (1) What is the motivation or function of this problem behavior? and (2) What more adaptive response does the individual need to learn to achieve this function? To consider the motivation of the problem behavior, the evaluator may wish to interview teachers and/or caregivers to identify the antecedents and consequences of the behavior. A rating scale such as that developed by Durand (1989) may expedite this process. Durand's scale poses 16 questions about the behavior. From this information, the evaluator is able to classify the function of the behavior as sensory, escape, attention, or tangible.

The second question concerning alternative adaptive responses may be addressed in two ways. Evans and Meyer (1985) suggested that the evaluator conduct a "discrepancy analysis" by comparing the individual's unacceptable responses to achieve a function to the way a nonhandicapped person of the same age would achieve it. Using the ecological inventory process described earlier, the evaluator would observe a peer group or would interview experts to identify the needed skills. For example, an adult with severe handicaps might refuse an undesired food by throwing the food or biting his or her arm and screaming. Observations of other adults placed in a similar situation would probably reveal that they say "no thank you" when offered an undesired food, or simply do not take the food from the choices available. Assessment would be needed of the skills the person with severe handicaps has to make choices and communicate a no response. The second way to identify alternative adaptive responses is to use indirect responses as described by Donnellan, Mirenda, Mesaros, and Fassbender (1984).

The benefits of assessing the function of problem behavior and addressing such alternative adaptive responses as communication have been described (Donnellan *et al.*, 1984; Gast & Wolery, 1987). More recently, research has emerged that demonstrates the benefits of assessing the function of problem behavior in developing educative and effective treatment (Durand & Kishi, 1987).

Direct Assessment

Direct assessment of a life skills curriculum cannot be conducted as a paper-and-pencil test. Because life skills assessment requires access to varied community environments and materials of daily living, it can become a time-consuming and expensive process if it is not well defined. If conducted first, indirect assessment will provide information on the skills a student has and priorities for improved independence. Direct assessment provides the means to identify specific treatment goals and to begin the measurement process that will be used for ongoing evaluation of progress.

Task Analytic Assessment

One of the most often used methods of assessment for daily living skills is task analytic assessment. Task analytic assessment is a variation of event recording that focuses on a chain of behavior rather than a single event. A skill, such as operating a vending machine, is broken down into the chain of responses that are required to perform the skill. To assess performance of the skill, the evaluator observes the individual while performing the skill and records whether each response in the chain is performed. Because performance of responses later in a chain may require completion of earlier responses, the evaluator may need to complete some of the responses to "set up" the materials for the next response. When performing the assessment, the evaluator does not guide the individual to perform the responses as would occur during teaching, but, rather, simply completes a step of the chain to allow for assessment of the next step. Sometimes the evaluator may terminate the assessment after the first error in the chain, especially if real-life events preclude proceeding after a mistake (e.g., failing to put money in the vending machine). An example of task analytic assessment is shown in Figure 3.

Numerous studies on daily living skills have reported excellent interrater agreement for task analytic assessment (e.g., Cronin & Cuvo, 1979; Snell, 1982; see Snell & Browder, 1986, for a review of this research). By contrast, little research exists on the design of the task analysis. Cuvo and his colleagues (Cronin & Cuvo, 1979; Johnson & Cuvo, 1981; Williams & Cuvo, 1986) described procedures to develop an analysis using social validation pro-

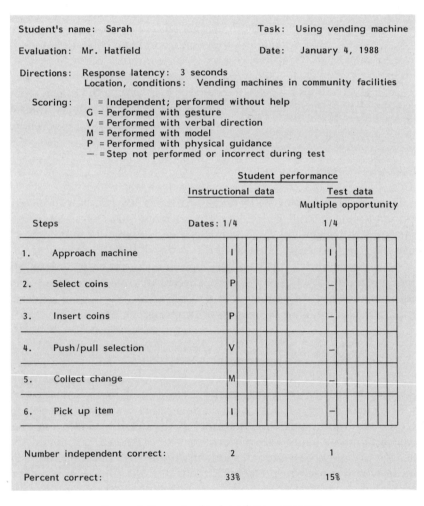

FIGURE 3. Example of task analytic assessment.

cedures. Browder (1987) described several steps to develop an analysis that are useful for initial and ongoing assessment. In a rare study on the development of the analysis itself, Crist, Walls, and Haught (1984) found some support for breaking the skill into more specific responses for learners with more severe handicaps. Further research is needed on how the development of the analysis itself influences assessment and treatment results.

Repeated Trial Assessment

Another method of assessment that has frequently been utilized in research with individuals with severe handicaps is a "test" in which the evaluator presents repeated opportunities to make the response. For example, the person is given repeated opportunities to label or request objects (Reichle & Brown, 1986). In this method of assessment, opportunities may be massed (presented in close temporal sequence, such as less than a minute between trials) or spaced (presented across naturally occurring opportunities to request objects during the day). They also may be distributed (several items presented together) or focused on one specific response (e.g., one object). While massed, distributed trials may be the most efficient way to assess skills, such as using a communication system to label and request objects. It should be noted that scheduling trials across the day may be more conducive to learning (Mulligan, Lacy, & Guess, 1982).

Observations in the Natural Environment

One of the criticisms of task analytic assessment is that it often does not indicate whether the student can make judgments required by the natural environment (Brown, 1987). Besides setting up a situation to test the student's skills in performing a chain of responses, or to test repeated opportunities to demonstrate such a response as communication, it may be important to observe the student's use of these skills in naturally occurring situations. Also, problem behaviors typically are assessed as they naturally occur. Assessment during observations may utilize task analyses adapted for variations in the natural environment, event recording, and descriptions of antecedents and consequences as described earlier in this chapter. Depending on the frequency, time sampling may be a more appropriate option than event recording for problem behavior. Another alternative for problem behavior is to assess further the function of the behavior by observing the antecedents and consequences to it. The function of the behavior may be discerned through the use of a scatterplot of the time and activity when the behavior occurs (Touchette, MacDonald, & Langer, 1985).

Because the natural environments for daily living skills extend beyond the classroom to include homes, public facilities, job environments, and other community sites, it also is important to obtain information on the individual's performance in these actual sites. Research on using classroom simulations of community activities has provided mixed results on an individual's generalization from a classroom simulation to the natural environment (Nietupski,

Hamre-Nietupski, Clancy, & Veerhusen, 1986). Thus, *in vivo* probes will be necessary. Sometimes generalization to one community site may still not reflect mastery of the skill across environments. Using a method of assessment and treatment known as "general case instruction" Horner and colleagues (Horner, Jones, & Williams, 1985; Sprague & Horner, 1984) have demonstrated an efficient way to evaluate stimulus and response generalization for daily living skills. Their method involves creating a "generic" task analysis and then defining how stimuli and responses will vary across the many examples of the task (e.g., vending machines with number selection buttons versus pull knobs). By selecting a few specific community sites that sample the range of variation, the evaluator can be more confident that the individual has mastered generalized use of the skill.

CONCLUSIONS AND SUMMARY

Probably one of the most important priorities for individuals working with persons with mental retardation is designing and implementing intervention procedures to assist these persons in acquiring skills that make daily living easier. This would include skills related to home, schools, community, and employment settings. Clearly, the methodology of behavioral assessment offers opportunities to assess directly and indirectly behavior that leads to the development of effective intervention strategies. Unlike more traditional assessment designed solely for classification purposes, behavioral assessment offers evaluation for a much broader range of purposes.

Although behavioral assessment has been widely applied across all levels of persons with mental retardation, there are specific adaptations necessary when assessment is conducted with persons whose handicaps are more severe. For these individuals, the indirect assessment methods of informant report (both interview and checklist/rating scales) play a very critical role in the process. Indeed, before effective direct observation procedures, such as task analysis, can be used to develop intervention procedures, accurate ecological inventories developed through informant reports must be obtained.

Clearly, behavioral assessment methodologies will continue to play significant parts in the evaluation of persons with mental retardation. Ongoing refinement of procedures and adaptations for assessing this client population will still be needed. In particular, the development of better and more accurate means of structured interviewing of persons with mental retardation appears to be a neglected area. Likewise, there have been few explorations of written self-reports with persons with mental retardation. Although there are obvious limitations in using these methods, particularly with a handicapped population, investigations of this method are certainly warranted. Likewise, there is much research needed on adaptations of behavioral assessment methods to persons with more severe handicaps. In particular, the need for empirically validated ecological inventories and task analyses is critical. Further, there is a need for the development of more standardized instruments specifically aimed for assessing persons with severe handicaps.

Despite the obvious needs for further development, behavioral assessment methodologies have provided a much needed link between assessment and intervention methods in determining intervention programs for persons with mental retardation. It is clear that there has been a substantial shift, in the field of those professionals who work with persons with mental retardation, from a focus on classification/identification through more traditional assessment measures, such as intelligence tests and tests of adaptive behavior, to an emphasis on treatment planning and socially valid assessment. As the methodology of behavioral assessment continues to grow from its childhood toward adulthood, continued contributions to adapting the methodology for assessing persons with mental retardation will likewise grow.

REFERENCES

Ackerman, A., & Shapiro, E. S. (1984). Self-monitoring and work productivity with mentally retarded adults. *Journal of Applied Behavior Analysis, 17*, 403–407.

Agran, M., & Martin, J. E. (1987). Applying a technology of self-control in community environments for individuals who are mentally retarded. In M. Hersen, R. M. Eisler, & P. M. Miller (Eds.), *Progress in behavior modification* (Vol. 21, pp. 108–151). Beverly Hills, CA: Sage Publications.

Aveno, A. (1987). A survey of activities engaged in and skills needed by adults in community residences. *Journal of the Association for Persons with Severe Handicaps, 12*, 125–130.

Barlow, D. H. (Ed.). (1981). *Behavioral assessment of adult disorders*. New York: Guilford Press.

Bijou, S., & Grimm, J. A. (1972) *Behavioral diagnosis and assessment in young handicapped children*. Washington, DC: Division of Research, Bureau of Education for the Handicapped.

Bornstein, M. T., Bellack, A. S., & Hersen, M. (1977). Social skills training for unassertive children: A multiple-baseline analysis. *Journal of Applied Behavior Analysis, 10*, 183–195.

Browder, D. (1987). *Assessment of individuals with severe handicaps*. Baltimore: Brookes.

Browder, D. M., & Shapiro, E. S. (1985). Applications of self-management to individuals with severe handicaps: A review. *Journal of the Association for Persons with Severe Handicaps, 10*, 200–208.

Brown, F. (1987). Meaningful assessment of people with severe and profound handicaps. In M. E. Snell (Ed.), *Systematic instruction of persons with severe handicaps* (3rd ed., pp. 39–63). Columbus, OH: Charles E. Merrill.

Brown, L., Branston, M. B., Hamre-Nietupski, S., Pumpian, I., Certo, N., & Gruenewald, L. (1979). A strategy for developing chronological-age-appropriate and functional curricular content for severely handicapped adolescents and young adults. *Journal of Special Education, 13*, 81–90.

Bruininks, R. H., Woodcock, R. W., Weatherman, R. F., & Hill, B. K. (1984). *Scales of independent behavior*. Allen, TX: Developmental Learning Materials.

Burgio, L., Whitman, T., & Johnson, M. (1980). A self-instructional package for increasing attending behavior in educable mentally retarded children. *Journal of Applied Behavior Analysis, 13*, 443–459.

Ciminero, A. R., Calhoun, K. S., & Adams, H. E. (Eds.). (1977). *Handbook of behavioral assessment*. New York: Wiley.

Ciminero, A. R., Nelson, R. O., & Lipinski, D. P. (1977). Self-monitoring procedures. In A. R. Ciminero, K. S. Calhoun, & H. E. Adams (Eds.), *Handbook of behavioral assessment* (pp. 195–232). New York: Wiley.

Cone, J. D. (1977). The relevance of reliability and validity for behavioral assessment. *Behavior Therapy, 88*, 411–426.

Cone, J. D. (1978). The behavioral assessment grid (BAG): A conceptual framework and a taxonomy. *Behavior Therapy, 9*, 882–888.

Cone, J. D. (1981). Psychometric considerations. In M. Hersen & A. S. Bellack (Eds.), *Behavioral assessment: A practical handbook* (2nd ed, (pp. 38–70). New York: Pergamon Press.

Cone, J. D. (1984). *The pyramid scales.* Austin, TX: Pro Ed.

Cone, J. D., & Hawkins, R. P. (Eds.) (1977). *Behavioral assessment: New directions in clinical psychology.* New York: Brunner/Mazel.

Conroy, J. W., & Bradley, V. J. (1985). *The Pennhurst longitudinal study: A report of five years of research and analysis.* Philadelphia: Temple University Developmental Disabilities Center.

Crist, K., Walls, R. T., & Haught, P. (1984). Degree of specificity in task analysis. *American Journal of Mental Deficiency, 89,* 67–74.

Cronbach, L. J., Gleser, G. S., Nanda, H., & Rajaratnam, N. (1972). *The dependability of behavioral measures.* New York: Wiley.

Cronin, K. A., & Cuvo, A. J. (1979). Teaching mending skills to retarded adolescents. *Journal of Applied Behavior Analysis, 12,* 401–406.

Cuvo, A. J., Jacobi, E., & Sipko, R. (1981). Teaching laundry skills to mentally retarded students. *Education and Training of the Mentally Retarded, 16,* 54–64.

Deno, S. L. (1985). Curriculum-based measurement: The emerging alternative. *Exceptional Children, 52,* 219–232.

Doll, E. A. (1953). *Measurement of social competence: A manual for the Vineland social maturity scale.* Minneapolis: Educational Publishers.

Donnellan, A. M., Mirenda, P. L., Mesaros, R. A., & Fassbender, L. L. (1984). Analyzing the communicative functions of aberrant behavior. *Journal of the Association for Persons with Severe Handicaps, 9*(3), 201–212.

Durand, M. (1989). The motivation assessment scale. In M. Hersen & A. S. Bellack (Eds.), *Dictionary of behavioral assessment techniques* (pp. 309–310). New York: Pergamon Press.

Durand, V. M., & Kishi, G. (1987). Reducing severe behavior problems among persons with dual sensory impairments: An evaluation of a technical assistance model. *The Journal of the Association for Persons with Severe Handicaps, 12,* 2–10.

Edelbrock, C. S. (1988). Informant reports. In E. S. Shapiro & T. R. Kratochwill (Eds.), *Behavioral assessment in schools: Conceptual foundations and practical applications* (pp. 351–383). New York: Guilford Press.

Eisler, R. M., Hersen, M., Miller, P. M., & Blanchard, E. B. (1975). Situational determinants of assertive behavior. *Journal of Consulting and Clinical Psychology, 43,* 330–340.

Evans, I. M., & Meyer, L. H. (1985). *An educative approach to behavior problems: A practical decision model for interventions with severely handicapped learners.* Baltimore: Paul H. Brookes Publishing Co.

Foster, R. W. (1974). *Camelot behavioral checklist.* Lawrence, KS: Camelot Behavior Systems.

Foxx, R. M., McMorrow, M. J., & Schloss, C. N. (1983). Stacking the deck: Teaching social skills to retarded adults with a modified table game. *Journal of Applied Behavior Analysis, 16,* 157–170.

Foxx, R. M., McMorrow, M. J., Bittle, R. G., & Ness, J. (1983). An analysis of social skills generalization in two natural settings. *Journal of Applied Behavior Analysis, 19,* 299–305.

Gast, D. L., & Wolery, M. (1987). Severe maladaptive behavior. In M. E. Snell (Ed.), *Systematic instruction of persons with severe handicaps.* Columbus, OH: Charles E. Merrill.

Gaylord-Ross, R., & Holvoet, J. (1985). *Strategies for educating students with severe handicaps.* Boston: Little, Brown.

Gresham, F. M. (1984). Behavioral interviews in school psychology: Issues in psychometric adequacy and research. *School Psychology Review, 13,* 17–25.

Hartmann, D. P., Roper, B. L., & Bradford, D. C. (1979). Some relationships between behavioral and traditional assessment. *Journal of Behavioral Assessment, 1,* 3–21.

Hay, W. M., Hay, L. R., Angle, H. V., & Nelson, R. O. (1979). The reliability of problem identification in the behavioral interview. *Behavioral Assessment, 1,* 107–118.

Hayes, S. C., & Nelson, R. O. (1986). Assessing the effects of therapeutic interventions. In R. O. Nelson & S. C. Hayes (Eds.), *Conceptual foundations of behavioral assessment* (pp. 430–460). New York: Guilford Press.

Hayes, S. C., Nelson, R. O., & Jarrett, R. B. (1986). Evaluating the quality of behavioral assessment. In R. O. Nelson & S. C. Hayes (Eds.), *Conceptual foundations of behavioral assessment* (pp. 461–504). New York: Guilford Press.

Hayes, S. C., Nelson, R. O., & Jarrett, R. B. (1987). The treatment utility of assessment: A functional approach to evaluating assessment quality. *American Psychologist, 42*, 963–974.

Haynes, S. N. (1978). *Principles of behavioral assessment*. New York: Gardner Press.

Haynes, S. N., & Wilson, C. C. (1979). *Behavioral assessment: Recent advances in methods, concepts, and applications*. San Francisco: Jossey-Bass.

Heal, L. W., & Chadsey-Rusch, J. (1985). The lifestyle satisfaction scale (LSS): Assessing individuals' satisfaction with residence, community setting, and associated services. *Applied Research in Mental Retardation, 6*, 475–490.

Hersen, M., & Bellack, A. S. (Eds.). (1987). *Behavioral assessment: A practical handbook* (3rd ed.). New York: Pergamon Press.

Hoge, R. D. (1983). Psychometric properties of teacher-judgment measures of pupil aptitudes, classroom behaviors, and achievement levels. *Journal of Special Education, 17*, 401–429.

Horner, R. H., Jones, D. N., & Williams, J. A. (1985). A functional approach to teaching generalized street crossing. *Journal of the Association for Persons with Severe Handicaps, 1*, 7–20.

Johnson, B. F., & Cuvo, A. J. (1981). Teaching mentally retarded adults to cook. *Behavior Modification, 5*, 187–202.

Kanfer, F. H., & Saslow, G. (1969). Behavioral diagnosis. In C. Franks (Ed.), *Behavior therapy: Appraisal and status* (pp. 417–444). New York: McGraw-Hill.

Kazdin, A. E. (1977). Assessing the clinical or applied importance of behavior change through social validation. *Behavior Modification, 1*, 427–452.

Lambert, N. M., Windmiller, M., & Cole, L. J. (1981). *ABS: AAMD adaptive behavior scale, school edition*. Washington, DC: American Association on Mental Deficiency.

Lentz, F. E., Jr. (1982). *An empirical examination of the utility of partial interval and momentary time sampling as measurements of behavior*. Unpublished doctoral dissertation, University of Tennessee.

Linehan, M. N. (1977). Issues in behavioral interviewing. In J. D. Cone & R. P. Hawkins (Eds.), *Behavioral assessment: New directions in clinical psychology* (pp. 30–51). New York: Brunner/Mazel.

Mace, F. C., & Kratochwill, T. R. (1985). Theories of reactivity in self-monitoring: A comparison of cognitive-behavioral and operant models. *Behavior Modification, 9*, 323–343.

Martin, J. E., Burger, D. L., Elias-Burger, S., & Mithaug, D. E. (1988). Applications of self-control strategies to facilitate independence. In N. W. Bray (Ed.), *International review of research in mental retardation* (Vol. 15). New York: Academic Press.

Mash, E., & Terdal, L. (Eds.). (1981). *Behavioral assessment of childhood disorders*. New York: Guilford Press.

Matson, J. L., Esveldt-Dawson, K., Andrasik, F., Ollendick, T. H., Petti, T. H., & Hersen, M. (1980). Direct, observational, and generalization effects of social skills training with emotionally disturbed children. *Behavior Therapy, 11*, 522–531.

McFall, R. M. (1977). Analogue methods in behavioral assessment: Issues and prospects. In J. D. Cone & R. P. Hawkins (Eds.), *Behavioral assessment: New directions in clinical psychology* (pp. 152–177). New York: Brunner/Mazel.

McGregor, G., Janssen, C., Larsen, L. A., & Tillery, W. L. (1986). Philadelphia's urban training model project: A statewide effort to integrate students with severe handicaps. *Journal of the Association for Persons with Severe Handicaps 11*, 61–67.

McLaughlin, J. A., & Lewis, R. B. (1986). *Assessing Special students* (2nd ed.). Columbus, OH: Merrill.

Meyers, C. E., Nihira, K., & Zetlin, A. (1979). The measurement of adaptive behavior. In N. R. Ellis (Ed.), *Handbook of mental deficiency, psychological theory and research* (pp. 431–481). Hillsdale, NJ: Lawrence Erlbaum.

Moon, S., Goodall, P., Barcus, M., & Brooke, V. (Eds.). (1985). *The supported work model of competitive employment for citizen with severe handicaps: A guide for job trainers*. Richmond: Virginia Commonwealth University, Rehabilitation Research and Training Center.

Mulligan, M., Lacy, L., & Guess, D. (1982). Effects of massed, distributed, and spaced trial sequencing on severely handicapped students' performance. *Journal of the Association for the Severely Handicapped, 7,* 48–61.

Nelson, R. O. (1977). Methodological issues in assessment via self-monitoring. In J. D. Cone & R. P. Hawkins (Eds.), *Behavioral assessment: New directions in clinical psychology* (pp. 217–240). New York: Brunner/Mazel.

Nelson, R. O. (1980). The use of intelligence tests within behavioral assessment. *Behavioral Assessment, 2,* 417–423.

Nelson, R. O. (1983). Behavioral assessment: Past, present, and future. *Behavioral Assessment, 5,* 195–206.

Nelson, R. O., & Hayes, S. C. (1979). The nature of behavioral assessment: A commentary. *Journal of Applied Behavior Analysis, 12,* 491–500.

Nelson, R. O., & Hayes, S. C. (1987). The nature of behavioral assessment. In R. O. Nelson & S. C. Hayes (Eds.), *Conceptual foundations of behavioral assessments* (pp. 3–41). New York: Guilford Press.

Nelson, R. O., Hay, L. R., & Hay, W. M. (1977). Comments on Cone's "the relevance of reliability and validity for behavioral assessment." *Behavior Therapy, 8,* 437–440.

Nietupski, J., Hamre-Nietupski, S., Clancy, P., & Veerhusen, K. (1986). Guidelines for making simulation an effective adjunct to in vivo community instruction. *Journal of the Association for Persons with Severe Handicaps, 11,* 12–18.

Nihira, K., Foster, R., Shellhaas, M., & Leland, H. (1969). *Manual for AAMD adaptive behavior scale.* Washington, DC: American Association on Mental Deficiency.

Ollendick, T. H., Shapiro, E. S., & Barrett, R. P. (1982). Effects of vicarious reinforcement in normal and severely disturbed children. *Journal of Consulting and Clinical Psychology, 50,* 63–70.

Powell, J., & Rockinson, R. (1978). On the inability of interval time sampling to reflect frequency of occurrence data. *Journal of Applied Behavior Analysis, 11,* 531–532.

Powell, J., Martindale, B., Kulp, S., Martindale, A., & Bauman, R. (1977). Taking a closer look: Time sampling and measurement error. *Journal of Applied Behavior Analysis, 10,* 325–332.

Powers, M. D., & Handleman, J. S. (1984). *Behavioral assessment of severe developmental disabilities.* Rockville, MD: Aspen Systems.

Prout, H. T., & Ferber, S. M. (1988). Analogue assessment: Traditional personality assessment measures in behavioral assessment. In E. S. Shapiro & T. R. Kratochwill (Eds.), *Behavioral assessment in schools: Conceptual foundations and practical applications* (pp. 322–350). New York: Guilford Press.

Reichle, J., & Brown, L. (1986). Teaching the use of a multipage direct selection communication board to an adult with autism. *Journal of the Association for Persons with Severe Handicaps, 11,* 68–72.

Rusch, F. R., Chadsey-Rusch, J., & Lagormarcino, T. (1987). Preparing students for employment. In M. E. Snell (Ed.), *Systematic instruction of persons with severe handicaps* (3rd ed.). Columbus, OH: Merrill.

Rusch, F., Schutz, R., & Agran, M. (1982). Validating entry-level survival skills for service occupations: Implications for curriculum development. *Journal of the Association for the Severely Handicapped, 7,* 32–41.

Schalock, R. L., Harper, R. S., & Carver, G. (1981). Independent living placement: Five years later. *American Journal of Mental Deficiency, 86,* 170–177.

Senatore, V., Matson, J. L., & Kazdin, A. E. (1982). A comparison of behavioral methods to train social skills to mentally retarded adults. *Behavior Therapy, 13,* 313–324.

Shapiro, E. S. (1984). Self-monitoring. In T. H. Ollendick & M. Hersen (Eds.), *Child behavior assessment: Principles and procedures* (pp. 148–165). New York: Pergamon Press.

Shapiro, E. S. (1987). *Behavioral assessment in school psychology.* Hillsdale, NJ: Lawrence Erlbaum.

Shapiro, E. S., & Ackerman, A. (1983). Increasing productivity rates in adult mentally retarded clients: The failure of self-monitoring. *Applied Research in Mental Retardation, 4,* 163–181.

Shapiro, E. S., & Barrett, R. P. (1983). Behavioral assessment of the mentally retarded. In J. L. Matson & F. Andrasik (Eds.), *Treatment issues and innovations in mental retardation* (pp. 159–212). New York: Plenum Press.

Shapiro, E. S., & Klein, R. D. (1980). Self-management of classroom behavior with retarded disturbed children. *Behavior Modification, 4*, 83–97.

Shapiro, E. S., & Kratochwill, T. R. (Eds.). (1988). *Behavioral assessment in schools: Conceptual foundations and practical applications.* New York: Guilford Press.

Shapiro, E. S., & Lentz, F. E., Jr. (1985). Assessing academic behavior: A behavioral approach. *School Psychology Review, 14*, 325–338.

Shapiro, E. S., & Lentz, F. E., Jr. (1986). Behavioral assessment of academic skills. In T. R. Kratochwill (Ed.), *Advances in school psychology* (Vol. 5, pp. 87–140). Hillsdale, NJ: Lawrence Erlbaum.

Shapiro, E. S., Barrett, R. P., & Ollendick, T. H. (1980). A comparison of physical restraint and positive practice overcorrection in treating stereotypic behavior. *Behavior Therapy, 11*, 227–233.

Shapiro, E. S., McGonigle, J. J., & Ollendick, T. H. (1980). An analysis of self-assessment and self-reinforcement in a self-managed token economy with mentally retarded children. *Applied Research in Mental Retardation, 1*, 227–240.

Shapiro, E. S., Browder, D. M., & D'Huyvetters, K. K. (1984). Increasing academic productivity of severely multi-handicapped children with self-management: Idiosyncratic effects. *Analysis and Intervention in Developmental Disabilities, 4*, 171–188.

Sigelman, C., Budd, E. C., Spanhel, C. L., & Schoenrock, C. J. (1981). When in doubt, say yes: Acquiescence in interviews with mentally retarded persons. *Mental Retardation, 19*, 53–58.

Snell, M. (1982). Teaching bedmaking to severely retarded adults through time delay. *Analysis and Intervention in Developmental Disabilities, 2*, 139–155.

Snell, M. (1987). *Systematic instruction of persons with severe handicaps.* Columbus, OH: Charles E. Merrill.

Snell, M., & Browder, D. (1986). Community-referenced instruction: Research and issues. *Journal of the Association for Persons with Severe Handicaps, 11*, 1–11.

Sparrow, S. S., Balla, D. A., & Cicchetti, D. V. (1984). *Vineland adaptive behavior scales. Interview edition: Survey form and expanded survey form.* Circle Pines, MN: American Guidance Service.

Sparrow, S. S., Balla, D. A., & Cicchetti, D. V. (1985). *Vineland adaptive behavior scales. Classroom edition.* Circle Pines: MN: American Guidance Service.

Sprague, J. R., & Horner, R. H. (1984). The effect of single instance, multiple instance, and general case training on a generalized vending machine use by moderately and severely handicapped students. *Journal of Applied Behavior Analysis, 17*, 273–278.

Strosahl, K. D., & Linehan, M. M. (1986). Basic issues in behavioral assessment. In A. R. Ciminero, K. S. Calhoun, & H. E. Adams (Eds.), *Handbook of behavioral assessment* (2nd ed., pp. 12–46). New York: Wiley.

Touchette, P., MacDonald, R., & Langer, S. (1985). A scatter plot for identifying stimulus control of problem behavior. *Journal of Applied Behavior Analysis, 18*, 343–351.

Van Hasselt, V. B., Hersen, M., & Bellack, A. S. (1981). The validity of role play tests for assessing social skills in children. *Behavior Therapy, 12*, 202–216.

Voeltz, L. M., Wuerch, B. B., & Bockhaut, C. H. (1982). Social validation of leisure activities training with severely handicapped youth. *Journal of the Association for the Severely Handicapped, 7*, 3–13.

Walls, R. T., Werner, T. J., Bacon, A., & Zane, T. (1977). Behavioral checklists. In J. D. Cone & R. P. Hawkins (Eds.), *Behavioral assessment: New directions in clinical psychology* (pp. 77–146). New York: Brunner/Mazel.

Wehman, P., Hill J. W., Wood, W., & Parent, W. (1987). A report on competitive employment histories of persons labeled severely mentally retarded. *Journal of the Association for Persons with Severe Handicaps, 12*, 11–17.

Williams, G. E., & Cuvo, A. J. (1986). Training apartment upkeep skills to rehabilitation clients: A comparison of task analytic strategies. *Journal of Applied Behavior Analysis, 19*, 39–51.

Williamson, D. A., Moody, S. C., Granberry, S. W., Lethermon, V. R., & Blouin, D. C. (1983). Criterion-related validity of a role-play social skills test for children. *Behavior Therapy, 14*, 466–481.

Witt, J. C., Cavell, T. A., Heffer, R. W., Carey, M. P., & Martens, B. K. (1988). Child self-report:

Interviewing techniques and rating scales. In E. S. Shapiro & T. R. Kratochwill (Eds.), *Behavioral assessment in schools: Conceptual foundations and practical applications* (pp. 384–454). New York: Guilford Press.

Wolf, M. M. (1978). Social validity: The case for subjective measurement, or how behavior analysis is finding its heart. *Journal of Applied Behavior Analysis, 11,* 203–214.

5

Principles of Behavior Modification

ENNIO CIPANI

The field of behavior modification, or applied behavior analysis, is distinguished from other approaches in several ways. The fundamental characteristics and properties of the behavioral approach were identified in an article appearing in the first issue of the *Journal of Applied Behavior Analysis* (Baer, Wolf, & Risley, 1968). One set of properties identified in this landmark article was the methodological requirements of applied behavior analysis. The methodology was characterized by four unique requirements. The empirical focus was on observable behavior, or rate of response, in contrast to inferred states of feelings. Second, the analytical orientation involving the experimental analysis of functional relationships between variables was the primary focus of research. Third, the utilization of within-subject analyses, controlling experimentally for potential confounding variables (in contrast to statistical control), was the preferred method of studying human behavior. Finally, the applied component of the field dictated that socially relevant problems be the subject of research, and that effective technologies be developed which produce practically significant changes in behavior (Kazdin, 1977; Wolf, 1978).

Although methodology has contributed substantially toward the definition of applied behavior analysis, a second set of principles involves the manipulation of environmental variables, guided by a theory of human behavior. Behavior is viewed as the result of the social and physical environment and heredity (Michael, 1987). Even though behavior analysts do not discredit the function of inherited characteristics on human behavior, they do not see it as a catch-all explanation for describing the conditions that produce behavior. Rather, the control and manipulation of environmental variables have constituted the basic empirical research paradigm.

There are two relations describing behavior and the environmental conditions surrounding it: respondent functional relations and operant functional relations (Michael, 1987). The overwhelming majority of applied research and clinical inquiry with people with mental retardation has studied operant behavior. Thus, this chapter will cover principles of operant behavior, but the author does recognize the importance of studying respondent relations in the development of present and future technologies.

ENNIO CIPANI • Department of Special Education, University of the Pacific, Stockton, California 95211.

Operant behavioral principles are based on the analysis and manipulation of observable environmental events involved in learning. Three temporally ordered events operationalize the observable elements of instruction: antecedent stimulus, operant response, and consequent stimulus. The (antecedent) stimulus is an object, event, or activity that precedes the response. An operant is a class of responses that are observable and measurable, and that operate on the environment in the same fashion (Catania, 1984). These responses are emitted in the presence of environmental antecedent stimuli. The consequence is an environmental event that follows a response, which alters the future probability, or level, of the operant behavior they follow. In the section that follows, we will provide a discussion of the basic theoretical principles as well as everyday examples illustrating such principles. Where appropriate, examples of basic and applied research will be offered to further illustrate such principles. We begin with two broad areas of discussion: response–consequence relations and stimulus–response relations.

RESPONSE–CONSEQUENCE RELATIONS

Contingencies

In part, behavior is a function of its consequences. This relationship between the operant response and the environmental consequence is termed a *contingency*. Contingencies occur in everyday situations; for example, saying "thank you" (consequence) after someone opens the door for you (behavior). Most everyday examples of contingencies are those that are socially mediated. But consequences can also be mediated by the physical environment; for example, the behavioral consequence of jumping into a pool of very cold water is the tightening of the muscles. Skinner (1957) identified two types of operants on the basis of the type of consequence following the response. Responses that are socially mediated are identified as *verbal behaviors* and responses mediated by the physical environment are termed *nonverbal behaviors*.

There are two types of consequent stimuli: reinforcing stimuli and punishing stimuli. Both sets of stimuli are operationally defined by their effects on behavior. Positive reinforcement occurs when an environmental event follows a behavior and, as a result of such a relationship, the future probability of that response is maintained or increased. Reinforcement cannot be operationalized as the provision of any specific event, activity, or object in a contingent fashion. By definition, reinforcement always serves to maintain or increase the behavior(s) it follows. This is not to say that certain applications of contingencies in certain situations are not successful in increasing behavior. However, in those situations, reinforcement did not occur; rather, some other phenomenon occurred.

Punishment is operationally defined as an environmental event that follows a behavior in a contingent fashion, and, as a function of this contingency, the behavior decreases in level or probability. Events that follow behavior that produce the opposite effect of reinforcers are termed *punishers*. As defined in the current context, event refers to either the addition of a consequent stimulus or the removal of a stimulus, thus negating the need for such terms as positive and negative punishment.

Behaviors can increase by two contingent operations: (1) by producing a stimulus (positive reinforcement), and (2) by removing a stimulus (negative reinforcement). Positive reinforcement has already been defined above and is typically referred to as reinforcement. Negative reinforcement is defined as the withdrawal of a response contingent upon the occurrence of a behavior, with the subsequent increase in the rate of that response (Reynolds, 1975). Two negative reinforcement paradigms can be created and are differentiated in the manner in which the response terminates or postpones the stimulus.

Escape conditioning involves the withdrawal of the stimulus (aversive) contingent upon the occurrence of the response. The response terminates an already present aversive stimulus, which eventually becomes discriminative for the escape response (Reynolds, 1975). For example, an alarm clock that sounds at 6:00 A.M. awakens a sleeper. The sleeper pushes a button that terminates the alarm. The withdrawal of the aversive sound is terminated upon the occurrence of the response. If the noise from the alarm clock is of sufficient aversion to this sleeper, he or she will become more adept at pushing the button quickly to avoid the sound for long durations. Escape responding typically will show decreases in the latency of the response (from the onset at the aversive stimulus) across training sessions.

Avoidance conditioning involves the avoidance or postponement of the presentation of the stimulus with the occurrence of the response. Avoidance conditioning can be an outgrowth of escape conditioning or it can be developed independently (Reynolds, 1975). In the example just used, the sleeper begins to wake up ahead of the alarm (discriminative stimulus), pushes the button (avoidance response), and avoids the noise (for at least that morning). Often, a neutral stimulus is presented prior to the onset of the aversive stimulus to serve as an additional discriminative stimulus and to facilitate the development of avoidance responding. In everyday examples of avoidance conditioning, the verbal stimulus "no" is usually the neutral stimulus that, it is hoped, produces the desired avoidance response, thus postponing the onset of the aversive consequence. When "no" does begin to control avoidance responding, then it has become a conditioned aversive stimulus (Reynolds, 1975).

Differential reinforcement is the process whereby some behaviors are followed by reinforcing stimuli, whereas other behaviors are not followed by such stimuli. This results in an increase in the frequency of behaviors that are followed by reinforcing stimuli, whereas the behaviors that are not followed by such stimuli undergo extinction. Extinction is the withdrawal of reinforcement for the occurrence of a previously reinforced operant, with subsequent reduction in the level of that operant (Reynolds, 1975). For example, differentially reinforcing a child for hand raising in class would increase the frequency

of such responding, while extinguishing other forms of attention-getting behavior (e.g., blurting out, whining) under specific stimulus conditions predictive of differential reinforcement for those sets of behavior.

A variety of procedures utilizing differential reinforcement principles
have been developed to decrease undesirable target behaviors (Repp &
Brulle, 1981):

1. Differential reinforcement of other behavior (DRO) involves the reinforcement of behaviors in a specified interval, given the absence of the
   target behavior within the interval.
2. Differential reinforcement of low rates of behavior (DRL) involves the
   reinforcement of a criterion level of low rates of undesirable target
   behavior in a given interval.
3. Differential reinforcement of high rates of behavior (DRH) involves
   the reinforcement of a criterion level of high rates of desirable
   behavior.
4. Differential reinforcement of incompatible behavior (DRI) involves the
   reinforcement of a select behavior that is physically incompatible with
   the target behavior.
5. Differential reinforcement of alternate behavior (DRA) involves the
   reinforcement of an alternate (appropriate) behavior that is not physically incompatible with the target behavior.

Factors Affecting Reinforcer Potency

The capability of a consequent event to function as a reinforcer is not a
static value; rather, its potency varies as a function of several conditions or
variables. The following factors ameliorate or strengthen a reinforcer's potency at a given point in time: (1) deprivation and satiation state with respect to
event, (2) magnitude of reinforcement per delivery, (3) immediacy of consequent event, and (4) schedule of reinforcement.

Deprivation and satiation are opposite phenomena. A reinforcer that is in
a deprived state will enhance the potency of the contingency being used at
that particular time. Therefore, the effect on behavior is to increase the rate of
behavior under the contingency. If access to a reinforcer is not restricted, then
the potency of the reinforcer is lessened. Increased access to a reinforcer leads
to satiation. For example, providing edible reinforcement for correct responses will maintain a stable rate of responding in a child who is hungry
(i.e., in a deprived state with respect to food). However, as the child gradually reaches a food satiety level, the ability of food to maintain or increase
correct responding becomes hindered.

A second factor influencing the potency of a contingent event is the
magnitude of the reinforcing event. The amount of the reinforcer delivered
(magnitude) has a curvilinear relationship with rate of response. As the
amount of a reinforcer given for a response increases, the rate of behavior

increases. However, at some point, which is defined individually, increasing the amount of the reinforcer delivered only results in decreased performance. This point can be defined as *satiation*.

The immediate delivery of a contingent event is very important, particularly when working with children or clients who are not under control of stimuli that serve as conditioned reinforcers (such as tokens) or instructions or rules about future contingencies. When the delivery of a consequent event is not immediate, the effect on the rate of response is to diminish acquisition. This is particularly true when other behaviors are allowed to occur in the interval between target response and consequence, and that subsequently get reinforced (Reynolds, 1975).

The effects of various schedules of reinforcement on altering rates of behavior were studied extensively in the animal laboratory (Ferster & Skinner, 1957). The schedule of reinforcement is an important factor in understanding the variables responsible for stimulus control. Recent research has demonstrated the importance of altering the schedule of reinforcement in effecting the transfer of stimulus control during fading procedures (Touchette & Howard, 1984). Reinforcement of behavior can occur either on a continuous schedule or on an intermittent schedule. A *continuous schedule* is defined as the reinforcement of each occurrence of the response. In contrast, *intermittent schedules* do not have a one-to-one relationship between response and consequence.

There are wide varieties of intermittent schedules. Two broad categories of simple reinforcement schedules are ratio and interval schedules. Ratio schedules require a certain number of responses to occur prior to the delivery of reinforcement. Interval schedules require certain amounts of time to elapse prior to the reinforcement of the occurrence of the first target response. For a more detailed description of more complex intermittent schedules, such as tandem, concurrent, or interlocking schedules, the reader should consult Reynolds (1975) or Catania (1984).

When developing a behavior of low frequency, a continuous schedule of delivery is most suited (Foxx, 1982; Reynolds, 1975). Once the behavior is acquired, intermittent schedules allow for rapid increases in the operant rate when "thinned" in a gradual manner. Fixed ratio schedules produce steady levels of behavior. Variable schedules produce the highest rates of responding, in that short interresponse times (IRTs) are highly likely to be reinforced (Reynolds, 1975). Particularly when the teacher/trainer is able to thin the reinforcement schedule to high variable ratio schedules (e.g., VR 48, VR 207, etc.), the effect on the student will be higher rates of behavior in contrast to continuous or dense fixed ratio schedules.

Intermittent schedules are also more resistant to extinction. Because the organism is accustomed to responding for long periods of time prior to delivery of reinforcement under intermittent schedules, it will take a longer period of time before the extinction schedule will be discriminably different from the previously instated intermittent reinforcement schedule. High variable schedules (ratio and interval) are the most resistant to extinction. In contrast, continuous schedules are affected easily by extinction procedures.

Shaping

Some teaching/training problems are not simply a matter of increasing or decreasing an existing operant. In many instructional situations, the response to be reinforced is not currently in the repertoire of the subject. Therefore, contingent access to some event or activity upon the occurrence of a behavior not in the repertoire of the client would not result in reinforcement of that response, since the behavior would probably not occur (Whitman, Scibak, & Reid, 1983). For example, using reinforcement contingencies alone in teaching a child with a profound handicap to wash his hands independently (given that the child is not currently capable of emitting any of the motor responses independently) would not result in skill acquisition on the part of the child. In these teaching situations, the problem is one of acquisition (Bailey & Bostow, 1981), and the behavior has to be shaped.

Shaping is the process of reinforcing successive behavioral approximations to a desired goal (Foxx, 1982; Popovich, 1983). Initially, many undergraduate psychology students come into contact with the process of shaping when they are required in an animal learning course to teach a rat to press the bar in the operant chamber. Most students eventually realize that just waiting for the rat to move to the bar and press it for reinforcement is not an efficient means of teaching such a response. The astute students learn quickly to reinforce behavioral approximations to the desired response. Shaping produces two results: (1) it increases the operant level of reinforced responses, and (2) it increases the variability of the topography of the response (Reynolds, 1975). It is the latter effect of reinforcement that allows the experimenter to alter the criteria for reinforcement, in that closer behavioral approximations of the desired target behavior begin to appear. The manipulation of the response criteria for reinforcement at various phases of the instructional program eventually "brings about" the independent occurrence of the desired behavior.

In reinforcing gradual approximations to a desired goal, a clear criterion at each phase should be set (Popovich, 1983). The initial form of the behavior to be reinforced has to be specified *a priori* so that anyone conducting the training can reinforce responses that reach the specified criterion (and also not reinforce responses that do not meet the criterion). A task analysis indicating successive behavioral approximations to the terminal skill is very important in determining the criterion for reinforcement at each phase of the program.

Shaping procedures have been used to bring eye contact to a child with severe handicaps under the control of the trainer's discriminative stimulus (Lovaas, Berberich, Perloff, & Schaeffer, 1966). Initially, the trainer reinforces the child for any head movements to the trainer's side of the table, within 30 seconds of the verbal cue "look at me." As this behavior occurs more frequently, the requirements for reinforcement are made more stringent. In the next phase, the child is reinforced only when he moves his head to face the trainer with 15 seconds of the command. Gradually, the time between verbal cue and occurrence of behavior is decreased, and the time required for maintaining eye contact is increased. The response required for reinforcement is changed across the various phases of the program until the criterion level of eye contact is occurring at an acceptable level.

Chaining

Many behaviors that are reinforced in everyday life are chains of behavior. Behavioral chains are comprised of multiple behaviors that occur in a sequence and lead to reinforcement upon completion of the chain. For example, going to work each day is comprised of a set of behaviors that ends in the person arriving at the work site (for argument's sake, this event is a conditioned reinforcer).

Behavioral chains illustrate how responses can serve as both discriminative stimuli (for the next response) and conditioned reinforcers (for the previous response). For example, the initial behavior of the chain of going to work is waking up. Waking up occurs in the presence of an alarm clock or a temporal discriminative stimulus (e.g., 6:30 A.M.). Waking up serves as the discriminative stimulus for the next behavior (e.g., getting out of bed). Getting out of bed is the conditioned reinforcer for waking up and then becomes the stimulus for the next behavior (e.g., going to the bathroom). This relationship between behaviors in the chain is continued throughout the entire chain until the terminal behavior occurs, which results in the delivery of reinforcement.

The use of stimulus prompts makes it easier to teach a chain of steps in sequence by providing additional "help" at points in the sequence in which the student's behavior is lacking. Extrastimulus prompts (Schreibman, 1975) that are utilized can be verbal, gestural, modeled, and physical. Such prompts can be removed with a time-delay fading technique. Fading allows for the behavior in the chain to come under stimulus control of the relevant discriminative stimulus. Generally, prompts are provided in the least intrusive fashion; that is, verbal and gestural are provided before modeled and physical prompts. Less intrusive prompts provide less help to the student regarding the desired performance. The sequence in which these prompts should be faded is the opposite sequence in which they were delivered. Generally, the more intrusive prompts are faded before prompts that are less intrusive.

Developing chains of behavior is accomplished by one of several types of chaining methods: backward chaining, forward chaining, and graduated guidance. All three methods utilize prompting and fading techniques to develop complex units of behavior (e.g., taking a bath, doing the laundry, tying shoelaces, and the like). The characteristics of each of these three chaining techniques are seen in Table 1.

Backward chaining procedures have been used to teach a wide variety of self-care skills (Baker, Brightman, Heifetz, & Murphy, 1976; Bensberg, Colwell, & Cassell, 1965). An example of backward chaining is found in a study that taught two female institutionalized residents with profound mental retardation to ascend stairs in an appropriate fashion (Cipani, Augustine, & Blomgren, 1982). Baseline data indicated that both residents would ascend

TABLE 1
Comparison of Behavioral Chaining Methods

Method	Delivery of reinforcement	Chain development	Target step(s)
Forward chaining	At end of target step	From front to back	First deficit step in front of chain
Backward chaining	At end of chain	From back to front	First deficit step from back of chain
Graduated guidance	At end of chain and throughout chain	All components of chain develop simultaneously	All deficit step(s)

stairs by using their hands and feet, without holding onto the guard rail, and also by climbing multiple steps in one leap. In the first phase, the resident was reinforced when she ascended two steps appropriately upon being placed two steps from the top of the stairway. The number of steps was gradually increased until the resident was ascending all the steps in the stairway appropriately. Generalization of this behavior occurred to a novel set of stairways.

Forward chaining methods have been used with a wide variety of self-care skills (Bender & Valletutti, 1976; Watson, 1978). Forward chaining involves the development of the chain from the initial steps of the sequence. As the client becomes independent in these initial target steps, the next steps in the sequence are targeted, until the entire chain is occurring independent of prompts.

Graduated guidance (Azrin & Armstrong, 1973; Azrin, Schaeffer, & Wesolowski, 1976) involves providing guidance wherever needed throughout the performance of the entire chain. A graduated guidance procedure was utilized in a state institution in teaching eight residents with moderate and mild handicaps independent toothbrushing skills (Horner & Keilitz, 1975). The training procedure utilized four levels of prompts with a 5-second latency between delivery of the prompts in the following order: (1) no help, (2) verbal instruction, (3) demonstration and verbal instruction, and (4) physical guidance and instruction. Each prompt level could be provided twice if incorrect or no responding occurred.

STIMULUS–RESPONSE RELATIONS

Stimulus–response relations examine the properties of the antecedent environment on the operant response. In this section, we will define and provide examples of the following terms: discriminative stimuli, discriminated behavior, stimulus control, and stimulus generalization. A discussion of stimulus control techniques will illustrate the application of stimulus–response relations to learning problems.

Discriminative Stimuli

As mentioned earlier, operant behaviors occur in the presence of certain stimuli. Stimuli do not elicit operant behaviors (unlike respondent behaviors). Rather, antecedent stimuli set the occasion, or evoke, certain operants, given the presence of a relevant motivative variable (Michael, 1987). A stimulus that (1) alters the momentary strength of a certain operant, and (2) sets the occasion for the reinforcement of such an operant(s) is termed a *discriminative stimulus* (Michael, 1987). Definitions that just refer to the relationship between stimulus and response then require another term (i.e., effective discriminative stimulus) to describe a stimulus that controls a response (Michael, 1987). But the above definition obviates this additional term by providing the relevant history in the definition (Michael, 1987).

Operants can be controlled by more than one discriminative stimulus. For example, stopping the car in the street should be controlled by multiple antecedent events: the presence of a red light at an intersection, the lane blocked by another car crossing the intersection, or a pedestrian crossing the street in front of the car.

In early operant research, the discriminative stimulus was presented for a period of time and then removed. Its absence set up the occasion for nonreinforcement of the selected response. The early researchers termed the absence of the discriminative stimulus the *nondiscriminative stimulus*. The nondiscriminative stimulus is a stimulus that sets the occasion for the lack of reinforcement of a certain response. The application to everyday examples is not as clear-cut. Nondiscriminative stimuli, which set the occasion for the nonreinforcement of a certain response, do set the occasion for reinforcement of some other response. It might be more useful to refer to all stimuli that evoke some operant response(s) as discriminative for some behavior, especially if one considers a lack of a response to be a "behavior," and avoid the use of the term nondiscriminative stimulus.

Discriminated Behavior

When a child is able to emit different responses to different discriminative stimuli, the child is demonstrating discriminative behavior. An example of discriminated behavior is a child who responds correctly to two different commands, such as "Touch your shoe!" and "Take off your shoe!" Discriminated operants come under the control of different discriminative stimuli through differential reinforcement. In the previous example, the occurrence of shoe-touching behavior is reinforced in the presence of the command "Touch your shoe!" Shoe-touching behavior would not be reinforced in the presence of the other command (i.e., "Take off your shoe!"). Similarly, taking off the shoe is reinforced in the presence of the respective command.

A common method of developing discriminated behavior is to present discriminative stimuli alternately. This procedure is termed a *discrimination task*. Using the previous example, the teacher would present the two commands (e.g., "Touch your shoe!" and "Take off your shoe!") in an alternate fashion. The correct response would result in reinforcement and an incorrect response would result in the withholding of reinforcement until the desired behavior occurs. In the formation of a discrimination (Reynolds, 1975), the teacher must alternate the presentation of at least two different discriminative stimuli, this procedure is termed a *two-choice discrimination task*. However, as the skill acquisition of the learner increases, a range of discrimination can be presented within a training session.

Stimulus Control

When a child's behavior can be reliably predicted given the presence of one stimulus or another, the behavior is said to be under stimulus control (Rodewald, 1979). Stimulus control denotes a high probability of a behavior in the presence of a given discriminative stimulus. Stimulus control can be seen in everyday examples (e.g., most people stop their cars at a red light; many children raise their hands in class when they want to speak; many people eat lunch at noon). Stimulus control is obtained through differential reinforcement of certain operants in the presence of discriminative stimuli.

Operants usually occur in the presence of discriminative stimuli with multiple elements. When the response reliably occurs in the presence of many discriminative stimulus elements, do all the elements of the stimulus control the operant? For example, one may see a dog approach its owner upon being called by name. The assumption of the observer might be that the stimulus, "Hey Rover, come here!" controls the running behavior of the dog. However, there are many more elements to this antecedent stimulus complex than just the command (i.e., the tone of voice used, possibly accompanying gestures, etc.). From a practical standpoint, one would like to believe that the specific command, "Hey Rover, come here!" controls the response. However, it is quite possible that the tone of voice (an irrelevant element) controls the dog's response of coming to its owner, regardless of the command given. In this case, stimulus control is restricted to an irrelevant element of the antecedent stimulus complex.

The identification of restricted stimulus control has important practical implications. From the previous example, one cannot assume that the relevant element of a stimulus complex controls the response. Understanding and analyzing the role of all the elements of the stimulus complex will lead to a more precise technology of teaching.

Lovaas and his colleagues found differential reinforcement alone to be an inadequate method for developing discriminated behavior in some children with autism (Lovaas, Koegel, & Schreibman, 1979). Their basic research on restricted stimulus control (which was termed *stimulus overselectivity*) attempted to provide an empirical explanation for the failure of autistic children to respond when a prompt is faded (Koegel & Rincover, 1976; Lovaas *et al.*, 1979; Lovaas, Schreibman, Koegel, & Rehm, 1971; Schreibman, 1975) and their failure to generalize across novel stimulus conditions. Errors, once previously thought to be random, must now be studied in order to identify controlling stimuli and provide data to program more effectively prompting and fading techniques that would lead to successful transfer of stimulus control.

Stimulus Generalization

When behavior that occurs under one stimulus occurs to a similar stimulus without previous exposure to reinforcement contingencies, the response is said to have generalized. *Generalization* is the transfer of stimulus control for a discriminative stimulus (in whose presence the response has been reinforced) to stimuli not having a previous history of reinforcement with such a response. Generalization occurs if a stimulus change decrement is not effected (Michael, 1987). It measures the spreading of the reinforcement effect. Of course, the response will be maintained to the novel stimulus only if reinforcement is contingent upon the generalized response.

Generalization has been studied in the operant laboratories for many years. A common experiment measuring generalization is to present three different colored keys (red, orange, and yellow) to a pigeon, while reinforcing responding only to one key (Reynolds, 1975). Reinforcing responding on the red key will increase the level of responses to this key while the other two keys show a stimulus change decrement (Michael, 1987). However, responding to the orange key remains at a higher level than the yellow key and extinguishes much more slowly. After generating extinction to the red key, it is again reinforced. Both nonreinforced responses to orange and to yellow show some recovery of response rate initially, but responding to yellow extinguished much quicker than responding to orange. In the presence of reinforcing responses to red, responding to orange does occur at some level higher than at another stimulus (yellow), thus showing some generalization effects.

Examples of generalization abound in everyday life. Children who are taught to say "thank you" at home and demonstrate such a response when given food at a restaurant exhibit generalization. Children who are trained to use the past tense form of the action verbs "-ed," often generalize such responding to special cases, such as in "win, winned" (i.e., generalizing when discriminating is required).

Stimulus control can transfer across novel settings, people, time, and other stimuli. Generalization across settings is often demonstrated when a child acquires a behavior at school, under given stimulus conditions, and exhibits the newly acquired behavior, under similar conditions, at home. In this particular case, generalization across novel people and time would also be demonstrated. The initial response was brought under control by the teacher, during the day, and then transferred to the parents, in the evening. In this example, the parents, although certainly having a history of reinforcing certain behaviors exhibited by their child, did not have a history of reinforcement with respect to the newly acquired behavior. Therefore, the occurrence of the behavior in the home constitutes a generalized response.

Generalization across stimuli is often desired by teaching staff. When the teacher develops reading skills in young children, he or she hopes that such behavior will not occur solely to the specific print of the words found in the primary training material (e.g., flashcards). Rather, the children should respond to these words in other and different forms of reading material (e.g., text, chalkboard).

A special case of generalization is response generalization in which stimulus control is not transferred across novel stimuli. Rather, the generalization is across responses not targeted under the designated contingencies. For example, reinforcing eye contact often brings an initial increase in other behaviors, such as proximity, and out-of-seat behavior, even though such behaviors are not directly reinforced.

Stimulus Control Strategies

Many learning problems involve transferring stimulus control from stimuli currently controlling the desired response to stimuli that currently do not control the response. The application of stimulus–response relations to these types of problems involves an analysis of stimulus control and programming methods that facilitates their transfer. Errorless learning paradigms involve gradual stimulus manipulations, with subsequent changes in the discriminative stimuli until all stimuli are at criterion level (Terrace, 1963). A three-category system for analyzing stimulus manipulations has been advanced (Cipani, 1987; Cipani & Madigan, 1987; Schilmoeller & Etzel, 1977a). These three programmatic strategies are stimulus shaping, stimulus fading, and superimposition. All three methods involve the initial alteration of the discriminative stimulus or stimuli, which produces immediate discriminated behavior on the part of the learner. Discriminated responding is then maintained throughout the changes in the initial presentation until the criterion level format is achieved.

Stimulus shaping involves a complete change in the topography of the initial presentation of the discriminative stimuli (Schilmoeller & Etzel, 1977). The stimulus configuration is gradually altered, or shaped, until the criterion level form of the discriminative stimulus or stimuli is presented. Stimulus-shaping programs involve many phases of stimulus changes. The instructional program requires much revision from the designer, utilizing evaluation data on the effectiveness of the stimulus-shaping sequence (Schilmoeller & Etzel, 1977).

Stimulus fading is the alteration of one or several elements of the criterion level stimulus or stimuli. Terrace (1963) utilized stimulus fading in developing discriminated responding to red- and green-colored keys by progressively altering the green key while maintaining a high rate of correct responses. The alteration of the green key was accomplished by changing the light intensity of the key (thereby changing the color of the green key from dark to bright green) and increasing the time length the green key was presented.

Superimposition is the addition of a superimposed prompt on the criterion level presentation of the discriminative stimulus. Prompts are additional discriminative stimuli that increase the probability of a correct response occurring to a stimulus that currently does not control the target response. Initially, these additional stimuli are presented simultaneously with the target discriminative stimulus, and the prompts are then faded. Fading is the gradual removal of the prompt, while maintaining the correct discriminated response during such stimulus changes.

The fading of superimposed prompts can be achieved either by a gradual withdrawal of its amount or intensity of the prompt or by a time delay of the prompt presentation. The manner in which a prompt is withdrawn cannot be specified *a priori*. Rather, the withdrawal of the prompt is a function of the particular learner's response rate.

An example of the first method of fading is illustrated in a study that sought to develop color discrimination behavior in a 16-year-old male with mental retardation, who was diagnosed organically blind (Stolz & Wolf, 1969). Baseline data indicated lack of color discrimination. The training procedure initially varied the size of the two different colored papers. The subject was allowed to touch each paper before choosing. The size of the papers was gradually altered until they were identical in size. At this point, the tactile cue was removed. The student was still able to continue responding correctly at a high level (statistically significant from chance level).

Time-delay fading has been used extensively in basic and applied research (Cipani, 1987; Cipani & Madigan, 1987; Gobbi, Cipani, Hudson, & Lapenta, 1986; Halle, Marshall, & Spradlin, 1979; Touchette, 1971; Smeets & Striefel, 1976; Striefel, Bryan, & Aikins, 1974). In utilizing a time-delay procedure, the prompt is faded by increasing the latency between its delivery and the presentation of the discriminative stimulus. As a result, the percentage of times the prompt is presented decreases across training until the learner is responding solely in the presence of the discriminative stimulus.

To a lesser extent in previous research publications, a technology of generalization has not developed a long standing history of research inquiry. And yet, many of the criticisms of behavioral treatment efforts dealt with the lack of generalization across varied relevant variables (e.g., time, settings, stimuli). Applied research efforts have begun to study procedures leading to a technology for producing generalization. Increases in such activity have come from criticisms that were leveled from others outside the field and the recognized need for a technology of generalization (Drabman, Hammer, & Rosenbaum, 1979; Stokes & Baer, 1977). Stokes and Baer (1977) identified a variety of strategies that could facilitate generalization. Strategies that planned for generalization *a priori* were seen as more capable of producing generalization in contrast to techniques that program generalization *post hoc* (Stokes & Baer, 1977).

A technology for programming generalization has been investigated in the design of direct instruction materials and principles (Becker & Engelmann, 1978; Engelmann & Carnine, 1982; Horner, Bellamy, & Colvin, 1984; Horner, Sprague, & Wilcox, 1982; P. Weisburg, Packer, & R. S. Weisburg,

1981). A large focus of their research and instructional development work has identified the juxtaposition of positive and negative examples in the instructional sequence as important variables in developing a generalized response across relevant elements (Carnine, 1980; Horner *et al.*, 1984; Horner, Eberhard, & Sheehan, 1986).

Current research has identified that the training of a sufficiently generalized response is a function of providing both the range of positive examples as well as minimally different negative examples. In teaching appropriate table-bussing skills, Horner *et al.* (1986) found that general case programming was effective in developing target skills to natural stimuli that should occasion such behavior. Through the use of negative training examples, the precision of the training program to develop the absence of table-bussing behaviors to stimuli that should not occasion such behaviors (e.g., when food was still on the plate, or while people were still eating) was also demonstrated.

This area of research has also examined the role of stimulus control by irrelevant features as a primary cause of faulty generalization (Horner *et al.*, 1984). This topic requires more attention than what is provided here, and the reader should consult further references in this fascinating area of research inquiry (Engelmann & Carnine, 1982).

SUMMARY

This chapter has provided a brief discussion of the basic principles of operant behavior. Two sets of relations between temporally ordered events were examined: response–consequence relations and stimulus–response relations. Both sets of relations identify the effects of environmental variables on the rate of response, the basic method of studying behavior.

Although methodology has certainly played a major role in distinguishing behavior analysis from other explanations of human behavior, the basic principles derived from laboratory research have guided practitioners in the design of effective treatment programs. The use of such principles leads to more efficient direct solutions to basic social problems, both current and future. In the chapters that follow, this basic analysis of behavior will be reflected as well as the methodological requirements of applied research. As behavior analysis looks to the future to solve continuing problems facing humanity, it will look to its "roots" in the basic principles of behavior to develop an effective technology for solving such problems.

REFERENCES

Azrin, N. H., & Armstrong, P. M. (1973). "The mini-meal": A method for teaching eating skills to the profoundly retarded. *Mental Retardation, 11,* 9–11.

Azrin, N. H., Schaeffer, R. M., & Wesolowski, M. D. (1976). A rapid method of teaching profoundly retarded persons to dress by a reinforcement-guidance method. *Mental Retardation, 14,* 29–33.

Baer, D. M., Wolf, M. M., & Risley, T. R. (1968). Some current dimensions of applied behavior analysis. *Journal of Applied Behavior Analysis, 1,* 91–97.

Bailey, J. S., & Bostow, D. E. (1981). *Research methods in applied behavior analysis.* Tallahassee, FL: Copy Grafix.

Baker, B. L., Brightman, A. J., Heifetz, L. J., & Murphy, D. N. (1976). *Steps to independence: A skills training series for children with special needs.* Champaign, IL: Research Press.

Becker, W. C., & Engelmann, S. (1974). *Achievement gains of disadvantaged children with IQ's under 80 in follow through* (Tech. Rep. No. 74-2). Eugene: University of Oregon Follow Through Project.

Becker, W. C. & Engelmann, S. E. (1978). Systems for basic instruction: Theory and applications. In A. Catania & T. Brigham (Eds.), *Handbook of applied behavior analysis: Social and instructional processes.* New York: Irvington.

Bender, M., & Valletutti, P. J. (1976). *Teaching the moderately and severely handicapped: Curriculum objectives, strategies and activities.* Baltimore: University Park Press.

Bensberg, G. J., Colwell, C. N. & Cassell, R. H. (1965). Teaching the profoundly retarded self-help activities by behavior shaping techniques. *American Journal of Mental Deficiency, 69,* 674–679.

Carnine, D. W. (1980). Three procedures for presenting minimally different positive and negative instances. *Journal of Educational Psychology, 72,* 452–456.

Catania, A. C. (1984). *Learning* (2nd ed.). Englewood Cliffs, NJ: Prentice-Hall.

Cipani, E. (1987). Errorless learning technology: Theory, research and practice. In J. L. Matson & R. P. Barett (Eds.), *Advances in developmental disorder* (pp. 237–275). Greenwich, CT: JAI Press.

Cipani, E., & Madigan, K. (1987). Errorless learning: Research and application for "difficult-to-teach" children. *Canadian Journal of Exceptional Children, 3,* 39–43.

Cipani, E., Augustine, A., & Blomgren, E. (1982). Teaching severely and profoundly retarded adults to ascend stairs safely. *Education and Training of the Mentally Retarded, 17,* 51–54.

Drabman, R. S., Hammer, D., & Rosenbaum, M. S. (1979). Assessing generalization in behavior modification with children: The generalization map. *Behavioral Assessment, 1,* 203–219.

Englemann, S., & Carnine, D. (1982). *Theory of instruction: Principles and applications.* New York: Irvington.

Ferster, C. B., & Skinner, B. F. (1957). *Schedules of reinforcement.* New York: Appleton-Century-Crofts.

Foxx, R. M. (1982). *Increasing behaviors of severely retarded and autistic persons.* Champaign, IL: Research Press.

Gobbi, L., Cipani, E., Hudson, C., & Lapenta, R. (1986). Developing "spontaneous requesting" among children with severe mental retardation. *Mental Retardation, 24,* 357–363.

Halle, J. W., Marshall, A. M. & Spradlin, J. E. (1979). Time delay: A technique to increase language use and facilitate generalization in retarded children. *Journal of Applied Behavior Analysis, 12,* 431–439.

Horner, R. D., & Keilitz, I. (1975). Training mentally retarded adolescents to brush their teeth. *Journal of Applied Behavior Analysis, 8,* 301–310.

Horner, R. H., Sprague, J., & Wilcox, B. (1982). Constructing general case programs for community activities. In B. Wilcox & T. Bellamy (Eds.), *Design of high school for severely handicapped students* (pp. 61–98). Baltimore: Brookes.

Horner, R. H., Bellamy, G. T. & Colvin, G. T. (1984). Responding in the presence of nontrained stimuli: Implications of generalization error patterns. *Journal of the Association for Persons with Severe Handicaps, 9,* 287–296.

Horner, R. H., Eberhard, J. M. & Sheehan, M. R. (1986). Teaching generalized table bussing: The importance of negative teaching examples. *Behavior Modification, 10,* 457–471.

Kazdin, A. E. (1977). Assessing the clinical or applied importance of behavior change through social validation. *Behavior Modification, 1,* 427–452.

Koegel, R. L., & Rincover, A. (1976). Some detrimental effects of using extra-stimuli to guide learning in normal and autistic children. *Journal of Abnormal Child Psychology, 4,* 59–71.

Lovaas, O. I., Berberich, J. P., Perloff, B. F., & Schaeffer, B. (1966). Acquisition of imitative speech by schizophrenic children. *Science, 151,* 705–707.

Lovaas, O. I., Schreibman, L., Koegel, R. L., & Rehm, R. (1971). Selective responding by autistic children to multiple sensory input. *Journal of Abnormal Psychology, 77*, 211–222.

Lovaas, O. I., Koegel, R. L., & Schreibman, L. (1979). Stimulus overselectivity in autism: A review of research. *Psychological Bulletin, 86*, 1236–1254.

Michael, J. (1987). *Advanced topics of behavior analysis.* San Mateo, CA: Northern Association for Behavior Analysis.

Popovich, D. (1983). *Effective educational and behavioral programming for severely and profoundly handicapped students: A manual for teachers and aides.* Baltimore: Brookes.

Repp, A. C., & Brulle, A. R. (1981). Reducing aggressive behavior of mentally retarded persons. In J. L. Matson & J. R. McCarthy (Eds.), *Handbook of behavior modification with the mentally retarded* (pp. 177–210). New York: Plenum Press.

Reynolds, G. S. (1975). *A primer of operant conditioning* (2nd ed.). Glenview: IL: Scott, Foresman.

Rodewald, H. K. (1979). *Stimulus control of behavior.* Baltimore: University Park Press.

Schilmoeller, K. J., & Etzel, B. C. (1977a). *A review of errorless stimulus control: Implications for a technology of errorless programming.* Unpublished manuscript, University of Kansas, Department of Human Development, Lawrence.

Schreibman, L. (1975). Effects of within-stimulus and extra-stimulus prompting on discrimination learning in autistic children. *Journal of Applied Behavior Analysis, 8*, 91–112.

Skinner, B. F. (1957). *Verbal behavior.* New York: Appleton-Century-Crofts.

Smeets, P. M., & Striefel, S. (1976). Acquisition of sign reading by transfer of stimulus control in a deaf retarded girl. *Journal of Mental Deficiency, 20*, 197–205.

Stokes, T. F., & Baer, D. M. (1977). An implicit technology of generalization. *Journal of Applied Behavior Analysis, 10*, 457–471.

Stolz, S. B., & Wolf, M. M. (1969). Visually discriminated behavior in a "blind" adolescent retardate. *Journal of Applied Behavior Analysis, 2*, 65–74.

Striefel, S., Bryan, K. S., & Aikins, D. A. (1974). Transfer of stimulus control from motor to verbal stimuli. *Journal of Applied Behavior Analysis, 7*, 123–135.

Terrace, H. S. (1963). Discrimination learning with and without errors. *Journal of the Experimental Analysis of Behavior, 6*, 1–27.

Touchette, P. E. (1971). Transfer of stimulus control: Measuring the moment of transfer. *Journal of the Experimental Analysis of Behavior, 15*, 347–354.

Touchette, P., & Howard, J. S. (1984). Errorless learning: Reinforcement contingencies and stimulus control transfer in delayed prompting. *Journal of Applied Behavior Analysis, 17*, 175–188.

Watson, L. S. (1978). *A management system approach to teaching independent living skills and managing disruptive behavior.* Tuscaloosa, AL: Behavior Modification Technology.

Weisburg, P., Packer, R. A. & Weisburg, R. S. (1981). Academic training. In J. L. Matson & J. R. McCartney (Eds.), *Handbook of behavior modification with the mentally retarded* (pp. 331–411). New York: Plenum Press.

Whitman, T. L., Scibak, J. W., & Reid, D. H. (1983). *Behavior modification with the severely and profoundly retarded: Research and application.* New York: Academic Press.

Wolf, M. M. (1978). Social validity: The case for subjective measurement, or how applied behavior analysis is finding its heart. *Journal of Applied Behavior Analysis, 11*, 203–214.

III

Treating Disruptive Behavior

6

Self-Injurious Behavior

STEPHEN R. SCHROEDER, JOHANNES ROJAHN,
JAMES A. MULICK, AND CAROLYN S. SCHROEDER

Defining self-injurious behavior (SIB) presents some difficulties. It has been broadly defined as behavior that produces injury to the individual's own body (Tate & Baroff, 1966a), and thus could be seen as including suicide, self-neglect, substance abuse, malingering, and so forth—all terms that infer some intent on the part of the client. The research literature on modification of SIB, however, has settled on a narrower definition: overt acts directed toward oneself that have restricted spatial and temporal topographies, whose rate of occurrence is reliably observable, and whose consequences are actual or threatened physical damage. Even this definition is not satisfactory, though. S. R. Schroeder, Mulick, and Rojahn (1980) have pointed out that it suffers from three flaws: (1) the consequences specified by the term do not pertain functionally to the reinforcing stimuli responsible for maintaining the behaviors; (2) researchers disagree about the membership of various topographies in the response class of SIB; and (3) no single intervention strategy is indicated for the particular "class" of SIB as opposed to other behaviors.

In this chapter, we will attempt to analyze critically the research literature on SIB in pursuit of answers to these questions. A brief review of the various etiological models of SIB will be followed by a discussion of antecedent conditions and the ecology of SIB, response-contingent management techniques, evaluation of treatment effects, and, finally, programmatic considerations with SIB. In updating this chapter, we will focus on research that has been published since 1981, when the first edition of this volume was published.

ETIOLOGICAL MODELS OF SIB

There are several excellent recent reviews of etiological models of SIB. Because Romanczyk (1986) provides a comprehensive analysis of 36 of these reviews that were published since 1971, only a summary of this work will be given here.

STEPHEN R. SCHROEDER, JOHANNES ROJAHN, AND JAMES A. MULICK • The Nisonger Center, Ohio State University, Columbus, Ohio 43201.   CAROLYN S. SCHROEDER • Department of Pediatrics, University of North Carolina, Chapel Hill, North Carolina 27514.

Studies of the etiology and pathogenesis of SIB suggest that it is not a unitary phenomenon. It is exhibited in a wide variety of behavioral topographies and environmental settings. At present, only two organic syndromes are known to have a high incidence of SIB as symptoms: Lesch–Nyhan and Cornelia de Lange syndromes. There exist several motivational conditions conductive to the development of SIB: arrested development, avoidance conditioning, stimulus discrimination for positive reward, stereotyped behavior related to arousal arising from disruption of homeostasis, and conditioned emotional responding elicited by anxiety-producing stimuli.

Medical Etiology

Lesch–Nyhan Syndrome

Physicians have developed increased interest in the physiological components of self-injurious behavior since the description of Lesch–Nyhan syndrome in 1964 (Lesch & Nyhan, 1964; Nyhan, 1967, 1968a,b). Lesch–Nyhan syndrome is a sex-linked disorder of purine metabolism in which the child demonstrates spasticity, choreoathetosis, possible mental retardation, elevated urine uric acid (the serum uric acid may also be elevated), self-mutilation, and aggressive behaviors. Mutilation, especially biting of the oral structures and fingers, is most common; this mutilation does cause pain, and the child may welcome restraints to prevent further injury. Patients can cause such severe self-mutilation that the mouth orifice is totally deformed or the fingers are lost.

The self-mutilation appears to be, at least in part, under voluntary control and may be partly related to attention-getting behaviors. However, in most cases, the patient's self-mutilation seems to be rather compulsive and uncontrollable. In addition, patients develop other forms of self-destruction, such as sticking their fingers in the spokes of their wheelchairs or throwing themselves off furniture, and may also show aggressive behaviors toward others. These other self-destructive and aggressive behaviors seem to be less compulsive and are geared more toward attention-getting.

It should be noted that the self-mutilation occurs in patients who are of near-normal intelligence and verbally communicative as well as in those with more severe intellectual and communication handicaps (Nyhan, 1976).

Lesch–Nyhan syndrome represents the first condition with a demonstrated biochemical defect in which very specific abnormal behaviors are described. However, the exact connection between the defect and the self-mutilation is unknown. Although the serum uric acid level may be elevated, reduction of the uric acid level with Allopurinol does not alter the neurological or behavioral phenomena. In addition, a survey of serum uric acid levels in an institutionalized mentally retarded population (Brandon Training School in Vermont) resulted in no definite correlation between serum uric acid levels and self-injurious responses. Thus, the uric acid level does not seem to be the determinant of the abnormal behavior. Although it is frustrating to know the specific biochemical defect in a condition and yet not be able to determine its relationship to behavior, it is to be hoped that this defect will be a clue toward an understanding of several different types of self-injurious behavior.

Recent neurobiological studies, especially animal models, suggest that dopamine depletion in the basal ganglia or an imbalance in neurotransmitter function in brain dopamine pathways that is due to their aberrant perinatal development may be a strong establishing condition for self-biting (see Baumeister, Frye, & S. R. Schroeder, 1984; Breese, Mueller, & S. R. Schroeder, 1986; and S. R. Schroeder, Breese, & Mueller, 1989, for a review of these models). This is an exciting new development, in that (1) it may pave the way for rational pharmacotherapy based on neuropharmacological theory rather than on trial and error, and (2) it may uncover methods for prevention of SIB (S. R. Schroeder, Bickel, & Richmond, 1986).

Cornelia de Lange Syndrome

Self-mutilation may also be a common accompaniment in Cornelia de Lange syndrome (Bryson, Sakati, Nyhan, & Fish, 1971; Marie, Royer, & Rappaport, 1967). This syndrome is characterized by low birth weight, retarded growth, hirsutism, a distinctive facies, and digital abnormalities. No specific genetic etiology has been demonstrated, no consistent chromosomal abnormalities have been found, and no biochemical defect has been identified. As a result, there is little apparent similarity between this syndrome and Lesch–Nyhan syndrome except for the tendency to self-mutilation. In Cornelia de Lange syndrome, the self-abusive behaviors include self-inflicted blunt trauma (hitting the face, extremities, trunk) as well as self-biting. Each patient appears to have individual stereotyped forms of self-abuse, and not all the case reports have noted the very destructive biting, which is always involved in Lesch–Nyhan syndrome. The compulsive quality of the self-injury, so striking in Lesch–Nyhan syndrome, is also absent. Operant programs have been noted as being effective in the management of both disorders (Duker, 1975b; Singh, 1981; Singh, Gregory, & Pullman, 1980).

Other Organic Theories

There are no other known physiological conditions with such a high incidence of self-injurious behavior. Patients with peripheral neuropathies, such as supersensitivity to or insensitivity to pain, also may demonstrate self-mutilation, but here the origin is more accidental and related to the lack of awareness of the damage being inflicted. These hypotheses, which have been reviewed recently by Cataldo and Harris (1982), Edelson (1984), and Levitt (1985), are based almost exclusively upon animal models that produce dysesthesias (i.e., unpleasant abnormal body experiences that might or might not be painful), such as peripheral neuropathies, somatosensory deafferentation, neurosensory deficits, and the like. The applicability of such animal models to human sensations that may cause SIB is not implausible, but it is also not very convincing at present. Proponents of this view would have to reconcile the following facts with their hypothesis: (1) the lack of incidence of SIB among traumatic brain-injured patients or among human subjects with experimentally induced paresthesias who are not retarded; and (2) the ruling out of other types of brain injury as causes of SIB among the severely and profoundly mentally retarded, where the prevalence of SIB is highest.

Psychodynamic Interpretations

Psychodynamic interpretations (e.g., Crabtree, 1967; Fitzherbert, 1950; Frederick & Resnik, 1971; Freud, 1954; Greenacre, 1954; Slawson & Davidson, 1964; Stinnett & Hollander, 1970) have viewed SIB as symbolic behavior related to infantile or fetal drives, or displacement upon oneself of one's anger and aggression toward others, or symbolic suicidal or masochistic tendencies, or self-stimulation related to parental rejection (see Lester, 1972, and Sandler, 1964, for review). What little research is available on these theories does not support such interpretations, and most psychotherapeutic methods have been ineffective in treating SIB. It is difficult to see how such interpretations apply to severely mentally retarded persons, in whom SIB is most prevalent, since these people to a large extent appear to have impaired symbolic thought processes as far as we know. In addition to these problems, they often lack expressive language to relate such thoughts, assuming that they occur.

Behavioral Motivational Interpretations

Behavioral motivational interpretations of SIB assume that it is behavior that is functionally related to consequences of reward in the subject's environment. There are at least five behavioral analyses, which are not mutually exclusive, of how SIB might come to be learned.

The Avoidance Hypothesis

The basic notion involved in the avoidance hypothesis was first proposed by Skinner (1953) and demonstrated very reliably with animals (Byrd, 1969; Kelleher, Riddle, & Cook, 1963; Sidman, Hernstein, & Conrad, 1957; Stretch, Orloff, & Dalrymple, 1968; M. Waller & P. Waller, 1963). It states that individuals might expose themselves to aversive stimulation—like SIB—in order to avoid more aversive consequences. This, of course, is a commonplace of everyday life and is known experimentally as avoidance learning. In avoidance learning, the behavior is associated with strong emotional response and is very resistant to extinction, even long after the avoidance stimulus has been withdrawn. Both of these characteristics are frequently observed with SIB.

This explanation of SIB requires a history or aversive stimulation and avoidance conditioning. Reported clinical studies of SIB that developed from conditioned avoidance of present or prior aversive stimulation are very few. Green (1968) reported a relationship between parental physical abuse and SIB among schizophrenic children. Thus, in some cases, SIB may develop to avoid more severe attacks. There is also some clinical justification for suggesting that SIB is related to avoidance of social contact. For instance, autistic children often display "tactile defensiveness" (i.e., they tend to avoid physical contact). The mentally retarded individual may often perform high rates of SIB upon release from restraint (Corte, Wolf, & Locke, 1971; R. F. Peterson & L. R. Peterson, 1968). Sometimes they even attempt to tie themselves down again (Tate, 1972). Social contact or particular caregivers may serve as aversive rather than positively rewarding stimuli. Nevertheless, there are many instances in which SIB in mentally retarded persons has developed in environments in which no primarily aversive social consequences could be identified. Although the avoidance hypothesis alone is inadequate to account for the pathogenesis of SIB, it does point out that the history of rewards and punishments is critical to the strategy for treatment.

Operant/Respondent Model

The operant/respondent model of SIB is an expansion of the operant model that attempts to account for the persistence and prepotency some stimuli have in eliciting SIB, such as is seen in avoidance conditioning (Romanczyk, 1986). It is suggested that SIB responses produce arousal stimuli or respondently conditioned emotional states that, when reduced, affect the stimulus complex presented to the client on subsequent occasions and thereby increase the probability of subsequent SIB. Such emotional states as arousal, hypertension, or depression become eliciting stimuli whose reductions are themselves reinforcing and tend, therefore, to increase the strength of SIB as an operant that produces them. Therapy would largely revolve around breaking this vicious cycle.

The operant/respondent model has much to recommend because of its comprehensive approach, but, at this point, there has not been a direct test of it. Relevant psychophysiological studies involving desensitization or biofeedback of arousal with SIB have generally shown a poor correlation between psychophysiological arousal and SIB probability. The relationship between conditioned emotional states or stimuli and situation specificity of some SIB topographies still remains to be explored. Nevertheless, they can be strong setting factors for SIB.

Stereotyped Response

In this view, SIB is considered an extreme case of the stereotypy frequently observed among mentally retarded persons, especially those who are institutionalized (Baumeister & Forehand, 1973). It is seen as an instrumental response developed from more benign types of stereotyped acts. For example, head banging might have had as its antecedents such activities as body rocking, body twirling, and hand waving, which were then shaped into head banging.

Again, this explanation is only a partial one. Stereotyped acts are repetitious, topographically invariant motor behaviors or action sequences in which reward is unspecified or noncontingent and the performance of which is considered pathological (S. Schroeder, 1970). SIB fits this definition in certain forms like head banging. However, many types of SIB are nonrhythmical, like gouging and digging, and are often unpredictable and highly variable in their occurrence. One current neurobiological theory (Barron & Sandman, 1983) suggests that some SIB which is stereotyped is mediated by different neural substrates than SIB which is not stereotyped.

In addition, when approaching SIB in terms of stereotyped behavior, one must deal with the uncertainties about the pathogenesis of stereotyped behavior (Baumeister, 1978; Berkson, 1967, 1983, 1987; Lewis & Baumeister, 1982; Lovaas, Newsom, & Hickman, 1987). The most widely accepted explanation of stereotyped behavior, however, is that it is a symptom of imbalance of internal homeostasis, perhaps central nervous system (CNS) arousal, which is precipitated by such things as sensory deprivation, sensory overload, and frustration (Berkson & Mason, 1964a,b; Green, 1967), and which is reinforced by response-produced sensory feedback. When applied to SIB, this would mean that environmental contingencies, such as parental neglect in infancy or lack of stimulation on a ward, could thus be the setting for homeostatic imbalance, and SIB a self-stimulatory mechanism for raising or lowering arousal to restore balance (Edelson, 1984; Lovaas, 1982). But this idea is difficult to document experimentally. Kohlenberg, Levin, and Belcher (1973) recorded skin conductance as a psychophysiological measure of arousal before, during, and after treatment of a severe case of SIB. They found that SIB resulted in increased levels of arousal after the client was removed from physical restraints, but before removal of restraints, there was no relationship between rates of SIB and amount of increase in skin conductance level. Furthermore, reduction in SIB after punishment produced effects on arousal different from those that were due to SIB itself. A simple homeostatic relationship of SIB to arousal levels did not occur and argues against the homeostatic and therefore the stereotyped behavior explanation of SIB.

Another argument against the general arousal hypothesis is that, as the subsequent literature review shows, SIB most often occurs in a specific context under specific environmental conditions. In addition, treatment of SIB does not generalize to other situations easily. This result would be unexpected if only internal homeostasis were involved. Although stimulus deprivation or stereotypy may be variables related to the pathogenesis of SIB, they cannot be considered an adequate explanation of it.

The Developmental Hypothesis

The developmental hypothesis is based on the assumption that SIB is a vestige of earlier motor behaviors that were adaptive (Lourie, 1949) for motor and personality development but that have never been outgrown (e.g., head banging in the crib). Perhaps head banging is maintained by coincidental reinforcement or persists after a disruption in child–caretaker relationships. There is some support for this view from animal studies of developmental insult related to maternal deprivation (Davenport & Berkson, 1963; Erwin, Mitchell, & Maple, 1973; Gluck & Sackett, 1974) and the significance of vestibular stimulation in infancy for later development (Clark, Kreutzberg, & Chee, 1977; Gregg, Haffner, & Korner, 1976; Sallustro & Atwell, 1978). The latter has been the stimulus for occupational therapy-oriented sensory integration programs designed to decrease SIB (Bittick, Fleeman, & Bright, 1978; Lemke & Mitchell, 1972; M. E. Wells & Smith, 1983). However, there is not enough research on the sensory integration hypothesis of SIB to evaluate it as yet. It is not known whether the need for vestibular stimulation can account for the occurrence of SIB, although this speculation is interesting.

The Discriminative Stimulus-Conditioned Reinforcer Hypothesis

One explanation of SIB, also posited by Skinner (1953), is based on the assumption that an aversive stimulus (SIB) might be paired with a positive reward that maintains it. This result has also been reliably demonstrated in animals and humans (Ayllon & Azrin, 1966; Brown, Martin, & Morrow, 1964; Holz & Azrin, 1961, 1962; Murray & Nevin, 1967; Stubbs & Silverman, 1972). Thus, under appropriate conditions, aversive stimulation during SIB could act as a signal informing the subject of impending positive rewards like attention, affection, and contact.

The discrimination hypothesis can account for a great deal of SIB that develops among mentally retarded persons. SIB is most prevalent among the severely and profoundly mentally retarded who also lack communication skills. For this type of individual, performing SIB, a response that cannot be ignored, could be tantamount to establishing communication and taking command of the environment. This view has been advanced cogently by Carr (1977) and his student (Durand, 1986) to great advantage for the past decade.

A number of studies involving treatment of SIB have noted that it occurred only under specific conditions of presentation or withdrawal of discriminative social stimuli (Corte et al., 1971; Lane & Domrath, 1970; Lovaas, Schaeffer, & Simmons, 1965; Lovaas & Simmons, 1969; R. F. Peterson & L. R. Peterson, 1968) and was maintained by its (SIB) consequences. Even though this explanation is suggestive, the necessary research differentiating it from competing hypotheses remains to be done. Many of the studies were conducted under conditions that did not permit adequate experimental control. That SIB is more than just intentional communication seems almost certain. If it were not, teaching language alone should suffice to eliminate SIB. Teaching discrimination and communication skills may be important, but it is usually not a sufficient condition by itself for the elimination of SIB over a long period of time. However, the discrimination hypothesis does point out the need to replace SIB with more appropriate alternative behaviors if it is to be eliminated successfully.

Summary

None of the above explanations is mutually exclusive and none alone accounts satisfactorily for the development of SIB. All of them are indirectly inferred from observation of current repertoires. It is likely that some or all of these conditions could be present in a single case of SIB. Research must be done that differentiates how each of these antecedents contributes to the development of SIB before an adequate and preferable treatment mode can be recommended. The ecobehavioral approach to be discussed in the next section focuses on methods that look more closely at a functional analysis of antecedent stimulus conditions.

ANTECEDENT CONDITIONS AND THE ECOLOGY OF SELF-INJURIOUS BEHAVIOR

Viewing self-injurious behavior as an operant response has had tremendous heuristic as well as practical value. It offers testable hypotheses, variables that are generally readily accessible, and a history of treatment procedures that permits optimism. Although in using this approach one cannot completely isolate antecedent stimuli from a response (or its parameters) or from the contingencies of reinforcement affecting the response, each of these interdependent aspects should be considered. In the next three sections, we shall discuss each of these aspects as they occur in SIB, particularly as they are relevant to treatment.

This section, which is concerned with a functional analysis of antecedent stimulus conditions and their importance for understanding the development and management of SIB, will present a compilation of some empirical data from the current literature from the points of view of (1) environmental conditions as setting occasions for SIB, (2) differential stimulus control of SIB, (3) interaction of environmental conditions with effectiveness of intervention, and (4) environmental conditions and response selection. Suggestions will also be offered on how these data relate to research and future directions. Before beginning, however, it will be helpful to mention some concepts that will be relevant to our discussion.

Ecology is a term shared by scientists in many fields. Its meaning, which varies greatly across disciplines, is still evolving with the purpose and perspective of the users (Rogers-Warren & Warren, 1977). At least two different but interdependent dimensions of ecology can be identified when it is applied to behavioral assessment of persons in small groups (Vyse, Mulick, & Thayer, 1984). The first refers to the system of *intrapersonal behavior,* in which the person is viewed as demonstrating a complex of interdependent behaviors. In this context, it is assumed that by changing one behavior, other behaviors of the same person will be affected. The second refers to a person within his or her *physical* and *social* context. Here, the arrangement of settings is seen as influencing a person's behavior, and this person is seen, in return, as affecting his or her environment (Rogers-Warren & Warren, 1977).

Ecological types of research with mentally retarded persons have been pursued mainly by experimental psychologists who have been influenced by ethology and who have carried out studies about complex nonverbal social behavior, such as territoriality, dominance, food sharing, social behavior with peers, and communication derived from theories of animal behavior (Berkson & Landesman-Dwyer, 1977). Researchers engaged in ecological psychology have not given much attention to research with the developmentally disabled (Schoggen, 1978), but the basic assumptions of this approach have been recognized and integrated into a more planned-control manner. Because of the increasing concern with stimulus conditions in natural environments and the need for a new rationale and technology, behavior analysts have begun to adapt technologies that attempt to describe carefully persons, environments, and their interactions. These methods show promise of revealing complex constellations of stimulus–response interrelationships involved in long-term behavior change.

This approach which has been labeled "ecobehavioral analysis" by Warren (1977), can be understood as the second step of the experimental behavior analysis beyond the operant animal laboratory. Applied behavior analysis has attempted to transfer the close control over stimulus–response functions from the controlled environment of the laboratory into the natural environment of human beings and the application of operant principles "to the problems of social importance" (Baer, Wolf, & Risley, 1968). The ecobehavioral approach holds the promise of providing a better understanding of how the environment and the behavior of its inhabitants impact on each other with respect to their long-term relationships. Already it has yielded important results with the emotionally disturbed (Wahler, House, & Stambaugh, 1976), with autistic children (Lichtstein & Wahler, 1976), and also with aberrant behaviors in mentally retarded persons (Axelrod, 1987; S. Schroeder et al., 1982; S. R. Schroeder et al., 1986; Vyse et al., 1984). The following review of how environmental antecedent conditions affect the occurrence of SIB will indicate the impact that the ecobehavioral approach can have on the treatment of SIB.

Analysis of Setting Occasions for SIB

Carr's (1977) influential review of the various sources of motivation for SIB turned researchers toward a functional analysis of antecedent factors affecting the occurrence of SIB. Another paper by Iwata, Dorsey, Slifer, Bauman, and Richman (1982) proposed standardized settings that would suggest different types of behavioral interventions for SIB. Thereafter, an increased interest in stimulus control of SIB grew, to the extent that Wieseler, Hanson, Chamberlain, and Thompson (1985) posited a functional taxonomy of SIB based on (1) positive environmental consequences, (2) task escape/avoidance, and (3) self-stimulation. Before we can accept such a taxonomy, we must examine some of the assumptions and the evidence for stimulus control of SIB.

Our first assumption is that there is a controlling stimulus for every SIB.

As Sidman (1978) stated, "behavior is never underdetermined." To be useful, therefore, a functional taxonomy must be exhaustive, mutually exclusive, and representative of the research literature on SIB. A second assumption is that the controlling stimuli can be defined. Few studies have demonstrated that stimuli defined by the therapist controlled SIB and that other stimuli did not. The only procedure known to the authors that demonstrates a functional taxonomy based on *differential* stimulus control is the scatter-plot technique of Touchette, MacDonald, and Langer (1985). In this study, it was found that SIB topographies happened at specific times of the day and week and not at others. Readjusting the clients' schedules nearly eliminated the SIB without manipulating any consequences. This demonstration is different from the standardized settings of Iwata *et al.* (1982), in which stimulus control is inferred from frequency of response across settings, and in which an intervention is hypothesized and tested. Such an intervention does not control for other antecedent stimuli, which are not specified by the therapist, but which could account in whole or in part for the outcome of an intervention. An example might be the client's emotional state. Most of the available research is of this latter type, in which control is demonstrated by successively presenting and removing a stimulus for SIB.

Situational Demands

Carr, Newsom, and Binkoff (1976) attempted to isolate situational demands that had controlled the SIB of a mildly mentally retarded autistic child. The subject was exposed to several demand and nondemand situations. Then the situations were changed so that demands occurred only in the context of positive social interaction between the child and the experimenter. The levels of SIB were high in demand situations and were decreased in nondemand conversational situations. In further support of the idea of the escape response function of self-hitting, the child abruptly stopped hitting himself when he was presented with the stimulus that normally signaled termination of a demand period. Other stimuli that were never related to the termination did not decrease SIB. In addition, SIB during demand sessions showed a scalloped pattern, the type of responding generally encountered of fixed-interval schedules of escape in lower organisms (cf. Carr, 1977). As indicated previously, several other authors have indicated that self-injury may function as an escape response from a variety of aversive situations (e.g., cf. Carr, 1977; Myers & Diebert, 1971; Wolf, Risley, Johnson, Harris, & Allen, 1967) or as conditioned avoidance of social contacts (Corte *et al.*, 1971; R. F. Peterson & L. R. Peterson, 1968).

Physical Self-Restraint

In one study, Favell, McGimsey, and Jones (1978) demonstrated the positively reinforcing function of physical restraint (rigid arm splints). Rapid and complete reduction of SIB was achieved when the subjects were physically restrained contingent on increasing periods without self-injury and on providing toys and attention during intervals between the wearing of restraints. When physical restraint was applied contingent on toy play, this response increased. Favell, McGimsey, Jones, and Cannon (1981) replicated these findings. Several interpretations were offered to explain the results. It was argued that (1) stimulus-change components of restraint might constitute positive reinforcement in nonstimulating environments; or that (2) restraint may be paired with a reduction in aversive stimuli, such as staff-imposed demands, and that self-injury in some individuals may function as an escape *into* restraint conditions; or that (3) restraint also could be paired with adult attention, and may therefore provide relative physical comfort. The points raised for the explanation of these somewhat paradoxical properties of restraints are well taken.

Self-Protective Devices

Sometimes when a client is emitting dangerous self-injurious behaviors for which behavior management or medication is not working, it is necessary for the client to wear a prosthetic device to allow wounds to heal, to protect the client from further self-harms, or to use as an adjunct until a behavior program becomes effective in controlling the SIB (Richmond, S. R. Schroeder, & Bickel, 1986). Frequent self-protective methods involve arm splints, mittens, protective padding, helmets, camisoles, and bed restraints.

When used as part of a treatment program and when faded out as soon as possible, self-protective devices have proven to be useful adjuncts to therapy (Dorsey, Iwata, Reid, & Davis, 1982; Hamad, Isley, & Lowry, 1983; Luiselli, 1986; Pace, Iwata, Edwards, & McGosh, 1986; Parrish, Aguerrevere, Dorsey, & Iwata, 1980). But there are many unwanted side effects, some of which have to do with stimulus control.

Using an ecobehavioral approach, Rojahn, Mulick, and S. R. Schroeder (1979) investigated the effects of restraints (a camisole and a fencing mask) on three mentally retarded persons with pica. Twenty-two client behaviors and six staff behaviors were simultaneously observed in a descriptive observational study. The study attempted an analysis of social dynamics in a special unit for profoundly mentally retarded clients with SIB (for the data collection system, see S. R. Schroeder, Rojahn, & Mulick, 1978a). Although this was not an attempt to replicate the study by Favell *et al.* (1978), the results lend support for their second explanation: the self-protective devices tended to decrease social interactions between the restrained subjects and their caretakers. Staff behaviors, such as nonprogrammatic positive attention, instructions, and reinforcement in the form of verbal praise for specific tasks, decreased for all three subjects during the time they were wearing restraints, relative to restraint-free periods; this pattern of responsiveness by the staff could reflect an increased demand situation for these clients when they were released from restraints. However, there was no indication with these three clients that the restraints had any reinforcing properties by themselves or provided an escape function of SIB (by performing pica). How much self-protective devices and their situational consequences lawfully contribute to the development and maintenance of such problem behaviors as SIB beyond their preventive function is an important question for ecobehavioral research.

Interaction of Environmental Conditions with Effectiveness of Intervention

When we analyze the functional relationship of aberrant behaviors and the conditions under which they occur, our primary concern is the control and deceleration of these behaviors. In the past, however, functional analysis has usually focused exclusively on the immediate consequences of such responses. This practice has led to the application of management procedures without taking into account other variables that are often powerful determinants in the natural environment. This neglect becomes evident when we look at problems like the often encountered lack of generalization across settings, response generalization to other behaviors, substitution, and the like. Even with perfectly executed management procedures, therapeutic interventions have to be designed not only to be adapted to the target behavior and its controlling conditions, but also to fit into the ecology of the client's habitat. Some procedures may be superior to others according to the prevailing conditions of the environment. Some environments are undoubtedly detrimental to the success of almost any therapeutic intervention.

Background Setting

Solnick, Rincover, and Peterson (1977) were emphasizing just this point when they investigated the importance of the background setting on the effectiveness of time-out. Their setting was either impoverished or enriched. In the impoverished setting, the client was presented with a discrimination task in which the correct response was either performed by the client or prompted by the experimenter. Edibles and praise plus a toy were given after each trial. The enriched setting involved the addition of music, new toys, and frequent prompting to play with the toys instead of engaging in the discrimination procedure. The time-out procedure involved a 90-second period of time during which the experimenter left the room. This contingency was applied to one and then two behaviors (head banging and spitting) in both types of settings. The context within which time-out occurred was found to be important. In the impoverished setting, the consequated target behaviors either increased or remained unchanged in frequency. In the enriched setting, the consequated target behaviors decreased in frequency. Time-out was effective only when time-in was enriched.

A subsequent study by Williams, S. R. Schroeder, Eckerman, and Rojahn (1983) was an attempt to assess the generality of the results of Solnick *et al.* (1977) in a group setting with four clients instead of one. The experiment evaluated which factors of the time-in environment were important. The findings lend partial support to the results of Solnick *et al.* (1977). Although suppression was seen in all settings with all four subjects, time-out was even more effective in the enriched environment for two clients. The clients met first in a custodial setting in which no toys were present and minimal supervision was offered; in another setting in which toys, but only minimal supervision, were offered; in a third setting in which the supervisor involved them in play, but without toys in the room; and finally in a setting in which there were toys as well as a supervisor actively involving them in play. The room was rearranged to create the four settings. Results showed that the four settings established different amounts of toy contact and interaction, and differentially effective time-outs. However, the rates of SIB and stereotypic behaviors were not greatly different during baselines. SIB and stereotyped responses that were already present were unaffected in frequency by noncontingently changing the environmental conditions of the setting. One way of conceptualizing these procedures is that new behaviors are reinforced in the presence of stimulus settings which previously had set the occasion for SIB. The functions of the controlling stimuli were changed. Of course, whether stimulus control of SIB was disrupted is still a moot point.

Availability of Alternative Behaviors

Another variable that interacts with the effectiveness of interventions is the availability of alternative behaviors that can be reinforced and can compete with stimuli that control SIB. This interaction was demonstrated in a study by Mulick, Hoyt, Rojahn, and S. Schroeder (1978) and replicated frequently (Favell, McGimsey, & Schell, 1982; Horner, 1980; Lockwood & Bourland, 1982). The subject was a 22-year-old, ambulatory, profoundly mentally retarded man with impaired vision that was due to bilateral cataracts. He was referred for treatment of excessive nail biting and finger picking. Screening observations revealed that the client spent most of his time sitting in his unit's large open dayroom. During unstructured periods, he remained seated, rocking back and forth, and intermittently biting small amounts of tissue from his fingertips, or he used his remaining fingernails to scratch at the tips of the fingers of the opposing hand until they were inflamed and infected. Nail biting and finger picking did not occur during structured fine-motor and tabletop activities. The client was extremely compliant with staff, and he readily had engaged in fine-motor tasks like stringing beads.

The intervention program was based on the simple assumption that if a variety of toys were located centrally and the client were taught to exchange old materials for new ones by a system of gradually faded prompts, then a rudimentary form of independent play might come to be substituted for hand-related SIB. Preliminary observations provided information about toy preference in the client. Relatively little investment of staff time and minor alterations in the environment resulted in dramatic increases in reinforced independent toy play and concomitant decreases in target behaviors.

Environmental Conditions and Response Selection

Sometimes environmental situations affect which responses are available for selection. There is very little research in this area. As Sidman (1978) has pointed out, the focus of the experimental analysis of behavior has been the investigation of reinforcement contingencies in controlled environments. We know much less about the technology of stimulus control in the environment. Naturalistic observational studies serve as a model for future research.

Sequential Relationships

MacLean and Baumeister (1979) used interactive analysis to study explicit sequential relationships among a variety of stereotyped topographies that were exhibited by a moderately retarded child as a function of environmental activities in an experimental preschool setting. They found that stereotypy was less frequent in settings in which the child was more actively engaged and closely supervised by the teacher. There was a significant suppression in one stereotyped topography (head shaking), but not in others, which was correlated with the teacher's approach and "negative contact" with the child. It is important to note that the teacher's behavior was *not* sequentially dependent upon the child's stereotyped behavior, but that the child's head shaking was temporarily decreased whenever any negative contact with the teacher occurred.

Complex Stimulus–Response Relationships

SIB is most prevalent among severely and profoundly mentally retarded and autistic persons who also tend to have a high incidence of organic dysfunction, long history of performing SIB, and frequent communication handicaps (S. R. Schroeder, C. Schroeder, Smith, & Dalldorf, 1978). However, their SIB topographies tend to be highly discriminated operants. In a study by S. R. Schroeder and MacLean (1987), the client reliably exhibited higher rates before and after unpleasant activities than after such pleasant activities as meals or snacks. Similarly, the selection of topography of SIB shifted dramatically depending on the activity in which the client was engaged.

Response–Response Relationships

It is necessary to study carefully not only complex stimulus–response relationships as seen in the study by S. R. Schroeder and MacLean (1987), but also simple response–response functions as seen in the study by MacLean and Baumeister (1979). Studies of such response–response relationships have shown the intra-individual ecobehavioral dynamics of response classes, hierarchical response chains, contrast effects, and natural covariations among responses. In the MacLean and Baumeister (1979) study, the interrelatedness of two stereotyped behaviors was demonstrated. Stereotyped hand flapping exhibited a relatively stable and significant sequential dependency with head shaking. The sequential analysis provided insight into the response complexity of these stereotypies of the subject. A similar result was achieved with the second subject of the study. Interactive analysis indicated that, given one form of stereotyped behavior, there were significant probabilities that another topography would follow immediately and continue. The results suggested a functional relationship between these two topographically different behaviors.

Response–response relationships were also found with multiple SIB topographies in a profoundly mentally retarded man (Rojahn, Mulick, McCoy, & S. R. Schroeder, 1978) through a *substitution effect*. The subject was a 30-year-old, nonambulatory, blind, profoundly mentally retarded male with a long history of SIB. At the time he was referred for treatment, he was demonstrating four different SIBs—two topographically related (head slapping with the palm of the hand and hitting the forehead with the knuckles of his fist) and two topographically unrelated (whipping his head toward his shoulder and wrapping his arms in his clothing until circulation of his blood was cut off). Treatment procedures consisted of a series of stimulus control procedures using a jacket with large sidepockets and/or a 10-cm foam-rubber neckbrace in systematic combinations. Interdependent patterns of head whipping and head banging or slapping resulted from wearing a prosthetic device.

Pearson correlation coefficients between head whipping and each of the two head-hitting behaviors across all treatments were $-.30$. Head banging and slapping were uncorrelated ($r = .01$). The internal relationship between the three SIB topographies was such that both head slapping and head banging, which were topographically similar, tended to preclude head whipping. But there was no functional dependency between head slapping and knuckles-to-forehead hitting, even though they were controlled by the same stimuli.

Arm wrapping was mutually exclusive to head slapping and head banging. Substitution occurred when the neckbrace was worn: head shipping decreased and head banging increased. The converse occurred when the neckbrace was removed and the jacket was worn. Findings of this nature are important for estimating prognosis of intervention and its long-term appropriateness for the client in his natural setting.

Silverman, Watanabe, Marshall, and Baer (1984) followed a similar rational in preventing SIB through strategic use of protective clothing. Use of the padded helmet substantially reduced face punching and arm self-restraint. Padded slippers reduced leg kicking and leg self-restraint. There were relationships between types of clothing used and their effects on SIB topography.

Summary

Antecedent conditions affect the occurrence of SIB in a variety of ways. SIB can come under differential stimulus control of situational demands, physical self-restraint, and daily routine activities. The client's habitat, the background setting, and the availability of alternative reinforcers all affect the success of behavioral interventions with SIB. Environmental conditions affect the development of multiple SIB topographies, their sequential interrelationships, and their natural covariation. This information on the occurrence and management of SIB is a rich array of findings. The challenge of future SIB research will be to elucidate the functional relationships among these antecedent conditions and to relate them to treatment effectiveness.

RESPONSE-CONTINGENT TECHNIQUES FOR MANAGING SIB

A variety of procedural options for treating SIB is well documented. The reader is referred to several review and analyses of the various intervention techniques with SIB (Baumeister & Rollings, 1976; Frankel & Simmons, 1976; Harris & Ersner-Hershfield, 1978; Johnson & Baumeister, 1978; Romanczyk, 1986; Singh, 1981). Few major new results have been reported since 1981. In this section, we shall first summarize and update what has been done in connection with each intervention technique.

Intervention Techniques for SIB

Punishment

Punishment consists of delivering an intense stimulus immediately contingent upon occurrence of SIB in order to suppress it. We emphasize that, according to Azrin and Holz (1966), the stimulus need not be aversive, but its presence must result in response suppression. If an aversive stimulus, when presented, results in an increase in the target response, it is, by definition, not a punisher. This is a point that is often confused in the literature, when aversive stimulation and punishment are considered synonymous. No stimulation is inherently aversive or punishing, but is so only in relation to its basic parameters (i.e., intensity, duration, and frequency, and their consequences on behavior).

Punishment of SIB has taken several forms: lemon juice (Sajwaj, Libet, & Agras, 1974); slapping (Duker, 1975a); tickling (Greene & Hoats, 1971); loud noises (Sajwaj & Hedges, 1971); noxious odors (Tanner & Zeiler, 1975); hairpulling (Griffin, Locke, & Landers, 1975); restraint (Saposnek & Watson, 1974); water mist (R. F. Peterson & L. R. Peterson, 1977); and electrical stimulation (Tate & Baroff, 1966a). Verbal reprimands have been ineffective except when used in conjunction with physical or electrical stimuli. Most punishment studies involve the use of electrical stimulation. However, the parameters of punishment of SIB have not yet been researched carefully. Very few studies have compared the different punishers (e.g., Rojahn, McGonigle, Curcio, & Dixon, 1987).

The suppressive effect of immediate contingent punishment is rapid and dramatic. When it occurs, it tends to be highly discriminated by the subject, and therefore generalization across settings is difficult to achieve. In Johnson and Baumeister's (1978) methodological review of 60 of the best-known studies of SIB, punishment procedures were used in 35, but failure was reported in only one study. The authors note that this effect probably reflects editorial bias in journals. In practice, punishment often fails to work. If it does work, it often loses its effectiveness (Birnbrauer, 1968; Romanczyk & Goren, 1975). There have been reports of suppression beyond a year with training of parents and teachers in the generalized setting (Merbaum, 1973). However, it is unlikely that SIB would be eliminated with punishment unless there were naturally reinforced alternative behaviors readily available in the client's environment and continued surveillance of SIB.

Harris and Ersner-Hershfield (1978) have thoroughly reviewed the side effects of punishment of SIB, such as generalized anxiety, withdrawal, counter aggression, escape behaviors, and symptom substitution, and concluded that they do not outweigh the positive effects, such as compliance, eye contact, and prosocial behaviors. These results are difficult to interpret, since few of the punishment studies were designed to evaluate carefully side effects, positive or negative. The main point is that many of the vaunted fears about serious negative side effects of a properly administered punishment procedure are generally unfounded. Other reviewers have come to similar conclusions (Carr & Lovaas, 1980; Foxx & Bechtel, 1983; Matson & DiLorenzo, 1984). Nevertheless, because caregivers find the practice repugnant (Pickering & Morgan, 1985) and administrators generally are reluctant to approve punishment except as a last resort, there has been a reduction in research on punishment of SIB and an increase in research on the other techniques.

Avoidance Conditioning

Avoidance conditioning has not received much attention in the SIB research, but it can be useful. For instance, Lovaas and Simmons (1969), after a number of SIB suppression trials in which "no" was paired with shock, found that "no" became sufficient to maintain suppression. Similarly, Tate and Baroff (1966b) noted that the buzz of the inductorium was enough to get a head banger to eat again after SIB had been suppressed and he was refusing to eat. Duker (1975a) compared punishment and avoidance conditioning on two SIB topographies of a mentally retarded woman. Both procedures were effective; however, while suppression of the punished behavior was lost, the SIB on the avoidance schedule continued to be suppressed.

Overcorrection

Overcorrection is a complex punishment procedure designed by Foxx and Azrin (1973) that attempts to capitalize on the suppressive effects of punishment while minimizing its negative side effects. Foxx (1978) has provided an excellent overview of overcorrection. The general rationale is "to require the misbehaving individual (a) to overcorrect the environmental effects of the inappropriate act, and (b) to practice overly correct forms of relevant behavior in those situations where the misbehavior commonly occurs." These two components are called *restitution* and *positive* practice. Epstein, Doke, Sajwaj, Sorell, and Rimmer (1974) have identified several components in overcorrection: (1) negative feedback, (2) time-out from positive reinforcement, (3) verbal reeducative instruction, (4) compliance training, such as gradual guidance or shadowing, and (5) negative reinforcement. Characteristics related to the success of acts are that they should (1) be directly related to the misbehaviors, (2) require effort, (3) be applied immediately following the misbehavior, (4) have a lengthy duration, and (5) be performed in a rapid, continued manner so as to be inhibiting.

Overcorrection is a good example of the often found advantage of combining the effective components of several procedures. But, like other forms of punishment, it is subject to both the same advantages (rapid, dramatic, and relatively enduring suppression of rate of SIB) and disadvantages (negative modeling, emotional conditioning, counteraggression, reinforcement of escape behavior, and substitution) (Harris & Ersner-Hershfield, 1978). The latter is especially true with strong, combative, noncompliant individuals. Foxx (1978) offers the guideline that if the overcorrection requires the involvement of two trainers instead of one, the danger of physical injury is greatly increased, and the procedure will not be feasible.

A bibliography by Matson and Ollendick on studies of overcorrection from 1971 to 1977 contains 77 items, of which only 10 studies are on SIB. The technique appears to hold a great deal of promise, but analysis of the effective ingredients remains to be performed (Ollendick & Matson, 1978). For instance, it is not always clear (1) when and how much restitution is necessary (Foxx, 1978); (2) how long the duration of positive practice needs to be: ranging from 40 seconds (Doleys, McWhorter, Williams, & Gentry, 1977; Jenner, 1984) up to 30 minutes (Foxx & Azrin, 1973; Gibbs & Luyben, 1985); (3) what the degree and topography of graduated guidance should be (Harris & Romanczyk, 1976; Ollendick & Matson, 1978); and (4) how overcorrection should be combined with such other procedures as rewarding alternative behaviors (DRO) (Azrin, Gottlieb, Hughart, Wesolowski, & Rahn, 1975). Foxx and Bechtel (1983) give a good analytic review of overcorrection procedures.

Contingent Restraint

Prolonged noncontingent physical restraint is a relatively sure way to prevent SIB, but, as Favell et al. (1978, 1981) have noted, it also may become reinforcing for the SIB client. Often release from restraints is a high-risk occasion for serious SIB. Favell et al. (1978) have shown that such clients will even perform other operant tasks for the opportunity to be returned to restraints.

However, brief contingent physical restraints have been used successfully to suppress head banging as time-out from positive reinforcement (Hamilton, Stephens, & Allen, 1967; Williams et al., 1983), as a punishment for pica (Bucher, Reykdal, & Albin, 1976), and in conjunction with biofeedback relaxation training (S. R. Schroeder, Peterson, Solomon, & Artley, 1977). In the latter case, the therapist applied and withdrew very brief periods of restraint with the clients contingent upon their level of muscle tension. Relaxation, a state incompatible with SIB, was reinforced. The therapist effectively faded out physical control when the client relaxed. This technique was very similar to the graduated guidance and shadowing techniques reported with overcorrection. Brief contingent restraint periods run less risk of becoming reinforcing than prolonged "safe" periods provided by noncontingent restraint as conventionally used.

Withdrawal of Positive Reinforcement

Withdrawal of positive reinforcement is another technique that has been used extensively to control SIB. The major forms are *extinction* (e.g., Bucher & Lovaas, 1968; Corte *et al.*, 1971; Lovaas & Simmons, 1969) and *time-out* (e.g., Hamilton *et al.*, 1967).

It is important to remember that extinction presupposes a history of rewarding patients for SIB (e.g., with differential attention or physical contact). Ignoring SIB of itself has little effect on frequency of SIB. In the Lovaas and Simmons (1969) study, the patient was released from restraint, and all attention to SIB was simply withdrawn. After 10 sessions and more than 9,000 instances of SIB, the behavior gradually disappeared. But in the Lovaas, Freitag, Gold, and Kassorla (1965) study, continued noncontingent attention to or ignoring of the SIB did not change its rate significantly. The possibility of adventitious reinforcement can be controlled by what Jones, Simmons, and Frankel (1974) call "noncontingent isolation" (i.e., removal to a special room). This procedure probably aided in controlling the number of stimuli that occasioned SIB and also helped observers and therapists to control their own reactions to SIB. Indeed, the subject in this experiment hit herself 34,000 times before SIB was suppressed.

Extinction, though effective, often poses great risks, because patients may seriously injure themselves during treatment. In addition, the initial withdrawal of reward may lead to an increase in SIB before a decrease occurs (Lovaas *et al.*, 1965). Also extinction depends greatly on the context in which reward for SIB has previously been delivered (Jones *et al.*, 1974). Thus, it has not always proven effective (Corte *et al.*, 1971). Studies with animals have shown that rate of extinction depends on conditioning history. Therefore, the longer the history of SIB, the longer it should take to extinguish. There has been no research with SIB on this latter point. Finally, as with punishment, problems with generalization, durability, and substitution have been observed with short-term extinction (Duker, 1975a; Jones *et al.*, 1974; Miron, 1971).

Sensory extinction is a new technique that was developed by Rincover (1978) and is based on the notion that SIB is self-stimulation maintained by sensory reinforcement. Noncontingent removal of the source of sensory reinforcement (e.g., by using a padded surface) should extinguish SIB. There is a small but compelling literature on sensory extinction for stereotyped behavior, but only a few studies on SIB (Luiselli, 1984; Rincover & Devaney, 1982). The sensory extinction hypothesis is an intriguing one, but it is also difficult to substantiate. Sensory reinforcement of SIB is essentially a hypothetical construct whose parameters are poorly established, especially in applied behavioral analysis. Considerably more work needs to be done to explore the conditions under which sensory extinction of SIB works.

Time-out—the withdrawal of access to reinforcement contingent on SIB—has been used much more successfully than extinction. A detailed analysis of the various forms of time-out is given in S. Schroeder, Mulick, and C. Schroeder (1979). Essentially, they are: contingent observation, withdrawal time-out, exclusion time-out, seclusion time-out, contingent restraint time-out, and response cost. All these forms vary on dimensions of intrusiveness of intervention, environmental demands, and the like. A recently developed technique, "facial screening," has shown promise as well (Lutzker, 1978; Winton, Singh, & Dawson, 1984; Zegiob, Alford, & House, 1978). In this instance, time-out consists of covering the client's face with a cloth bib or some other opaque material as a visual screen (McGonigle, Duncan, Cordisco, & Barrett, 1982).

MacDonough and Forehand (1973) have reviewed several of the parameters of time-out, most of which have not been investigated at all, let alone among SIB cases. Lucero, Frieman, Spoering, and Fehrenbacher (1976) compared the effects of food withdrawal and attention withdrawal on SIB at mealtime in three profoundly mentally retarded girls and found food withdrawal more effective. Whether this effect held beyond mealtime was not mentioned. Effective time-out durations have varied from 90 seconds to 30 minutes (White, Nielsen, & Johnson, 1972; Williams et al., 1983). Investigation of optimal durations appears to be based on the interpretation of time-out as punishment, rather than a choice by the client of time-out or time-in so as to maximize reinforcement (Leitenberg, 1965). It appears that time-out parameters cannot be isolated from time-in parameters. Probably elements of both punishment and maximization of reinforcement are involved in most time-out procedures.

Birnbrauer (1976) has suggested that a main effect of time-out may be disruption of an ongoing chain of inappropriate behavior, and that the effective duration may interact with other parameters, such as inhibition of responses during time-out, contingent release, and the reinforcing nature of the time-in environment. This line of reasoning receives indirect support from the experiments of Favell et al. (1978, 1981, 1982), in which alternative activities were chosen as distractors in order to disrupt and replace SIB in the client's repertoire. It is also supported by the experiments of Azrin, Besalel, and Wisotzek (1982) and Slifer, Iwata, and Dorsey (1984) who used a contingent response interruption technique and differential reinforcement of incompatible functional behaviors contingent upon SIB in two severely self-injurious adult males. Undoubtedly, a significant component of the physical restraint procedure and of the facial screening procedure also is response interruption.

Rewarding Alternative Behaviors (DRO)

The term *DRO* was coined in operant animal research (Reynolds, 1961) to reflect the pigeon's withholding of a pecking response for a criterion period that was followed by reinforcement. It has occasionally been known in the behavior therapy literature as "omission training" (Weihar & Harman, 1975). Presumably whatever "other" response was occurring at the time of reinforcement was strengthened. Thus, an SIB client may be rewarded for other non-SIB behaviors for longer and longer periods of time (DRO). If SIB occurs before a specific time period is completed, the time period is recycled, and reward is withheld until the criterion time period has elapsed. Good examples of this technique are described by Brawley, Harris, Allen, Fleming, and Peterson (1969), Lovaas et al. (1965), Tierney (1986), and Weihar and Harman (1975). Poling and Ryan (1982) provide a recent review of DRO studies. DRO procedures are typically used in conjunction with other methods, such as extinction or time-out from positive reinforcement (Repp & Deitz, 1974). This technique makes an evaluation of the DRO contingency alone difficult to assess because of the confounding effects of time-out (Baumeister & Rollings, 1976).

The mere reinforcement of alternative behaviors may not be sufficient to suppress SIB (Young & Wincze, 1974). Tarpley and S. Schroeder (1979) performed an experiment with three profoundly mentally retarded head bangers, comparing extinction, DRO, and DRI (differential reinforcement of incompatible behavior) in a multiple-schedule design. Another dimension of this study was that three forms of prompting incompatible behavior were used: manual guidance, manual and verbal prompts, and verbal prompts only. DRI suppressed SIB more than DRO, which suppressed SIB more than extinction. The degree of prompting incompatible behavior affected clients differently. For a compliant subject, verbal prompts were sufficient to make DRI effective. In another experiment involving biofeedback, S. R. Schroeder et al. (1977) showed that relaxation training with two severe head bangers resulted in a physiological state that was incompatible with the performance of SIB. Thus, the receptive state of the client and the degree of incompatibility of the alternative behavior are probably related to the effectiveness of reinforcement for alternative behavior.

As with punishment, generalizability and substitution with differential reinforcement procedures seem to be a problem, although there is not as much research available here. Durability seems to be a little better, but again not enough is known about the relevant parameters to make a conclusive statement.

Exercise

Recently, there have been two studies that have shown a decrease in SIB among persons by engaging them in vigorous exercise (Baumeister & MacLean, 1984; Lancioni, Smeets, Ceccarini, Capodaglio, & Campanari, 1984). In the Baumeister and MacLean (1984) study, there was a parametric negative relationship between SIB and noncontingent exercise. The alternative of stressing wellness and exercise to prevent SIB is an appealing treatment that needs exploration.

Satiation

Techniques based on *reinforcement alone* have not been very effective in suppressing SIB. However, there have been three case reports involving reinforcement of SIB that deserve mention. There are two reports of head banging in nonretarded persons (Mogel & Schiff, 1967; Wooden, 1974). In Wooden (1974), a nocturnal head banger was reinforced for negative practice of SIB, which resulted in quick, permanent suppression. Every night before sleeping he was told to grind his head into his pillow until he could no longer stand the pain. SIB stopped after four nights. Holburn and Dougher (1985) successfully used satiation techniques to treat aerophagia. An attempt at satiation in a severely retarded girl (Duker, 1975b) with head banging was unsuccessful. However, Jackson, Johnson, Ackron, and Crowley (1975) and Libby and Phillips (1979) have used food satiation very successfully to decelerate rumination. In the Jackson *et al.* study, the client was given a thick milkshake about 90 minutes after mealtime. Presumably this method averted the initial link in the chain of regurgitation leading to rumination and reconsumption of the vomitus. This study is one of a few demonstrations (see also Kohlenberg, 1970; Lang & Melamed, 1969) that shows intervention early in the chained sequence can prevent SIB.

Recent satiation experiments by Rast, Johnston, Drum, and Conrin (1981) and Rast, Johnston, and Drum (1984) allowed their profoundly mentally retarded ruminators to eat large meals until they refused any more food. Rast *et al.* (1981, 1984) were able to demonstrate a parametric inverse relationship between amount of rumination and amount eaten. All clients stopped ruminating completely if allowed to eat until satiety. Surprisingly, the amount eaten was three to eight times their single baseline normal adult portions. The portions were in the form of starches, including potatoes, rice, grits, cream of wheat, and bread. Since all of the subjects were underweight, the anticipated weight-gain resulting from the satiation procedure was not an issue in the Rast *et al.* (1981, 1984) studies. Dietary studies involving biochemical variables concerning the nutritional properties of different foods and their effects on the digestive system are now in progress, so that this promising procedure can be of more general use in the treatment of chronic rumination.

Summary of Response-Contingent Techniques for Reducing SIB

There now exist at east 100 well-controlled studies with SIB clients using several intervention techniques. The most frequently used techniques have incorporated punishment. This procedure has been used effectively with nearly all SIB topographies, except biting among Lesch–Nyhan patients (Anderson, Dancis, & Alpert, 1978) for whom it has aggravated SIB. Most punishment techniques do not generalize and maintain treatment effects as well as overcorrection. The latter method has been used effectively with nearly all SIB topographies, particularly self-hitting and pica. Time-out can be used effectively to suppress self-hitting and especially self-biting; but it is probably less advised for nonsocial consummatory types of SIB like pica, ruminative vomiting, and coprophagy, since its effectiveness depends primarily on the preexistence of a reinforcing time-in environment. Brief contingent restraint has been used effectively with self-hitting and pica. A caution with contingent restraint is necessary, lest the restraint should provide "safe" periods that themselves become reinforcing for the SIB client. Rewarding alternative behaviors has been used primarily with self-hitting and ruminative vomiting. DRI is likely to be more effective when it differentially provides reinforcement of alternative behaviors that are specifically incompatible with topographies of SIB and/or the contingencies reinforcing SIB. Although extinction has been used successfully with self-hitting, it is generally considered risky. The technique occasionally has been successful when punishment has failed, for instance, with self-biting among Lesch–Nyhan syndrome patients or as noncontingent social isolation for self-hitting. Satiation has been used effectively only with chronic ruminative vomiting and aerophagia. New treatments that merit exploration are response interruption techniques, exercise, and sensory extinction.

Our analysis of the response-contingent techniques illustrated in Figure 1 may convey a false sense of simplicity with regard to the clinical decision to apply them to the individual case. The application of these techniques never occurs in a vacuum. Therefore, the choice of technique must be mitigated by several qualifiers.

Response-dependent decelerative procedures may temporarily remove a reinforcer, as in response cost and time-out, or provide negative stimulus following each response, as in punishment. Both procedures lead to direct reductions in the rate of target behaviors. The other two cells represent response-dependent procedures that lead to an increase in the rate of a target

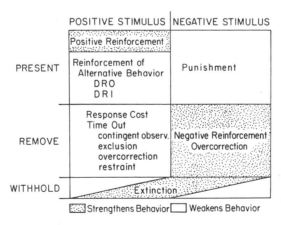

FIGURE 1. Contingency table showing the methods and consequences of strengthening and weakening behavior that have been used with self-injurious behavior.

behavior. Treatment procedures that derive from such *strengthening effects* on behavior depend upon substitution of a new behavior for an old one. Thus, differential positive reinforcement may be provided for topographically incompatible behaviors, or for the absence of SIB itself as in differential reinforcement of other behavior (or DRO). Negative reinforcement may also be used to strengthen competing behavior, as Lovaas *et al.* (1965) have shown, by increasing the social approach in autistic children through the use of contingent termination of electrical stimulation. Similarly, it is believed that the overcorrection procedure, as described by Foxx and Azrin in 1973, utilizes negative reinforcement to strengthen competing behavior, but also involves a period of time-out from other reinforcers and is, therefore, classified in more than one cell (Epstein *et al.*, 1974; K. Wells, Forehand, & Hickey, 1977). However, since these relationships have not yet been clearly demonstrated, this classification in Figure 1 must be viewed with caution.

The effects of noncontingently withholding a stimulus—or using an extinction procedure—will depend on whether the self-injurious behavior was dependent upon the presentation or the removal of the stimulus (Carr, 1977). In practice, the use of extinction to treat SIB usually involves withholding positive consequences that are thought to maintain the behavior. But the difficulty of identifying and controlling all sources of positive reinforcement and the gradual decrease in the responding characteristic of extinction (Lovaas & Simmons, 1969) preclude its use in many cases.

An overall treatment strategy is beginning to emerge that stems in part from an analysis of what happens when procedures from more than one cell are combined (Gaylord-Ross, Weeks, & Lipner, 1980; Parrish, Iwata, Dorsey, Bunck, & Slifer, 1985). As already alluded to in the case of overcorrection, it is recognized that immediate suppressive effects and their long-run durability are enhanced when decelerative procedures are combined with attempts to increase systematically, and ultimately substitute, setting-appropriate behaviors. The goal is then to arrange conditions so that appropriate behaviors come to occupy functional positions in the individual's habitual repertoire of daily activities.

The strategy is sound enough. The difficulty comes in actually selecting the components of an individualized treatment plan. One problem is that decelerative procedures differ in their intrusiveness and aversiveness, and no experimental analysis of these procedures as they relate to client characteristics or the severity and nature of the problem behavior yet exists. Because of additional questions, such as (1) the restrictiveness of the procedure and the treatment environment, (2) what constitutes a success or failure, (3) what procedures fit the capabilities of the resource system where the treatment will be used and maintained, or (4) what SIB is severe enough to warrant intrusive treatment, decisions to treat SIB are the province of Human Rights Committees and Internal Review Boards. These issues center around the reaction of the environment to behavior changes of the client before, during, and after intervention. To evaluate such factors, an ecobehavioral assessment of the treatment is needed.

Ecobehavioral Assessment

Ecobehavioral analysis extends traditional views of behavior modification tactics from the unidimensional to the multidimensional aspects of intervention. It reflects the complexity of behavior changes by observing behaviors of one person as he or she interacts with the group rather than by being preoccupied with the behavior of one person who is not adapting to the environment. Perhaps environments could be altered on several levels to fit the needs of their inhabitants and thereby reduce occasions for SIB. Interventions in such environments are also more likely to be successful.

Environmental Organization

Environmental organization should be based on objective behavior analysis (Risley, 1977; S. R. Schroeder et al., 1978a). For example, Rojahn et al. (1979) showed that the use of self-protective devices with SIB residents not only decreased but also social interactions with caretakers. This finding is an important consideration, because such clients depend so heavily on caregivers for the development of their adaptive skills. An unintended side effect of the noncontingent prevention of SIB may be the reinforcement of using more physical restraints by caregivers, simply because they require less effort than arduous surveillance and behavior management of a severe case of SIB.

Effects of Medication

Another important area of ecobehavioral assessment is evaluation of the effects of medication on SIB (Singh & Millichamp, 1985). Lipman (1970) and Sprague and Baxley (1978) have estimated that over one half of the residents in state facilities across the United States receive regular psychotropic drugs, 58% of which are large doses of the neuroleptic tranquilizers sustained over long periods of time (e.g., thioridazine and chlorpromazine) for behavioral control. A recent national survey by Hill, Balow, and Bruininks (1985) suggests that prevalence has been decreasing in recent years but is still high (39.7% in public and 25.4% in community residential facilities). Although earlier studies showed marginal efficacy of psychopharmacological treatment for SIB, recent treatments based on neuropharmacological theory offer more hope (S. R. Schroeder et al., 1987). S. R. Schroeder et al. (1978a) demonstrated how ecobehavioral assessment can be used to study caretaker reactivity in drug treatment of SIB. While a client's SIB and tantrums were being modified by a time-out procedure, his medication was changed independent in double-blind fashion. As the client improved, caretakers' positive responses to him increased. The course of improvement followed the time-out intervention, whereas the change in medication had a suppressive effect on all behaviors. If multiple behaviors of client and caretakers had not been recorded, a false conclusion could have been reached that thioridazine had brought tantrum behavior under control.

Side Effects

Ecobehavioral assessments have proven useful for examining covariation among collateral behaviors when intervention with target behaviors occurs. The problem of unwanted "side effects" became an issue with the use of intrusive punishment for the management of SIB. A second type of covariation is transitional change in target behaviors as a function of changes in stimulus conditions, for instance, behavioral contrast (Reynolds, 1961). A change in behavior is called a *contrast* when the change in the rate of responding during the presentation of one stimulus is in a direction away from the rate of responding generated during the presentation of a different stimulus (e.g., as in baseline rebound effects following a reinforcing intervention). When a new undesirable behavior emerges as a function of suppression of other behaviors, this type of covariation is called *response substitution* (Baumeister & Rollings, 1976). Originally found mainly with punishment of SIB, substitution has been observed with nearly every suppression technique (S. Schroeder *et al.*, 1979), even stimulus control procedures (Rojahn *et al.*, 1978). The multicategory system used in ecobehavioral assessment is designed to detect such "side effects."

Site Specificity

In addition to environment and medication, another area of stimulus control with SIB that could be investigated successfully with ecobehavioral technology is site specificity (Schoggen, 1978). This term refers to the notion that certain place-behavior systems are rather strictly organized and fixed, so that behaviors and environmental demands remain fairly constant within and across individuals. Examples would be school behaviors, home behaviors, ward behaviors, church behaviors, mealtime etiquette, and the like. Questions of interest from an ecological standpoint would be: (1) Are certain SIB topographies specific to certain places? (2) What are the antecedents and consequences for SIB in different sites? (3) Do different sites promote different degrees of adaptive behavior and communication that affect occasions (i.e., are pathogenic) for SIB? Some of the pertinent literature has been reviewed in previous sections, but this is a vastly unresearched area in behavior management of SIB.

Summary

Ecobehavioral analysis attempts to look at not only SIB target behaviors but also their covariants, setting characteristics, their patterns, sequential dependencies, and so forth, over extended periods of an intervention program. In the future, research is likely to focus on complex organism–environment interactions. A substantial technology already exists and has developed greatly in the past decade. It is hoped that such technology will improve the quality of treatment and the prevention of SIB among mentally retarded persons.

Some Programmatic Considerations with SIB

The reader is warned that the present section lacks the firm data base of the previous sections. The system of service delivery with which behavior management specialists must interface is at least as important as the intervention itself if a program is to be carried out and successfully maintained (Altmeyer *et al.*, 1987). Behavior management is usually only part of a treatment package (e.g., the individualized educational plan [IEP]). Behaviorists often consider behavior analysis the "bottom line" in an IEP; but, if they are honest, they recognize that behavior analysis data must go through several transformations, such as defining behaviors, getting interobserver agreement, and choosing units of measurement and validating them before the data can be adapted for use in a particular setting (Cone & Hawkins, 1977). They also make use of other sources of information besides direct observations (e.g., self-reports, daily logs, subjective impressions, etc.) (Hersen, 1978). The need for a systems model for clinical decision making has been recognized repeatedly by behavior analysts (Baer, 1977; Gaylord-Ross, 1978; Rogers-Warren & Warren, 1977). Reviews about SIB (Carr, 1977; Harris & Ersner-Hershfield, 1978; Romanczyk, 1986) contain a series of questions as the basis of a functional analysis for selecting particular interventions. Matson (1986) has argued that self-injury should be conceptualized within accepted diagnostic schemes, such as are described in the DSM-III. Most of these schemes address broader programming issues of which behavior management is a component. In this section, we address these issues more from a perspective of pointing out the need for research in the future rather than with a view toward answering any of the difficult questions posed.

Legal and Ethical Issues

Because of the high-risk nature of SIB, and because it is managed most frequently in restrictive settings like residential institutions or among persons who are usually severely or profoundly intellectually handicapped, program review committees play a vital role in deciding what, when, where, and how to modify behavior. Program review committees are basically legally mandated so that no behavior analyst can independently specify the most effective or least restrictive treatment. It should be remembered that program decisions should not only be shared with clients to the fullest extent possible but also with their families and their support systems.

The most common mechanism for program review is the internal review board, which is composed primarily of members of the institution (Cooke, Tannenbaum, & Gray, 1977). Although internal review boards serve an important function in protecting human rights, it must be recognized that they also have a vested interest in self-protection. Thus, a treatment strategy can be chosen out of caution and not necessarily because of effectiveness. As a consequence, external review boards composed of persons employed outside of the institutional have come into vogue.

External review boards are also very important to delivery of services. However, their role and impact on service systems have rarely been the subject of research. In many states these review boards are now mandated by law for residential facilities. The same type of monitoring should be mandated for other service settings, such as school programs and developmental day care, as well. S. R. Schroeder, Rojahn, and Mulick (1978b) have outlined a behavioral analysis of the roles of members on an external review board in a program for managing SIB in a state residential facility. The service professionals on the board acted mainly as problem solvers, whereas administrators dealt primarily with administrative or political matters, and legal professionals were primarily interested in detecting abuse of rights. Although all of these roles are useful for good program review, their balanced representation on the review board can be important to the success of the behavior management specialist. For instance, if the primary mandate of the review board is to prevent abuse and if there is little apparent danger of abuse in the program, members' attendance at meetings will diminish, the board's mandate will be compromised, and programming will be impeded. However, if the primary mandate is the enhancement of patients' rights, the review board can be another resource for improving development, implementation and maintenance of programs as well.

Recent Legal and Ethical Challenges to the Use of Aversive Treatment for SIB

As we had predicted in 1981, there has been an increased focus on the use of positive procedures to treat SIB, especially as people with severe SIB are being retained or moved back into community settings. Unfortunately, some organizations (Association for Retarded Citizens, 1987; The Association for Persons with Severe Handicaps, 1987) have coordinated this effort with an attack on the use of all aversive procedures on the grounds that they are ineffective (Guess, Helmstetter, Turnbull, & Knowlton, 1987), a conclusion considerably at variance with the present review. Turnbull *et al.* (1986) have even concluded that the use of shock to punish SIB is *immoral*. There have been attempts to make entitlement to federal grant and entitlement funds contingent upon the use of exclusively nonaversive procedures. The debate over the use of aversive procedures is still far from resolution (Mulick & Kedesdy, 1988). Whatever the legal ramifications and outcomes, it is likely that these procedures will be used less in the future than they have in the past. It is unknown what effect this decision will have on the effectiveness of treatments for SIB, more complete habilitation, place of residence options, and the use of psychotropic medication instead of behavior management of SIB.

Service Delivery Systems

There are few behavior management programs that require more arduous, continuous, and direct "hands-on" intervention than those for SIB.

This means that the demands on any service system will be a severe drain on manpower and financial resources. For an inefficient service delivery system, managing SIB may be impossible. The need for a vertically organized administration with adequate accountability seems to be recognized in the current trend to institutionalize SIB clients in "high control" units in residential facilities. There are many risks involved in such a programming strategy, for instance, modeling others' inappropriate behaviors, aperiodic reward and punishment of SIB, and lack of generalization beyond that specialized setting, to say nothing of the increased danger of physical injury. However, in our experience, accountability in the community is often far worse than in the institution. Some states now have the legal mandate to close *all* of their large public residential facilities and serve all clients in community settings. As Landesman and Butterfield's review (1987) shows, the empirical evidence to support this drastic step, especially for severe cases of SIB and aggression, is not convincing. Therefore, the nature of the service delivery system can have a profound effect on whether a behavior management program for SIB will be implemented competently in one setting, regardless of its proven effectiveness in another setting.

Programming Structures

Nearly all service delivery systems require that each client have an individualized program plan. Yet the program structures under which this mandate is implemented may vary tremendously. In an organization whose habilitation plans are strongly influenced by the medical model, the accepted methods of managing SIB may be psychotropic medication and self-protective restraint devices like camisoles, helmets, and fencing masks. In a behaviorally oriented establishment, just the opposite extreme may be in effect. Perhaps the so-called lack of generalization among SIB clients may really be adaptive discrimination of programming structures in different settings. Whatever the case, the role of the behavior analyst in both structures is usually that of a consultant.

The role of the behavioral consultant on a treatment team is primarily that of the ecobehavioral analyst. Not only is his or her task the management of the client's SIB, but also the management of the primary caregiver's behavior. Therefore, the behavioral consultant's primary client is usually the caregiver, not the SIB client. Unfortunately, a behavioral analysis of consultation is a rarely researched area, and thus poorly understood.

The beginnings of a behavioral analysis of consultation have been made by C. Schroeder (1978), C. Schroeder and Miller (1975), and C. Schroeder and S. Schroeder (1979). The model is adapted from the familiar behavior-analysis cycle of defining behavior, gathering baseline, planning programs, doing follow-up, and giving feedback—but to caregivers instead of the clients themselves. Each step in this cycle contains important issues for the consultant. The first step is consultant entry. C. Schroeder and Miller (1975) discuss several entry patterns and their relative advantages for developing with the consultee a joint ownership of the consulting problem. The next step is taking baseline on the consultee to discover skill levels, strengths, and weaknesses. Often a consultee may begin by requesting a simple information- or task-oriented consultation and end up really wanting training consultation (e.g., workshops and courses, or collaborative long-term consultation). Each type of consultation requires different contingencies and different levels of effort by the consultant. The consultant's role in planning interventions, doing follow-up, and giving feedback occurs only in collaborative consultation. The best contingencies in collaborative consultation are written contingency contracts with the consultee and written consultant reports. C. Schroeder and S. Schroeder (1979) have given a brief outline and analysis of the contingencies in using consultant reports.

The vicissitudes of the consultant's role on a team managing SIB are striking. Often consultees change because of staff turnover. Very often referral agents look upon the behavior management specialist as simply another resource to solve their staffing problems. If the consultant gives in to the pressure to "take over" noncontingently, rather than share ownership of the problem, the intervention program will be transferred later with even greater difficulty. More than likely, it will be discontinued once the consultant withdraws regardless of whether it has been effective or not.

Staffing Considerations

Little is known about the proper selection, entering competencies, motivation, skills, and reasons for rapid turnover of direct caregivers for the severely and profoundly handicapped. Only recently has this area become of interest to behavioral researchers (Zaharia & Baumeister, 1978). Obviously, staff development must be a continuing operation for caregivers dealing with SIB, because (1) a continued high level of competence in behavior management is required to deal effectively with SIB; (2) staff support to maintain focus on program objectives and new techniques is necessary because of the risky nature of SIB and the "high-pressure" circumstances under which behavioral intervention takes place; and (3) the arduous nature of the daily regimes required for effective management is emotionally draining. The latter factor leads to sickness, absenteeism, and eventually turnover if some respite for staff is not periodically arranged.

Staff Training

Bernstein (1982) has published an excellent conceptual review of the training of behavior change agents. Her conceptualization revolves around four questions: (1) What problems must behavior change agents be able to solve? (2) What skills are most likely to lead to solutions to those problems? (3) What techniques should be used to teach those skills? and (4) What procedures are most likely to assure generalization of those skills? Her review of the literature shows that the answers depend upon the type of change agent being trained.

After several years of experience with formal education of direct caregiving staff in certification programs, continuing-education programs, and the like, we have concluded that most formal training, such as lectures, coursework, and demonstration workshops, are good public relations, but they are relatively useless for creating new skills. An analysis of the contingencies affecting staff performance makes the reasons apparent: (1) state personnel policies often fail to provide the necessary financial incentives for direct care staff to undergo the hardships of continuing education; (2) the level of expertise required to develop and implement adequate programs to manage problems as severe as SIB requires extensive education and training. Although most direct care staff have skills in patient care, they are not qualified to design programs or exert quality control of behavior intervention programs.

The only staff training that has been effective in our work with SIB has been where direct caregivers referred a client with SIB to us and then the client's program was developed jointly with them to meet a specific need that they had. Once this bridge was crossed, more general topics related to intervention tactics could be addressed with a view toward further training. This approach is more difficult for the consultant than traditional staff-training models, but it is also most efficient, because it concentrates only on those staff persons who have strong incentives to participate and use their training.

CONCLUSION

Since 1981, there have been well over 50 research and over 20 review papers on the etiology and management of SIB. About half of them have to do with behavioral management techniques and about half with the neurobiological etiology and management of SIB. Recent accounts of SIB have given a much more balanced behavioral approach, stressing a functional analysis of a variety of etiological factors related to intervention. Behavior management techniques will likely be increasingly oriented toward nonaversive interventions more acceptable to parents and advocates in community settings—a trend which we had predicted in 1981. An exciting new development has been the major focus on the neurobiological substrates of SIB, which shows promise of improving hope for a rational approach to the pharmacotherapy of SIB.

REFERENCES

Altmeyer, B. K., Locke, B. J., Griffin, J. C., Ricketts, R., Williams, D. E., Mason, M., & Stark, M. E. (1987). Treatment strategies for self-injurious behavior in a large service delivery network. *American Journal of Mental Deficiency, 91*, 333–340.

Anderson, L., Dancis, J., & Alpert, M. (1978). Behavioral contingencies and self-stimulation in Lesch-Nyhan disease. *Journal of Consulting and Clinical Psychology, 46*, 529–536.

Association for Retarded Citizens (ARC). (1987). Position statement on behavior management. *TASH Newsletter, 13*, 3.

Axelrod, S. (1987). Functional and structural analyses of behavior: Approaches leading to reduced use of punishment procedures? *Research in Developmental Disabilities, 8*, 165–178.

Ayllon, T., & Azrin, N. (1966). Punishment as a discriminative conditioned reinforcer with humans. *Journal of the Experimental Analysis of Behavior, 9*, 411–419.

Azrin, N. H., & Holz, W. C. (1966). Punishment. In W. K. Honig (Ed.), *Operant behavior: Areas of research and application*, (pp. 380–447). New York: Appleton-Century-Crofts.

Azrin, N. H., Gottlieb, L., Hughart, L., Wesolowski, M. D., & Rahn, T. (1975). Eliminating self-injurious behavior by educative procedures. *Behaviour Research and Therapy, 13*, 101–111.

Azrin, N. H., Besalel, V. A., & Wisotzek, I. E. (1982). Treatment of self-injurious behaviors by a reinforcement plus interruption procedure. *Analysis and Intervention in Developmental Disabilities, 2*, 105–113.

Baer, D. M. (1977). Some comments on the structure of the intersection of ecology and applied behavior analysis. In A. Rogers-Warren & S. Warren (Eds.), *Ecological perspectives in behavior analysis*. Baltimore: University Park Press.

Baer, D. M., Wolf, M. M., & Risley, T. (1968). Some current dimensions of applied behavior analysis. *Journal of Applied Behavior Analysis, 1*, 91–97.

Barron, J., & Sandman, C. (1983). Relationship of sedative-hypnotic response to self-injurious behavior and stereotypy by mentally retarded clients. *American Journal of Mental Deficiency, 88*, 177–186.

Baumeister, A. A. (1978). Origins and control of stereotyped movements. In C. E. Meyers (Ed.), *Quality of life in severely and profoundly mentally retarded people: Research foundations for improvement* (pp. 353–384). Washington, DC: AAMD Monograph, No. 3.

Baumeister, A. A., & Forehand, R. (1973). Stereotyped acts. In N. R. Ellis (Ed.), *International review of research in mental retardation* (Vol. 6, pp. 55–96). New York: Academic Press.

Baumeister, A. A., & MacLean, W. E., Jr., (1984). Deceleration of self-injurious and stereotypic responding by exercise. *Applied Research in Mental Retardation, 5*, 385–394.

Baumeister, A. A., Rollings, J. P. (1976). Self-injurious behavior. In N. R. Ellis (Ed.), *International review of research in mental retardation* (Vol. 9, pp. 55–96). New York: Academic Press.

Baumeister, A. A., Frye, G. R., & Schroeder, S. R. (1984). Neurochemical correlates of self-injurious behavior. In J. A. Mulick & B. L. Mallory (Eds.), *Transitions in mental retardation: Advocacy, technology and science* (pp. 207–228). Norwood, NJ: Ablex.

Berkson, G. (1967). Abnormal stereotyped acts. In J. Zubin & H. Hunt (Eds.), *Comparative psychopathology* (pp. 76–94). New York: Grune & Stratton.

Berkson, G. (1983). Repetitive stereotyped behaviors. *American Journal of Mental Deficiency, 88*, 239–246.

Berkson, G. (1987, August). *Three approaches to an understanding of abnormal stereotyped behaviors.* Paper presented at the 105th Annual Convention of the American Psychological Association, New York.

Berkson, G., & Landesman-Dwyer, S. (1977). Behavioral research on severe and profound retardation (1955–1974). *American Journal of Mental Deficiency, 81*, 428–454.

Berkson, G., & Mason, W. A. (1964a). Stereotyped movements of mental defectives: III. Situational effects. *Perceptual and Motor Skills, 19*, 635–652.

Berkson, G., & Mason, W. A. (1964b). Stereotyped movements of mental defectives: IV. The effects of toys and the character of the acts. *American Journal of Mental Deficiency, 68*, 511–524.

Bernstein, G. S. (1982). Training behavior change agents: A conceptual review. *Behavior Therapy, 13*, 1–23.

Birnbrauer, J. S. (1968). Generalization of punishment effects: A case study. *Journal of Applied Behavior Analysis, 1*, 201–211.

Birnbrauer, J. S. (1976). Mental retardation. In H. Leitenberg (Ed.), *Handbook of behavior modification and behavior therapy* (pp. 361–404). New York: Appleton-Century-Crofts.

Bittick, K., Fleeman, W., & Bright, T. (1978, March). *Reduction of self-injurious behavior utilizing sensory integration techniques.* Paper presented at the Gatlinburg Conference on Mental Retardation, Gatlinburg, TN.

Brawley, E., Harris, F., Allen, K., Fleming, R., & Peterson, R. (1969). Behavior modification of an autistic child. *Behavioral Science, 4*, 87–97.

Breese, G. R., Mueller, R. A., & Schroeder, S. R. (1986). The neurochemical basis of symptoms in the Lesch-Nyhan syndrome. In E. Schopler & G. Mesibov (Eds.), *Neurobiological issues in autism* (pp. 145–160). New York: Academic Press.

Brown, J. S., Martin, R., & Morrow, M. (1964). Self-punitive behavior in the rat: Facilitative effects of punishment on resistance to extinction. *Journal of Comparative and Physiological Psychology, 57*, 127–133.

Bryson, Y., Sakati, N., Nyhan, W., & Fish, C. (1971). Self-mutilative behavior in the Cornelia de Lange Syndrome. *American Journal of Mental Deficiency, 76,* 319–324.

Bucher, B., & Lovaas, O. I. (1968). Use of aversive stimulation in behavior modification in mental retardation. In M. R. Jones (Ed.), *Miami symposium on the prediction of behavior: Aversive stimulation.* Coral Gables, FL: University of Miami Press.

Bucher, B., Reykdal, B., & Albin, J. (1976). Brief physical restraint to control pica. *Journal of Behavior Therapy and Experimental Psychiatry, 1* 137–140.

Byrd, L. (1969). Responding in the rat maintained under response-independent electric shock and response-produced electric shock. *Journal of the Experimental Analysis of Behavior, 12,* 1–10.

Carr, E. G. (1977). The motivation of self-injurious behavior: A review of some hypotheses. *Psychological Bulletin, 84,* 800–816.

Carr, E. G., & Lovaas, O. I. (1980). Contingent electric shock as a treatment for severe behavior problems. In S. Axelrod & J. Apsche (Eds.), *Punishment: Its effects on human behavior.* Lawrence, KS: H & H Enterprises.

Carr, E. G., Newsom, C. D., & Binkoff, J. A. (1976). Stimulus control of self-destructive behavior in a psychotic child. *Journal of Abnormal Child Psychology, 4,* 139–153.

Cataldo, M. F., & Harris, J. (1982). The biological basis for self-injury in the mentally retarded. *Analysis and Intervention in Developmental Disabilities, 2,* 21–39.

Clark, D., Kreutzberg, J. R., & Chee, F. (1977). Vestibular stimulation influence on motor development in infants. *Science, 196,* 1228.

Cone, J., & Hawkins, R. (1977). Current status and future directions in behavioral assessment. In J. Cone & R. Hawkins (Eds.), *Behavioral assessment* (pp. 381–392). New York: Brunner/Mazel.

Cooke, R., Tannenbaum, A., & Gray, B. (1977). *A survey of institutional review boards and research involving human subjects.* (Contract No. NO1-HU-6-2110). Ann Arbor: University of Michigan, Institute for Social Research.

Corte, H. E., Wolf, M. M., & Locke, B. J. (1971). A comparison of procedures for eliminating self-injurious behavior of retarded adolescents. *Journal of Applied Behavior Analysis, 4,* 201–213.

Crabtree, L. H. (1967). A psychotherapeutic encounter with a self-mutilating patient. *Psychiatry, 30*(1), 91–100.

Davenport, R., & Berkson, G., (1963). Stereotyped movements of mental defectives: II. Effects of novel objects. *American Journal of Mental Deficiency, 67,* 879–882.

Doleys, D., McWhorter, A., Williams, S., & Gentry, W. (1977). Encopresis: Its treatment and relation to nocturnal enuresis. *Behavior Therapy, 8,* 77–82.

Dorsey, M., Iwata, B. A., Reid, D., & Davis, P. (1982). Protective equipment: Continuous and contingent application in the treatment of self-injurious behavior. *Journal of Applied Behavior Analysis, 15,* 217–230.

Duker, P. C. (1975a). Behaviour therapy for self-injurious behavior: Two case studies. *Research Exchange and Practice in Mental Retardation, 1,*(4), 223–232.

Duker, P. C. (1975b). Behaviour control of self-biting in a Lesch-Nyhan patient. *Journal of Mental Deficiency Research, 19,*(11), 11–19.

Durand, V. M. (1986). Self injurious behavior as intentional communication. In K. Gadow (Ed.), *Advances in learning and behavioral disabilities* (Vol. 5, pp. 141–155). Greenwich, CT: JAI Press.

Edelson, S. M. (1984). Implications of sensory stimulation in self-destructive behavior. *American Journal of Mental Deficiency, 80,* 140–145.

Epstein, H., Doke, L., Sajwaj, T., Sorell, S., & Rimmer, B. (1974). Generality and side effects of overcorrection. *Journal of Applied Behavior Analysis, 7,* 385–390.

Erwin, J., Mitchell, G., & Maple, T. (1973). Abnormal behavior in non-isolate reared monkeys. *Psychological Reports, 33,* 515–523.

Favell, J. E., McGimsey, J. F., & Jones, M. L. (1978). The use of physical restraint in the treatment of self-injury and as positive reinforcement. *Journal of Applied Behavior Analysis, 11,* 225–241.

Favell, J. E., McGimsey, J. F., Jones, M. L., & Cannon, P. R. (1981). Physical restraint as positive reinforcement. *American Journal of Mental Deficiency, 85,* 425–432.

Favell, J. E., McGimsey, J. F., & Schell, R. M. (1982). Treatment of self-injury by providing alternate sensory activities. *Analysis and Intervention in Developmental Disabilities, 2,* 83–104.

Fitzherbert, J. (1950). The origin of head-banging: A suggested explanation with an illustrative case history. *Journal of Mental Science, 96,* 793–795.

Foxx, R. (1978). An overview of overcorrection. *Journal of Pediatric Psychology, 3*, 97–101.

Foxx, R. M., & Azrin, N. H. (1973). The elimination of self-stimulatory behavior of autistic and retarded children by overcorrection. *Journal of Applied Behavior Analysis, 6*, 1–14.

Foxx, R. M., & Bechtel, D. R. (1983). Overcorrection: A review and analysis. In S. Axelrod & J. Apsche (Eds.), *The effects of punishment on human behavior.* (pp. 227–288). New York: Academic Press.

Frankel, F., & Simmons, J. Q. (1976). Self-injurious behavior in schizophrenic and retarded children. *American Journal of Mental Deficiency, 80*, 512– 522.

Frederick, C. J., & Resnik, H. L. P. (1971). How suicidal behaviors are learned. *American Journal of Psychotherapy, 25*, 37–55.

Freud, A. (1954). Self-mutilative behavior. *Psychoanalytic Study of the Child, 8*, 9–19.

Gaylord-Ross, R. (1978). *A decision model for the treatment of aberrant behaviors in applied settings.* Unpublished manuscript.

Gaylord-Ross, R. J., Weeks, M., & Lipner, C. (1980). An analysis of antecedent, response, and consequence events in the treatment of self-injurious behavior. *Education and Training of the Mentally Retarded, 15*, 35–42.

Gibbs, J. W., & Luyben, P. D. (1985). Treatment of self-injurious behavior: Contingent versus non-contingent positive practice overcorrection. *Behavior Modification, 9*, 3–21.

Gluck, J., & Sackett, G. (1974). Frustrations and self-aggression in social isolate rhesus monkeys. *Journal of Abnormal Psychology, 83*, 331–334.

Green, A. (1967). Self-mutilation in schizophrenic children. *Archives of General Psychiatry, 17*, 234–244.

Green, A. (1968). Self-destructive behavior in physically abused schizophrenic children. *Archives of General Psychiatry, 19*, 171–179.

Greenacre, P. (1954). Certain relationships between fetishism and faulty development of the body image. *Psychoanalytic Study of the Child, 8*, 78–98.

Greene, R. J., & Hoats, D. L. (1971). Aversive tickling: A simple conditioning technique. *Behavior Therapy, 2*, 389–393.

Gregg, C., Haffner, M., & Korner, A. (1976). The relative efficacy of vestibular-proprioceptive stimulation and the upright position in enhancing visual pursuit in neonates. *Child Development, 40*, 309.

Griffin, J. C., Locke, B. J., & Landers, W. F. (1975). Manipulation of potential punishment parameters in the treatment of self-injury. *Journal of Applied Behavior Analysis, 8*, 458–464.

Guess, D., Helmstetter, E. Turnbull, H. R., & Knowlton, S. (1987). Use of aversive procedures with persons who are disabled: An historical review and critical analysis. *Monograph of the Association for Persons with Severe Handicaps, 2*, 1–68.

Hamad, C. D., Isley, E., & Lowry, M. C. (1983). The use of mechanical restraint and response incompatibility to modify self-injurious behavior: A case study. *Mental Retardation, 21*, 213–217.

Hamilton, H., Stephens, L., & Allen, P. (1967). Controlling aggressive and destructive behavior in severely retarded institutionalized residents. *American Journal of Mental Deficiency, 71*, 852–856.

Harris, S., & Ersner-Hershfield, R. (1978). Behavioral suppression of seriously disruptive behavior in psychotic and retarded patients: A review of punishment and its alternatives. *Psychological Bulletin, 85*, 1352–1375.

Harris, S. L., & Romanczyk, R. G. (1976). Treating self-injurious behavior of a retarded child by overcorrection. *Behavior Therapy, 7*, 235–239.

Hersen, M. (1978). Do behavior therapists use self-reports as major criteria? *Behavior Analysis and Modification, 2*, 328–334.

Hill, B. K., Balow, E. B., & Bruininks, R. H. (1985). A national study of prescribed drugs in institutions and community residential facilities for mentally retarded people. *Psychopharmacology Bulletin, 21*, 279–284.

Holburn, C. S., & Dougher, M. J. (1985). Behavioral attempts to eliminate air-swallowing in two profoundly mentally retarded clients. *American Journal of Mental Deficiency, 89*, 524–536.

Holz, W., & Azrin, N. (1961). Discriminative properties of punishment. *Journal of the Experimental Analysis of Behavior, 4*, 225–232.

Holz, W., & Azrin, N. (1962). Interactions between the discriminative and adversive properties of punishment. *Journal of the Experimental Analysis of Behavior, 5*, 229–234.

Horner, R. D. (1980). The effects of an environmental "enrichment" program on the behavior of institutionalized profoundly retarded adolescents. *Journal of Applied Behavior Analysis, 13*, 473–492.

Iwata, B. A., Dorsey, M. F., Slifer, K. J., Bauman, K. E., & Richman, G. S. (1982). Towards a functional analysis of self-injury. *Analysis and Intervention in Developmental Disabilities, 2*, 3–20.

Jackson, G. M., Johnson, C. R., Ackron, G. S., & Crowley, R. (1975). Good satiation as a procedure to decelerate vomiting. *American Journal of Mental Deficiency, 80*, 223–227.

Jenner, S. (1984). The effectiveness of abbreviated overcorrection-based treatments. *Behavioral Psychotherapy, 12*, 175–187.

Johnson, W., & Baumeister, A. (1978). A self-injurious behavior: A review and analysis of methodological details of published studies. *Behavior Modification, 2*, 465–484.

Jones, F. H., Simmons, J. Q., & Frankel, F. (1974). An extinction procedure for eliminating self-destructive behavior in a 9-year-old autistic girl. *Journal of Autism and Childhood Schizophrenia, 4*, 241–250.

Kelleher, R., Riddle, W., & Cook, L. (1963). Persistence of behavior maintained by unavoidable shocks. *Journal of the Experimental Analysis of Behavior, 6*, 507–517.

Kohlenberg, R. (1970). The punishment of persistent vomiting: A case study. *Journal of Applied Behavior Analysis, 3*, 241–245.

Kohlenberg, R. J., Levin, M., & Belcher, S. (1973). Skin conductance changes and the punishment of self-destructive behavior: A case study. *Mental Retardation, 11*, 11–13.

Lancioni, G. E., Smeets, P. M., Ceccarini, P. S. Capodaglio, L., & Campanari, G. (1984). Effects of gross motor activities on the severe self-injurious tantrums of multihandicapped individuals. *Applied Research in Mental Retardation, 5*, 471–482.

Landesman, S., & Butterfield, E. C. (1987). Normalization and deinstitutionalization of mentally retarded individuals: Controversy and facts. *American Psychologist, 42*, 809–816.

Lane, R. G., & Domrath, R. P. (1970). Behavior therapy: A case history. *Hospital and Community Psychiatry, 21*, 150–153.

Lang, P., & Melamed, B. (1969). Case report: Avoidance conditional therapy of an infant with chronic ruminative vomiting. *Journal of Abnormal Psychology, 74*, 1–8.

Leitenberg, H. (1965). Is time-out from positive reinforcement an aversive event? A review of the experimental evidence. *Psychological Bulletin, 64*, 428–441.

Lemke, H., & Mitchell, R. (1972). Controlling the behavior of a profoundly retarded child. *American Journal of Occupational Therapy, 26*, 261–264.

Lesch, M., & Nyhan, W. (1964). A familial disorder of uric acid metabolism and central nervous system function. *American Journal of Medicine, 36*, 561– 570.

Lester, D. (1972). Self-mutilating behavior. *Psychological Bulletin, 78*, 119–128.

Levitt, M. (1985). Dysesthesies and self-mutilation in humans and subhumans: A review of clinical and experimental studies. *Brain Research Reviews, 10*, 247–290.

Lewis, M. H., & Baumeister, A. A. (1982). Stereotyped mannerisms in mentally retarded persons: Animal models and theoretical analyses. In N. R. Ellis (Ed.), *International review of research in mental retardation* (Vol. 12, pp. 123–161). New York: Academic Press.

Libby, D., & Phillips, E. (1979). Eliminating rumination behavior in a profoundly retarded adolescent: An exploratory study. *Mental Retardation, 17*, 94–95.

Lichtstein, K., & Wahler, R. (1976). The ecological assessment of an autistic child. *Journal of Abnormal Child Psychology, 4*, 31–54.

Lipman, R. (1970). The use of psychopharmacological agents in residential facilities for the retarded. In F. Menolascino (Ed.), *Psychiatric approaches to mental retardation* (pp. 387–398). New York: Basic Books.

Lockwood, K., & Bourland, G. (1982). Reduction of self-injurious behaviors by reinforcement and toy use. *Mental Retardation, 20*, 169–173.

Lourie, R. (1949). The role of rhythmic patterns in childhood. *American Journal of Psychiatry, 105*, 653–660.

Lovaas, O. I. (1982). Comments on self-destructive behaviors. *Analysis and Intervention in Developmental Disabilities, 2*, 115–124.

Lovaas, O. I., & Simmons, J. Q. (1969). Manipulation of self-destruction in three retarded children. *Journal of Applied Behavior Analysis, 2,* 143–157.

Lovaas, O. I., Freitag, G., Gold, V. J., & Kassorla, I. C. (1965). Experimental studies in childhood schizophrenia: Analysis of self-destructive behavior. *Journal of Experimental Child Psychology, 2,* 67–84.

Lovaas, O. I., Schaeffer, R., & Simmons, J. Q. (1965). Experimental studies in childhood schizophrenia: Building a social behavior in autistic children by the use of electric shock. *Journal of Experimental Research in Personality, 1,* 99–109.

Lovaas, O. I., Newsom, C., & Hickman, C. (1987). Self-stimulatory behavior and perceptual development. *Journal of Applied Behavior Analysis, 20,* 45–68.

Lucero, W. J., Frieman, J., Spoering, K., & Fehrenbacher, J. (1976). Comparison of three procedures in reducing self-injurious behavior. *American Journal of Mental Deficiency, 80,* 548–554.

Luiselli, J. K. (1984). Use of sensory extinction in treating self-injurious behavior—A cautionary note. *Behavior Therapist, 7,* 142.

Luiselli, J. K. (1986). Modification of self-injurious behavior: An analysis of the use of contingently applied protective equipment. *Behavior Modification, 10,* 191–204.

Lutzker, J. R. (1978). Reducing self-injurious behavior by facial screening. *American Journal of Mental Deficiency, 82,* 510–513.

MacDonough, T., & Forehand, R. (1973). Response-contingent time-out: Important parameters in behavior modification with children. *Journal of Behavior Therapy and Experimental Psychiatry, 4,* 231–236.

MacLean, W., & Baumeister, A. A. (1979, April). *An environmental analysis of stereotyped behavior of developmentally delayed children.* Paper presented at the Twelfth Annual Gatlinburg Conference on Research in Mental Retardation, Gulf Shores, AL.

Marie, C., Royer, P., & Rappaport, R. (1967). Congenital hyperuricemia with neurological renal and hematologic problems. *Archives Françaises de Pediatrie, 24*(5), 501–510.

Matson, J. L. (1986). Self-injury and its relationship to diagnostic schemes in psychopathology. *Applied Research in Mental Retardation, 7,* 223–227.

Matson, J. L., & DiLorenzo, T. (1984). *Punishment and its alternatives.* New York: Springer.

McGonigle, J. J., Duncan, D., Cordisco, L., & Barrett, R. P. (1982). Visual screening: An alternative method for reducing stereotypic behavior. *Journal of Applied Behavior Analysis, 15,* 461–467.

Merbaum, M. (1973). The modification of self-destructive behavior by a mother-therapist using aversive stimulation. *Behavior Therapy, 4,* 442, 447.

Miron, N. B. (1971). Behavior modification techniques in the treatment of self-injurious behavior in institutionalized retardates. *Bulletin of Suicidology, 8,* 64–69.

Mogel, S., & Schiff, W. (1967). Extinction of a head bumping symptom of eight years duration in 2 minutes: A case report. *Behaviour Research and Therapy, 5*(2), 131–132.

Mulick, J. A., & Kedesdy, J. H. (1988). Self-injurious behavior, its treatment, and normalization. *Mental Retardation, 26,* 223–229.

Mulick, J., Hoyt, R., Rojahn, J., & Schroeder, S. (1978). Reduction of a "nervous habit" in a profoundly retarded youth by increasing toy play: A case study. *Journal of Behavior Therapy and Experimental Psychiatry, 9,* 381–385.

Murray, M., & Nevin, J. (1967). Some effects of correlation between response-contingent shock and reinforcement. *Journal of the Experimental Analysis of Behavior, 10,* 301–309.

Myers, J. J., Jr., & Diebert, A. N. (1971). Reduction of self-abusive behavior in a blind child by using a feeding response. *Journal of Behavior Therapy and Experimental Psychiatry, 2,* 141–144.

Nyhan, W. L. (1967). The Lesch-Nyhan syndrome: Self-destructive biting, mental retardation, neurological disorder and hyperuricaemia. *Developmental Medicine and Child Neurology, 9,* 563–572.

Nyhan, W. L. (1968a). Clinical features of the Lesch-Nyhan syndrome: Introduction—Clinical and genetic features. *Federation Proceedings, 27*(4), 1027–1033.

Nyhan, W. L. (1968b). Summary of clinical features. *Federation Proceedings, 27*(4), 1034–1041.

Nyhan, W. L. (1976). Behavior in the Lesch-Nyhan syndrome. *Journal of Autism and Childhood Schizophrenia, 6,* 235–252.

Ollendick, T., & Matson, J. (1978). Effectiveness of hand overcorrection for topographically similar and dissimilar self-stimulatory behavior. *Journal of Experimental Child Psychology, 25,* 396–403.

Pace, G. M., Iwata, B. A., Edwards, G. L., & McGosh, K. C. (1986). Stimulus fading and transfer in the treatment of self-restraint and self-injurious behavior. *Journal of Applied Behavior Analysis, 19,* 381–390.

Parrish, J. M., Aguerrevere, L., Dorsey, M. F., & Iwata, B. A. (1980). The effects of protective equipment on self-injurious behavior. *Behavior Therapist, 3,* 28–29.

Parrish, J. M., Iwata, B. A., Dorsey, M. F., Bunck, J. J., & Slifer, K. J. (1985). Behavior analysis, program development, and transfer of control in the treatment of self-injury. *Journal of Behavior Therapy and Experimental Psychiatry, 16,* 159–168.

Peterson, R. F., & Peterson, L. R. (1968). The use of positive reinforcement in the control of self-destructive behavior in a retarded boy. *Journal of Experimental Child Psychology, 6,* 351–360.

Peterson, R. F., & Peterson, L. R. (1977). Hydropsychotherapy: Water as a punishing stimulus in the treatment of problem parent-child relationships. In B. C. Etzel, J. M. LeBlanc, & D. M. Baer, (Eds.), *New developments in behavioral research, therapy, and applications.* Hillsdale, NJ: Lawrence Erlbaum.

Pickering, D., & Morgan, S. B. (1985). Parental ratings of treatments of self-injurious behavior. *Journal of Autism and Developmental Disorders, 15,* 303–314.

Poling, A., & Ryan, C. (1982). Differential-reinforcement-of-other-behavior schedules: Therapeutic applications. *Behavior Modification, 6,* 3–21.

Rast, J., Johnston, J. M., Drum, C., & Conrin, J. (1981). The relation of food quantity to rumination behavior. *Journal of the Experimental Analysis of Behavior, 14,* 121–130.

Rast, J., Johnston, J. M., & Drum, C. (1984). A parametric analysis of the relationship between food quantity and rumination. *Journal of the Experimental Analysis of Behavior, 41,* 125–134.

Repp, A. C., & Deitz, S. M. (1974). Reducing aggressive and self-injurious behavior of institutionalized retarded children through reinforcement of other behavior. *Journal of Applied Behavior Analysis, 7,* 313–325.

Reynolds, G. S. (1961). Behavioral contrast. *Journal of the Experimental Analysis of Behavior, 4,* 57, 71.

Richmond, G., Schroeder, S. R., & Bickel, W. (1986). Tertiary prevention of attrition related to self-injurious behavior. In K. Gadow (Ed.), *Advances in learning and behavioral disabilities* (pp. 97–108). Greenwich, CT: JAI Press.

Rincover, A. (1978). Sensory extinction: A procedure for eliminating self-stimulatory behavior in autistic and retarded children. *Journal of Abnormal Child Psychology, 6,* 695–701.

Rincover, A., & Devaney, J. (1982). The application of sensory extinction principles to self-injury in developmentally disabled children. *Analysis and Intervention in Developmental Disabilities, 2,* 67–86.

Risley, T. (1977). The ecology of applied behavior analysis. In A. Rogers-Warren & S. Warren (Eds.), *Ecological perspectives in behavior analysis.* Baltimore: University Park Press.

Rogers-Warren, A., & Warren, S. (1977). *Ecological perspectives in behavior analysis.* Baltimore: University Park Press.

Rojahn, J., Mulick, J. A., McCoy, D., & Schroeder, S. R. (1978). Setting effects, adaptive clothing, and the modification of head banging and self-restraint in two profoundly retarded adults. *Behavioral Analysis and Modification, 2,* 185–196.

Rojahn, J., Mulick, J., & Schroeder, S. R. (1979, April). *Analysis of generalization and setting effects during overcorrection to control pica in two retarded adults.* Paper presented at the Twelfth Annual Gatlinburg Conference on Mental Retardation, Gulf Shores, AL.

Rojahn, J., McGonigle, J. J., Curcio, C., & Dixon, M. J. (1987). Suppression of pica by water mist and aromatic ammonia. *Behavior Modification, 11,* 65–74.

Romanczyk, R. G. (1986). Self-injurious behavior: Conceptualization, assessment, and treatment. In K. Gadow (Ed.), *Advances in learning and behavioral disabilities* (pp. 29–56). Greenwich, CT: JAI Press.

Romanczyk, R. G., & Goren, E. (1975). Self injurious behavior: The problem of clinical control. *Journal of Clinical Psychology, 43,* 730–739.

Sajwaj, T., & Hedges, D. (1971, April). *"Side effects" of a punishment procedure in an oppositional retarded child.* Paper presented at Western Psychological Association, San Francisco, CA.

Sajwaj, T., Libet, J., & Agras, S. (1974). Lemon juice therapy: The control of life-threatening rumination in a six-month-old infant. *Journal of Applied Behavior Analysis, 1,* 557–566.

Sallustro, F., & Atwell, C. (1978). Body rocking, head banging, and head rolling in normal children. *Journal of Pediatrics, 93,* 704–708.

Sandler, J. (1964). Masochism: An empirical analysis. *Psychological Bulletin, 62,* 197, 204.

Saposnek, D. T., & Watson, L. S., Jr. (1974). The elimination of the self-destructive behavior of a psychotic child: A case study. *Behavior Therapy, 5,* 79–89.

Schoggen, P. (1978). Ecological psychology and mental retardation. In G. Sackett (Ed.), *Observing behavior* (Vol. 1, pp. 33–66). Baltimore: University Park Press.

Schroeder, C. (1978, September). *The psychologist's role in P.L. 94-142: Consultation strategies with peer groups of handicapped children.* Paper presented at the Annual Convention of the American Psychological Association, Toronto, Canada.

Schroeder, C., & Miller, F. T. (1975). Entry patterns and strategies in consultation. *Professional Psychology, 2,* 182–186.

Schroeder, C., & Schroeder, S. (1979, May). *A behavioral model to school consultation.* Paper presented at the Annual Convention of the American Association on Mental Deficiency, Miami, FL.

Schroeder, S. (1970). Usage of stereotypy as a descriptive term. *Psychological Record, 29,* 457–464.

Schroeder, S., Mulick, J., & Schroeder, C. (1979). Management of severe behavior problems of the retarded. In N. Ellis (Ed.), *Handbook of mental deficiency* (2nd ed., pp. 341–366). New York: Lawrence Erlbaum.

Schroeder, S., Kanoy, R., Thios, S., Mulick, J., Rojahn, J., Stephens, M., & Hawk, B. (1982). Antecedent conditions affecting management and maintenance of programs for the chronically self-injurious. In J. Hollis & C. E. Meyers (Eds.), *Life-threatening behavior* (pp. 105–160). Washington, DC: AAMD Monograph Series No. 5.

Schroeder, S. R., & MacLean, W. (1987). If it isn't one thing, it's another: Experimental analysis of covariation in behavior management data of severely disturbed retarded persons. In S. Landesman-Dwyer & P. Vietze (Eds.), *Living environments and mental retardation* (pp. 315–338). Washington, DC: AAMD Monograph Series.

Schroeder, S. R., Peterson, C. R., Solomon, L. J., & Artley, J. J. (1977). EMG feedback and the contingent restraint of self-injurious behavior among the severely retarded: Two case illustrations. *Behavior Therapy, 8,* 738–741.

Schroeder, S. R., Rojahn, J., & Mulick, J. A. (1978a). Ecobehavioral organization of developmental day care for the chronically self-injurious. *Journal of Pediatric Psychology, 3,* 81–88.

Schroeder, S. R., Rojahn, J., & Mulick, J. (1978b). A behavioral analysis of consent committee performance. *North Carolina Journal of Mental Health, 8,* 25–30.

Schroeder, S. R., Schroeder, C., Smith, B., & Dalldorf, J. (1978). Prevalence of self-injurious behavior in a large state facility for the retarded. *Journal of Autism and Childhood Schizophrenia, 8,* 261–269.

Schroeder, S. R., Mulick, J. A., & Rojahn, J. (1980). The definition, taxonomy, epidemiology, and ecology of self-injurious behavior. *Journal of Autism and Developmental Disorders, 10,* 417–432.

Schroeder, S. R., Bickel, W. K., & Richmond, G. (1986). Primary and secondary prevention of self-injurious behavior. In K. Gadow & I. Bialer (Eds.), *Advances in learning and behavioral disabilities* (Vol. 5, pp. 65–87). Greenwich, CT: JAI Press.

Schroeder, S. R., Breese, G. R., & Mueller, R. A. (1989, in press). Dopaminergic mechanisms in self-injurious behavior. In D. K. Routh & M. Wolraich (Eds.), *Advances in developmental and behavioral pediatrics.* Greenwich, CT: JAI Press.

Sidman, M. (1978). Remarks. *Behaviorism, 6,* 265–268.

Sidman, M., Hernstein, R., & Conrad, D. (1957). Maintenance of avoidance behavior by unavoidable shocks. *Journal of Comparative and Physiological Psychology, 50,* 558–562.

Silverman, K., Watanabe, K., Marshall, A. M., & Baer, D. M. (1984). Reducing self-injury and corresponding self-restraint through the strategic use of protective clothing. *Journal of Applied Behavior Analysis, 17,* 545–552.

Singh, N. N. (1981). Self-injurious behavior. In L. A. Barnes (Ed.), *Advances in pediatrics* (Vol. 28, pp. 337–440). Chicago: Yearbook Medical Publishers.

Singh, N. N., & Millichamp, C. J. (1985). Pharmacological treatment of self-injurious behavior in mentally retarded persons. *Journal of Autism and Developmental Disorders, 15,* 257–267.

Singh, N. N., Gregory, P. R., & Pulman, R. M. (1980). Treatment of self-injurious behavior: A three-year follow-up. *New Zealand Psychologist, 9*, 65–67.

Skinner, B. F. (1953). *Science and human behavior.* New York: Macmillan.

Slawson, P. F., & Davidson, P. W. (1964). Hysterical self-mutilation of the tongue. *Archives of General Psychiatry, 11*(6), 581–588.

Slifer, K. J., Iwata, B. A., & Dorsey, M. F. (1984). Reduction of eye gouging using a response interruption procedure. *Journal of Behavior Therapy and Experimental Psychiatry, 15*, 369–375.

Solnick, J. V., Rincover, A., & Peterson, C. R. (1977). Some determinants of the reinforcing and punishing effects of time out. *Journal of Applied Behavior Analysis, 10*, 415–424.

Sprague, R. L., & Baxley, G. B. (1978). Drugs used for the management of behavior in mental retardation, with comments on some legal aspects. In J. Wortis (Ed.), *Mental retardation* (Vol. 10, pp. 92–129). New York: Brunner/Mazel.

Stinnett, J. L., Hollander, J. H. (1970). Compulsive self-mutilation. *Journal of Mental and Nervous Diseases, 150*, 371–375.

Stretch, R., Orloff, E., & Dalrymple, S. (1968). Maintenance of responding by fixed-interval schedules or electric shock presentation in squirrel monkeys. *Science, 162*, 583–586.

Stubbs, D., & Silverman, P. (1972). Second-order schedules: Brief shock at the completion of each component. *Journal of the Experimental Analysis of Behavior, 17*, 201–212.

Tanner, B. A., & Zeiler, M. (1975). Punishment of self-injurious behavior using aromatic ammonia as the aversive stimulus. *Journal of Applied Behavior Analysis, 8*, 53–57.

Tarpley, H., & Schroeder, S. (1979). A comparison of DRO and DRI procedures in the treatment of self-injurious behavior. *American Journal of Mental Deficiency, 84*, 188–194.

Tate, B. (1972). Case study: Control of chronic self-injurious behavior by conditioning procedures. *Behavior Therapy, 3*, 72–83.

Tate, B. G., & Baroff, G. S. (1966a). Aversive control of self-injurious behavior in a psychotic boy. *Behaviour Research and Therapy, 4*, 281–287.

Tate, B. G., & Baroff, G. S. (1966b, March). *The application of reinforcement theory to modification of self-mutilation behavior.* Paper presented at the meeting of the Southeastern Psychological Association, New Orleans, LA.

The Association for Persons with Severe Handicaps (TASH). (1987). TASH resolution on the cessation of intrusive interventions. *TASH Newsletter, 13*, 3.

Tierney, D. W. (1986). The reinforcement of calm sitting behavior: A method used to reduce the self-injurious behavior of a profoundly retarded boy. *Journal of Behavior Therapy and Experimental Psychiatry, 17*, 47–50.

Touchette, P. E., MacDonald, R. F., & Langer, S. N. (1985). A scatter plot for identifying stimulus control of problem behavior. *Journal of Applied Behavior Analysis, 18*, 343–351.

Turnbull, H. R., Guess, D., Backus, L., Barber, P., Fiedler, C., Helmstetter, E., & Summers, J. A. (1986). A model for analyzing the normal aspects of special education and behavioral interventions: The moral aspects of aversive procedures. In P. Dokecki & R. Zaner (Eds.), *Ethics and decision making for persons with severe handicaps: Toward an ethically relevant research agenda* (pp. 167–210). Baltimore, MD: Brookes.

Vyse, S., Mulick, J. A., & Thayer, B. (1984). An ecobehavioral assessment of a special education classroom. *Applied Research in Mental Retardation, 5,* 395–408.

Wahler, R. G., House, A. E., & Stambaugh, E. E. (1976). *Ecological assessment of child problem behavior.* New York: Pergamon Press.

Waller, M., & Waller, P. (1963). The effects of unavoidable shocks on a multiple schedule having an avoidance component. *Journal of the Experimental Analysis of Behavior, 6*, 29–37.

Warren, S. (1977). A useful ecobehavioral perspective for applied behavior analysis. In A. Rogers-Warren & S. Warren (Eds.), *Ecological perspectives in behavior analysis.* Baltimore: University Park Press.

Weihar, R. G., & Harman, R. E. (1975). The use of omission training to reduce self-injurious behavior in a retarded child. *Behavior Therapy, 6*, 261–268.

Wells, K., Forehand, R., & Hickey, K. (1977). Effects of a verbal warning and overcorrection on stereotyped and appropriate behaviors. *Journal of Abnormal Child Psychology, 5*, 387–403.

Wells, M. E., & Smith, D. W. (1983). Reduction of self-injurious behavior of mentally retarded persons using sensory-integration techniques. *American Journal of Mental Deficiency, 87,* 664–666.

White, G., Nielsen, G., & Johnson, S. (1972). Time-out duration and the suppression of deviant behavior in children. *Journal of Applied Behavior Analysis, 5,* 111–120.

Wieseler, N. A., Hanson, R. H., Chamberlain, J. P., & Thompson, T. (1985). Functional taxonomy of stereotypic and self-injurious behavior. *Mental Retardation, 23,* 230–234.

Williams, J., Schroeder, S. R., Eckerman, D. A., & Rojahn, J. (1983). An ecological analysis of time-out from positive reinforcement in the mentally retarded. In S. Brenning & J. L. Matson (Eds.), *Advances in research in mental retardation and developmental disabilities* (Vol. 1, pp. 199–236). Greenwich, CT: JAI Press.

Winton, A. S., Singh, N. N., & Dawson, M. J. (1984). Effects of facial screening and blind fold on self-injurious behavior. *Applied Research in Mental Retardation, 5,* 29–42.

Wolf, M., Risley, T., Johnson, M., Harris, F., & Allen, E. (1967). Application of operant conditioning procedures to the behavior problems of an autistic child. A follow-up and extension. *Behaviour Research and Therapy, 5,* 103–111.

Wooden, H. E. (1974). The use of negative practice to eliminate nocturnal headbanging. *Journal of Behavior Therapy and Experimental Psychiatry, 5,* 81–82.

Young, J. A., & Wincze, J. P. (1974). The effects of the reinforcement of compatible and incompatible alternative behaviors on the self-injurious and related behaviors of a profoundly retarded female adult. *Behavior Therapy, 5,* 614–623.

Zaharia, E., & Baumeister, A. (1978). Technician turnover and absenteeism in public residential facilities. *American Journal of Mental Deficiency, 82,* 580–593.

Zegiob, L., Alford, G. S., & House, A. (1978). Response suppressive and generalization effects of facial screening on multiple self-injurious behavior in a retarded boy. *Behavior Therapy, 9,* 688.

7

Stereotyped Behavior

JOHANNES ROJAHN AND LORI A. SISSON

INTRODUCTION

Stereotyped behaviors, movements, and acts, stereotypies, autisms, self-stimulatory behaviors, idiosyncratic mannerisms, or blindisms are synonymous terms that refer to a set of clinically conspicuous, socially undesirable, and topographically heterogeneous behaviors. Stereotyped behavior, which will be the preferred term for this chapter, is characteristic of severely and profoundly mentally retarded individuals. It is a key diagnostic feature of childhood autism, and also occurs in blind persons, in the mentally ill, and in geriatric patients. Typical forms are body rocking, mouthing, complex hand and finger movements, repetitive vocalizations, and gazing. The diversity of these behaviors is strikingly illustrated in a review by LaGrow and Repp (1984), who identified 50 different categories in 60 treatment studies.

Stereotyped behavior is generally considered inappropriate, maladaptive, and even harmful for the individual as it is incompatible with learning (e.g., Koegel & Covert, 1972) and appropriate behavior (e.g., Epstein, Doke, Sajwaj, Sorrell, & Rimmer, 1974). During the past 25 years, behavior modification has been the most frequently employed treatment modality for this kind of behavior. The purpose of this chapter is to present a critical review of the behavior modification literature for stereotyped behavior, with special emphasis on outcome research between 1977 and 1987.* Also, three other relevant forms of treatment, pharmacotherapy, structural rearrangements of

---

*The basis of this review, besides a computerized literature search (MEDLARS) and the review of relevant book chapters, is the manual screening of all papers which appeared between January 1977 and July 1987 in the following 17 scientific journals: *American Journal of Mental Deficiency, Analysis and Intervention in Developmental Disabilities, Applied Research in Mental Retardation* (now *Research in Developmental Disabilities*), *Behavioral Assessment, Behavior Modification, Behaviour Research and Therapy, Behavior Therapy, British Journal of Mental Subnormality, Journal of Abnormal Child Psychology, Journal of Applied Behavior Analysis, Journal of Autism and Developmental Disabilities, Journal of Behavioral Assessment and Psychopathology, Journal of Behaviour Therapy and Experimental Psychiatry, Journal of Child and Family Behavior Therapy, Journal of Consulting and Clinical Psychology, Mental Deficiency Research,* and *Mental Retardation.*

JOHANNES ROJAHN • The Nisonger Center, Ohio State University, Columbus, Ohio 43201. LORI A. SISSON • Western Psychiatric Institute and Clinic, University of Pittsburgh School of Medicine, Pittsburgh, Pennsylvania 15238.

the environment, and physical exercise, will be briefly reviewed. Before we turn to the intervention literature, however, pertinent issues regarding the definition, taxonomy, and the origin of stereotyped behaviors shall be addressed.

DEFINITION OF STEREOTYPED BEHAVIOR

Although behaviorally oriented scientists often are less concerned with categorical definitions of clinical phenomena, there is no question that they are extremely important for clinical communication and scientific progress. For instance, when we generalize from the literature about the effectiveness of a certain treatment procedure for stereotyped behavior, we need to know for exactly which behaviors this extrapolation is warranted. At first glance, stereotyped behaviors appear to be easily recognized and identified, because they are so unusual, bizarre, and idiosyncratic in their appearance that they are a primary distinguishing feature between the handicapped and the non-handicapped individual (O'Brien, 1981). Yet the validity of a categorical definition reflects the state of the art of our knowledge about the subject. Because our understanding of the origins and functional properties of stereotyped behavior is still rudimentary, so are our attempts to define such behavior.

According to Berkson's early definition (1967), stereotyped behaviors are associated with mental retardation, mental illness, and blindness in children. They consist of repetitive or nonrepetitive movements, postures, and repetitive utterances of meaningless sounds. Berkson also explicitly distinguished stereotyped movements from other movement disorders with a specific and well-recognized neuropathology, such as parkinsonian symptoms or tardive dyskinesia, and from tics and compulsive rituals, which he considered to be idiosyncratic with a complex symbolic basis. Researchers following an operant approach have addressed external controlling variables, adding that they are often unknown or unspecified (Baumeister & Forehand, 1973; Schroeder, 1970). Others have speculated that a majority of stereotyped behaviors appear to be controlled by proprioceptive, internal reinforcers (Lovaas, Newsom, & Hickman, 1987).

Schroeder (1970) compared different usages of the term *stereotypy* for semantic clarification. He identified four commonly used characteristics of stereotyped behavior as they were known in clinical psychology: Stereotyped behavior (1) occurs more than once, (2) involves the same topography at each occurrence, (3) has unspecified reinforcement contingencies or an unknown etiology, and (4) is related to pathology. Despite some important findings since Schroeder's paper, characteristic (3) still remains the critical differential feature in distinguishing stereotyped behaviors from other movement disorders, such as tardive dyskinesia, Tourette's syndrome, or Huntington's chorea. This leaves a definition by default. Consistent with this logic, the *Diagnostic and Statistical Manual of Mental Disorders* (DSM-III) assigned stereotyped behaviors into a residual category (Atypical Stereotyped Movement Disorders), which is to be distinguished from better understood Specific Stereotyped Movement Disorders, such as the Transient and Chronic Motor Tic and Tourette's Disorders (American Psychiatric Association, 1980). In DSM-III-R (American Psychiatric Association, 1987), this category is called Stereotypy/Habit Disorder. Strictly speaking, stereotyped behaviors are defined by exclusion from known movement disorders, rather than by their generic explanatory elements similar for all stereotypies. It is, however, a legitimate question to ask whether such diverse behaviors as light gazing, object twirling, or posturing actually belong in one group.

CHARACTERISTICS OF STEREOTYPED BEHAVIORS

Rhythmicity of Stereotyped Behavior

Most movement stereotypies, such as body rocking, are performed in a rhythmic fashion; others, such as hand posturing and grimacing, are not. The terminology regarding the distinction of rhythmic versus nonrhythmic performance modes is often inexact. The terms *repetitive, repetitious, invariant,* or *recurring* usually refer to the reappearance of fixed movements or action patterns. The same topography consistently appears with only small variations in an on-or-off fashion (Berkson, 1983). Repetitive occurrence, however, does not imply rhythmicity. Only some forms of stereotypy are rhythmical. Rhythm is a perceptible kinesthetic quality, which is distinguishable by a highly consistent, oscillating movement pattern, which ranges from about half a second to three seconds (e.g., Hollis, 1968; Maris, 1971). Lewis and Baumeister (1982) described rhythmicity as a largely fixed temporal structure or period of the behavior. Thelen (1981) defined it even more precisely as repeated movements, which are executed in the same form at least three times during regular, short intervals of about a second or less. The average frequency of body rocking in 17 severely and profoundly mentally retarded subjects was observed to range between 0.42 to 1.0 Hz (Lewis *et al.*, 1984).

There are indications that rhythmical and arrhythmical stereotypies may have different functional and etiological characteristics. Because early on rhythmic movements have been regarded to serve basic needs necessary for the release of tensions (Langford, 1953; Lourie, 1949), more recently, Berkson (1983) hypothesized that rhythmic movements may be reinforcing in a self-stimulatory sense. Also there is some preliminary evidence that rhythmic stereotyped movements are related to aberrant neurobiologic mechanisms of the dopamine and endorphin systems (see below). These hypotheses have been mostly limited to rhythmical forms of stereotypies and have not been mentioned with behaviors, such as posturing or self-restraint. Most importantly, however, Young and Clements (1979) found differences in the physiological correlates of rhythmical and arrhythmical stereotypies. They studied complex hand movements and rocking behavior in three subjects with mental retardation. It was determined that periods in which the subjects were engaged in complex hand movements were associated with significantly decreased heart rate variability (HRV) as compared to periods of inactivity or gross motor behavior. A reverse effect was observed during periods of body rocking, which was associated with increased HRV levels. These findings suggest that different forms of stereotyped behaviors may have different functional properties depending on whether they are performed in a rhythmic fashion or not.

Stereotyped versus Self-Injurious Behavior

Whether self-injurious behavior (SIB) is a special form of stereotyped behavior, or whether SIB constitutes a separate class of behaviors is occasionally a matter for debate. From a practical point of view, there is no question that it is feasible to distinguish between SIB and stereotyped topographies, because SIB is clinically much more dramatic. SIB also presents a much more serious problem with regard to community placement and risk of reinstitutionalization (e.g., Scheerenberger, 1981). From a scientific perspective, however, the issue is less clear. For instance, it is a widely held position that stereotyped behavior can be self-injurious (American Psychiatric Association, 1987; Carr, 1977; Schroeder, 1970), and also that SIB is an exacerbated form of stereotyped behavior, with a common etiologic basis (e.g., Baumeister & Forehand, 1973). Barron and Sandman (1983) investigated drug response to sedative medication in persons of a mental retardation residential facility. They concluded that persons displaying stereotyped and self-injurious behaviors might have a common biological substrate, which was responsible for the paradox drug response of this group, and which distinguishes them from those residents without either one or only one of these behaviors. There are a few studies that have addressed this issue of classification.

The first type of study deals with the classification of behaviors according to their functional properties. Wieseler, Hanson, Chamberlain, and Thompson (1985) conducted such a study for stereotyped behaviors and SIB based on direct care staff information. They concluded that, in general, stereotypies and SIBs had different functional properties and therefore belonged to different response classes. The vast majority of stereotyped behaviors (92%) were assumed to be motivated by some self-stimulatory effects, whereas most SIB was believed to produce more external, observable rewards, such as attention or escape from an unpleasant task. Unfortunately, stereotyped and self-injurious behaviors were presented as global categories, and it is therefore unclear which specific types of stereotyped or self-injurious behaviors were actually evaluated.

The second type of study deals with topographic classifications of behaviors. Leudar, Fraser, and Jeeves (1984) conducted a factor-analytic study in Scotland on the typology of disturbed behavior in mentally retarded individuals from adult training centers ($n = 247$). Out of 51 problem behavior items, six factors were extracted (idiosyncratic mannerisms, self-injury, aggressive conduct, mood disturbance, antisocial conduct, and communicativeness). By and large, stereotyped behavior and SIB loaded on two separate and independent factors. This indicates that SIB and stereotyped behavior are relatively unrelated phenomena. However, this result has to be viewed with some caution, since SIB and stereotypy were again represented by only one global item each.

Aman, Singh, Stewart, and Field (1985) surveyed maladaptive behaviors in 927 long-stay residents in New Zealand. The problem behaviors were categorized by factor analysis, and it was found that SIB clustered together with other problem behaviors on a factor that was designated "Irritability, Agitation, and Crying." Stereotypies formed a factor on their own. It was found that the correlation between these two behaviors was very weak, signifying relative independence between these domains. In a subsequent study, Aman, Richmond, Stewart, Bell, and Kissel (1987) used the same behavioral items to rate 531 residents of an institution in North Carolina. They found the same pattern of SIB and stereotypy loading on two different factors.

In order to investigate the relationship between SIB and stereotyped behavior, Barron and Sandman (1984) assigned 100 mentally retarded, institutionalized adolescents to four groups; those with self-injurious and stereotyped behaviors, those with SIB only, those with stereotyped behavior, and those without either one. They used the Fairview Problem Behavior Checklist, which lists examples of 22 SIB and 21 types of stereotypy. No differences in demographic characteristics were found among the four groups, offering no evidence for a typological distinction between persons who display stereotyped behaviors and/or SIB. Instead, the authors suggested that these behaviors rather should be classified according to their motivational characteristics as stereotyped SIB and withdrawal stereotypy. However, the lack of reliability estimates and the questionable subject sampling procedure leave some questions open regarding the validity of the results.

Finally, Rojahn (1986) conducted a nationwide SIB survey in noninstitutionalized mentally retarded individuals and identified 431 individuals with that behavior. Information was solicited by staff members through a mail survey on 15 self-injurious and 4 stereotyped categories. Multivariate statistical analyses revealed that *some* forms of SIB were associated with *some* forms of stereotyped behavior, whereas other forms of SIB appeared to be unrelated to stereotyped behaviors. For instance, body rocking was only related to the SIBs head hitting and body slapping; self-restraint was only significantly correlated with pinching. These findings were similar to Barron and Sandman's results (1984) in that there was no evidence in the data to suggest a global taxonomic distinction between SIBs and stereotyped behaviors.

In summary, although studies using global rather than operationalized categories indicate some independence between SIB and stereotypic behavior, it seems that a taxonomic distinction along an "injurious-noninjurious" dimension is not warranted, because neither SIB nor stereotyped behavior is topographically or functionally homogeneous. Research also suggests that some forms of stereotyped and some forms of self-injurious behaviors are related to each other, suggesting that they have a common etiology or similar functional properties.

Prevalence and Incidence

Incidence data on the occurrence of stereotyped behavior in mentally retarded persons are rare. We know, however, that the onset of abnormal stereotyped behavior is generally not reported before the second year (Berkson, McQuiston, Jacobson, Eyman, & Borthwick, 1985). Prevalence estimates usually vary between one and two thirds of the mentally retarded population (Berkson & Davenport, 1962; Dura, Mulick, & Rasnake, 1987; Kaufmann & Levitt, 1965; Rojahn, 1986). On the other hand, Jacobson (1982) found a considerably lower prevalence rate of only 5.8% in a population of over 30,000 people from the state of New York. This comparatively low rate may be accounted for by the restrictive assessment criterion employed by Jacobson. Only "stereotypic/repetitive movements" that were regarded as a behavioral impediment to independent functioning were assessed. Thus, prevalence figures of stereotyped behavior vary widely depending on a number of variables, such as the type of population (e.g., institution versus community), mental and chronological age, and assessment criteria.

Chronological Age and Developmental Level

Data collected by Berkson et al. (1985) indicate that stereotyped behavior is related to chronological age in an inverse U-shaped function. Prevalence of stereotyped behaviors increases until the teenage years and then slowly diminishes. In the profoundly mentally retarded population, the peak prevalence rates occur relatively later in life as compared to less severely mentally retarded people. Interestingly, Thompson and Berkson (1985) reported that stereotyped behaviors in children and young adolescents *without* object involvement (e.g., body rocking, head rolling, or postures) did correlate positively with age, whereas stereotyped behaviors *with* objects (e.g., shake, twirl, or pat) did not.

The prevalence of problem behaviors is generally higher in persons with more severe forms of intellectual impairment. The same finding is true for stereotyped behavior (Eyman & Call, 1977; Jacobson, 1982; Thompson & Berkson, 1985). Eyman and Call (1977), for instance, found in a three state survey involving almost 7,000 individuals that stereotypy was detected in 52% of the profoundly, 34% of the severely, and 14% of the mildly/moderately mentally retarded population.

Residential Setting

Concern over the behavior deteriorating effects of restrictive environments has been voiced repeatedly. The issue of a causal relationship between restrictiveness of the environment and maladaptive behavior of its residents is a difficult one. To resolve it in an empirical fashion seems almost impossible, because the multitude of variables involved. We can safely assume, however, that problem behaviors in general and stereotyped behavior in particular tend to be more prevalent among institutionalized residents than in those living under less restrictive conditions (Borthwick, Meyers, & Eyman, 1981). For instance, Jacobson's (1982) data reveal that serious forms of stereotypic/repetitive movements in persons living in the community was 4% (among a total of over 16,500 persons) as compared to 9% in persons accommodated in developmental centers. Eyman and Call (1977) found stereotyped behavior in 44% of hospitalized individuals, in 21% of the persons living in community living arrangements, and 17% living at home. However, both the restrictiveness of the setting as well as the prevalence of stereotypy are related to level of mental retardation. Eyman and Call's data (1977) confirm this assumption, specifically for the group of individuals who were 12 years and older.

Mental Illness

The notion that mentally retarded children and adolescents are at a much higher risk for emotional and behavioral disturbances than the nonretarded population was first established in the Isle of Wight study (Rutter, Graham, & Yule, 1970; Rutter, Tizard, Yule, Graham, & Whitmore, 1976). Until recently, very little was known about psychiatric disorders in mental retardation, and the identification of psychiatric disorders in mentally handicapped persons still presents considerable diagnostic problems (Costello, 1982; Matson & Barrett, 1982; Reid, Ballinger, & Heather, 1978; Reiss & Szyszko, 1983). The question has been raised whether stereotyped behaviors are associated with psychiatric disorders, or whether they represent a separate, population-specific form of psychopathology.

Reid *et al.* (1978) developed a diagnostic framework for the severely/profoundly mentally retarded population by investigating the natural relationships of general psychiatric symptoms and behavioral disturbances associated with mental retardation. The data were collected via nursing staff ratings, record searches, and a standardized psychiatric patient interview (Goldberg, Cooper, Eastwood, Kedward, & Shephard, 1970). The data of 100 severely and profoundly mentally retarded, hospitalized adults were entered into a cluster analysis. Eight types of individuals were distinguished. One cluster was especially characterized by stereotyped behavior, whereas the other one represented the most severely disturbed subgroup of patients with multiple behavioral abnormalities. Fraser, Leudar, Gray, and Campbell (1986) related psychiatric diagnosis to behavior problems by stepwise multiple regression, including idiosyncratic mannerisms. Again, no significant relationships between any of the eight factors of psychiatric disturbance and idiosyncratic mannerisms were found. Stereotyped behaviors do not appear to predict mental illness. This result is also supported by Jacobson's (1982) finding that the prevalence of stereotyped behavior among mentally retarded persons with and without emotional disturbances was similar (7.3% versus 6%). In summary, there is little empirical evidence in support of the assumption that stereotyped behavior is linked to special forms of psychiatric illness.

ORIGIN AND MAINTENANCE OF STEREOTYPED BEHAVIOR

Stereotyped behavior has been a challenge for researchers from different orientations and scientific approaches, and a large amount of data has been accumulated both in human beings and in subhuman species. Numerous factors associated with stereotyped behavior have been found, animal models have been developed, and complex, yet largely unsubstantiated theories of the origin of stereotyped behavior have been proposed. Some recent neurochemical research findings have opened promising new perspectives and have given older data new meaning. In the current context, only the most relevant theories and observations regarding treatment will be presented. However, etiological theories have recently been treated in more detail in several excellent reviews (Baumeister, 1978; Berkson, 1983; Lewis & Baumeister, 1982).

Physiological Theories

Theory of Homeostatic Balance

The underlying assumption is that organisms strive for the maintenance of a balanced level of central nervous system (CNS) activation. Many mentally retarded and autistic individuals are believed to exhibit a chronically increased level of arousal. In their case, monotonous stereotyped movements block external stimulation and thus lower the arousal level (cf. Lovaas *et al.*, 1987). In support of this hypothesis, stereotyped behavior has been observed to increase with the administration of amphetamines (Klawans, Moses, & Beaulieu, 1974; Randrup & Munkvad, 1967; cf. Lewis & Baumeister, 1982). As was described above, there may also be functional differences between different stereotyped topographies regarding their effects on CNS arousal (Young & Clements, 1979). In general, the empirical evidence related to the arousal hypothesis in human beings is limited.

Central Oscillator Hypothesis

The rhythmical nature of some stereotyped topographies led to the view that they might be controlled by a neural oscillator mechanism in the CNS. Support for this assumption was found in biorhythm research on temporal patterns of rhythmic stereotyped topographies in the retarded (e.g., Lewis *et al.*, 1984; Lewis, MacLean, Johnson, & Baumeister, 1981; Pohl, 1977).

The importance of both physiological theories is that they refer to internal mechanisms that can function in absence of peripheral feedback. This might account for the difficulties in achieving enduring elimination of stereotyped behavior through the control of external variables.

Neurochemical Theories

Behavioral Dopaminergic Supersensitivity

The behavioral dopaminergic supersensitivity theory suggests that the biological basis of stereotyped behavior is a depletion of the neurotransmitter dopamine in postsynaptic cells in the basal ganglia. It is assumed that supersensitivity of the receptors acts as a compensatory mechanism, in that even low levels of dopamine transmission cause an excess response. Depletion of dopamine at postsynaptic receptor sites can be produced by a blockage of dopamine receptor sites caused by the chronic administration of neuroleptic medication, by denervation of dopamine pathways, and by stress. Lewis and Baumeister (1982) hypothesized that such supersensitivity in persons with mental retardation is most plausibly caused by lesions and/or disuse of dopaminergic pathways. Dopamine antagonistic drugs (neuroleptics) have proven to reduce stereotyped behavior, whereas dopamine agonists, such as L-dopa and amphetamines, can exacerbate preexisting stereotypies and even produce new forms in some populations.

Endorphin Hypothesis

Endorphin release in the brain is related, among others, to mild physical stress and intense stereotyped behavior. Endorphin release presumably results in euphoric sensations, and can potentially act as an internal reinforcer (Lewis & Baumeister, 1982). The endorphin hypothesis assumes that stereotyped behavior is maintained by internal reinforcement in the form of endorphin release.

Further research is needed to substantiate these findings. Important information might result from the administration of opiate antagonists, such as naloxone or naltrexone, substances which counteract the endorphin action in the brain. Such results in human SIB research are mixed. The only study in which the effects of naloxone on a stereotypic behavior was observed was published by Sandman et al. (1983). Although the target behavior was SIB, one out of two persons showed a temporary decrease in stereotypic self-restraint during a brief period of time shortly after drug administration.

Behavioral Models

The most important theoretical models for behavior modification are those that consider stereotyped behavior as a learned response. At least three behavioral models of motivation can be distinguished.

Conditional Escape/Avoidance or Negative Reinforcement

The escape/avoidance model assumes a history of successful escape from or avoidance of unpleasant situations by exhibiting stereotyped behavior that maintains that behavior. For instance, stereotyped body rocking is negatively reinforced when it is followed by the termination of a demand to engage in an uninspiring developmental task. Thus, it is likely to occur again. Durand and Carr (1987) found evidence in support of the escape/avoidance hypothesis of stereotyped behavior. They showed that hand flapping and body rocking in four developmentally disabled children increased with the introduction of difficult academic tasks. It was also demonstrated that removal of these tasks contingent upon stereotyped behavior resulted in increased rates of these behaviors. In general, however, the escape/avoidance hypothesis appears to be more relevant for SIB rather than stereotyped behaviors.

Schedule-Induced Stereotyped Behavior

The second behavioral model is based on the observation that repetitive collateral behaviors appear in animals under conditions of low rate reinforcement (DRL) in laboratory situations. The schedule-induced behavior is seemingly nonfunctional (producing no external reward) and therefore reminiscent of stereotyped behavior in developmentally disabled individuals (Lewis & Baumeister, 1982). Although this analog model may offer some interesting and testable questions, its relevance in applied research with the mentally retarded has not been investigated.

Positive Reinforcement or Discriminant Stimulus Control

Under this paradigm, stereotyped behavior is assumed to be maintained by external positive reinforcement. However, such typical rewards as the attention of a caregiver have seldom been observed to follow stereotyped behavior. Related to this model is the *self-stimulation hypothesis,* a theory comprehensively reformulated by Lovaas *et al.* (1987), who stated that stereotyped behaviors are operants that are automatically reinforced by perceptual stimuli produced by the behavior. These reinforcing stimuli can be exteroceptive (e.g., lights, sounds), interoceptive (e.g., vestibular stimulation), or both. Repetitive movement is widespread among infants during the first year of life, which led some theorists to assume that rhythmic movements are innate substrates of more complex motor behavior. Berkson (1983) argued that rhythmic movement itself may be a reinforcer. The self-stimulation theory has served as the conceptual basis of sensory extinction procedures (see below). Although the self-stimulation model has strong face validity, its merits as a scientific theory are questionable. Demonstrating the functional property of an interoceptive stimulus on stereotyped behavior seems beyond empirical verification at this point. In any case, stereotyped behavior often appears to be a highly preferred activity to engage in. The opportunity to engage in

stereotyped behavior has been shown to be an effective reinforcing conse-
quence for the acquisition of low probability behaviors (e.g., Hung, 1978;
Wolery, Kirk, & Gast, 1985), and for the elimination of inappropriate behavior
(Foxx, McMorrow, Fenlon, & Bittle, 1986; see below).

Restricted Environmental and Social Conditions

Intriguing similarities have been noticed between abnormal stereotyped
behavior in mentally retarded individuals and aberrant behavior patterns
exhibited by *isolation-reared* monkeys and apes, particularly in stressful situations (e.g., Berkson & Mason, 1964; Davenport & Berkson, 1963). *Cage-pacing*
behavior of wild animals in captivity has also been considered a model of
stereotyped behavior in mentally retarded people (Berkson, 1983; Lewis &
Baumeister, 1982). As a result of these observations, stereotypic behavior has
been considered to be a behavioral consequence of deprived environmental
conditions.

Ecological Factors Associated with Stereotyped Behavior

Stereotyped behavior appears to be largely influenced by "internal" organismic events, but it is not independent from environmental variables. For
instance, stereotyped behavior has been observed to *increase* with novel restricted environments (Berkson & Mason, 1963) and unfamiliar therapists
(Runco, Charlop, & Schreibman, 1986), television (Gary, Tallon, & Stangl,
1980), prior movement restraint (Forehand & Baumeister, 1970), or the removal of a preferred toy (Greer, Becker, Saxe, & Mirabella, 1985). Wolery *et al.*
(1985) reported that the modeling of a person's stereotypies by another individual can trigger the stereotypic behavior. *Decreases* in stereotyped behavior
are often related to opportunities for alternative behavior (Berkson & Mason,
1963; Goodall & Corbett, 1982), the availability of toys (Davenport & Berkson,
1963), particularly in combination with staff interaction (Berkson & Mason,
1964; Moseley, Faust, & Reardon, 1970), to training in how to engage in toy
play (Greer *et al.*, 1985; Mulick, Hoyt, Rojahn, & Schroeder, 1978), and to
prior rigorous physical exercise (Allen, 1980; Kern, Koegel, & Dunlap, 1984;
Kern, Koegel, Dyer, Blew, & Fenton, 1982; Watters & Watters, 1980). In the
classroom, short intertrial intervals during teaching procedures were also
associated with lower rates of stereotypies as compared to long intervals
(Dunlap, Dyer, & Koegel, 1983).

Regarding the effects of environmental stimuli on stereotyped behaviors,
there are also inconsistencies that might be due partly to insufficiently operationalized behaviors, unprecisely defined independent variables, and the
small number of subjects investigated. For instance, normal volume popular
music was reported to increase stereotyped behaviors in 12 adult retarded
persons with body rocking (Tierney, McGuire, & Walton, 1978), whereas
normal easy listening radio also played at "normal volume" did not increase

stereotyped behaviors in four individuals (Adams, Tallon, & Stangl, 1980). Similar contradiction exists with regard to the rate effect of rhythmic cuing on the tempo of stereotyped behavior (Christopher & Lewis, 1984; Soraci, Deckner, McDaniel, & Blanton, 1982; Stevens, 1971).

Many of the studies cited above used few subjects and investigated only a limited number of ecological variables at a time. However, there is a much higher order of complexity in the interrelationship between setting events and different topographies of stereotyped behaviors than the above listed variables might suggest. For instance, Winnega and Berkson (1986) found that, in a group of 10 subjects, stereotypies were displayed significantly more often during a music condition as compared to meal time, although this difference was not found for stereotyped movements involving objects. Also, Frankel, Freeman, Ritvo, and Pardo (1978) found that the level of environmental stimulation had a differential effect on the stereotyped behavior of autistic children, depending on their level of functioning. Free or controlled naturalistic ecobehavioral correlation studies with multiple response measures might be the better means to reveal some of these intricate stimulus–response and interresponse relationships (e.g., MacLean & Baumeister, 1981; Reese, Schroeder, & Gullion, in press; Rogers-Warren & Warren, 1977; Schroeder, Rojahn, & Mulick, 1978; Schroeder, Schroeder, Rojahn, & Mulick, 1981; Thompson & Berkson, 1985).

BEHAVIORAL ASSESSMENT AND ANALYSIS

Data Collection

Behavioral assessment with mentally retarded persons mostly relies on direct observation by which relative frequency or duration (time spent engaging in stereotyped behavior) can be obtained (Rojahn & Schroeder, 1983). For basic research, in which more precise measures of specific response parameters are required, automated recording devices have been used. For instance, Maris (1971) developed the "rockometer," a device that automatically transformed rhythmical movement into analog waveforms on moving paper (described by Baumeister & Forehand, 1973). A similar instrument was described by Aman (1980) and Aman, White, and Field (1984), who had modeled it after an apparatus by Hollis (1968). Later Hollis (1978) built equipment that used a photocell and a light beam to count back-and-forth movements of body rocking. Lewis *et al.* (1984) used a standard physiograph interfaced with a microcomputer to investigate the synchronicity of body rocking and cardiac activity. Body rocking was recorded with a commercially available single plane accelerometer, which was vertically positioned on the subject's shoulders. Back-and-forth movements were converted into electric signals for recording.

The evaluation of behavior modification techniques for stereotyped behavior is typically performed by means of single subject experimental design (Hersen & Barlow, 1976; Kazdin, 1982). In the psychological literature, treatment evaluations frequently take the form of group studies in which one group receives treatment, a second group receives no treatment or a different treatment, and the two groups are compared on a set of outcome measures. There are no such group studies investigating the relative efficacy of interventions for stereotypy in mentally retarded persons. Group research is often prohibitive in this population because of the extreme heterogeneity in the nature and degree of mental impairment (as well as associated sensory and physical disabilities) and the type of self-stimulatory behavior exhibited. Single-case experimental designs overcome the above mentioned difficulties inherent in group designs because each subject serves as his or her own control. These strategies also allow for comparison of treatment efficacy, although they have been used for this purpose infrequently.

Functional and structural analysis is essential for the selection of appropriate behavior management techniques (Kanfer & Phillips, 1970; Kanfer & Saslow, 1965). Functional analysis is supposed to identify behavior-maintaining contingencies in the natural environment, while structural analysis reveals antecedent stimuli and setting events that are associated with the occurrence of the target behavior. Functional and structural analysis can be performed by informal or systematic observations in the natural environment and by interviewing parents or staff persons familiar with the client's behavior. For these interviews, simple questionnaires or rating scales could be used.

Axelrod (1987) suggested that such formalized procedures of functional and structural analysis might decrease the employment of aversive treatment procedures.

Functional Analysis

Wieseler *et al.* (1985) developed a six-item questionnaire on the motivation of SIB, to be completed by staff members. Two items each addressed one of three controlling consequences of SIB (positive environmental consequences, escape/avoidance, and self-stimulation). A similar instrument was developed by Durand and Crimmins (1983) for different problem behaviors, including stereotyped behavior. It consisted of 16 items (e.g., "Does this behavior occur when you stop attending to him on her?"), each of which represented one of four rewarding consequences (attention, escape, self-stimulation, and tangible reward). Answers were to be given on a seven-point scale, ranging from "always never" to "almost always." Psychometric properties were highly satisfactory. A 56-item functional assessment questionnaire was developed by Hauck (1985) that reflected four consequences (self-stimulation, attention seeking, alleviating pain, and escape/avoidance). Item development, selection, and categorization into subscales of these instruments were based on current motivational theories of SIB (e.g., Carr, 1977). The validity of these scales is still untested.

Functional analysis can also be conducted empirically by procedures, such as the one proposed by Iwata and his research group, that were developed for SIB (Iwata, Dorsey, Slifer, Bauman, & Richman, 1982; Iwata, Pace,

Cataldo, Kalsher, & Edwards, 1984; Parrish, Iwata, Dorsey, Bunck, & Slifer, 1985). In these procedures, the person is repeatedly placed in different, well-defined analog environments, each of which is designed to inhibit differentially or increase the rate of the target behavior according to certain hypotheses. Differential responding of the client in different settings indicates the relevance of particular motivational factors that can determine treatment selection. Iwata *et al.* (1982) designed four environments. In the first, social disapproval was provided for the target behavior, challenging the social reinforcement hypothesis of stereotyped behavior. High rates of self-injury in this condition would be an indication for DRO, DRI, or extinction procedures (a detailed description of these procedures follows below). A second setting tested for escape/avoidance functions of the target behavior by involving the person in educational or other demand-related activities. Proposed treatment recommendations for escape/avoidance behavior were response shaping and guided compliance. Third, being unattended without access to toys was expected to exacerbate SIB that is primarily controlled by its self-stimulatory properties. Treatment could consist of sensory extinction and sensory reinforcement of alternative behaviors. An unstructured play situation was supposed to act as a simulated "environmental enrichment" (Horner, 1980) control condition. The data indicate that there was a considerable amount of between- and within-person variability, suggesting that SIB often has multiple functional properties. However, more research is needed to evaluate the validity and utility of these procedures in applied settings.

Structural Analysis

Touchette, MacDonald, and Langer (1985) introduced the scatter plot technique, a simple but effective observational data recording system, which is intended to reveal functional antecedents graphically. The target behavior is monitored and recorded throughout the client's waking hours by staff or parents. The data sheet consists of a grid box, in which the lines represent time units (30 minutes), and the columns, days. Behavior is recorded categorically as either having not occurred during the past 30-minute time period, as having occurred once, or more than once. The data sheet thus becomes a graph in which occurrence patterns of the target behavior, either during certain times of the day or across days, can be readily identified.

MANAGEMENT OF STEREOTYPED BEHAVIOR

The majority of treatment research with stereotyped behavior among mentally retarded persons involved behavior modification techniques. However, before we discuss behavioral techniques, three other treatment modalities deserve being mentioned. These are physical exercise, psychotropic medication, and environmental rearrangements.

Nonbehavioral Forms of Treatment

Physical Exercise

Physical exercise not only has beneficial effects for mentally retarded persons' cardiovascular efficiency, physical fitness, and general health (cf. Tomporowski & Ellis, 1984), it can also reduce stereotyped behaviors. Positive effects of noncontingent exercise were observed with two severely mentally retarded, institutionalized persons (Baumeister & MacLean, 1984) as well as with autistic children (Kern et al., 1982, 1984; Watters & Watters, 1980). The explanation of the effects of exercise programs on stereotyped behavior are speculative at this point. Simple fatigue can be ruled out to account for all the observed effects (Baumeister & MacLean, 1984). It is likely that physical exercise causes complex physiological and neurochemical changes which, in turn, have an impact on stereotyped behavior. Schroeder, Bickel, and Richmond (1986) argue that dopamine supersensitivity of brain dopamine receptors is responsible for stereotyped behavior, which might come about through lack of use. Exercise, like other mild forms of stress, is known to increase levels of the dopamine metabolite norepinephrine, and thus might counterbalance neurochemically the usual lack of dopamine transmission in the brain.

Psychotropic Medication

Despite the fact that psychotropic medication in general and anti-psychotic drugs in particular can have serious physical and psychological side effects (Aman & Singh, 1980; Gualtieri, Quade, Hicks, Mayo, & Schroeder, 1984), their use for "behavior control" is widespread both in institutional (Radinsky, 1984; Silva, 1979; Sprague, 1977) and in community settings (Agran & Martin, 1982; Gadow & Kalachnik, 1981; Radinsky, 1984). The effects of medication on stereotyped behavior have been investigated in several studies. Reviews of the literature suggest that the only types of medication that appear to reduce stereotyped behavior are the neuroleptics (Aman & Singh, 1986; Aman et al., 1984; Davis, 1971; Hollis, 1968; Hollis & St. Omer, 1972). But the response of stereotyped behaviors to neuroleptics seems to be more complex than that. Singh and Aman (1981) found that lower dosages of thioridazine (2.5 mg/kg) were just as effective as much higher, individually titrated ones in suppressing stereotyped behavior. A subsequent study found that doses of haloperidol, which were functionally half of those used in the thioridazine study, resulted in increased levels of stereotypy (Aman, Teehan, White, Turbott, & Vaithiananthan, 1989). Furthermore, it was found that nondrug stereotypy levels interacted with clinical response to haloperidol: Subjects with low levels of stereotypy tended to show a poorer response to the drug, whereas those with high levels of stereotypy were more likely to show a favorable reaction.

In any case, the practice of medicating mentally retarded persons for such problem behaviors is still far from a satisfactory state, and frequent evaluations of drug regimens would be necessary to assure optimal treatment. For instance, Millichamp and Singh (1987) reported that even substantial reductions of maintenance dosages of neuroleptics did not result in clinically significant increments of stereotyped responding in six profoundly mentally retarded persons. Drug treatment is not particularly popular among some staff members and parents, and the concern about serious side effects and the restrictiveness of treatment are pervasive. Aman, Singh, and White (1987) found that even for staff persons who would carry the burden of management difficulties resulting from withdrawal programs, behavior modification was considered to be a viable alternative for most cases of self-injurious and stereotyped behavior. In another study, mothers of mildly or moderately mentally retarded children who were seeking training in behavior modification were questioned about the acceptability of various treatment procedures (Singh, Watson, & Winton, 1987). The mothers indicated that they preferred positive reinforcement procedures over drug therapy and punishment (time-out), without showing a different opinion between the latter two forms of intervention.

Environmental Modifications

Research has suggested that environmental variables, such as population density, noise, issues related to the daily routine, or availability of "things to do," can have a systematic impact on maladaptive behavior. Structural analysis, as described above, and ecobehavioral research (e.g., Schroeder et al., 1982) can help generate ideas for simple structural rearrangements of the environment, which can be tried prior to initiating more involved forms of intervention. These approaches also provide the necessary assessment methodology. For instance, Gallagher and Berkson (1986) were able to reduce significantly hand gazing in two nearsighted developmentally disabled children by providing corrective lenses. In addition, the posture of these children became upright, and they were more attuned to the surroundings. Mulick et al. (1978) reduced finger picking and nail biting in providing access to toys. Many more examples of such simple and minimally intrusive types of intervention can be found in the literature. Usually, however, such rearrangements do not eliminate stereotyped behavior, but they can play a significant role in combination with more direct forms of intervention.

Behavior Modification

The following section deals with behavior modification techniques for stereotyped behavior, primarily focusing on the literature of the past 10 years (1977–1987). Each of the treatment techniques will consist of the discussion of selected treatment studies, highlighting both the current state of the art and their effectiveness.

Presentation of Positive Reinforcement

Training Adaptive Behavior. As mentioned earlier, researchers noted that stereotyped behavior decreased when novel objects were made available to mentally retarded subjects (Davenport & Berkson, 1963) and when toys were handed to them (Berkson & Mason, 1964). Recently, several investigators have attempted to develop these observations into practical treatments. In one study (Eason, White, & Newsom, 1982), six mentally retarded and autistic children were trained to play with a variety of toys via prompts and reinforcement with edibles, music, or tickles. No consequences were applied to stereotyped behavior. During baseline, toy play seldom was observed, and subjects frequently engaged in stereotyped behavior. However, training increased toy play to high rates and decreased stereotyped behavior to negligible levels. It is significant that these results were seen in settings other than the treatment room, when the trainer was not available, and during 2-month follow-up probes.

Results of the Eason *et al.* (1982) study were replicated and extended by Greer *et al.* (1985). In this investigation, toy play by three severely retarded adults were shaped via prompts, modeling, physical guidance, and reinforcement (edibles). After training, toy play was observed more frequently, while stereotyped behavior occurred less often in free play sessions. Furthermore, gains were maintained across a 6-month follow-up period.

These two studies showed that increases in toy play were accompanied by decreases in stereotypy, even when the stereotyped repertoires were not incompatible with play (Greer *et al.*, 1985). Extrinsic reinforcement can explain why there were initial changes in rates of target behaviors. However, if this were the only variable responsible for the results, it would be expected that the two behaviors would have reversed back to baseline levels when reinforcement was not available. Yet behavioral improvements were observed when the trainer was absent, even after extended follow-up periods. Eason *et al.* (1982) suggested that increased performance of toy play may have introduced the subjects to "natural maintaining contingencies of reinforcement" (Stokes & Baer, 1977). First, caretakers and peers may have begun to reinforce appropriate toy play in other settings, once it began occurring at a sufficiently high, salient rate. Playing with toys would likely elicit positive social interactions, especially as compared to high-rate stereotyped behavior. Alternatively, toy play may have provided sensory reinforcement that was subjectively "better" in quantity and/or quality than that provided by self-stimulatory behavior. Establishing high-level appropriate play may have been necessary to expose subjects to this new form of sensory reinforcement. No matter what the explanation, results of these studies suggest that it may be quite cost efficient to train adaptive behaviors in an effort to control maladaptive stereotyped behavior.

Differential Reinforcement Procedures. Differential reinforcement procedures represent a second noninvasive approach to the treatment of stereotyped behavior in mentally retarded persons and consist of differential reinforcement of other behavior, incompatible behavior, and reinforcement of low rates of stereotyped behavior.

Differential reinforcement of other behavior (DRO) is a format for delivery of a reinforcer after a period of time has elapsed in which a specified target behavior has not occurred. Results of early investigations examining the effectiveness of DRO in reducing stereotyped behavior were mixed, with some studies finding no meaningful effects at all (Luiselli, 1975), others reporting marginal success (Mulhern & Baumeister, 1969), and still others demonstrating marked and rapid effects (Repp, Deitz, & Speir, 1974). This inconsistency led researchers to conclude that the primary value of DRO was as an adjunct to aversive techniques (LaGrow & Repp, 1984).

Two recent efforts conducted by Luiselli and his colleagues are significant in that they support the effectiveness of DRO in managing self-stimulatory behavior and incorporate carefully designed fading phases to facilitate maintenance of treatment gains. In the first study (Luiselli, Colozzi, & O'Toole, 1980), a moderately retarded child received tokens for the absence of inappropriate responding during prescribed intervals measured by a mechanical timer. Tokens were exchanged for access to a play area. Following stable suppression of target responses, maintenance procedures were implemented. First, token reinforcers were gradually eliminated; second, the timer was removed; and third, intervals of reinforcement were increased from 1 minute at the start of the study to 30 minutes at the end of the investigation. Self-stimulatory behaviors failed to increase during the application of maintenance-facilitating procedures, and they remained at low levels at a 2-month follow-up. By the time of this follow-up, treatment contingencies had been faded completely.

In the second investigation evaluating DRO (Luiselli, Myles, Evans, & Boyce, 1985), a young, severely mentally retarded, multihandicapped child gained access to a favorite toy for 1 minute contingent on the absence of stereotyped eye pressing for increasing durations of time. Reinforcement intervals were gradually increased from 1 to 5 minutes across the first phase of the study and from 5 to 25 minutes across the second experimental phase and follow-up. A 3-month follow-up probe showed that treatment gains were maintained with continued use of DRO.

DRO is a cumbersome procedure usually requiring high levels of staff involvement to (1) observe the subject continuously during the intervals, (2) set and reset a timing apparatus, and (3) deliver reinforcers at frequent intervals. In fact, DRO was terminated prematurely by one group of investigators because of staff resistance to its implementation (Tierney, McGuire, & Walton, 1979). Thus, the effectiveness of a modified DRO procedure, which requires less effort on the part of the attending adult, has been investigated. In *momentary DRO* reinforcement is delivered if responding is not occurring at a particular moment of observation (Repp, Barton, & Brulle, 1983). Typically, an event or auditory cue signals time of observation/reinforcement. Harris and Wolchik (1979) used the momentary DRO procedure to reduce self-stimulatory behaviors exhibited by four autistic, mentally retarded boys. Reinforcement was provided following every second academic trial in a school setting, or at 25-second intervals in a play setting. Momentary DRO was found to be moderately effective in decreasing the behavior of one boy, to have no effects with two others, and to increase stereotyped behavior in the fourth. In all four cases, aversive techniques were necessary to achieve clinically significant results.

Although momentary DRO procedures may not reliably reduce stereotyped behavior, they appear to be effective in maintaining improvements once behaviors have been decelerated through traditional DRO schedules. Barton, Brulle, and Repp (1986) exposed nine severely mentally retarded, multihandicapped children to DRO schedules that were designed to decrease maladaptive responding. In seven of these cases, the targets were self-stimulatory in nature. DRO was effective in decreasing occurrences of these behaviors. Following treatment, three maintenance procedures were evaluated: DRO, momentary DRO, and no treatment. Results were that DRO and momentary DRO maintained response suppression at comparable levels whereas rates of behavior increased under baseline conditions.

Differential reinforcement of low rates of behavior (DRL) is another method of programming reinforcement to reduce maladaptive responding. DRL is similar to DRO except that reinforcement is delivered for rates of behavior that are lower than baseline levels rather than for the total absence of the behavior. Singh, Dawson, and Manning (1981) employed DRL in the modification of stereotyped behavior in three profoundly retarded adolescents by providing praise contingent on a target response if it followed the previous stereotyped behavior by at least 12 seconds. Subsequent to suppression of stereotypy, the interresponse time was increased to 30, 60, and then 180 seconds. DRL reduced (but did not eliminate) stereotyped behavior. In addition, social interactive behavior increased although no specific contingencies were applied.

Finally, differential reinforcement of incompatible behavior (DRI) is a procedure in which a specific behavior that competes with stereotyped behavior is shaped by contingent reinforcement. This approach is intuitively appealing because reinforcement follows a predefined adaptive alternative to stereotyped behavior. However, few researchers have evaluated the efficacy of DRI with stereotyped behavior, and results are inconclusive. When used to maintain toy play, DRI reduced the stereotypies of three mentally retarded children (Favell, 1973). Reinforcement for operation of a hand switch also decreased stereotyped hand mouthing in a multihandicapped boy (McClure, Moss, McPeters, & Kirkpatrick, 1986). However, in another investigation (Denny, 1980), reinforcement of toy play eliminated stereotyped behavior in only one of three profoundly mentally retarded subjects, with the remaining individuals requiring the addition of an aversive consequence. Finally, Cavalier and Ferretti (1980) found DRI to be of no use in reducing stereotyped behavior in a profoundly retarded child. Again, punishment procedures were necessary to achieve clinically significant results. Yet, in comparison to DRO, DRI was more effective in reducing self-induced vomiting (Mulick, Schroeder, & Rojahn, 1980) and SIB (Tarpley & Schroeder, 1979).

Although differential reinforcement procedures are preferable to aversive techniques in managing stereotyped behavior, the available literature suggests that they often are insufficient when used alone. Several explanations for this fact are possible. First, it is well known that identification of preferred stimuli is difficult with many mentally retarded clients (Pace, Ivancic, Edwards, Iwata, & Page, 1985). It is possible that investigators have failed to employ potent reinforcers in their work. Second, DRO represents an atypical use of reinforcement in which the contingency is based on the absence of a response rather than on response occurrence. The response-reinforcer relationship may be difficult for the subject to ascertain. Third, DRI is based on the assumption that stereotyped responding will decrease when topographically incompatible responses are increased (Berkson & Mason, 1964; Davenport & Berkson, 1963). However, this relationship is not always straightforward (Klier & Harris, 1977). Because of the inconsistent findings of studies evaluating differential reinforcement procedures, many investigators have used reinforcement in combination with other behavior reduction programs, such as physical restraint (Azrin & Wesolowski, 1980; Barkley & Zupnick, 1976; Barton, Repp, & Brulle, 1985; Cinciripini, Epstein, & Kotanchik, 1980), overcorrection (Coleman, Whitman, & Johnson, 1979; Johnson, Baumeister, Penland, & Inwald, 1982; Kelly & Drabman, 1977), or a slap (Cavalier & Ferretti, 1980; Lancioni, Smeets, Ceccarani, & Goossens, 1983). Use of such treatment "packages" has proven to be quite effective.

Reinforcer Displacement

Another reason why differential reinforcement procedures may not be optimally effective in reducing stereotyped behavior is that this response may be maintained by some historic and inaccessible partial schedule of reinforcement. Laboratory research and anecdotal classroom observations show that behaviors that have been maintained on partial schedules of reinforcement, in contrast to those receiving continuous reinforcement, are highly resistant to extinction. Because DRO and DRI do not provide direct consequences for stereotyped behavior, they rely partly on extinction for their effectiveness. These observations have led several groups of experimenters to gain control of stereotypies by deliberately reinforcing each occurrence of the behavior of interest, thus changing the schedule of reinforcement from an unidentified partial to an explicit continuous one (CRF). Then, reinforcement is abruptly stopped in an extinction phase (EXT). Using this CRF/EXT sequence to reduce existing behavior has been called "reinforcer displacement" (Neisworth, Hunt, Gallop, & Madle, 1985) or "interpolated reinforcement" (Schmid, 1986).

A recent study by Neisworth *et al.* (1985) provided support for a beneficial CRF/EXT effect. Two severely mentally retarded youths were given CRF (edibles) contingent on self-stimulatory behaviors that were being maintained by unplanned reinforcers. Following a number of sessions in this condition, an EXT phase was initiated. Both subjects showed decreases in rate of responding below initial baseline rates when CRF was discontinued. Treatment effects for one participant were maintained over a 2-week follow-up. Schmid

(1986) essentially replicated this effect with six mentally retarded individuals, although target behaviors in this study were not necessarily self-stimulatory in nature.

Foxx *et al.* (1986) described an interesting program whereby the absence of genital stimulation by a severely retarded adolescent male was reinforced with opportunity to engage in stereotyped behavior (DRO). In addition, each instance of the stereotyped behavior during the reinforcement period was followed by delivery of a preferred edible. Later, edible reinforcement was discontinued in an effort to reduce the rate of stereotypy. The results were that genital stimulation was nearly eliminated with the DRO procedure, but CRF/EXT had little effect in reducing the stereotyped behavior. However, reduction in genital stimulation was maintained via DRO, with edibles rather than with stereotyped behavior as the reinforcer. Clearly, more research with the reinforcer displacement technique is needed before any firm conclusions can be drawn about its effectiveness in an applied setting.

Removal of Positive Reinforcement

Social Extinction. Several early investigators hypothesized that social consequences were responsible for maintaining stereotyped behavior in some mentally retarded individuals. It follows, then, that ignoring the subject contingent upon the target response should reduce the level of stereotypy. One study that evaluated social extinction to decrease stereotyped behavior was conducted by Laws, Brown, Epstein, and Hocking (1971) with two mentally retarded children who were involved in a language-training program. Both children engaged in high-frequency stereotyped movements. Ignoring (looking away until stereotypy was terminated) was made contingent upon the target responses. A study reduction in stereotyped behavior was observed over sessions. Using a similar procedure, Sachs (1973) instructed a therapist to turn his back for 30 seconds on a subject on each occasion of spinning or head weaving. Again, this procedure virtually eliminated stereotyped responding. Despite these compelling results, social extinction alone is rarely advocated as a treatment for stereotyped behavior. The reason is because there are many individuals in the wards of institutions who engage in high rates of stereotyped responding with no obvious social stimuli controlling their behaviors. Indeed, one often gets the impression that many of these persons, while engaged in their stereotypy, are "tuned out" and quite oblivious to social events (Baumeister, 1978). This observation was also confirmed by the above-mentioned staff survey by Wieseler *et al.* (1985), which found staff believing that over 90% of stereotyped behavior was performed for self-stimulation. Thus, the primary use of social extinction currently is as part of differential reinforcement procedures.

Time-Out. Time-out is a related procedure whereby all accessible positive reinforcement is withheld for some period as a response consequence. Often, time-out involves removal of the individual to a quiet area contingent on occurrence of the target behavior. There are several reports suggesting that this procedure effectively suppresses stereotyped behavior (e.g., Hamilton, Stephens, & Allen, 1967; Pendergrass, 1972; Wolf, Risley, Johnston, Harris, & Allen, 1967). However, results of a more recent investigation are in conflict with early findings (Clarke & Thomason, 1984). In this study, hand gesturing by an autistic-retarded subject was treated with a 1-minute time-out with virtually no effects. Use of aversive procedures was necessary to eliminate self-stimulatory behavior.

Two variations of time-out from positive reinforcement deserve mention as procedures with potential efficacy in managing stereotyped behavior. In *nonexclusionary time-out*, the target behavior is followed by removal of a discriminative cue (e.g., a ribbon tied to the arm of the client). Although the client is not physically removed from the ongoing activity, absence of the cue provides a signal to both the individual and caretakers that reinforcement will not be delivered. The cue is reintroduced when the target behavior has been suppressed for a period of time. At this time, ongoing positive reinforcement is resumed. McKeegan, Estill, and Campbell (1984) provide data to support the efficacy of nonexclusionary time-out in reducing table slapping in a profoundly mentally retarded adult.

Whether exclusionary or nonexclusionary time-out is used, the importance of the time-in environment cannot be underestimated. Time-in must be highly reinforcing in order that the time-out condition is perceived to be relatively undesirable. Murphy, Nunes, and Hutchings-Ruprecht (1977) ensured the reinforcing properties of time-in by providing continual access to vibratory stimulation for two profoundly retarded young adults. However, when stereotyped hyperventilation or mouthing occurred, the vibrator was removed for the duration of the behavioral episode. This procedure, called *contingent-interrupted stimulation*, was effective in reducing target stereotyped behaviors. Strawbridge, Sisson, and Van Hasselt (1987) have recently replicated this effect by using contingent-interrupted auditory stimulation to eliminate loud, repetitive vocalizations exhibited by a young girl who was profoundly mentally retarded and visually impaired.

Sensory Extinction. Rincover (1978) has suggested that self-stimulatory responses are performed primarily for their sensory input rather than for external consequences. Following this rationale, he developed a treatment that involved removing the sensory feedback from the inappropriate behavior. This intervention is referred to as *sensory extinction*. In one study, Rincover (1978) tested the efficacy of this procedure with an autistic child who spun objects on a table repetitively. It was assumed that the major mode of stimulation was auditory. Thus, auditory input was removed by carpeting the top of the table. Once the carpeting was applied, the child stopped twirling the objects.

Rincover, Cook, Peoples, and Packard (1979) replicated this effect with four other children. With the first subject, proprioceptive stimulation produced by hand flapping was masked by taping a small vibrator to the backs of his hands. In the second case, auditory feedback was removed for a client's plate spinning by carpeting the top of the table. The third child was blindfolded to eliminate the visual consequences of floating objects in the air. Finally, in the case of the fourth child, both proprioceptive and visual input of finger and arm movements were interrupted by vibration and dimming the lights. Stereotyped responding was significantly reduced with these sensory extinction procedures. In an interesting extension of these results, the investigators then trained toy play by carefully selecting toys to provide the type of stimulation offered by the self-stimulatory behavior. For example, a music box was used to produce auditory stimulation, and a bubble-blowing kit was introduced for visual stimulation. Following training in use of these objects, toy play was recorded at high levels, and stereotypies were significantly reduced in three of the four subjects.

Independent replications by other researchers have confirmed the effectiveness of sensory extinction in controlling maladaptive stereotyped behavior. Aiken and Salzberg (1984) used white noise, programmed through earphones, to mask auditory stimuli resulting from aberrant vocalizations that were exhibited by two mentally retarded children. They found dramatic decreases in self-stimulatory responding with application of this technique. Similarly, Maag, Wolchik, Rutherford, and Parks (1986) used visual and kinesthetic sensory extinction procedures to reduce stereotyped finger gazing and manipulating string by two severely retarded boys. Results showed that targeted maladaptive behaviors decreased when sensory extinction procedures were identified and applied. In addition, Maag *et al.* found that results generalized to an untreated topographically similar stereotyped behavior in one child and did not generalize to a topographically dissimilar behavior in the second subject.

As a treatment for stereotyped behavior, sensory extinction has several advantages over many other procedures: for example, it (1) breaks existing contingencies rather than setting up new ones, (2) identifies reinforcers the client selects that can be used to build appropriate behavior, and (3) involves no aversive properties (LaGrow & Repp, 1984). However, although sensory extinction has been effective in reducing a variety of stereotyped behaviors, the practical application of some of the sensory masking procedures must be questioned. Specifically, cumbersome apparatus is often necessary to suppress targeted behaviors, which may restrict the individual's ability to participate in activities outside of carefully controlled environments (Maag *et al.*, 1986). Furthermore, it is difficult to eliminate all the sensory consequences inherent in many commonly occurring stereotyped responses, such as rocking or clapping (Aiken & Salzberg, 1984). Given these problems, researchers should examine both its long-term suppressive effects and ways of making the sensory extinction procedure easier to administer.

Aversive Contingencies

Interruption. Verbal reprimands and/or physical prompts have frequently been used as mildly annoying consequences to reduce stereotyped behavior. In a study conducted by Azrin and Wesolowski (1980), an interruption plus reinforcement procedure was used to decrease stereotyped behavior. During baseline, seven mentally retarded students were involved in a number of activities and were praised for completing tasks. During intervention, praise and edibles were provided for completing tasks while stereotyped behavior was interrupted. The interruption procedure entailed the verbal command, "No, don't . . . ," and guiding the student's hand to his lap or to the table for a 2-minute period. Although the trainer did not hold the child's hands on his lap or on the table (as in studies using immobilization), the child was required to keep his hands down. Gradually, the interruption was faded to 1 second. Results showed that reinforcement plus interruption was effective in decreasing stereotyped behavior to a near zero level for a 35-day period.

Using interruption to reduce hand mouthing also was investigated by Richmond (1983) and Richmond and Bell (1983). In these studies, interruption, which entailed guiding individuals' hands down to their laps for 2 to 3 seconds, was effective in reducing hand mouthing for 3 subjects for 6 months (Richmond, 1983) and for 4 subjects for 12 months (Richmond & Bell, 1983). Chock and Glahn (1983) and Fellner, LaRoche, and Sulzer-Azaroff (1984) found similar procedures to be effective in managing a variety of stereotyped behaviors displayed by developmentally disabled children. In the latter study experimental effects were maintained for 4 months. Several new forms of stereotypy that had appeared as the target behaviors diminished decreased rapidly when interruption was applied to them, and independent toy play increased as a by-product of the treatment.

Immobilization. Other investigators have evaluated the efficacy of response-contingent immobilization techniques in reducing stereotyped behaviors. With this approach, stereotyped behavior is prevented from occurring by interrupting the sequence of responding and by briefly restraining the body part involved in the response. Bitgood, Crowe, Suarez, and Peters (1980) modified the disruptive and self-stimulatory arm-flapping, clapping, pounding, and head-slapping behaviors of four mentally retarded children using immobilization. Each time the target behavior occurred, an experimenter grasped the child by the forearms and held the child's arms at his or her sides, using only the force necessary to keep the arms touching the side of the body. No prompt or verbal caution preceded the application of this treatment. The immobilization lasted 15 seconds. This study is notable in that the investigators carefully recorded the occurrence of several self-stimulatory and disruptive behaviors exhibited by each child in addition to the response receiving treatment. Interestingly, although target behaviors were reduced by the immobilization procedure in all four cases, nontarget stereotypies decreased in three cases but increased in one.

Reid, Tombaugh, and Heuvel (1981) treated body rocking by seven profoundly mentally retarded persons using a 1-minute immobilization procedure. These researchers reported that the effectiveness of immobilization depended in part at which point, in the sequence of the target behavior, treatment was applied. The most effective application was when the subject was bent over in the middle of the response sequence rather than while sitting upright at the end of the response sequence. In another evaluation of immobilization, Luiselli (1981) found a 10-second restraint to be more effective than reinforcement methods in managing self-stimulatory arm-and-hand movements in two multihandicapped children.

Finally, Rolider and Van Houten (1985) adapted a corner time-out procedure by adding immobilization for the treatment of stereotyped behaviors exhibited by three mentally retarded young adults. In particular, whenever stereotypies were observed, subjects were told to go immediately to a corner and were assisted in going there as quickly as possible. Then, if the individual engaged in stereotyped movements while in time-out, the trainer said "Don't move" and pressed the subject firmly into the corner by placing one hand against his upper back between the shoulder blades. This procedure lasted approximately 3 minutes. This modified time-out was found to be more effective than traditional corner time-out or isolation time-out in all three cases. Stereotyped behavior was reduced to negligible levels in two of the three subjects. The effectiveness of immobilization time-out was attributed to the fact that subjects were unable to engage in stereotyped responding while under the time-out contingency.

Overcorrection. Frequently used in the treatment of stereotyped behavior, overcorrection is a more intrusive procedure. It typically involves components of interruption and immobilization. In addition, overcorrection requires clients to perform a sequence of repetitive behaviors as a consequence of the stereotyped act. The behaviors required by the overcorrection rationale are of two types: restitution and positive practice. In *restitutional overcorrection*, the individual must restore him- or herself or the environment to a state that is much improved over what existed before the undesirable act occurred. In *positive practice overcorrection*, the emphasis is placed upon extensive practice of behaviors that are often, but not always, physically incompatible with the inappropriate behavior.

Foxx and Azrin (1973) and Azrin, Kaplan, and Foxx (1973) described the first systematic applications of overcorrection to self-stimulatory behaviors in mentally retarded individuals. These studies provided the impetus for a large literature that addresses the efficacy of both restitutional and positive practice overcorrection in managing a variety of self-stimulatory behaviors across a wide range of settings (see reviews by O'Brien, 1981; Ollendick & Matson, 1978). For example, Doke and Epstein (1975) used contingent teeth brushing to reduce thumb sucking by a developmentally delayed child in day care; Barrett and Linn (1981) required toe tapping whenever toe standing or toe walking was emitted by a multihandicapped child during physical therapy sessions; and Maag, Rutherford, Wolchik, and Parks (1986) guided mentally retarded subjects' hands and arms through a series of exaggerated movements following each instance of stereotyped finger play and clapping during a classroom instructional period.

As these examples indicate, the overcorrection exercises generally are chosen to be topgraphically related to the offending behavior. Yet a number of early investigations revealed that many stereotypies could be suppressed with overcorrection activities that were not topographically similar to them.

In one investigation (Epstein *et al.*, 1974), a positive practice requirement involving individuals' hands and arms was applied to foot stereotyped behavior as well as to vocal stereotyped behavior. The target stereotypy was decreased in both cases. Similarly, when hand overcorrection exercises were used to reduce two hand stimulation behaviors (hand shaking and nose touching) and two behaviors not involving hands (laughing and head weaving), all four stereotyped behaviors decreased (Ollendick, Matson, & Martin, 1978). However, the two hand stimulation behaviors were reduced more quickly, and they remained at lower levels after treatment than the two behaviors that were unrelated to the hand overcorrection exercises.

The duration of overcorrection exercises has ranged from 30 seconds (Barrett & Linn, 1981) to 20 minutes (Foxx & Azrin, 1973), with the majority of studies reporting positive effects with procedures lasting from 2 to 5 minutes (e.g., Matson & Stephens, 1981; Wells, Forehand, Hickey, & Green, 1977). In a few studies, the duration of overcorrection was examined for individuals whose inappropriate behaviors were not eliminated by initial brief overcorrection procedures. In these studies, increasing the duration of overcorrection resulted in an increase in effectiveness (Czyzewsky, Barrera, & Sulzer-Azaroff, 1982; Foxx & Azrin, 1973; Ollendick & Matson, 1976).

Even at short durations, overcorrection is sometimes difficult to apply on account of staffing constraints in clinical settings or uncooperative clients (Sisson, Van Hasselt, Hersen, & Aurand, 1988). Thus, issues of generalization of treatment effects across conditions and maintenance of treatment gains across time become extremely relevant issues. An early investigation (Martin, Weller, & Matson, 1977) reported that object manipulation that was suppressed with overcorrection in the classroom also decreased on the hospital ward, although no treatment occurred there. However, most studies of overcorrection consequences for stereotyped behavior have demonstrated little transfer of suppression. Foxx and Azrin (1973) noted that while overcorrection virtually eliminated mouthing of objects by one client in a day-care program, parents reported that mouthing increased in the home.

Rollings, Baumeister, and Baumeister (1977) demonstrated a client's ability to discriminate between safe and punishment conditions on the basis of the proximity of the trainer to the client. These results were extended in a later study (Rollings & Baumeister, 1981), in which discrimination training using the overcorrection technique was carried out under conditions in which a light on one end of a series of five lights signaled the presence of the punishment contingency and a light on the other end was associated with the absence of punishment. Tests for generalization of inhibition of stereotypy were made to all five lights in the series. Sharp generalization gradients were found, indicating that the two subjects (one severely and one profoundly retarded) easily discriminated the stimulus conditions under which punishment occurred. In a third study (Matson & Stephens, 1981), overcorrection was used to treat the wall-patting behavior of a severely mentally retarded adult in three hallways. These researchers found that the subject clearly discriminated safe hallways from those in which overcorrection was used and that this subject and three similar subjects clearly discriminated the trainer from three other persons in terms of the amount of stereotyped responding emitted in the presence of each.

The effects of overcorrection appear to be limited not only by their failure to transfer across situations but also by their lack of durability over time. In three studies, the self-stimulatory behaviors treated with overcorrection had returned to baseline levels by the time of 6- (Rollings *et al.*, 1977), 9- (Czyzewski *et al.*, 1982), and 12-month (Matson, Ollendick, & Martin, 1979) follow-up probes. Foxx and Azrin (1973) and Barrett and Linn (1981) facilitated maintenance of treatment gains by instituting a verbal warning phase once control over the target behavior was obtained. In this procedure, subjects were given a verbal warning on the first instance of stereotyped behavior during a session of prespecified length. If stereotyped behavior ceased immediately, overcorrection was not implemented. However, the verbal warning plus overcorrection was carried out whenever any additional stereotyped behaviors occurred. In another attempt to promote treatment durability, Matson and Stephens (1981) systematically positioned the trainer farther away from the subject while continuing to administer the overcorrection treatment on each occurrence of the target behavior. It appears that generalization and maintenance of treatment effects must be programmed to occur through training in more than one environment, by using as many different trainers as possible, and by continuing to use overcorrection, albeit in a modified form.

Unfortunately, several researchers have found that the use of overcorrection sometimes increases nontarget stereotyped behaviors (Harris & Wolchik, 1979; Rollings & Baumeister, 1981; Rollings *et al.*, 1977). More importantly, Rollings *et al.* (1977) noted the emergence of troublesome self-injurious behaviors not previously seen, including self-pinching, head banging, and self-scratching. On the other hand, Foxx and Azrin (1973) mentioned that, in addition to decreasing stereotyped behavior, overcorrection serves to teach the adaptive behaviors included in the positive practice or restitution requirement. There has been much debate surrounding this claim (Doke & Epstein, 1975; Hobbs, 1976). When one group of investigators (Wells *et al.*, 1977) incorporated appropriate playing with toys in the positive-practice requirement for decreasing object manipulation, hand movements, and mouthing, they noted an increase in appropriate toy play for one of their two autistic clients. However, in a second study (Roberts, Iwata, McSween, & Desmond, 1979), overcorrection responses remained stable or decreased when they were effectively applied for various stereotyped behaviors.

Positive concurrent effects unrelated to the target or overcorrection responses have been observed. Matson and Stephens (1981) recorded an increase in smiling and verbal communications when they decreased wall patting with overcorrection. Czyzewski *et al.* (1982) reported that social interactions improved whereas tantrum behavior declined when a variety of stereotypies were treated with overcorrection procedures. Thus, studies that decreased stereotyped behavior with overcorrection have reported both negative and positive side effects on other behaviors. Although concurrent behavior changes should be expected whenever a target response is modified, these early accounts have alerted clinicians and researchers to monitor such changes when decreasing self-stimulatory behavior. Development of deceleration techniques for inappropriate concurrent behaviors and reinforcement strategies for desirable concurrent behaviors may be necessary to increase overall adaptive responding.

Facial and Visual Screening. Facial screening is a procedure that involves the use of a terry cloth bib to cover the subject's entire face, for a brief time period, contingent on the occurrence of a target behavior (Lutzker, 1974; Zegiob, Jenkins, Becker, & Bristow, 1976). It is the newest treatment for stereotyped behavior. Like visual sensory extinction (Rincover, 1978) described earlier, facial screening is thought to be effective because visual input is blocked. However, in the first investigation in which facial screening was applied to a self-stimulatory behavior (Barmann & Murray, 1981), the target behavior was a topographically dissimilar one (i.e., it did not provide visual stimulation). The subject was a severely mentally retarded adolescent who exhibited frequent public genital stereotyped behavior. The facial screening procedure was applied for 5 seconds contingent on each instance of this behavior. Public masturbation was rapidly eliminated at school, on the school bus, and at home. Further, treatment gains were durable across a 6-month follow-up period.

A variation of this procedure has been investigated in three subsequent studies. The technique, termed *visual screening*, differs from facial screening in that the therapist uses his or her hand rather than a bib to cover the individual's eyes. In the first investigation (McGonigle, Duncan, Cordisco, & Barrett, 1982), a variety of visual and auditory self-stimulatory behaviors exhibited by moderately and profoundly mentally retarded children were successfully modified. Results indicated that visual screening was equally effective for topographically similar and dissimilar stereotypies. In the second study (Barrett, Staub, & Sisson, 1983), repetitive shoe-related activities (touching, kissing, fondling shoes) were reduced with visual screening. Finally, Dick and Jackson (1983) found visual screening to be effective in eliminating stereotyped screaming by a mentally retarded preschool child. In all cases, behavioral gains were seen for at least 6 months following termination of treatment. Watson, Singh, and Winton (1986) demonstrated with two subjects that visual screening was slightly more superior to facial screening in terms of consistency and degree of suppression.

Other Aversive Consequences. The preceding review has presented the most frequently used techniques to modify stereotyped behavior in mentally retarded persons. Sometimes these strategies are ineffective, and, in such cases, more intrusive procedures have been applied with apparent success. Alternatively, researchers have turned to other aversive techniques to preclude problems of resistance expected with such procedures as immobilization and overcorrection. These procedures include electric shock (Baumeister & Forehand, 1972; Lovaas, Schaeffer, & Simmons, 1965), aromatic ammonia (Clarke & Thomason, 1984), slapping (Romanczyck, 1977), contingent lemon juice, vinegar, or water mist (Friman, Cook, & Finney, 1984), all of which have been shown to reduce stereotyped responding in severely and profoundly mentally retarded subjects. Some contingencies had inconsistent effects; for instance, contingent imitation of the target behavior by the therapist decreased tongue protrusion (Kauffman, Hallahan, & Ianna, 1977), but increased a child's yelping (Kauffman, LaFleur, Hallahan, & Chanes, 1975).

Although these procedures are usually effective, their use with mentally retarded individuals (The Association for Persons with Severe Handicaps, 1986), and particularly for stereotyped behavior which does not inflict physical harm (Hobbs & Goswick, 1977), has been questioned by some professionals on ethical grounds.

Treatment Packages

Combinations of Behavioral Components. In order to gain rapid success in treatment, clinical research and practice frequently has used intervention "packages" (Paniagua, Braverman, & Capriotti, 1986). These packages consist of two or more techniques likely to be effective alone or in combination in managing the target response. Typically, these treatment packages include a reinforcement strategy plus an aversive contingency. For example, in two studies mentioned previously (Richmond, 1983; Richmond & Bell, 1983), DRO (one spoonful of ice cream delivered on a DRO 1- to 5-minute schedule) plus interruption (moving the individuals' hands to their laps for 2 to 3 seconds) was effective in eliminating hand mouthing in several profoundly retarded women. In the second study (Richmond & Bell, 1983), a component analysis for two subjects indicated that DRO alone had little effect on the level of mouthing, whereas interruption alone resulted in a substantial reduction in occurrence of the target behavior. Indeed, the additive effect of combining DRO with interruption was small.

DRO (M&M candies given according to an increasing DRO schedule) plus immobilization (holding the subject's arms at her sides) resulted in a significant decrease in stereotyped body contortions in a mentally retarded girl (Barkley & Zupnick, 1976). In a similar effort, Barton *et al.* (1985) treated a number of stereotypies exhibited by four severely or profoundly mentally retarded students with a combined DRO and immobilization approach. In the latter investigation, both DRO and immobilization intervals were increased systematically, depending on the subject's performance across a 1-day period.

Treatment packages described in the literature have most frequently included a reinforcement program coupled with overcorrection. Denny (1980) combined DRI (praise contingent on toy play) with positive practice overcorrection (wheelchair-mobility training) to modify successfully a variety of stereotyped behaviors displayed by three multihandicapped youths. With effective treatment for stereotyped behavior, toy play increased, although subjects did not achieve proficiency in propelling their wheelchairs. Follow-up probes at 1 and 2 months showed that effects were durable. Other investigators also have reported that reinforcement (praise and/or edibles given according to DRO or DRI schedules) plus overcorrection (manipulation through various exercises) efficiently reduced stereotyped behavior (Coleman *et al.*, 1979; Kelly & Drabman, 1977; Paniagua *et al.*, 1986; Sisson *et al.*, 1988). Sisson *et al.* (1988) found that momentary DRO alone decreased stereotyped behavior somewhat in one multihandicapped child but had no effect on level of stereotypy in a second subject. In both cases, the addition of overcorrection was necessary to achieve near-zero rates of maladaptive stereotyped behavior. All studies reported that transfer of treatment effects did not occur automatically but had to be programmed by having a variety of trainers carry out procedures across relevant settings. Sisson *et al.* (1988) found low levels of stereotypy at 5-month follow-up assessment. However, this result was achieved only through careful fading of DRO and overcorrection treatments over an extended time period.

Stereotyped behavior of severely to profoundly mentally retarded subjects also has been decreased through the use of treatment packages that included DRI plus slapping (Cavalier & Ferretti, 1980; Lancioni *et al.*, 1983) and DRI plus water mist (Lancioni *et al.*, 1983). In both studies, reinforcement alone proved insufficient in managing stereotyped behavior.

Combinations of Behavioral and Pharmacological Treatments. Combined treatment with behavior modification and neuroleptic medication in mental retardation is often a clinical reality, yet only a few studies have been conducted to investigate the possibility of complementary treatment effects. There are indications that simultaneous pharmacological and behavioral treatment can be superior to unimodal interventions (e.g., Campbell *et al.*, 1978; Durand, 1982). The interaction between behavioral and pharmacological treatments for stereotyped behavior have been evaluated in only two efforts. In a group study, Schalock, Foley, Toulouse, and Stark (1985) found that using behavior management programs allowed reduction in neurologic and antidepressant medications without loss of behavioral control of stereotypies and noncompliance. As indicated by the authors, several methodological shortcomings limit the generalizability of the results. In the second study, an anticonvulsant drug was not found to contribute to the effectiveness of a behavior modification package. Cinciripini *et al.* (1980) reported that DRI plus immobilization decreased hand stereotyped behavior and increased on-task behavior in a multihandicapped child. Medication (carbamazepine) was added, but then withdrawn, since it produced no added benefits. An 8-month follow-up showed maintenance of behavioral gains even though no behavioral contingencies were in effect at the time.

Treatment Comparisons

The previous review demonstrates that stereotyped behavior has been suppressed by a variety of different procedures based on the principles of reinforcement, extinction, and punishment. In a few cases, researchers have utilized several procedures, one after the other, in an attempt to achieve control over problematic behavior. When this has occurred, findings were that reinforcement was insufficient when used alone to manage stereotypy, and the addition of interruption (Richmond & Bell, 1983), immobilization (Barton *et al.*, 1985), overcorrection (Sisson *et al.*, 1988), or other aversive procedures was necessary to achieve behavioral control (Lancioni *et al.*, 1983). In light of these results, it is tempting to conclude that punishment procedures are more effective than reinforcement strategies in reducing stereotyped behavior.

However, there are few direct comparisons of treatments for stereotyped behavior. In a recent investigation, McKelvey, Sisson, Van Hasselt, and Hersen (1987) used a withdrawal design to compare two treatment procedures for mouthing of objects by a severely handicapped deaf-blind girl. In the first phase of the study, baseline observations were carried out to ascertain the level of mouthing observed in each of three settings. Then, in one setting only, DRO was applied in which the subject was given a preferred edible reinforcer following increasing intervals without mouthing. DRO had no readily apparent effects on the target behavior. Next, brief immobilization was added. In this condition, DRO continued; in addition, whenever mouthing occurred, the child's hands were grasped firmly by the trainer and held at her sides for 3 seconds. DRO plus immobilization substantially reduced mouthing. In accordance with the requirements of the withdrawal design, DRO plus immobilization was withdrawn and DRO alone was reinstituted. During this phase, levels of mouthing increased to those observed under previous DRO contingencies. Then, when the treatment package was applied again, behavioral control was achieved. This sequence of experimental conditions allowed the conclusion that DRO plus immobilization was superior to DRO alone in reducing object mouthing in this multihandicapped girl. Experimental control was demonstrated further by extending treatment to the other two settings, in multiple-baseline fashion. Treatment effects were durable for 4 months.

In another study using an alternating treatments design, Barrett, Matson, Shapiro, and Ollendick (1981) treated high-rate stereotyped responding in two moderately mentally retarded children with DRO and punishment. For one child, the study was initiated by taking baseline data on rate of stereotypy (finger sucking) under three conditions that were identical except for discriminative cues that signaled potential consequences for stereotyped behavior. During the alternating treatments phase, three response consequences were evaluated: no treatment (a control condition), DRO, and visual screening. Within a few sessions, the differential effectiveness of these procedures became apparent, with visual screening resulting in marked reduction of the target behavior. Visual screening was then instituted in the other two conditions, in sequential fashion, and was effective in both. This study showed that visual screening was more effective than no treatment and DRO procedures. Treatment was extended throughout the child's day, and effects were durable for 6 months. Similar alternating treatment evaluations have found that (1) depression of the tongue with a wood blade reduced tongue protrusion more efficiently than DRO and no treatment in one multihandicapped child (Barrett *et al.*, 1981); (2) immobilization and positive practice overcorrection were equally effective in decreasing mouthing in three severely retarded children

(Shapiro, Barrett, & Ollendick, 1980); and (3) although immobilization and positive practice overcorrection were both superior to no treatment in the modification of stereotypies in three mentally retarded, behaviorally disordered children, the active treatments were differentially effective for different subjects.

These initial efforts to determine empirically the relative efficacy of treatments for stereotyped behavior are encouraging. However, because of the paucity of such studies, we are reluctant to make summary statements with regard to the most efficacious interventions. Clearly, future investigative endeavors must address the impact of differential treatment. Such studies are warranted in order to direct clinical management of stereotyped behavior in mentally retarded persons.

CONCLUDING REMARKS

Stereotyped behavior among persons with mental retardation is a fascinating clinical phenomenon that has attracted the curiosity of many scientists in basic and applied research. Yet we still know relatively little about the origin, the functional properties, and the taxonomy of these different forms of stereotyped behaviors. Research suggests that there is no strong evidence for a taxonomic distinction between SIB and stereotyped behavior. Also, stereotyped behavior does not appear to be predictive of special types of psychiatric illness.

Neurochemical research has advanced new and interesting perspectives in recent years, offering insight on the biological basis of stereotyped behavior. It remains to be seen whether better understanding of biological substrates will lead to new generations of safer drugs with fewer side effects and to pharmacotherapy for stereotyped behavior with a satisfactory rationale. At this point, pharmacotherapy is still in its initial stages (Aman, 1986). It seems as if the neuroleptics are the only currently available drugs that can systematically decrease stereotyped behavior. Much more research is needed in this area.

Noncontingent exercise programs and environmental rearrangements were discussed as simple, noninvasive procedures, which also warrant further research. Although their effects are probably too small and nonspecific for a clinically valid treatment program *per se* for stereotyped behavior, they appear to be beneficial when accompanying more systematic and focused interventions.

As far as management is concerned, behavior modification has continued to be the most effective type of treatment of stereotyped behavior over the past 10 years. Almost the entire spectrum of techniques has been employed for stereotyped behaviors in one study or another, ranging from relatively benign procedures, such as selective reinforcement to increase appropriate responding, to restrictive, aversive programs that are aimed at quick suppression of stereotyped behavior. Some of these techniques, specifically, removal of reinforcement and aversive contingencies (overcorrection, immobilization, visual and facial screening), are often highly effective, but only for short-term control. Negative side effects of these techniques are less of a problem than often implied by some researchers, who oppose aversive procedures on philosophical rather than scientific grounds. In fact, some of the studies featuring aversives or "mild punishment" procedures, as they are sometimes called, found even positive side effects. The main problems of most of the procedures involving aversives and/or reinforcement removal are a lack of transfer of treatment effects to other settings and a limited time of maintenance. Other forms of behavioral intervention, such as reinforcement techniques, are mostly useful as components in treatment packages, including response reduction techniques. Usually, elimination of stereotyped behavior will not be achieved by reinforcement of some other behaviors alone. Clinicians are therefore confronted with the dilemma either to select a potent, but invasive and ethically questionable procedure or to relinquish complete suppression of the target behavior as a treatment goal.

In reviewing the treatment literature, it occurred to us that a word of caution about the treatment indication for stereotyped behaviors might be appropriate. The clinical rationale for some of the reviewed studies was occasionally difficult to discern. In justifying intervention, the authors generally refer to the literature that stereotyped behavior is supposedly harmful for the individual because it interferes with learning (e.g., Koegel & Covert, 1972), adaptive functioning (Epstein *et al.*, 1974), and with desirable interaction with the environment. Rarely do we find empirical demonstration of the clinical necessity for treatment prior to intervening with a given individual. Similarly, it is rare to find evidence that an increase of appropriate behavior actually resulted as a function of the suppression of stereotyped behavior. Further research may reveal that not all individuals with stereotyped behaviors will benefit from elimination of their stereotyped mannerisms, because they are not that disadvantaged by their stereotyped behavior to begin with. An excellent case in point is the experimental study by Watkins and Konarski (1987), who found that not all subjects showed a detrimental impact of their stereotyped behavior on learning. Their data suggested that only the low-functioning subjects with high-level stereotypies were adversely affected in their learning.

REFERENCES

Adams, G. L., Tallon, R. J., & Stangl, J. M. (1980). Environmental influences on self-stimulatory behavior. *American Journal of Mental Deficiency, 85,* 171–175.

Aiken, J. M., & Salzberg, C. L. (1984). The effects of a sensory extinction procedure on stereotypic sounds of two autistic children. *Journal of Autism and Developmental Disabilities, 14,* 291–299.

Allen, J. J. (1980). Jogging can modify disruptive behaviors. *Teaching Exceptional Children, 12,* 66–70.

Agran, M., & Martin, J. E. (1982). Use of psychotropic drugs by mentally retarded adults in community programs. *Journal of the Association for the Severely Handicapped, 7,* 54–59.

Aman, M. G. (1980). Mechanism for testing operant conditioning and body rocking in developmental disabilities. *Perceptual and Motor Skills, 58,* 751–756.

Aman, M. G. (1986). Drugs in mental retardation: Treatment or tragedy? *Australia and New Zealand Journal of Developmental Disabilities, 10,* 215–226.

Aman, M. G., & Singh, N. N. (1980). The usefulness of thioridazine for treating childhood disorders—fact or folklore? *American Journal of Mental Deficiency, 84,* 331–338.

Aman, M. G., & Singh, N. N. (1986). A critical appraisal of recent drug research in mental retardation: The Coldwater studies. *Journal of Mental Deficiency Research, 30,* 203–216.

Aman, M. G., White, A. J., & Field, C. (1984). Chlorpromazine on stereotypic and conditioned behavior of severely retarded patients—a pilot study. *Journal of Mental Deficiency Research, 28,* 253–260.

Aman, M. G., Singh, N. N., Stewart, A. W., & Field, C. T. (1985). The aberrant behavior checklist: A behavior rating scale for the assessment of treatment effects. *American Journal of Mental Deficiency, 89,* 485–491.

Aman, M. G., Richmond, G., Stewart, A. W., Bell, J. C., & Kissel, R. C. (1987). The aberrant behavior checklist: Factor structure and the effect of subject variables in American and New Zealand facilities. *American Journal of Mental Deficiency, 91,* 570–578.

Aman, M. G., Singh, N. N., White, A. J. (1987). Caregiver perceptions of psychotropic medication in residential facilities. *Research in Developmental Disabilities, 8,* 449–465.

Aman, M. G., Teehan, C. J., White, A. J., Turbott, S. H., & Vaithianathan, C. (1989). Haloperidol treatment with chronically medicated residents: Dose effects on clinical behavior and reinforcement contingencies. *American Journal of Mental Retardation, 93,* 452–460.

American Psychiatric Association. (1980). *Diagnostic and statistical manual of mental disorders* (3rd ed.). Washington, DC: Author.

American Psychiatric Association. (1987). *Diagnostic and Statistical Manual of Mental Disorders* (3rd ed., rev.). Washington, DC: Author.

Axelrod, S. (1987). Functional and structional analysis of behavior: Approaches leading to reduced use of punishment procedures? *Research in Developmental Disabilities, 8,* 165–178.

Azrin, N. H., & Wesolowski, M. D. (1980). A reinforcement plus interruption method of eliminating behavioral stereotypy of profoundly retarded persons. *Behaviour Research and Therapy, 18,* 113–119.

Azrin, N. H., Kaplan, S. J., & Foxx, R. M. (1973). Autism reversal: Eliminating stereotypic self-stimulation of retarded individuals. *American Journal of Mental Deficiency, 78,* 241–248.

Barkley, R. A., & Zupnick, S. (1976). Reduction of stereotypic body contortions using physical restraint and DRO. *Journal of Behavior Therapy and Experimental Psychiatry, 7,* 167–170.

Barmann, B. C., & Murray, W. J. (1981). Suppression of inappropriate sexual behavior by facial screening. *Behavior Therapy, 12,* 730–735.

Barrett, R. P., & Linn, D. M. (1981). Treatment of stereotyped toe-walking with overcorrection and physical therapy. *Applied Research in Mental Retardation, 2,* 13–21.

Barrett, R. P., Matson, J. L., Shapiro, E. S., & Ollendick, J. H. (1981). A comparison of punishment and DRO procedures for treating stereotypic behavior of mentally retarded children. *Applied Research in Mental Retardation, 2,* 247–256.

Barrett, R. P., Staub, R. W., & Sisson, L. A. (1983). Treatment of compulsive rituals with visual screening: A case study with long-term follow-up. *Journal of Behavior Therapy and Experimental Psychiatry, 14,* 55–59.

Barron, B., & Sandman, C. A. (1983). Relationship of sedative hypnotic response to self-injurious behavior and stereotypy by mentally retarded clients. *American Journal of Mental Deficiency, 88,* 177–186.

Barron, B., & Sandman, C. A. (1984). Self-injurious behavior and stereotypy in an institutionalized mentally retarded population. *Applied Research in Mental Retardation, 5,* 499–511.

Barton, L. E., Repp, A. C., & Brulle, A. R. (1985). Reduction of stereotypic behaviours using differential reinforcement procedures and momentary restraint. *Journal of Mental Deficiency Research, 29,* 71–79.

Barton, L. E., Brulle, A. R., & Repp, A. C. (1986). Maintenance of therapeutic changes by momentary DRO. *Journal of Applied Behavior Analysis, 19,* 277–282.

Baumeister, A. A. (1978). Origins and control of stereotyped movements. In C. E. Meyers (Ed.), *Quality of life in mentally retarded people: Research foundations for improvements* (pp. 353–384). Washington, DC: American Association on Mental Deficiency.

Baumeister, A. A., & Forehand, R. (1972). Effects of contingent shock and verbal command on body rocking of retardates. *Journal of Clinical Psychology, 28,* 586–590.

Baumeister, A. A., & Forehand, R. (1973). Stereotyped acts. In N. R. Ellis (Ed.), *International review of research in mental retardation* (Vol. 6, pp. 55–96). New York: Academic Press.

Baumeister, A. A., & MacLean, W. E. (1984). Deceleration of SIB and stereotypic responding by exercise. *Applied Research in Mental Retardation, 5,* 385–394.

Berkson, G. (1967). Abnormal stereotyped motor acts. In J. Zubin & H. F. Hunt (Eds.), *Comparative psychopathology—animal and human* (pp. 76–94). New York: Grune & Stratton.

Berkson, G. (1983). Repetitive stereotyped behaviors. *American Journal of Mental Deficiency, 88,* 239–246.

Berkson, G., & Davenport, R. K. (1962). Stereotyped movements in mental defectives. *American Journal of Mental Deficiency, 66,* 849–852.

Berkson, G., & Mason, W. A. (1963). Stereotyped movements of mental defectives: III. Situational effects. *American Journal of Mental Deficiency, 68,* 409–412.

Berkson, G., & Mason, W. A. (1964). Stereotyped movements of mental defectives: IV. The effects of toys and the character of the acts. *American Journal of Mental Deficiency, 68,* 511–524.

Berkson, G., McQuiston, S., Jacobson, J. W., Eyman, R., & Borthwick, S. (1985). The relationship between age and stereotyped behavior. *Mental Retardation, 23,* 31–33.

Bitgood, S. C., Crowe, M. J., Suarez, Y., & Peters, R. D. (1980). Immobilization: Effects and side-effects on stereotyped behavior in children. *Behavior Modification, 4,* 187–208.

Borthwick, S. A., Meyers, C. E., & Eyman, R. K. (1981). Comparative adaptive and maladaptive behavior of mentally retarded clients of five residential settings in three Western states. In R. H. Bruinincks, C. E. Meyers, B. B. Sigford, & K. C. Lakin (Eds.), *Deinstitutionalization and community adjustment of mentally retarded people* (AAMD Monograph No. 4, pp. 351–359). Washington, DC: American Association on Mental Deficiency.

Campbell, M., Anderson, L. T., Meier, M., Cohen, I. L., Small, A. M., Samit, C., & Sachar, E. J. (1978). A comparison of haloperidol and behavior therapy and their interaction in autistic children. *Journal of the American Academy of Psychiatry, 12,* 640–655.

Carr, E. (1977). The motivation of self-injurious behavior. *Psychological Bulletin, 84,* 800–816.

Cavalier, A. R., & Ferretti, R. D. (1980). Stereotyped behavior, alternative behavior and collateral effects: A comparison of four intervention procedures. *Journal of Mental Deficiency Research, 24,* 219–230.

Chock, P. N., & Glahn, T. J. (1983). Learning and self-stimulation in mute and echolalic autistic children. *Journal of Autism and Developmental Disabilities, 13,* 365–381.

Christopher, R., & Lewis, B. (1984). The effects of auditory tempo changes on rates of stereotypic behavior in handicapped children. *Mental Retardation and Disability Bulletin, 12,* 105–114.

Cinciripini, P. M., Epstein, L. H., & Kotanchik, N. L. (1980). Behavioral intervention for self-stimulatory, attending, and seizure behavior in a cerebral palsied child. *Journal of Behavior Therapy and Experimental Psychiatry, 11,* 313–316.

Clarke, J. C., & Thomason, S. (1984). The use of an aversive smell to eliminate autistic self-stimulatory behavior. *Child and Family Behavior Therapy, 3,* 51–61.

Coleman, R. S., Whitman, T. L., & Johnson, M. R. (1979). Suppression of self-stimulatory behavior of a profoundly retarded boy across staff and settings: An assessment of situational generalization. *Behavior Therapy, 10,* 266–280.

Costello, A. (1982). Assessment and diagnosis of psychopathology. In J. L. Matson & R. P. Barrett (Eds.), *Psychopathology in the mentally retarded* (pp. 37–52). New York: Grune & Stratton.

Czyzewski, M. J., Barrera, R. D., & Sulzer-Azaroff, B. (1982). An abbreviated overcorrection program to reduce self-stimulatory behaviors. *Journal of Behavior Therapy and Experimental Psychiatry, 13,* 55–62.

Davenport, R. K., & Berkson, G. (1963). Stereotyped movements of mental defectives: II. Effects of novel objects. *American Journal of Mental Deficiency, 67,* 879–882.

Davis, K. V. (1971). The effect of drugs on stereotyped and nonstereotyped operant behaviors in retardates. *Psychopharmacologia, 22,* 195–213.

Denny, M. (1980). Reducing self-stimulatory behavior of mentally retarded persons by alternative positive practice. *American Journal of Mental Deficiency, 84,* 610–615.

Dick, D. M., & Jackson, H. J. (1983). The reduction of stereotypic screaming in a severely retarded boy through a visual screening procedure. *Journal of Behavior Therapy and Experimental Psychiatry, 14,* 363–367.

Doke, L. A., & Epstein, L. H. (1975). Oral overcorrection: Side-effects and extended applications. *Journal of Experimental Child Psychology, 20,* 496–511.

Dunlap, G., Dyer, K., & Koegel, R. L. (1983). Autistic self-stimulation and intertrial interval duration. *American Journal of Mental Deficiency, 88,* 194–202.

Dura, J. R., Mulick, J. A., & Rasnake, L. K. (1987). Prevalence of stereotypy among institutionalized nonambulatory profoundly mentally retarded people. *American Journal of Mental Deficiency, 91,* 548–549.

Durand, V. M. (1982). A behavioral/pharmacological intervention for the treatment of severe self-injurious behavior. *Journal of Autism and Developmental Disorders, 12,* 243–251.

Durrand, V. M., & Carr, E. G. (1987). Social influences on "self-stimulatory" behavior: Analysis and treatment application. *Journal of Applied Behavior Analysis, 20,* 119–132.

Durand, V. M., & Crimmins, D. B. (1983, October). *The motivation assessment scale: A preliminary instrument which assesses the functional significance of children's deviant behavior.* Paper presented at the meeting of the Berkshire Association of Behavior Analysis and Therapy, Amherst, MA.

Eason, L. J., White, M. G., & Newsom, C. (1982). Generalized reduction of self-stimulatory behavior: An effect of teaching appropriate play to autistic children. *Analysis and Intervention in Developmental Disabilities, 2,* 157–169.

Epstein, L. H., Doke, L. A., Sajwaj, T. E., Sorrell, S., & Rimmer, B. (1974). Generality and side effects of overcorrection. *Journal of Applied Behavior Analysis, 7,* 285–390.

Eyman, R. K., & Call, T. (1977). Maladaptive behavior and community placement. *American Journal of Mental Deficiency, 82,* 137–144.

Fellner, D. J., LaRoche, M., & Sulzer-Azaroff, B. (1984). The effects of adding interrupting to differential reinforcement on targeted and novel self-stimulatory behaviors. *Journal of Behavior Therapy and Experimental Psychiatry, 4,* 315–321.

Favell, J. E. (1973). Reduction of stereotypies by reinforcement of toy play. *Mental Retardation, 11,* 21–23.

Forehand, R., & Baumeister, A. A. (1970). Body rocking and activity level as a function of prior movement restraint. *American Journal of Mental Deficiency, 74,* 608–610.

Foxx, R. M., & Azrin, N. H. (1973). The elimination of autistic self-stimulatory behavior by overcorrection. *Journal of Applied Behavior Analysis, 6,* 1–14.

Foxx, R. M., McMorrow, M. J., Fenlon, S., & Bittle, R. G. (1986). The reductive effects of reinforcement procedures on the genital stimulation and stereotypy of a mentally retarded adolescent male. *Analysis and Intervention in Developmental Disabilities, 6,* 239–248.

Frankel, F., Freeman, B. J., Ritvo, E., & Pardo, R. (1978). The effect of environmental stimulation upon the stereotyped behavior of autistic children. *Journal of Autism and Developmental Disorders, 8,* 389–394.

Fraser, W. I., Leudar, I., Gray, J., & Campbell, I. (1986). Psychiatric and behaviour disturbance in mental handicap. *Journal of Mental Deficiency Research, 30,* 49–57.

Friman, P. C., Cook, J. W., & Finney, J. W. (1984). Effects of punishment procedures on the self-stimulatory behavior of an autistic child. *Analysis and Intervention in Developmental Disabilities, 4,* 39–46.

Gadow, K. D., & Kalachnik, J. (1981). Prevalence and pattern of drug treatment for behavior and seizure disorders of TMR students. *American Journal of Mental Deficiency, 85,* 588–595.

Gallagher, R. J., & Berkson, G. (1986). Effect of intervention techniques in reducing stereotypic hand gazing in young severely disabled children. *American Journal of Mental Deficiency, 91,* 170–177.

Gary, L. A., Tallon, R. J., & Stangl, J. M. (1980). Environmental influences on self-stimulatory behavior. *American Journal of Mental Deficiency, 85,* 171–175.

Goldberg, D. P., Cooper, B., Eastwood, M. R., Kedward, H. B., & Shephard, M. (1970). A standardized psychiatric interview for use in community surveys. *British Journal of Preventive and Social Medicine, 24,* 18–23.

Goodall, E., & Corbett, J. (1982). Relationships between sensory stimulation and stereotyped behavior in severely mentally retarded and autistic children. *Journal of Mental Deficiency Research, 26,* 163–175.

Greer, R. D., Becker, B. J., Saxe, C. D., & Mirabella, R. F. (1985). Conditioning histories and setting stimuli controlling engagement in stereotypy or toy play. *Analysis and Intervention in Developmental Disabilities, 5,* 269–284.

Gualtieri, C. T., Quade, D., Hicks, R. E., Mayo, J. P., & Schroeder, S. R. (1984). Tardive dyskinesia and other clinical consequences of neuroleptic treatment in children and adolescents. *American Journal of Psychiatry, 141,* 20–23.

Hamilton, H., Stephens, L., & Allen, P. (1967). Controlling aggressive and destructive behavior in severely retarded institutionalized residents. *American Journal of Mental Deficiency, 71,* 852–856.

Harris, S. L., & Wolchick, S. A. (1979). Suppression of self-stimulation: Three alternative strategies. *Journal of Applied Behavior Analysis, 12,* 185–198.

Hauck, F. (1985). Development of a behavior-analytic questionnaire precising four functions of self-injurious behavior in the mentally retarded. *International Journal of Rehabilitation Research, 8,* 350–352.

Hersen, M., & Barlow, D. H. (1976). *Single case experimental designs.* New York: Pergamon Press.

Hobbs, S. A. (1976). Modifying stereotyped behaviors by overcorrection: A critical review. *Rehabilitation Psychology, 23,* 1–11.

Hobbs, S. A., & Goswick, R. (1977). Behavioral treatment of self-stimulation: An examination of alternatives to physical punishment. *Journal of Clinical Child Psychology, 6,* 20–23.

Hollis, J. H. (1968). Chlorpromazine: Direct measurement of differential behavioral effects. *Science, 159,* 1487–1489.

Hollis, J. H. (1978). Analysis of rocking behavior. In C. E. Meyers (Ed.), *Quality of life in severely and profoundly mentally retarded people: Research foundations for improvement* (pp. 1–53). Washington, DC: American Association on Mental Deficiency.

Hollis, J. H., & St. Omer, V. V. (1972). Direct measurement of psychopharmacologic response: Effects of chlorpromazine on motor behavior of retarded children. *American Journal of Mental Deficiency, 76,* 580–587.

Horner, R. D. (1980). The effects of an environmental "enrichment" program on the behavior of institutionalized profoundly retarded children. *Journal of Applied Behavior Analysis, 13,* 437–491.

Hung, D. W. (1978). Using self-stimulation as reinforcement for autistic children. *Journal of Autism and Childhood Schizophrenia, 8,* 355–366.

Iwata, B. A., Dorsey, M. F., Slifer, K. J., Bauman, K. E., & Richman, G. S. (1982). Toward a functional analysis of self-injury. *Analysis and Intervention in Developmental Disabilities, 2,* 3–20.

Iwata, B. A., Pace, G. M., Cataldo, M. F., Kalsher, M. J., & Edwards, G. L. (1984). A center for the study and treatment of self-injury. In J. C. Griffin, M. T. Stark, D. E. Williams, B. K. Altmeyer, & H. K. Griffin (Eds.), *Advances in the treatment of self-injurious behavior* (pp. 27–39). Austin: Department of Health and Human Services, Texas Planning Council for Developmental Disabilities.

Jacobson, J. W. (1982). Problem behavior and psychiatric impairment within a developmentally disabled population: I. Behavior frequency. *Applied Research in Mental Retardation, 3,* 121–139.

Johnson, W. L., Baumeister, A. A., Penland, M. J., & Inwald, C. (1982). Experimental analysis of self-injurious, stereotypic, and collateral behavior of retarded persons: Effects of overcorrection and reinforcement of alternative responding. *Analysis and Intervention in Developmental Disabilities, 2,* 41–66.

Kanfer, F. H., & Phillips, J. S. (1970). *Learning foundations of behavior therapy.* New York: Wiley.

Kanfer, F. H., & Saslow, G. (1965). Behavioral diagnosis. *Archives of General Psychiatry, 12,* 529–538.

Kauffman, J. M., LaFleur, N. K., Hallahan, D. P., & Chanes, C. M. (1975). Imitation as a consequence for children's behavior: Two experimental case studies. *Behavior Therapy, 6,* 535–542.

Kauffman, J. M., Hallahan, D. P., & Ianna, S. (1977). Suppression of retardate's tongue protrusion by contingent imitation. *Behaviour Research and Therapy, 15,* 196–197.

Kaufman, M. E., & Levitt, H. A. (1965). A study of three stereotyped behaviors in institutionalized mentally defectives. *American Journal of Mental Deficiency, 69,* 467–473.

Kazdin, A. E. (1982). *Single-case research design.* New York: Oxford University Press.

Kelly, J. A., & Drabman, R. S. (1977). Generalizing response suppression of self-injurious behavior through an overcorrection punishment procedure: A case study. *Behavior Therapy, 8,* 468–472.

Kern, L., Koegel, R. L., Dyer, K., Blew, P. A., & Fenton, L. R. (1982). The effect of physical exercise on self-stimulation and appropriate responding in autistic children. *Journal of Autism and Developmental Disabilities, 12,* 399–419.

Kern, L., Koegel, R. L., & Dunlap, G. (1984). The influence of vigorous versus mild exercise on autistic stereotyped behaviors. *Journal of Autism and Developmental Disorders, 14,* 57–67.

Klawans, H. L., Moses, H., Beaulieu, D. M. (1974). The influence of caffeine on *d*-amphetamine and apomorphine-induced stereotyped behavior. *Life Sciences, 14,* 1493–1500.

Klier, J., & Harris, S. L. (1977). Self-stimulatory behavior and learning in autistic children: Physical or functional incompatibility. *Journal of Applied Behavior Analysis, 10,* 311.

Koegel, R. L., & Covert, A. (1972). The relationship of self-stimulation to learning in autistic children. *Journal of Applied Behavior Analysis, 5,* 381–387.

LaGrow, S. J., & Repp. A. C. (1984). Stereotypic responding: A review of intervention research. *American Journal of Mental Deficiency, 88,* 595–609.

Lancioni, G. E., Smeets, P. M., Ceccarani, P. S., & Goossens, A. J. (1983). Self-stimulation and task-related responding: The role of sensory reinforcement in maintaining and extending treatment effects. *Journal of Behavior Therapy and Experimental Psychiatry, 14,* 33–41.

Langford, W. S. (1953). Psychopathological problems. In L. E. Holt & R. McIntosh (Eds.), *Holt's diseases of infancy and childhood* (12th ed.). New York: Appleton-Century-Crofts.

Laws, D. R., Brown, R. A., Epstein, J., & Hocking, N. (1971). Reduction of inappropriate social behavior in disturbed children by an untrained paraprofessional therapist. *Behavior Therapy, 2,* 519–533.

Leudar, I., Fraser, W. I., & Jeeves, M. A. (1984). Behaviour disturbance and mental handicap: Typology and longitudinal trends. *Psychological Medicine, 14,* 923–935.

Lewis, M., MacLean, W. E., Bryson-Brockman, W., Arendt, R., Beck, B., Fidler, P. S., & Baumeister, A. A. (1984). Time-series analysis of stereotyped movements: Relationship of body-rocking to cardiac activity. *American Journal of Mental Deficiency, 89,* 287–294.

Lewis, M. H., & Baumeister, A. A. (1982). Stereotyped mannerisms in mentally retarded persons: Animal models and theoretical analyses. In N. R. Ellis (Ed.), *International review of research in mental retardation* (Vol. 11, pp. 123–161). New York: Academic Press.

Lewis, M. H., MacLean, W. E., Johnson, W. L., & Baumeister, A. A. (1981). Ultradian rhythms in stereotyped and self-injurious behavior. *American Journal of Mental Deficiency, 85,* 601–610.

Lourie, R. S. (1949). The role of rhythmic pattern in childhood. *American Journal of Psychiatry, 105,* 653–660.

Lovaas, I. O., Schaeffer, B., & Simmons, J. (1965). Building social behavior in autistic children by use of electric shock. *Journal of Experimental Research in Personality, 1,* 99–109.

Lovaas, O. I., Newsom, C., & Hickman, C. (1987). Self-stimulatory behavior and perceptual reinforcement. *Journal of Applied Behavior Analysis, 20,* 45–68.

Luiselli, J. K. (1975). The effects of multiple contingencies on the rocking behavior of a retarded child. *Psychological Record, 25,* 559–565.

Luiselli, J. K. (1981). Evaluation of a response-contingent immobilization procedure for the classroom management of self-stimulation in developmentally disabled children. *Behavior Research of Severe Developmental Disabilities, 2,* 67–78.

Luiselli, J. K., Colozzi, G. A., & O'Toole, K. M. (1980). Programming response maintenance of differential reinforcement effects. *Child Behavior Therapy, 2,* 65–73.

Luiselli, J. K., Myles, E., Evans, T. P., & Boyce, D. A. (1985). Reinforcement control of severe dysfunctional behavior of blind, multihandicapped students. *American Journal of Mental Deficiency, 90,* 328–334.

Lutzker, J. R. (1978). Reducing self-injurious behavior by facial screening. *American Journal of Mental Deficiency, 82,* 510–513.

Maag, J. W., Rutherford, R. B., Wolchick, S. A., & Parks, B. T. (1986). Comparison of two short overcorrection procedures on the stereotypic behavior of autistic children. *Journal of Autism and Developmental Disabilities, 16,* 83–87.

Maag, J. W., Wolchik, S. A., Rutherford, R. B., & Parks, B. T. (1986). Response covariation on self-stimulatory behaviors during sensory extinction procedures. *Journal of Autism and Developmental Disabilities, 16,* 119–132.

MacLean, W. E., & Baumeister, A. A. (1981). Observational analysis of the stereotyped mannerisms of a developmentally delayed infant. *Applied Research in Mental Retardation, 2,* 257–262.

Maris, R. S. (1971). *Stereotyped body-rocking in severely retarded patients: A study of rhythm and topography.* Unpublished doctoral dissertation. University of Alabama.

Martin, J., Weller, S., & Matson, J. (1977). Eliminating object transferring by a profoundly retarded female by overcorrection. *Psychological Reports, 40,* 779–782.

Matson, J. L., & Barrett, R. P. (1982). *Psychopathology in the mentally retarded.* New York: Grune & Stratton.

Matson, J. L., & Stephens, R. M. (1981). Overcorrection treatment of stereotyped behaviors. *Behavior Modification, 5,* 491–502.

Matson, J. L., Ollendick, T. H., & Martin, J. E. (1979). Overcorrection revisited: A long-term follow-up. *Journal of Behavior Therapy and Experimental Psychiatry, 10,* 11–14.

McClure, J. T., Moss, R. A., McPeters, J. W., & Kirkpatrick, M. A. (1986). Reduction of hand mouthing by a boy with profound mental retardation. *Mental Retardation, 24,* 219–222.

McGonigle, J. J., Duncan, D., Cordisco, L., & Barrett, R. P. (1982). Visual screening: An alternative method for reducing stereotypic behaviors. *Journal of Applied Behavior Analysis, 15,* 461–467.

McKeegan, G. F., Estill, K., & Campbell, B. M. (1984). Use of nonexclusionary timeout for the elimination of a stereotyped behavior. *Journal of Behavior Therapy and Experimental Psychiatry, 15,* 261–264.

McKelvey, J. L., Sisson, L. A., Van Hasselt, V. B., & Hersen, M. (1987, November). *Multiple-component behavioral intervention to reduce mouthing in a blind multihandicapped child.* Paper presented at the Annual Conference of the Association for Advancement of Behavior Therapy, Boston, MA.

Millichamp, C. J., & Singh, N. N. (1987). The effects of intermittent drug therapy on stereotypy and collateral behaviors of mentally retarded persons. *Research in Developmental Disabilities, 8,* 213–227.

Moseley, A., Faust, M., & Reardon, D. M. (1970). Effects of social & nonsocial stimuli on the stereotyped behaviors of retarded children. *American Journal of Mental Deficiency, 74,* 809–811.

Mulhern, T., & Baumeister, A. A. (1969). An experimental attempt to reduce stereotypy by reinforcement procedures. *American Journal of Mental Deficiency, 74,* 69–74.

Mulick, J. A., Hoyt, P., Rojahn, J., & Schroeder, S. R. (1978). Reduction of a "nervous" habit in a profoundly retarded youth by increasing toy play. *Journal of Behavior Therapy and Experimental Psychiatry, 9,* 381–385.

Mulick, J. A., Schroeder, S. R., & Rojahn, J. (1980). Chronic ruminative vomiting: A comparison of four treatment procedures. *Journal of Autism and Developmental Disorders, 10,* 203–213.

Murphy, R., Nunes, D., & Hutchings-Ruprecht, M. (1977). Reduction of stereotyped behavior in profoundly retarded individuals. *American Journal of Mental Deficiency, 82,* 238–245.

Neisworth, J. T., Hunt, F. M., Gallop, H. R., & Madle, R. A. (1985). Reinforcer displacement: A preliminary study of the clinical application of the CRF/EXT effect. *Behavior Modification, 9,* 102–115.

O'Brien, F. (1981). Treating self-stimulatory behavior. In J. L. Matson & J. R. McCartney (Eds.), *Handbook of behavior modification with the mentally retarded.* New York: Plenum Press.

Ollendick, T. H., & Matson, J. L. (1976). An initial investigation into the parameters of overcorrection. *Psychological Reports, 39,* 1139–1142.

Ollendick, T. H., & Matson, J. L. (1978). Overcorrection: An overview. *Behavior Therapy, 9,* 830–842.

Ollendick, T. H., Matson, J. L., & Martin, J. E. (1978). Effectiveness of hand overcorrection for topographically similar and dissimilar self-stimulatory behavior. *Journal of Experimental Child Psychology, 25,* 296–403.

Ollendick, T. H., Shapiro, E. S., & Barrett, R. P. (1981). Reducing stereotypic behaviors: An analysis of treatment procedures utilizing an alternating treatments design. *Behavior Therapy, 12,* 570–577.

Pace, G. M., Ivancic, M. J., Edwards, G. L., Iwata, B. A., & Page, T. J. (1985). Assessment of stimulus preference and reinforcer value with profoundly retarded individuals. *Journal of Applied Behavior Analysis, 18,* 249–255.

Paniagua, F. A., Braverman, C., & Capriotti, R. M. (1986). Use of a treatment package in the management of a profoundly mentally retarded girl's pica and self-stimulation. *American Journal of Mental Deficiency, 90,* 550–557.

Parrish, J. M., Iwata, B. A., Dorsey, M. F., Bunck, T. J., & Slifer, K. J. (1985). Behavior analysis, program development, and transfer of control in the treatment of self-injury. *Behavior Therapy and Experimental Psychiatry, 16,* 159–168.

Pendergrass, V. E. (1972). Timeout from positive reinforcement following persistent, high rate behavior in retardates. *Journal of Applied Behavior Analysis, 5,* 85–91.

Pohl, P. (1977). Tempo changes during body rocking. *Developmental Medicine and Child Neurology, 19,* 485–488.

Radinsky, A. M. (1984). *A descriptive study of psychotropic and antiepileptic medication use with mentally retarded persons in three residential environments.* Unpublished doctoral dissertation, University of Pittsburgh.

Randrup, A., & Munkvad, I. (1967). DOPA and other naturally occurring substances as causes of stereotypy and rage in rats. *Acta Psychiatrica Scandinavica, 42,* 193–199.

Reese, R. M., Schroeder, S. R., & Gullion, C. M. (in press). Ecobehavioral-architectural design variabilities affecting staff and peer interactions in facilities for the developmentally disabled. In J. A. Mulick, & R. F. Antonak (Eds.), *Transitions in mental retardation.* Norwood, NJ: Alex Publishing Corp.

Reid, A. H., Ballinger, B. R., & Heather, B. B. (1978). Behavioural syndromes identified by cluster analysis in a sample of 100 severely and profoundly retarded adults. *Psychological Medicine, 8,* 399–412.

Reid, J. G., Tombaugh, T. N., & Heuvel, K. V. (1981). Application of contingent physical restraint to suppress stereotyped body rocking of profoundly mentally retarded persons. *American Journal of Mental Deficiency, 86,* 78–85.

Reiss, S., & Szyszko, J. (1983). Diagnostic overshadowing and professional experience with mentally retarded persons. *American Journal of Mental Deficiency, 87,* 361–367.

Repp, A. C., Deitz, S. M., & Speir, N. (1974). Reducing stereotypic responding of retarded persons by the differential reinforcement of other behavior. *American Journal of Mental Deficiency, 78,* 279–284.

Repp, A. C., Barton, L. E., & Brulle, A. R. (1983). A comparison of two procedures for programming the differential reinforcement of other behaviors. *Journal of Applied Behavior Analysis, 16,* 435–445.

Richmond, G. (1983). Evaluation of a treatment for hand-mouthing stereotypy. *American Journal of Mental Deficiency, 87,* 667–669.

Richmond, G., & Bell, J. C. (1983). Analysis of a treatment package to reduce a hand-mouthing stereotypy. *Behavior Therapy, 14,* 576–581.

Rincover, A. (1978). A procedure for eliminating self-stimulatory behavior in psychotic children. *Journal of Abnormal Child Psychology, 6,* 299–310.

Rincover, A., Cook, R., Peoples, A., & Packard, D. (1979). Sensory extinction and sensory reinforcement principles for programming multiple adaptive behavior change. *Journal of Applied Behavior Analysis, 12,* 221–233.

Roberts, P., Iwata, B. A., McSween, T. E., & Desmond, E. F. (1979). An analysis of overcorrection movements. *American Journal of Mental Deficiency, 83,* 588–594.

Rogers-Warren, A., & Warren, S. F. (1977). (Eds.). *Ecological perspectives in behavior analysis.* Baltimore: University Park Press.

Rojahn, J. (1986). Self-injurious and stereotypic behavior of noninstitutionalized mentally retarded people: Prevalence and classification. *American Journal of Mental Deficiency, 91,* 268–276.

Rojahn, J., & Schroeder, S. R. (1983). Behavioral assessment. In J. L. Matson & J. A. Mulick (Eds.), *Handbook of mental retardation* (pp. 227–243). New York: Pergamon Press.

Rolider, A., & Van Houten, R. (1985). Movement suppression time-out for undesirable behavior in psychotic and severely developmentally delayed children. *Journal of Applied Behavior Analysis, 18,* 275–288.

Rollings, J. P., & Baumeister, A. A. (1981). Stimulus control of stereotypic responding: Effects on target and collateral behavior. *American Journal of Mental Deficiency, 86,* 67–77.

Rollings, J. P., Baumeister, A. A., & Baumeister, A. A. (1977). The use of overcorrection procedures to eliminate the stereotyped behaviors of retarded individuals: An analysis of collateral behaviors and generalization of suppressive effects. *Behavior Modification, 1,* 29–46.

Romanczyk, R. G. (1977). Intermittent punishment of self-stimulation: Effectiveness during application and extinction. *Journal of Consulting and Clinical Psychology, 45,* 53–60.

Runco, M. A., Charlop, M. J., & Schreibman, L. (1986). The occurrence of autistic children's self-stimulation as a function of familiar versus unfamiliar stimulus conditions. *Journal of Autism and Developmental Disorders, 16,* 31–44.

Rutter, M., Graham, P., & Yule, W. (1970). *A neuropsychiatric study in childhood.* London: Heinemann/SIMP.

Rutter, M., Tizard, J., Yule, W., Graham, P., & Whitmore, K. (1976). Isle of Wight studies, 1964–1974. *Psychological Medicine, 6,* 313–332.

Sachs, D. A. (1973). The efficacy of time-out procedures in a variety of behavior problems. *Journal of Behavior Therapy and Experimental Psychiatry, 4,* 237–242.

Sandmann, C. A., Datta, P. C., Barron, J., Hoehler, F. K., Williams, C., & Swanson, J. M. (1983). Naloxone attenuates self-abusive behavior in developmentally disabled clients. *Applied Research in Mental Retardation, 4,* 5–11.

Schalock, R. L., Foley, J. W., Toulouse, A., & Stark, J. A. (1985). Medication and programming in controlling the behavior of mentally retarded individuals in community settings. *American Journal of Mental Deficiency, 89,* 503–509.

Scheerenberger, R. C. (1981). Deinstitutionalization: Trends and difficulties. In R. H. Bruininks, C. E. Meyers, B. B. Sigford, & K. C. Lakin (Eds.), *Deinstitutionaliztion and community adjustment of mentally retarded people* (Monograph No. 4, pp. 3–13). Washington, DC: American Association on Mental Deficiency.

Schmid, J. (1986). Reducing inappropriate behavior of mentally retarded children through interpolated reinforcement. *American Journal of Mental Deficiency, 91,* 286–293.

Schroeder, S. R. (1970). Usage of stereotypy as a descriptive term. *Psychological Record, 20,* 337–342.

Schroeder, S. R., Rojahn, J., & Mulick, S. R. (1978). Ecobehavioral organization of developmental day care for the chronically self-injurious. *Journal of Pediatric Psychology, 3,* 81–88.

Schroeder, S. R., Schroeder, C. S., Rojahn, J., & Mulick, J. A. (1981). Self-injurious behavior: An analysis of behavior modification techniques. In J. L. Matson & J. R. McCartney (Eds.), *Handbook of behavior modification with the mentally retarded* (pp. 61–115). New York: Plenum Press.

Schroeder, S. R., Bickel, W. A., & Richmond, G. (1986). Primary and secondary prevention of self-injurious behaviors: A life-long problem. In K. D. Gadow (Ed.), *Advances in learning and behavioral disabilities* (Vol. 5, pp. 63–85). Greenwich, CT: JAI Press.

Schroeder, S. R., Kanoy, R. C., Mulick, J. A., Rojahn, J. R., Thios, S. J., Stephens, M., & Hawk, B. (1982). Environmental antecedents which affect management of programs for self-injurious behavior. In J. H. Hollis & C. E. Meyers (Eds.), *Life-threatening behavior* (pp. 105–159). Washington, DC: American Association on Mental Deficiency.

Shapiro, E. S., Barrett, R. P., & Ollendick, T. H. (1980). A comparison of physical restraint and positive practice overcorrection in treating stereotypic behavior. *Behavior Therapy, 11,* 227–233.

Silva, D. A. (1979). The use of medication in a residential institution for mentally retarded persons. *Mental Retardation, 17,* 285–288.

Singh, N. N., & Aman, M. G. (1981). Effects of thioridazine dosage on the behavior of severely mentally retarded persons. *American Journal of Mental Deficiency, 85,* 580–587.

Singh, N. N., Dawson, M. J., & Manning, P. (1981). Effects of spaced responding DRL on the stereotyped behavior of profoundly retarded persons. *Journal of Applied Behavior Analysis, 14,* 521–526.

Singh, N. N., Watson, J. E., & Winton, A. S. W. (1987). Parents' acceptability ratings of alternative treatments for use with mentally retarded children. *Behavior Modification, 11,* 17–26.

Sisson, L. A., Van Hasselt, V. B., Hersen, M., & Aurand, J. C. (1988). Tripartite behavioral intervention to reduce stereotypic and disruptive behaviors in young multihandicapped children. *Behavior Therapy, 19,* 503–526.

Soraci, S., Deckner, C. W., McDaniel, C., & Blanton, R. L. (1982). The relationship between rate of rhythmicity and the stereotypic behaviors of abnormal children. *Journal of Music Therapy, 19,* 46–54.

Sprague, R. L. (1977). Overview of psychopharmacology for the retarded in the U.S. In P. Mittler (Ed.), *Research to practice in mental retardation: Biomedical aspects* (Vol. 3, pp. 350–364). Baltimore: University Park Press.

Stevens, E. A. (1971). Some effects of tempo changes on stereotyped rocking movements of low-level mentally retarded subjects. *American Journal of Mental Deficiency, 76,* 76–81.

Stokes, T. F., & Baer, D. M. (1977). An implicit technology of generalization. *Journal of Applied Behavior Analysis, 10,* 349–367.

Strawbridge, L. A., Sisson, L. A., & Van Hasselt, V. B. (1987). Reducing disruptive behavior in the classroom using contingent-interrupted auditory stimulation. *Journal of the Association for Persons with Severe Handicaps, 12,* 199–204.

Tarpley, H., & Schroeder, S. R. (1979). A comparison of DRO and DRI procedures in the treatment of self-injurious behavior. *American Journal of Mental Deficiency, 84,* 188–194.

The Association for Persons with Severe Handicaps (TASH). (1986, July). Resolution on intrusive intervention. *TASH Newsletter,* p. 8.

Thelen, E. (1981). Rhythmical behavior in infancy: An ethological perspective. *Developmental Psychology, 17,* 237–257.

Thompson, T. J., & Berkson, G. (1985). Stereotyped behavior of severely disabled children in classroom and free-play settings. *American Journal of Mental Deficiency, 89,* 580–586.

Tierney, I. R., McGuire, R. J., Walton, H. J. (1978). The effect of music on body-rocking manifested by severely mentally deficient patients in ward environments. *Journal of Mental Deficiency Research, 22,* 255–261.

Tierney, I. R., McGuire, R. J., & Walton, H. J. (1979). Reduction of stereotyped body-rocking using variable time reinforcement: Practical and theoretical implications. *Journal of Mental Deficiency Research, 23,* 175–185.

Tomporowski, P. D., & Ellis, N. R. (1984). Effects of exercise on the physical fitness, intelligence, and adaptive behavior of institutionalized mentally retarded adults. *Applied Research in Mental Retardation, 5,* 329–337.

Touchette, P. E., MacDonald, R. F., & Langer, S. N. (1985). A scatter plot for identifying stimulus control of problem behaviors. *Journal of Applied Behavior Analysis, 18,* 343–351.

Watson, J., Singh, N. N., & Winton, A. S. W. (1986). Suppressive effects of visual and facial screening on self-injurious finger sucking. *American Journal of Mental Deficiency, 90,* 526–534.

Watkins, K. M., Konarski, E. A. (1987). Effect of mentally retarded persons' level of stereotypy on their learning. *American Journal of Mental Deficiency, 91,* 361–365.

Watters, R. W., & Watters, W. E. (1980). Decreasing self-stimulatory behavior with physical exercise in a group of autistic boys. *Journal of Autism and Developmental Disorders, 10,* 378–387.

Wells, K. C., Forehand, R., Hickey, K., & Green, K. D. (1977). Effects of a procedure derived from the overcorrection principle on manipulated and nonmanipulated behaviors. *Journal of Applied Behavior Analysis, 10,* 679–687.

Wieseler, N. A., Hanson, R. H., Chamberlain, T. P., & Thompson, T. (1985). Functional taxonomy of stereotypic and self-injurious behavior. *Mental Retardation, 5,* 230–234.

Winnega, M., & Berkson, G. (1986). Analyzing the stimulus properties of objects used in stereotyped behavior. *American Journal of Mental Deficiency, 91,* 277–285.

Wolery, M., Kirk, K., & Gast, D. L. (1985). Stereotypic behavior as a reinforcer: Effects and side effects. *Journal of Autism and Developmental Disorders, 15,* 149–161.

Wolf, M. M., Risley, T., Johnston, M., Harris, F., & Allen, E. (1967). Application of operant conditioning procedures to the behavior problems of an autistic child: A follow-up and extension. *Behaviour Research and Therapy, 5,* 103–111.

Young, R., & Clements, J. (1979). The functional significance of complex hand movement stereotypies in the severely retarded. *British Journal of Mental Subnormality, 25,* 79–87.

Zegiob, L., Jenkins, J., Becker, J., & Bristow, A. (1976). Facial screening: An analysis of clinical applicability. *Journal of Behavior Therapy and Experimental Psychiatry, 7,* 355–357.

8

Aggression and Related Conduct
Difficulties

WILLIAM I. GARDNER AND CHRISTINE L. COLE

INTRODUCTION

It is well documented that one of the more prevalent, chronic, and socially disruptive problems among those with mental retardation is that of aggressive behavior and related difficulties of conduct. Eyman and Call (1977), for example, investigated the prevalence of maladaptive behaviors among groups of individuals with mental retardation living in institutions, in community facilities, and with their parents. They reported that 45% of the institutionalized sample, 20% of persons in community facilities, and 20% of those living with their parents threatened to or actually did engage in physical violence to other people. Evidence of the durability of aggression and related conduct difficulties is provided by Eyman, Borthwick, and Miller (1981). These researchers evaluated the changes in maladaptive behaviors (e.g., threatens or does physical damage to others, damages own or others' property, uses profane or hostile language) over a 2-year period in groups of persons with mental retardation residing either in residential facilities or in various community placements. As is typical, the institutional group exhibited more maladaptive behaviors than did the community groups. Also, the less severe the level of mental retardation, the more severe the maladaptive behavior in the institutional group. Of most interest was the finding that "whatever maladaptive behavior was present at the time of the individual's referral for service did not significantly change over a two-year-period for any of the subgroups of clients studied" (Eyman et al., 1981, p. 476). Further support of this observation is provided by Koller, Richardson, Katz, and McLaren (1983) who reported that 33% of individuals studied in childhood and later as young adults presented recurring aggressive conduct disorders.

Physical violence toward others and to property, explosive outbursts, temper tantrums, and other disruptive actions, such as taunting peers, verbal

WILLIAM I. GARDNER • Behavioral Research Unit, Waisman Center on Mental Retardation and Human Development, University of Wisconsin, Madison, Wisconsin 53706.   CHRISTINE L. COLE • School Psychology Program, Lehigh University, Bethlehem, Pennsylvania 18015.

and nonverbal threats of violence, screaming, and extreme negativism, all
interfere with the development and occurrence of adaptive behaviors, including desired social relationships and interactions. As chronic difficulties of
conduct are aversive to others and represent actual or potential safety haz-
ards, these behaviors often result in dismissal or exclusion from educational,
recreational, rehabilitation, community residential, and vocational programs.

The list that follows centers upon the more specific effects of chronic
conduct difficulties of persons with mental retardation:

1. *Referral for mental health services.* Reiss (1982) and Benson (1985) reported that aggression and oppositional behaviors represent the most frequently occurring problems (30%) that are referred to a metropolitan mental
health program serving those with mental retardation. Similarly, Szymanski
and Leaverton (1980) identified aggression as the problem most frequently
referred for psychiatric consultation among groups of persons with mental
retardation who are attending special education programs.

2. *Management concerns in educational programs.* In studying behavior problems among the more severely mentally retarded persons attending educational programs in residential and community settings, Wehman and
McLaughlin (1979) found aggression, temper tantrums, and property destruction not only to be prevalent but also to create the greatest management
concerns among staff.

3. *Failure in competitive employment.* Studies reveal that acting-out and
related conduct difficulties contribute significantly to the competitive employment failures of persons with mental retardation (Greenspan & Shoultz,
1981).

4. *Increased likelihood of abuse.* Rusch, Hall, and Griffin (1986) presented
data that suggest there is an increased likelihood among those persons who
present problems of aggression and other conduct difficulties of becoming a
victim of physical abuse from institutional staff members.

5. *Initial institutional placement.* It is well documented that the presence of
conduct difficulties has been associated with initial placement in an institutional setting (Thorsheim & Bruininks, 1979).

6. *Difficulties in being selected for community placement.* Borthwick-Duffy,
Eyman, and White (1987) reported that among those remaining in institutional settings instead of being selected for placement into less restrictive
community living are persons who present difficult problems of conduct.
These current findings are consistent with those personal barriers to deinstitutionalization reported a decade ago by Eyman and Call (1977) who
noted that "chronic problems of self-violence, violence to others, and damag-
ing property represent the types of behaviors that will surely persist as obstacles to community placement for large numbers of retarded individuals"
(p. 143).

7. *Community failure and reinstitutionalization.* Conduct difficulties represent a major factor in community adjustment failure of those persons who
have been placed from institutional settings (Heal, Sigelman, & Switsky,
1978; Schalock, Harper, & Genung, 1981).

Additionally, persons with conduct difficulties are less likely to be selected by community residential facilities and are more likely to be dismissed for reinstitutionalization (Hill & Bruininks, 1981). In a national study of admissions and readmissions to state residential facilities, Lakin, Hill, Hauber, Bruininks, and Heal (1983) reported such frequently occurring characteristics as "injures others," "damages property," "disruptive behavior," and "refuses routine."

8. *Social intolerability*. Direct care staff members of institutional and community residential facilities in the United States and in Israel ranked the social tolerability of 84 types of behaviors displayed by persons with mental retardation. Physical violence toward self, others, and property was viewed as the most intolerable of behaviors along with such socially unacceptable behaviors as incontinence, sexual improprieties, and playing with feces and urine (Isett, Roszkowski, & Spreat, 1983).

Thus, these and similar data emphasize the need for effective psychological treatment approaches to ensure that those with mental retardation and conduct disorders do experience a more independent and personally satisfying life.

The purpose of this chapter is to describe the recent behavior therapy literature devoted to this problem. Examples are provided of studies that investigate factors correlated with the acquisition, instigation, and maintenance of aggression, as well as studies that report the effectiveness of various behavioral intervention procedures on reducing the rate of occurrence of clinically significant problems of aggression. Although not comprehensive in coverage, examples are provided of intervention procedures that are used with persons with mental retardation who vary in age, severity of handicapping conditions, and in the severity levels of aggression and related aberrant behaviors.

The usefulness of a range of behavioral procedures has been demonstrated in treatment of clinically significant problems of aggression and related problems of conduct presented by persons with mental retardation (Gardner & Cole, 1984; Matson & Gorman-Smith, 1986; Repp & Brulle, 1981). From the 1950s, when clinical researchers initially began investigating behavioral methods of treatment of problems of aggression among those with mental retardation, through the 1970s, the primary focus of treatment has been to reduce or eliminate aggression and related problem behaviors through contingent aversive consequences. As noted by Carr and Durand (1985), this focus reflects a "consensus among researchers and clinicians that the elimination of behavior problems is an important first step in remediation" (p. 111). In support of this view are comments by Repp and Brulle (1981) that "the behavioral study of aggressive behavior has been to this date primarily a study of how to consequate behavior so that it will be rapidly reduced" (p. 206) and by Bornstein, Bach, and Anton (1982) that "for the severely and profoundly retarded person, aversive procedures, and, to a lesser extent, time-out may be the treatment of choice" (p. 263).

Even though the published literature of the 1980s continues to focus excessively on deceleration through aversive procedures (e.g., Foxx, McMorrow, Bittle, & Bechtel, 1986; Rolider & Van Houten, 1985), a distinct shift in focus is occurring that is characterized by (1) increased attention to behavioral diagnosis (Gardner & Cole, 1983, 1984, 1985, 1987) as a basis for selecting specific intervention procedures, and (2) investigation of treatment procedures designed specifically to teach alternative skills to replace the aggressive mode of behaving (Carr & Durand, 1985; Cole, Gardner, & Karan, 1985). This changing focus is consistent with current legal guidelines for least restrictive treatment and reflects a basic ethical commitment to providing the most humane and normalizing treatment available. It also is consistent with the positions articulated by various professional organizations, such as the American Association on Mental Retardation (Berkowitz, 1987) and The Association for Persons with Severe Handicaps (Guess, Helmstetter, Turnbull, & Knowlton, 1987). Finally, from both theoretical and pragmatic perspectives, this changing focus avoids some of the basic problems associated with excessive reliance on suppression of aggression through use of aversive consequences and concurrently offers greater promise of producing behavior change of a more durable nature (Axelrod, 1987; Matson & DiLorenzo, 1984).

BEHAVIORAL DIAGNOSIS

The completion of a diagnostic assessment prior to developing and implementing a behavioral treatment program recognizes that no single or simple psychological mechanism underlies recurring problems of aggression (Gardner & Cole, 1988). Because aggressive behaviors are predominantly interpersonal, they are best understood and treated in the context of social interactions. Thus, diagnostic activities should include the assessment of interpersonal/environmental influences and unique personal characteristics. Additionally, as chronic problems of aggression may accompany various other aberrant physical and psychological conditions, behavioral assessment should closely interface with medical and psychiatric diagnostic efforts. When associated with other psychiatric or physical disorders, such as schizophrenia, mania, agitated depression, generalized anxiety, seizure activity, and akathisia, treatment of these underlying clinical conditions may result in a concomitant decrease in aggression (Sovner & Hurley, 1986).

The objective of a behavioral diagnostic assessment is to obtain information from which a client-specific behavioral intervention program can be devised. This represents a three-step process of (1) gathering information relative to those variables that potentially contribute to the likelihood of the occurrence of aggression, (2) developing client-specific hypotheses following analysis and interpretation of assessment information relative to contributing factors, and (3) developing client-specific treatment procedures consistent with these hypotheses. Assessment information may be obtained through direct observation of and interaction with the client in the actual situations in which the target behaviors occur; interviews of the client, staff, family members, and peers; review of case records; and exposure to analog conditions. The reader is encouraged to consult Mace, Page, Ivancic, and O'Brien (1986) for illustration of this latter procedure.

To guide the activities involved in the diagnostic assessment and related treatment program development, a multicomponent model for assessment and treatment of aggression, depicted in Figure 1, has been described by Gardner (1989) and Gardner and Cole (1983, 1984, 1985, 1987). This model, based on constructs and empirical data from various contemporary behavioral and related systems, includes assessment of those variables involved in the *instigation* of aggressive behaviors as well as those contributing to the *acquisition* and *persistent recurrence* of the problem behaviors.

Step 1: Gather Assessment Data

External Factors Correlated with Aggression

An initial focus of assessment and intervention of aggression and related difficulties involves those preceding external environmental events that may instigate or otherwise increase the likelihood of occurrence of these problem behaviors. These events include those of a *psychosocial* and a *physical* nature. Assessment seeks to identify the specific discriminative events for aggressive behavior (e.g., a workshop supervisor reprimanding the client in the presence of peers) as well as other general sources of environmental stimulation that may contribute to aggressive actions (e.g., high noise level, overcrowd-

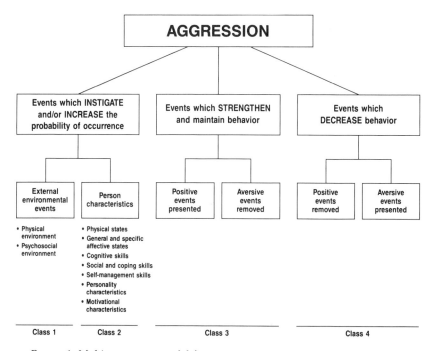

FIGURE 1. Multicomponent model for assessment and treatment of aggression.

ing, excessively demanding performance standards, or aggressive peer models).

Illustrations of the research support for a relationship between aspects of the environment and aggression are provided by Boe (1977) and by Rago, Parker, and Cleland (1978), who investigated the amount and type of physical space available in a residential unit to persons with mental retardation (population density) and the incidence of aggressive behavior. Boe (1977) demonstrated a significant reduction in the number of aggressive episodes on a residential unit of children and adolescents with severe and profound levels of mental retardation by increasing the amount of dayroom space available to the group. Boe speculated that the additional space available to each resident decreased the number of contacts each person had with others, thereby reducing the number of opportunities to be aggressive. Rago *et al.* (1978) also reported an association between an increase in physical playroom space and a decrease in the frequency of aggression in a group of males with profound mental retardation. These researchers offered the additional observation that crowding represented a stress variable and that the additional space provided a source of psychological relief for the residents that, in turn, served to reduce aggression.

A related approach to investigating the relationship between external environmental events and aggression is represented by Levy and McLeod (1977). In this study, the effects on aggression of providing an enriched physical environment (i.e., the creation of a gross motor activity area consisting of a carpeted pyramid, slide, and tunnel, and a fine motor activity area including tables for crafts) was evaluated. The enriched environment resulted in an overall decrease in socially undesirable behaviors. Although aggression toward others was at a low pretreatment level and remained so throughout the study, aggression toward self decreased from 41% to 8% and aggression toward objects decreased from 42% to 17% of the time residents were observed. Other reported benefits of the enriched environment included a decrease in neutral or stereotypic behavior and an increase in appropriate social interaction behaviors.

As a final example, Murphy and Zahm (1978), by improving the physical and the psychosocial environments, demonstrated a significant decrease in frequency and intensity of aggressive behaviors in groups of adolescents with severe and profound levels of mental retardation. These researchers hypothesized that the environmental changes may have functioned to eliminate the eliciting and reinforcing stimuli for the aggressive behavior that had existed prior to the changes.

A significant psychosocial influence involves the behaviors of others to whom a person is exposed. A number of studies with nonhandicapped persons report that individuals exposed to the aggressive behaviors of others are prone to engage in similar aggressive actions (e.g., Bandura, 1973; Zillmann, 1979). Aggressive actions of others may serve as cues that instigate aggressive behaviors in those persons who are inclined toward aggression. Bandura (1973) suggested also that aggressive provocation is most likely to produce aggressive behavior when the person being provoked has an impoverished repertoire of coping skills. This relationship between environmental variables and person characteristics emphasizes the need to consider both when assessing aggression in persons with mental retardation.

Talkington and Altman (1973) demonstrated that aggressive behaviors of persons with mental retardation could be influenced by exposure to aggressive models. Individuals were shown either (1) a film of aggressive behavior, (2) an affectual film, or (3) no film. When observed after the treatment condition, all subjects in the aggressive film group exhibited significantly greater imitative aggressive behaviors. These data are consistent with Bandura's (1973) comment that "models can serve as teachers, as elicitors, as disinhibitors, as stimulus enhancers, and as emotion arousers" (p. 130).

The discriminative events for any specific person's aggressive behaviors obviously are person-specific and can be identified only through systematic and objective observation of the individual in those particular situations in which aggressive behavior occurs. These conditions may include such factors as reduction in the frequency of staff attention (Carr & Durand, 1985), presentation of demands (Carr, Newsom, & Binkoff, 1980), social disapproval (Mace *et al.*, 1986), peer taunting (Cole *et al.*, 1985), and removal of positive conditions (Mace, Kratochwill, & Fiello, 1983). Assessment must be individualized, as emphasized by findings reported by Mace and colleagues (1986) and Carr and Durand (1985), revealing obvious individual differences among persons with developmental disabilities in the types of antecedent conditions that serve to instigate aggressive and related disruptive behaviors. Social disapproval, adult demands, and reduced social attention resulted in varying effects on the aberrant behaviors of different children. These findings emphasize that treatment should be preceded by client-specific assessment designed to identify the specific antecedent conditions presumed to instigate aggression.

Subject Characteristics Correlated with Aggression

A number of subject characteristics have been suggested as influential variables in occurrence of aggression, including conditions that, in isolation or in combination with external events, instigate or increase the likelihood of problem behaviors. Examples of these include transitory as well as more enduring *physical/sensory factors* (e.g., fatigue, chronic pain, hearing impairment, and premenstrual pain), *affective states* (e.g., anger, generalized anxiety, and chronic sadness), and *cognitive variables* (e.g., provocative, covert verbal rumination, and paranoid ideation). Also included is consideration of *deficit skill areas*, such as social communication, self-management, and related problem-solving and coping skills that, because of their low strength or absence, increase the likelihood of problems in those inclined to engage in aberrant behaviors.

Evidence that supports a relationship between an increased inclination toward aggressive responding and various subject characteristics comes from a variety of sources. As illustrations, Podboy and Mallery (1977) demonstrated a relationship between levels of caffeine intake and aggressive incidents among persons with severe mental retardation residing in an institu-

tional setting. Reduction in caffeine level, through substitution of decaffein-
ated coffee, correlated with a reduction in aggression as well as the number of
nocturnal awakenings. Rapport, Sonis, Fialkov, Matson, and Kazdin (1983)
noted that the physical aggression, consisting of grabbing, biting, kicking,
and hair pulling, of a young adolescent client was related to prodromal and
postictal seizure activity. Talkington and Riley (1971) reported a relationship
between an imposed reduction diet and aggressive incidents among institutionalized adults with mild and moderate levels of mental retardation. Following imposition of the reduction diet, the number of aggressive incidents
toward peers and staff increased substantially. These results were interpreted
within a frustration–aggression hypothesis. In a study of persons with mental
retardation and differing levels of communication skills, Talkington, Hall,
and Altman (1971) found that those with severe communication difficulties
engaged in more destructive outbursts, such as breaking windows, overturn-
ing furniture, and ripping clothing, than did matched peers who had adequate communication skills. These researchers speculated that the aggressive
acts of these individuals served to reduce their arousal level. Gardner, Clees,
and Cole (1983) described the potential role that verbal ruminations assumed
in producing an increased inclination for disruptive outburst in an adult with
moderate mental retardation.

A final variable of significance in understanding chronic problem behaviors is the individual's *motivational features.* Knowledge of events that serve as
positive reinforcers (adult approval, peer acceptance, having control over
others, aggravating others), as well as the variety or relative influence of
aversive events that influence the person's behaviors (rejection by peers,
difficult task demands, adult reprimand), are of importance in behavioral
assessment and related treatment planning. In sum, some personal characteristics, such as excessive negative emotional arousal, may *by their presence*
increase the likelihood of aggressive behaviors. Other variables, such as communication skills and motivation to please others, *by their absence or low
strength* render the person more vulnerable to inappropriate behaviors under
conditions of provocation.

Setting Events: Combining External and Internal Influences

In assessing events that serve to instigate aggression, it would be highly
unusual for aggressive behavior always to follow the occurrence of any specific
stimulus. In most cases, a *stimulus complex* sets the occasion for aggressive
reactions. This complex frequently involves sources of internal as well as
external stimulation. For example, an adolescent with mild mental retardation
who is likely to engage in aggression under conditions of provocation may
behave appropriately, when in a state of positive emotional arousal, if taunted
by a peer. When aroused negatively, this same adolescent under the same
external provocation may behave aggressively. This diagnostic information
would suggest that the critical variable requiring treatment is the person's lack
of coping skills under the dual conditions of negative emotional arousal and
peer teasing.

Gardner, Cole, Davidson, and Karan (1986) described an expanded behavioral assessment model that highlights this stimulus complex. The traditional applied behavior analysis assessment model, consisting of immediately
preceding stimulus events-behavior-consequences, was expanded to include
an assessment of *setting events*. These events are defined as those immediate
circumstances that influence which specific stimulus–response relationships
would occur out of all those currently comprising a person's behavioral repertoire. These setting events may consist of (1) *physiological conditions,* such as
sleep deprivation or the presence/absence of drugs; (2) *durational events,* such
as the presence of a specific staff member or specific work requirements in a
vocational training program; and (3) *behavioral histories* that represent temporally distant stimulus–response interactions wholly separate in space and
time from current stimulus conditions, such as an argument with mother
prior to arriving at school (Bijou, 1976; Bijou & Baer, 1961). The effects of
setting events are presumed to either *facilitate* or *inhibit* the occurrence of
current stimulus–response functions.

Setting events are not constant across persons and thus must be individually defined and identified. For example, the mere presence of a large
male staff member (as a durational setting event) may serve to inhibit aggressive behavior in a client who is likely to behave aggressively when reprimanded by other staff. However, this same event may have no such "setting"
effect on another client under the same stimulus conditions.

Expansion of the applied behavior analysis assessment and intervention
model to include consideration of setting events (i.e., setting event-immedi-
ate antecedent-behavior-consequence) holds promise of providing a more
complete and functional description of the combination of physiological, durational, temporally historical, and temporally immediate events that influence aggressive and related conduct difficulties of persons with mental retardation. Studies reported by Brown, Gardner, and Davidson (1989), Davidson,
Gardner, and Brown (1989), and Gardner *et al.* (1986) support the usefulness
of this expanded assessment protocol. With groups of persons with lengthy
histories of aggressive and related conduct difficulties and mild to profound
levels of mental retardation, the identification of person-specific setting
events resulted in significant improvement in predicting the occurrence of
aberrant behaviors. In each case, the conduct problems were more likely to
occur in the presence of specific discriminative conditions when occurring in
combination with a setting event than in the absence of this event. Thus,
including assessment of setting events greatly increased the predictability
that conduct problems would occur in the presence of the immediately preceding discriminative event. The identification of these conditions that contribute to the likelihood of aggression offers a number of intervention strategies (Gardner *et al.,* 1986).

The final set of variables evaluated are those that may serve to strengthen
and thus maintain the aggression. Consequences assessed include both potentially positive events presented following behavior (positive reinforcement) and unpleasant events removed following these actions (negative reinforcement). Recent studies (e.g., Carr & Newsom, 1985) support our own

clinical experience that negative reinforcement influences are at least partially involved in strengthening and maintaining chronic problem behaviors. Thus, this potential influence should be assessed to ensure adequate behavioral diagnosis.

Step 2: Develop Hypotheses Based on Assessment

The assessment data form the basis for developing a series of hunches about current factors that contribute to the person's aggression and related problems. Hypotheses are developed about (1) current environmental conditions (e.g., task demands and threats from peers), (2) personal characteristics (e.g., deficit communication skills, chronic fatigue, and anger) that increase the likelihood of aggressive behavior, and (3) the functions served by the behavior (e.g., aggression results in removal of task demands, aggression produces staff distress and peer approval). In most instances of chronic aggression, multiple hypotheses are developed about contributing factors in each of these areas.

Step 3: Select Client-Specific Treatment Procedures

Hypotheses about contributing factors are used to select the specific procedures comprising a behavioral treatment program that addresses these client-specific influences. An adolescent, for example, who demonstrates an increased set to aggress following nonattainment of a valued reward, and whose assessment data reveal deficit coping skills, would be provided a program designed to teach alternative means of coping with this failure.

The selection of punishment procedures in treatment of aberrant behaviors poses some particular problems for the behavioral diagnostician. In most cases, punishment procedures are selected for the purpose of suppressing excessively occurring aberrant behaviors. Their selection, however, is not based on diagnostic information relative to factors that contribute to the instigation or strength of the person's undesired actions. On the contrary, the use of punishment as a behavior treatment procedure most frequently is based on the supposition that the aversive properties will be sufficient to suppress the problem behavior by overcoming the effects of whatever may be producing or maintaining the behavior. Typically, the rationale used for selection of punishment procedures, especially those involving strong aversive stimuli, is that (1) the aberrant behavior poses a distinct danger to self or others and interferes significantly with the person's involvement in his or her social and habilitation environments, and that (2) other less intrusive treatment procedures have been attempted and were found to be ineffective. In practice, it is not unusual for the therapist to justify the use of highly intrusive punishment procedures based on the *a priori* conclusion that the personnel resources are not available to evaluate effectively the treatment efficacy of other procedures, such as a combined differential reinforcement of other behaviors (DRO) and extinction. In any event, the criteria of severity of the problem behaviors and the relative effectiveness and efficiency of punishment procedures typically are used in justifying the use of these approaches rather than selecting them on the basis of conceptually based diagnostic information.

BEHAVIOR TREATMENT, BEHAVIOR MANAGEMENT, AND BEHAVIOR CONTROL

Prior to discussion of the behavioral intervention literature relating to aggression, a distinction is made between behavioral procedures designed to produce enduring behavior change and those designed to manage the occurrence or intensity/duration of a specific aggressive episode. Additionally, a distinction is made between these behavioral procedures and those nonbehavioral ones that are used to control specific aggressive episodes.

Behavior Treatment

Behavior treatment refers to those procedures designed to *reduce* the frequency, duration, and/or intensity of excessive behaviors (e.g., self-injury, pica, psychogenic vomiting, aggression) and to *increase* the strength of positive alternative behavioral skills. The major objective of treatment is to produce *enduring* behavior change that will persist across time and situations. The treatment program is designed to change the person's responsiveness to external and internal conditions that instigate aggression, and to teach new socially appropriate emotional and behavioral skills that will replace the aggressive acts. The specific treatment procedures selected should have conceptual and, whenever available, empirical support for enduring behavior change. As an example, a young man with moderate mental retardation who engages in frequent aggressive outbursts may be provided a skills training program designed to teach him to cope with peer conflict (Cole *et al.*, 1985). As a second example, children with severe developmental disabilities may be taught communication skills as replacements for tantrum, self-abusive, and aggressive behaviors for use under instructional demand situations (Carr & Durand, 1985).

Behavior Management

Behavior management refers to those procedures that (1) eliminate or minimize specific stimulus conditions that are likely to instigate problem behaviors, (2) present or emphasize specific stimulus conditions that increase the likelihood of competing prosocial behaviors, (3) present or emphasize specific stimulus conditions that inhibit the occurrence of aggressive behaviors, and (4) minimize the duration and intensity of aggressive acts following their initiation. The initial three procedures are *proactive* in nature because they involve changing antecedents that precede problem behavior and are designed to encourage alternative prosocial actions. The fourth management procedure is *reactive* in nature as it is initiated following the occurrence of aggression. Even though reactive, this management procedure may prove quite valuable in minimizing the effects of any specific aggressive act. As a group these management procedures are supportive of active treatment efforts, but differ critically in function and in effect because they do not, in isolation, produce durable changes in behavior strength.

In the first proactive approach, management procedures are initiated that serve to *remove* or *minimize* the effects of specific preceding conditions that instigate aggression (e.g., reassigning a staff member who consistently provokes a particular trainee) (Gardner *et al.*, 1986).

In the second proactive behavior management approach, stimulus conditions are presented that increase the likelihood of competing prosocial adaptive, instead of aggressive, behaviors. As an example, Carr *et al.* (1980) demonstrated that providing strongly preferred reinforcers for correct responding under aversive demand conditions resulted in an increase in prosocial behavior and a concomitant abrupt decrease to a low level in the previously observed high-rate aberrant behaviors. The reinforcers were discriminative events that served to instigate prosocial behaviors that successfully competed with the aberrant responses.

In the third proactive behavior management procedure, inappropriate behaviors are inhibited by the presentation of stimulus conditions that signal the potential occurrence of aversive consequences contingent on aggression. For example, a reminder that the occurrence of a specific behavior will result in the loss of valued privileges may serve to inhibit the occurrence of the aberrant behavior.

The final behavior management procedure is reactive in nature and is used after aggressive behavior has begun. This procedure is designed to terminate or decrease the duration and/or intensity of the current episode. Such specific approaches as redirection, removing the provoking conditions, ignoring the behavior when acknowledging it would serve to intensify it, and removing the person from the source of provocation (e.g., removing the person to a quiet area away from the provoking noisy environment) illustrate the types of reactive tactics that may serve this management function.

As indicated, the primary purpose of behavior management procedures is not to teach alternative competency skills or to produce durable behavior change across time and changing conditions. As an example, a behavioral diagnostic assessment of aggression in children who are severely developmentally delayed may reveal an increased likelihood of aggression under conditions of specific task demands or under conditions of reduced social attention (Carr & Durand, 1985). With this diagnostic information, the occurrence of disruptive behaviors may be reduced or even eliminated by removing these controlling conditions; that is, by never presenting task demands and/or by providing a rich schedule of social attention. Under these conditions of managing the specific stimulus conditions that produce the aggression, the inappropriate behavior may not occur. However, when the controlling stimulus events of task demands and reduced social attention are reintroduced, the problem behavior reappears. Thus, the strength of aggression in the presence of these controlling stimulus condition has not been altered by the use of the management procedures. Durable changes could be expected only when active treatment procedures are included that teach alternative responses to these controlling events.

As a second example, behavioral diagnostics may reveal that a person's episodes of agitation and aggression could be minimized in intensity and duration if, immediately following initial signs of agitation, the person is redirected into alternative activities. The strength of these problem behaviors is not altered by this management procedure; rather, its disruptive features are minimized. With consistent use of this management procedure, the person more quickly becomes available to participate in whatever treatment experiences are provided. This behavior management program would be improved considerably by adding treatment procedures that, for example, would teach the person (1) to recognize his own early signs of agitation and then (2) to self-initiate alternative activities that would reduce or remove the agitation and the subsequent aggression.

Behavior Control

Behavior control refers to those procedures designed to be used in a behavioral crisis to deal with out-of-control behaviors that represent a potential danger to the person and/or those in the environment. These control procedures include the use of various *physical restraints* (e.g., isolating the person in a locked space, physically holding the person, and using such mechanical devices as leather belts or cuffs) and *chemical restraints* (e.g., use of Haldol to physiologically immobilize the person). These procedures are used in emergency situations for the sole purpose of immobilizing the individual for the duration of a current crisis, and are used only after other behavior treatment and management procedures have failed. The purpose is neither to produce durable behavior change (i.e., to serve as a reinforcement or punishment behavior treatment procedure) nor to reduce the likelihood that a current behavior episode will escalate to out-of-control status (i.e., to serve as a behavior management procedure). Rather, behavior control procedures are used to protect the person who is no longer in control by restraining his or her actions to minimize the possibility of self-injury or injury to others. It is, of course, possible that some behavior control procedures for some individuals (e.g., placing an out-of-control person in a locked isolation room or physically restraining a person's movement by holding him or her on the floor until control is regained) may have a treatment effect (i.e., a reinforcing or punishing effect) of increasing, or reducing, the future probability of the out-of-control behavior. However, a particular control procedure used with a specific person is neither selected nor used to produce this effect.

Interrelations of Procedures

Behavioral intervention programs for aggression should have the dual objectives of teaching and/or strengthening the discriminated occurrence of personally satisfying and socially appropriate adaptive behaviors and of reducing or eliminating excessively occurring aberrant behaviors. To accomplish these objectives, active treatment programs most frequently will include, in addition to therapeutic procedures designed to produce durable change, (1) those supportive behavior management procedures designed to facilitate occurrence of desired behavior and to minimize occurrence of problem behavior, and, when needed for those persons who are inclined to demonstrate out-or-control behaviors, (2) behavior control components. With effective treatment procedures, however, these supportive management and control components will be faded as treatment goals are accomplished and as the person is able to adapt appropriately under the normal or usual conditions of his or her everyday living environment.

BEHAVIORAL INTERVENTION

As suggested, aggressive behavior may be strengthened and maintained by the effects of both positive reinforcement (i.e., reinforcement-motivated aggression) and negative reinforcement (i.e., escape-motivated aggression). When the types(s) and source(s) of reinforcement can be identified, behavioral interventions that remove or reduce these sources of reinforcement can be effective in modifying the strength of aggression.

Behavioral Intervention for Reinforcement-Motivated Aggression

Aggression and related conduct difficulties may be functional for some individuals because they result in the occurrence or increase in positive consequences. Consequences suggested by various researchers as positive reinforcers for aggression include (1) various aspects of the victim's behavior, (2) various aspects of the behavior of others in the social environment who may verbally or physically intervene or otherwise react, and (3) either attaining or avoiding loss of material reinforcers or other items or activities of value, such as winning a fight or regaining a denied reinforcer. This hypothesis suggests intervention approaches consisting of (1) removing the functionality of the aggression through extinction, (2) teaching the person specific alternative (functionally equivalent) ways of obtaining the same or similar reinforcers, (3) strengthening alternative behaviors through providing reinforcement for the nonoccurrence of aggressive behaviors, and (4) suppressing the aberrant behavior through contingent use of punishment procedures.

Extinction

Feshbach (1964) suggested that signs from a victim of inflicted pain, injury, and/or distress may represent possible sources of social reinforcement for aggressive and other disruptive acts. Martin and Foxx (1973) further suggested that such social feedback as lectures, concern, or defensive reactions actually may be reinforcing to the aggressor and thus ensure future aggression. These researchers emphasized the potential strong reinforcing influence of aggression-produced social attention in such settings as institutions in which there are few reinforcers available for appropriate behavior. Thus, the staff's "reasonable reaction to an aggressive act such as disgust, lectures, physical restraint, isolation or giving intramuscular injections may serve as social reinforcement for the attention-deprived resident" (p. 162).

This observation emphasizes that consequences are defined by their effects on contingent behavior and not by the intent of the person presenting the consequences. Contingent staff reprimand, which to most would represent an aversive consequence, may in fact exert a positive reinforcement effect for a particular individual. Negative attention from a valued adult for some persons with mental retardation may be the most available and predictable alternative to little or no positive social feedback. In fact, as suggested, reprimands or other forms of negative attention may serve to increase rather than inhibit aggressive behavior. Mace *et al.* (1986) demonstrated this effect in their analysis of the environmental determinants of aggressive behaviors of three children with developmental disabilities. When provided reprimand in the form of social disapproval following the occurrence of aggression, each showed an increase rather than a decrease in aggression when exposed to this seemingly aversive condition.

Additional illustration that aggressive behavior in individuals with mental retardation may be maintained and extinguished by the contingent presentation and removal of social attention is provided by Martin and Foxx (1973). These therapists demonstrated that the presence or absence of social feedback or reactions of a victim to the physically aggressive behavior of an adult female with moderate mental retardation served either to maintain or to eliminate the aggressive behavior. Whenever the victim ignored the physical attacks, they gradually extinguished. But when the victim reacted to an attack, subsequent attacks were more likely to occur.

Although instructive in its demonstration that physically aggressive behavior may be controlled by the contingent occurrence and withdrawal of victim social attention, this obviously is not a feasible intervention procedure because of the passive role that victims must assume during attacks. Additionally, the initiation of an extinction procedure may result in a temporary increase in the frequency, duration, and/or intensity of aggressive actions. This is especially evident if the removed positive reinforcer is quite valuable to the person and if the person has limited functional alternative means of obtaining the reinforcer. The social environment may be unable, or unwilling, to tolerate such an increase. In commenting on the extinction procedure described above, Martin and Foxx (1973) noted:

It is not feasible, in cases similar to Gail, to arrange for the ward staff to withdraw
social reinforcement for aggressive behavior. The treatment is much too dangerous
for individuals functioning as victims because of the passive role they must assume
during attacks. (p. 165)

Thus, use of an extinction procedure in isolation in instances of severe
forms of aggression may not be a preferred intervention approach. However,
whenever possible, presumed sources of positive reinforcement, which are
hypothesized to strengthen and maintain aggressive actions, should be removed or minimized as other behavior change procedures are implemented.

This is not to suggest, though, that an extinction procedure may not be
useful with less severe forms of conduct difficulties. Forehand (1973) provided an illustration of its successful use in treating high-rate spitting behavior in a 6-year-old boy with mild mental retardation who was attending an
educational program. The teacher hypothesized that the attention the boy
received for spitting was maintaining the behavior and instructed her aides to
completely ignore it. The behavior decreased and eventually was eliminated.

Reinforcement of Functionally Equivalent Behaviors

When a person's aggression or related conduct difficulties are hypothesized to be maintained by contingent positive consequences, the behavioral
treatment program may include approaches that are designed to teach and/or
increase the strength of skills that would serve as alternatives to aggression.
This approach reflects a *skill deficit* perspective. The person is taught a functionally equivalent prosocial skill that can be used to produce the same or
similar reinforcing consequences.

Carr and Durand (1985) demonstrated through behavioral diagnostics of
children with developmental disabilities, who were attending an instructional
school program, that aberrant behaviors were more likely under conditions of
low levels of social attention than when provided frequent social attention.
Based on the assumption that the children were deficit in alternative skills of
gaining attention, each was taught to solicit increased attention through a
relevant communicative behavior. Following the use of this new mode of
communication, disruptive behaviors decreased significantly.

Differential Reinforcement and Extinction

Extinction may be combined with a procedure of differential reinforcement of other behaviors (DRO). In DRO, reinforcement is provided if the
client does not engage in the target aberrant behavior(s) for a specified time
period. The time interval is reinitiated following (1) each reinforcement or (2)
the occurrence of an aggressive behavior and is increased gradually until
reinforcement is no longer required for nonoccurrence of aggression.

After demonstrating in an individualized diagnostic behavioral assessment that aggression in a 15-year-old developmentally disabled male increased under a social disapproval contingency, Mace *et al.* (1986) selected a
treatment program consisting of DRO and extinction procedures. During

treatment, social attention in the form of conversation was provided on a variable 160-second schedule contingent on the absence of aggression during the preceding 10 seconds. Incidents of aggression were ignored. Treatment resulted in levels of aggression that were approximately one third of those that were observed when aggression was followed by social disapproval.

DRO Paired with Punishment

Friman, Barnard, Altman, and Wolf (1986) provided an example of an effective treatment program in which a DRO procedure was combined with a mildly aversive one consisting of response prevention. The treatment program was designed to reduce the aggressive pinching, both at home and in the classroom, of a 10-year-old girl with severe mental retardation and a deteriorating neurological condition. The child could not self-feed, had no speech, and was not toilet trained. At program initiation, both the mother's and the teachers' arms had scratch marks, scabs, and bruises resulting from the child's pinching. Although a formal diagnostic analysis was not conducted, the pinching behavior appeared to be maintained by the physical and social feedback that this behavior produced. Previous punishment procedures used unsuccessfully in home and school settings included reprimands, hand slapping, and blowing hot air from a blow dryer into the child's face whenever she pinched.

Initial treatment by the mother in the home setting during play sessions using a 10- to 20-second DRO schedule, with reinforcement consisting of praise and gentle touching, produced only temporary reduction in the pinching. The DRO procedure was next combined with a 5-minute time-out procedure which, again, produced only temporary reduction in the target behavior. Finally, the DRO procedure was combined with a response prevention procedure in which the child's hands were held stationary for 2 minutes after each pinch. This procedure, designed to prevent repeated pinching, consisted of a gentle holding technique which emphasized using the least amount of pressure necessary to keep the child's hands stationary. This program, used in the home and in the school, produced a rapid reduction in pinching in both settings. Follow-up in the home at 3 and at 15 months revealed maintenance of these gains.

Reinforcement of Incompatible Behavior

In designing a treatment program to reduce pinching during mealtimes for the child described above, Friman et al. (1986) used a treatment procedure consisting of providing differential reinforcement for a behavior that was physically incompatible (DRI) with the pinching. During this treatment condition, the mother brought food or drink to the child's mouth only when both of the child's hands were on or below the table. Whenever the child's hands were not on or below the table, the mother stated "hands down and kept food and drink completely out of reach until the child's hands were down. Prior to treatment, pinching occurred during nearly 100% of sessions. Following treatment initiation, pinching reduced rapidly to near zero level and remained at these rates at 3- and 15-month follow-up.

Punishment Procedures

As suggested above, even though diagnostic assessment reveals that aggression and related disruptive behaviors may be maintained by contingent social attention, some clinicians contend that under certain conditions use of a DRO and/or extinction procedure would not be appropriate. As an example, Mace *et al.* (1986) selected a time-out procedure in the treatment of the chronic and high-rate disruptive behaviors of a young girl with mild mental retardation, after a diagnostic assessment had revealed that the behaviors were maintained because of the disapproving comments of parents and other supervising adults. Diagnostic logic would have suggested that an extinction procedure be paired with differential reinforcement procedures designed to provide the child with valued social attention and to strengthen alternative socially appropriate skills of soliciting or otherwise obtaining positive social feedback. These clinicians reasoned, however, that (1) the child's disruptive behaviors were too severe to ignore, because they had previously resulted in physical injury and property destruction, and (2) that time-out involving a standard reprimand (e.g., "No spitting, go to time-out") would establish reprimands as aversive rather than reinforcing events. Use of a 2-minute time-out contingency did produce a significant reduction in the disruptive behaviors. In our view, the program would have been improved significantly, and would have been more consistent with a diagnostic behavioral approach, with the addition of procedures designed to teach the family to provide more frequent social attention, both noncontingently as well as contingent upon desired behaviors, and to teach the child alternative means of gaining desired social attention.

Behavioral Intervention for Escape-Motivated Aggression

Aggression and related conduct difficulties may be functional for some individuals in reducing or terminating sources of aversiveness as, for example, in the case of disliked or difficult task demands. In this case, aggression represents a form of escape-motivated behavior that is maintained by negative reinforcement (Carr & Newsom, 1985; Carr *et al.*, 1980; Sailor, Guess, Rutherford, & Baer, 1968; Weeks & Gaylord-Ross, 1981). This hypothesis suggests various intervention approaches consisting of (1) proactive behavior management procedures of completely removing the controlling aversive condition or of reducing the aversiveness of the event and thus reducing its discriminative control over aggressive responding, and (2) procedures removing the functionality of the aberrant behaviors through extinction or by teaching the person specific skills that can be used to eliminate or minimize the effects of the aversive conditions.

Proactive Behavior Management Approaches

Carr *et al.* (1980) and Carr and Newsom (1985) demonstrated management of aggression and tantrums in developmentally disabled children by
removing the conditions that instigated the behaviors. When instructional
demands in a classroom setting were placed on boys, who had a diagnosis of
mental retardation with autistic features, each engaged in high-rate aggressive behaviors, such as scratching, hitting, kicking, biting, pinching, and
hair pulling. When these demands were removed, the aggressive acts reduced immediately to near zero level of occurrence, even though the teacher
remained in close physical proximity to the child. Thus, the teacher was able
to manage the occurrence of the aggressive behaviors by removal of the
aversive conditions that instigated the aggression. However, when similar
demands were presented again, aggression returned to the rate previously
observed.

Weeks and Gaylord-Ross (1981) also demonstrated this effect with a child
with profound mental retardation whose aberrant behavior consisted of striking others with an open hand and of crying frequently. The child was exposed to the following situations: (1) no demands, (2) easy task demands, and
(3) difficult task demands. Greater rates of aberrant behavior occurred in
demand situations than in situations in which no demands were made of the
child, and noticeably greater rates of aberrant behavior occurred during difficult tasks than during easy tasks.

Carr *et al.* (1980) and Carr and Newsom (1985) provided a variation of this
proactive behavior management procedure by reducing the aversiveness of a
situation through the introduction of strongly preferred reinforcers for competing prosocial behaviors. After an initial demonstration that developmentally disabled children engaged in high-rate tantrum behaviors when instructional demands were presented in a classroom setting, the teacher provided
strongly preferred food reinforcers for each correct response (i.e., compliance
with teacher demand). Tantrums reduced to a negligible level under the
demand plus food condition, and compliance improved significantly (e.g.,
from 11% of trials to 65% in the Carr and Newsom study). Again, the instructor was able to manage the tantrum behaviors under the specific condition of
availability of highly preferred reinforcers, a condition that apparently attenu-
ated the aversiveness of the demand situation and thus reduced the functionality of the aggressive behaviors. However, as in the previously described
behavior management procedure, once the highly preferred food contingency
for compliance behavior is removed, one could expect the demand condition
to be discriminative once again for aberrant behaviors.

Behavioral Treatment Approaches

In contrast to these behavior management approaches to escape-motivated aggression are those behavioral treatment procedures that produce
more enduring behavior change. Procedures involving (1) removal of main-

taining conditions, that is, extinction (Carr *et al.*, 1980), and (2) teaching alternative skills that are functionally equivalent to the aggression, have been reported (Carr & Durand, 1985; Carr *et al.*, 1980). This latter approach represents the previously described skill deficit perspective. In escape-motivated behavior, the aggression is assumed to occur because the person does not have alternative functionally equivalent prosocial skills to cope successfully with the instigating aversive conditions.

Extinction. The use of extinction of aggression maintained by negative reinforcement (i.e., escape extinction) was demonstrated by Carr *et al.* (1980). High-rate aggressive behaviors of a severely developmentally disabled adolescent, which occurred in a demand situation, was virtually eliminated after the aggressive behavior became nonfunctional in producing escape. As is typical of an extinction procedure, aggressive behaviors occurred at a high rate during the early phase of the extinction experience. When aggression was again negatively reinforced (i.e., produced escape from the demand situation), the rate of aggression immediately increased. However, when extinction conditions were reintroduced, aggression abruptly fell to a near zero level. With each repetition of this sequence, aggression occurred at a progressively decreasing level during escape conditions. These researchers speculated that this decrease might have been attributable to the cumulative effects of prolonged exposure to the aversive situation—a possible habituation effect. Following this habituation, the adolescent, whose previous levels of aggression rendered it impossible for him to participate in an instructional task, was successful in learning a number of imitation discriminations.

Teaching Alternative Coping Skills. In an initial demonstration of decreasing aggressive behaviors when an alternative nonaggressive behavior is strengthened, Carr *et al.* (1980) taught a severely handicapped adolescent a nonaggressive tapping response as a means of escaping from an aversive demand situation. Previously observed high rates of aggressive behaviors reduced significantly whenever this alternative behavior became functional. In a follow-up demonstration of this procedure of teaching a functionally equivalent, but appropriate, means of escape from aversive conditions, Carr and Durand (1985) initially exposed children with both developmental disabilities and chronic problems of aggression and related disruptive behaviors to an instructional program that varied in task difficulty and in the level of teacher attention. They demonstrated that both low level of teacher attention and high level of task difficulty were discriminative for aberrant behaviors. Of interest were the findings that (1) the specific conditions that served to instigate misbehavior differed across children, and (2) that similar aberrant behaviors of a specific child could be escape motivated under certain conditions and reinforcement motivated under others.

Based on these individualized assessment data, children were provided training in functional communication designed to teach each child those communicative phrases that served to alter the stimulus conditions that controlled their problem behaviors (viz., deprivation of adult social attention or difficulty of task demands). As described earlier, children who were more likely to exhibit aggression under low levels of adult attention were taught to solicit praise through a relevant communicative response. Similarly, children who demonstrated an increased likelihood of aggression under difficult task demands were taught to solicit assistance by simply saying "I don't understand." Following training and consistent use of these communicative phrases, disruptive behavior was reduced to low levels. Thus, the communicative phrase was functionally equivalent to the aggressive behavior in reducing the aversiveness of the academic tasks.

Behavioral Intervention for Aggression of Uncertain Origin

In many instances, it is difficult to establish the specific preceding discriminating events that serve to instigate or increase the likelihood of acts of aggression. Thus, neither the previously discussed diagnostically based proactive behavior management procedures of removing or minimizing the discriminative events nor the behavioral treatment procedures of teaching the person to adapt to or remove/reduce these conditions or to engage in alternative coping skills in the presence of these controlling events are available for use. Additionally, in the natural settings of living and program environments, it frequently is not possible to establish the specific functionality of aggression and related disruptive behaviors. As a result, diagnostically based behavioral treatment procedures of extinction or shifting the specific reinforcement contingencies from aggression to competing prosocial behaviors become less precise.

In these instances, the varieties of differential reinforcement and skill development procedures represent potentially effective behavior treatment approaches. A number of recent studies have demonstrated reduction of aggression through developing and/or strengthening alternative social, coping, and self-management skills. In these studies, a skill deficit rationale guides the selection of the intervention procedures.

Differential Reinforcement of Other Behaviors

Luiselli and Slocumb (1983) demonstrated the successful use of a DRO procedure in reducing the aggressive behaviors of a 9-year-old girl with severe mental retardation and a dual diagnosis of autism and childhood psychosis. In the classroom, her behaviors, which consisted of hitting, kicking, hair pulling, spitting, and tantrumming, were directed at peers and instructional staff, and occurred in the absence of any clearly discernible antecedent events. Systematic use of a planned ignoring procedure and a behavior control approach (designed to protect staff and peers from repeated assaults) of physically immobilizing the child's movements during violent aggressive tantrumming until a period of nonagitation was achieved produced no effects during a 21-day baseline period. During DRO treatment, the child was provided praise ("Good girl, you kept hands to yourself and mouth dry") and a piece of favorite edible following a 7-minute period of no aggression. The DRO interval was gradually increased to 24 minutes. At the 34-week follow-up, the target behaviors had decreased to 1 per day compared to a preintervention rate of 17.8 per day.

Social Skills Training

Social skills training programs for individuals with mental retardation have combined components of modeling, instruction, feedback, and/or role playing. Matson and Zeiss (1978) compared the effects of two social skills training packages on interpersonal and chronic explosive behaviors of 12 severely disturbed psychiatric inpatients, 8 of whom had additional diagnoses of mental retardation. A training program containing instructions, modeling, and performance feedback was compared to a second program that included the additional component of *in vivo* role playing. Results indicated that both social skills training approaches increased appropriate interpersonal behaviors and decreased fighting and arguing, although clients trained with *in vivo* role playing improved more quickly.

In a second social skills training study, Matson and Stephens (1978) used social skills training to increase conversational skills and reduce arguing and fighting in four explosive institutionalized females with mixed diagnoses of chronic psychosis and mental retardation. The training program included instructions, modeling, role playing, and feedback.

In a similar vein, socialization games were used by Edmonson and Han (1983) to increase prosocial behavior and decrease aggressive behavior in 19 moderately and severely retarded institutionalized women (with chronological ages of 19–32). Simple games were selected that required group members to sit or stand close to one another, to notice some characteristics of the other players, and to provide positive reinforcement to one another in an enjoyable structured situation. During each training session, participants were reinforced for prosocial behaviors. In addition to fewer incidents of aggression, the social skills training procedure resulted in more prosocial interaction, a lower rate of inactivity, and closer proximity to peers.

Self-Management Training in Structured Environments

Although of recent origin, an increasing number of studies have begun investigating the therapeutic value of combining various self-management procedures with more traditional approaches in the treatment of severe conduct difficulties of adults with mental retardation. A skill deficit rationale underlies these studies, with the assumption made that skills of self-management would serve as alternatives to the impulsive aggressive reactions to sources of provocation.

Harvey, Karan, Bhargava, and Morehouse (1978) used various external and self-managed procedures to eliminate violent outbursts in a 38-year-old woman with moderate mental retardation. More recently, Gardner, Cole, Berry, and Nowinski (1983) and Gardner *et al.* (1983) used a multicomponent self-management package to reduce high-rate conduct problems in institutionalized adults with moderate mental retardation. As a final example, Cole *et al.* (1986) evaluated the therapeutic value of a self-management intervention program with mildly and moderately mentally retarded adults whose chronic and severe conduct difficulties prevented their participation in community vocational rehabilitation programs. The treatment package included the self-management skills of self-monitoring, self-evaluation, and self-consequation of their own appropriate and inappropriate work-related behaviors. In addition, these adults were taught to self-instruct prosocial behaviors that served as alternatives to aggression under conditions of provocation. In addition to a significant reduction of verbal and physical aggression, two collateral behaviors not specifically treated (on-task behavior and work productivity) showed positive effects. The 9-month follow-up revealed continued maintenance of treatment gains.

Self-Management Training in Open Environments

Most studies demonstrating the effectiveness of self-management treatment of aggression have been completed in closed or highly structured settings, such as institutions, classrooms, and workshops. In these environments, it is possible to monitor behaviors closely, to control the types of conditions present, and to provide immediate consequences following behaviors. In contrast, behavioral programming in open community settings, such as group homes, may present difficulties because of the reduced structure and the reduction in the number of staff available to monitor the program.

In these open setting, programs that include various self-management procedures offer considerable potential as the clients themselves manage components of the program. Reese, Sherman, and Sheldon (1984) evaluated the potential efficacy of a multicomponent behavioral treatment program that included a major self-management component. Young adults, in the mild to moderate range of mental retardation, were taught to self-record the occurrence or nonoccurrence of agitated/disruptive behaviors during previous time periods varying from 1 to 6 hours. This procedure was used in a program that also included token reinforcement, response cost, and social skills training. This latter training involved teaching alternatives to disruption and relaxation. The self-recorded DRO procedure proved to be effective in producing a significant reduction in the target behaviors. These therapists concluded that the major value of the self-recording procedure was to set the occasion for peers to give the client valued positive social feedback, such as praise, attention, or approval for more acceptable behaviors.

Benson (1986) and Benson, Rice, and Miranti (1986) provided a final example of a self-control intervention program. The program, which is called *anger management training*,

> teaches clients self-control skills which will enable them to handle anger-arousing situations in socially acceptable ways. Clients are taught not only to modify their outward behaviors (e.g., hitting someone), but also to modify the cognitions (thoughts which accompany those behaviors). (p. 51)

Although only preliminary data supporting its efficacy in producing positive behavior change in clients trained are provided, this cognitive behavioral program offers considerable potential for teaching those alternative prosocial skills required for increased independence.

SUMMARY AND CONCLUSIONS

During the late 1970s and throughout the 1980s, the behavior therapy literature devoted to treatment of aggression and related conduct difficulties among individuals with mental retardation has shown some significant shifts in focus. First, an increasing number of studies are investigating the efficacy of treatment procedures selected on the basis of client-specific diagnostic information. Second, intervention procedures are being designed specifically to teach alternative coping skills to replace aggressive reactions. This approach is in contrast to a major focus, historical and current, of evaluating the suppressive effects on aberrant behaviors of various contingent aversive consequences.

Even though the research literature is not sufficient in scope to provide unequivocal support for these diagnostic and skill development approaches, the available studies do provide encouraging results. Severe behavior difficulties have responded positively to programs that, viewing aggression as reflecting skill deficits, are designed to teach the person functionally equivalent alternative skills. Finally, this diagnostic and skill development focus is highly compatible with the legal and ethical guidelines articulated by various professional and advocacy groups (e.g., the American Association on Mental Retardation, The Association for Persons with Severe Handicaps).

ACKNOWLEDGMENTS. This chapter was supported in part by Research Grant G008300148 from the National Institute of Disability and Rehabilitation Research, Department of Education, Washington, DC 20202.

REFERENCES

Axelrod, S. (1987). Functional and structural analyses of behavior: Approaches leading to reduced use of punishment procedures? *Research in Developmental Disabilities, 8,* 165–178.

Bandura, A. (1973). *Aggression: A social learning theory.* Englewood Cliffs, NJ: Prentice-Hall.

Benson, B. A. (1985). Behavioral disorder and mental retardation: Association with age, sex, and levels of functioning in an outpatient clinic sample. *Applied Research in Mental Retardation, 6,* 79–85.

Benson, B. A. (1986). Anger management training. *Psychiatric Aspects of Mental Retardation Reviews, 5,* 51–55.

Benson, B. A., Rice, C. J., & Miranti, S. V. (1986). Effects of anger management training with mentally retarded adults in group treatment. *Journal of Counseling and Clinical Psychology, 54,* 728–729.

Berkowitz, A. J. (1987). The AAMD position statement on aversive therapy. *Mental Retardation, 25,* 118.

Bijou, S. W.(1976). *Child development III: Basic stage of early childhood.* Englewood Cliffs, NJ: Pren-tice-Hall.

Bijou, S. W., & Baer, D. M. (1961). *Child development I: A systematic and empirical theory.* Englewood Cliffs, NJ: Prentice-Hall.

Boe, R. B. (1977). Economical procedures for the reduction of aggression in a residential setting. *Mental Retardation, 15,* 25–28.

Bornstein, P. H., Bach, P. J., & Anton, B. (1982). Behavioral treatment of psychopathological disorders. In J. L. Matson & R. P. Barrett (Eds.), *Psychopathology on the mentally retarded* (pp. 253–292). New York: Grune & Stratton.

Borthwick-Duffy, S. A., Eyman, R. K., & White, J. F. (1987). Client characteristics and residential placement patterns. *American Journal of Mental Deficiency, 92,* 24–30.

Brown, M. G., Gardner, W. I., & Davidson, D. P. (1989). *A setting event analysis of aggression in persons with profound mental retardation.* Manuscript submitted for publication.

Carr, E. G., & Durand, V. M. (1985). Reducing behavior problems through functional commu-nication training. *Journal of Applied Behavior Analysis, 18,* 111–126.

Carr, E. G., & Newsom, C. (1985). Demand-related tantrums conceptualization and treatment. *Behavior Modification, 9,* 403–426.

Carr, E. G., Newsom, C. D., & Binkoff, J. A. (1980). Escape as a factor in the aggressive behavior of two retarded children. *Journal of Applied Behavior Analysis, 13,* 101–117.

Cole, C. L., Gardner, W. I., & Karan, O. C. (1985). Self-management training of mentally retarded adults presenting severe conduct difficulties. *Applied Research in Mental Retardation, 6,* 337–347.

Davidson, D. P., Gardner, W. I., & Brown, M. G. (1989). *Factors influencing conduct difficulties in person with mental retardation: A setting event analysis.* Manuscript submitted for publication.

Edmonson, B., & Han, S. (1983). Effects of socialization games on proximity and prosocial behavior of aggressive mentally retarded institutionalized women. *American Journal of Mental Deficiency, 85,* 473–477.

Eyman, R. K., Borthwick, S. A., & Miller, C. (1981). Maladaptive behavior and community placement of mentally retarded persons. *American Journal of Mental Deficiency, 85,* 473–477.

Eyman, R. K., & Call, T. (1977). Maladaptive behavior and community placement of mentally retarded persons placed in community and institutional settings. *American Journal of Mental Deficiency, 82,* 137–144.

Feshbach, S. (1964). The function of aggression and the regulation of aggressive drive. *Psycholog-ical Review, 71,* 257–272.

Forehand, R. (1973). Teacher recording of deviant behavior: A stimulus for behavior change. *Journal of Behavior Therapy and Experimental Psychiatry, 4,* 39–40.

Foxx, R. M., McMorrow, M. J., Bittle, R. G., & Bechtel, D. R. (1986). The successful treatment of a dually-diagnosed deaf man's aggression with a program that included contingent electric shock. *Behavior Therapy, 17,* 170–186.

Friman, P. C., Barnard, J. D., Altman, K., & Wolf, M. M. (1986). Parent and teacher use of DRO and DRI to reduce aggressive behavior. *Analysis and Intervention in Developmental Disabilities, 6,* 319–330.

Gardner, W. I. (1989). Behavior therapies: Past, present, and future. In J. Stark, F. Menolascino, M. Albarelli, & V. Gray (Eds.), *Mental retardation and mental health: Classification, diagnosis, treatment, services* (pp. 161–172). New York: Springer.

Gardner, W. I., & Cole, C. L. (1983). Selecting intervention procedures: What happened to behavioral assessment? In O. C. Karan & W. I. Gardner (Eds.), *Habilitation practices with the developmentally disabled who present behavioral and emotional disorders* (pp. 91–119). Madison, WI: Rehabilitation Research and Training Center in Mental Retardation.

Gardner, W. I., & Cole, C. L. (1984). Aggression and related conduct difficulties in the mentally retarded: A multicomponent behavior model. In S. E. Breuning, J. L. Matson, & R. P. Barrett (Eds.), *Advances in mental retardation and developmental disabilities: A research annual* (Vol. 2, pp. 41–84). Greenwich, CT: JAI Press.

Gardner, W. I., & Cole, C. L. (1985). Acting out disorders. In M. Hersen (Ed.), *Practice of inpatient behavior therapy: A clinical guide* (pp. 203–230). New York: Grune & Stratton.

Gardner, W. I., & Cole, C. L. (1987). Managing aggressive behavior: A behavioral diagnostic approach. *Psychiatric Aspects of Mental Retardation Reviews, 6*, 21–25.

Gardner, W. I., & Cole, C. L. (1988). Conduct disorders: Psychological therapies. In J. L. Matson (Ed.), *Handbook of treatment approaches in childhood psychopathology* (pp. 163–194). New York: Plenum Press.

Gardner, W. I., Clees, T. J., & Cole, C. L. (1983). Self-management of disruptive verbal ruminations by a mentally retarded adult. *Applied Research in Mental Retardation, 4*, 41–58.

Gardner, W. I., Cole, C. L., Berry, D. L., & Nowinski, J. M. (1983). Reduction of disruptive behavior in mentally retarded adults: A self-management approach. *Behavior Modification, 7*, 76–96.

Gardner, W. I., Cole, C. L., Davidson, D. P., & Karan, O. C. (1986). Reducing aggression in individuals with developmental disabilities: An expanded stimulus control, assessment, and intervention model. *Education and Training of the Mentally Retarded, 21*, 3–12.

Greenspan, S., & Shoultz, B. (1981). Why mentally retarded adults lose their jobs: Social competence as a factor in work adjustment. *Applied Research in Mental Retardation, 2*, 23–38.

Guess, D., Helmstetter, E. Turnbull, H. R., & Knowlton, S. (1987). Use of aversive procedures with persons who are disabled: An historical review and critical analysis. *Monograph of the Association for Persons with Severe Handicaps, 2*(1).,

Harvey, J. R., Karan, O. C., Bhargava, D., & Morehouse, N. (1978). Relaxation training and cognitive behavioral procedures to reduce violent temper outbursts in a moderately retarded woman. *Journal of Behavior Therapy and Experimental Psychiatry, 9*, 347–351.

Heal, L. W., Sigelman, C. K., & Switzky, H. N. (1978). Research on community residential alternatives for the mentally retarded. In N. R. Ellis (Ed.), *International review of research in mental retardation* (Vol. 9, pp. 209–249). New York: Academic Press.

Hill, B. K., & Bruininks, R. H. (1981). *Physical and behavioral characteristics and maladaptive behavior of mentally retarded people to residential facilities.* Minneapolis: University of Minnesota, Department of Psychoeducational Studies.

Isett, R., Roszkowski, M., & Spreat, S. (1983). Tolerance for deviance: Subjective evaluation of the social validation of the focus of treatment on mental retardation. *American Journal of Mental Deficiency, 87*, 458–461.

Koller, H., Richardson, S. A., Katz, M., & McLaren, J. (1983). Behavior disturbance since childhood among a 5-year birth cohort of all mentally retarded young adults in a city. *American Journal of Mental Deficiency, 87*, 386–395.

Lakin, K. C., Hill, B. K., Hauber, F. A., Bruininks, R. H. & Heal, L. W. (1983). New admissions and readmissions to a national sample of public residential facilities. *American Journal of Mental Deficiency, 88*, 13–20.

Levy, E., & McLeod, W. (1977). The effects of environmental design on adolescents in an institution. *Mental Retardation, 15*, 28–32.

Luiselli, J. K., & Slocumb, P. R. (1983). Management of multiple aggressive behaviors by differential reinforcement. *Journal of Behavior Therapy and Experimental Psychiatry, 14*, 343–347.

Mace, F. C., Kratochwill, T. R., & Fiello, R. A. (1983). Positive treatment of aggressive behavior in a mentally retarded adult: A case study. *Behavior Therapy, 14*, 689–696.

Mace, F. C., Page, T. J., Ivancic, M. T., & O'Brien, S. (1986). Analysis of environmental determinants of aggression and disruption in mentally retarded children. *Applied Research in Mental Retardation, 7*, 203–221.

Martin, P. L., & Foxx, R. M. (1973). Victim control of aggression of an institutionalized retardate. *Journal of Behavior Therapy and Experimental Psychiatry, 4*, 161–165.

Matson, J. L., & DiLorenzo, T. M. (1984). *Punishment and its alternatives.* New York: Springer.

Matson, J. L., & Gorman-Smith, D. (1986). A review of treatment research for aggressive and disruptive behavior in the mentally retarded. *Applied Research in Mental Retardation, 7*, 95–103.

Matson, J. L., & Stephens, R. M. (1978). Increasing appropriate behavior of explosive chronic psychiatric patients with a social skills training package. *Behavior Modification, 2*, 61–76.

Matson, J. L., & Zeiss, R. A. (1978). Group training of social skills in chronically explosive, severely disturbed psychiatric patients. *Behavioral Engineering, 5*, 41–50.

Murphy, M. J., & Zahm, D. (1978). Effect of improved physical and social environment on self-help and problem behaviors of institutionalized retarded males. *Behavior Modification, 2*, 193–210.

Podboy, J. W., & Mallery, W. A. (1977). Caffeine reduction and behavior change in the severely retarded. *Mental Retardation, 15*, 40.

Rago, W. V., Parker, R. M., & Cleland, C. C. (1978). Effect of increased space on the social behavior of institutionalized profoundly retarded male adults. *American Journal of Mental Deficiency, 82*, 554–558.

Rapport, M. D., Sonis, W. A., Fialkov, M. J., Matson, J. L., & Kazdin, A. E. (1983). Carbamazepine and behavior therapy for aggressive behavior: Treatment of a mentally retarded, postencephalatic adolescent with seizure disorders. *Behavior Modification, 7*, 255–265.

Reese, R. M., Sherman, J. A., & Sheldon, J. (1984). Reducing agitated-disruptive behavior of mentally retarded residents of community group homes: The role of self-recording and peer-prompted self-recording. *Analysis and Intervention in Developmental Disabilities, 4*, 91–107.

Reiss, S. (1982). Psychopathology and mental retardation: Survey of a developmental disabilities health program. *Mental Retardation, 20*, 128–132

Repp, A. C., & Bruelle, A. R. (1981). Reducing aggressive behavior of mentally retarded persons. In J. L. Matson & J. R. McCartney (Eds.), *Handbook of behavior modification with the mentally retarded* (pp. 177–210). New York: Plenum Press.

Rolider, A., & Van Houten, R. (1985). Movement suppression time-out for undesirable behavior in psychotic and severely developmentally delayed children. *Journal of Applied Behavior Analysis, 18*, 275–288.

Rusch, R. G., Hall, J. C., & Griffin, H. C. (1986). Abuse-provoking characteristics of institutionalized mentally retarded individuals. *American Journal of Mental Deficiency, 90*, 618–624.

Sailor, W., Guess, D., Rutherford, G., & Baer, D. M. (1968). Control of tantrum behavior by operant techniques during experimental verbal training. *Journal of Applied Behavior Analysis, 1*, 237–243.

Schalock, R. L., Harper, R. S., & Genung, T. (1981). Community integration of mentally retarded adults: Community placement and program success. *American Journal of Mental Deficiency, 85*, 478–488.

Sovner, R., & Hurley, A. (1986). Managing aggressive behavior: A psychiatric approach. *Psychiatric Aspects of Mental Retardation, 5*, 16–21.

Szymanski, L. S., & Leaverton, D. R. (1980). Mental health consultations to educational programs for retarded persons. In L. S. Szymanski & P. E. Tanguay (Eds.), *Emotional disorders of mentally retarded persons* (pp. 243–253). Baltimore: University Park Press.

Talkington, L. W., & Altman, R. (1973). Effects of film-mediated aggressive and affectual models on behavior. *American Journal of Mental Deficiency, 77*, 420–425.

Talkington, L., & Riley, J. (1971). Reduction diets and aggression in institutionalized mentally retarded patients. *American Journal of Mental Deficiency, 76*, 370–372.

Talkington, L., Hall, S., & Altman, R. (1971). Communication deficits and aggression in the mentally retarded. *American Journal of Mental Deficiency, 76*, 235–237.

Thorsheim, M. J., & Bruininks, R. H. (1979). *Admissions and readmissions of mentally retarded people to residential facilities.* Minneapolis: University of Minnesota, Department of Psychoeducational Studies.

Weeks, M. & Gaylord-Ross, R. (1981). Task-difficulty and aberrant behavior in severely handicapped students. *Journal of Applied Behavior Analysis, 14*, 449–463.

Wehman, P., & McLaughlin, P. J. (1979). Teachers perceptions of behavior problems with severely and profoundly handicapped students. *Mental Retardation, 17*, 20–21.

Whitman, T. L., Scibak, J. W., & Reid, D. H. (1983). *Behavior modification with the severely and profoundly retarded: Research and application.* New York: Academic Press.

Zillmann, D. (1979). *Hostility and aggression.* New York: Lawrence Erlbaum.

IV

Treating Self-Help Problems

9

Toilet Training

JOHN R. McCARTNEY

INTRODUCTION

The introduction to the first edition of this chapter (McCartney & Holden, 1981) emphasized the importance of training toileting skills in mentally retarded persons. Absent or inadequate toileting skills were described as a basic problem in the habilitation of severely and profoundly mentally retarded persons, one that has a significant impact on their quality of life.

The relative importance of toilet training mentally retarded persons is supported by the amount of research the problem has generated over the last two decades. Konarski and Diorio (1985) found that toileting was the most frequently studied self-help skill with severely and profoundly mentally retarded persons between 1962 and 1982. They presented cumulative frequency curves demonstrating the steady growth of the toilet training research literature over that time interval. The continuing interest in this area will be illustrated by the review of recent research presented later in this chapter.

The 1981 review (McCartney & Holden, 1981) yielded mixed results on the state of the knowledge base regarding operant conditioning methods of toilet training mentally retarded persons. Much had been learned, for example, operant principles worked to some degree, improvement was possible with practically all clients, and the more intense approaches produced more fully independent toileters. However, perhaps because the research was still in an early phase of development, there were many questions left to be answered. We suggested that an increase in methodological rigor was needed. Some of the major changes recommended were: (1) more attention to describing subject samples for the purposes of replication and to allow practitioners to make judgments about the appropriateness of the procedures for their clients; (2) the use of more appropriate dependent variables, including, in most cases, the number of self-initiated uses of the toilet; (3) the addition or upgrading of control procedures to ensure that the specified treatment was responsible for improvement; (4) an increased emphasis on long-term follow-up to determine the longevity of the new skills; and (5) the direct comparison of different

JOHN R. McCARTNEY • Alabama Department of Mental Health and Mental Retardation, Applied Research Bureau, University of Alabama, Tuscaloosa, Alabama 35486.

training programs and component analyses of successful training programs to determine the most beneficial, cost-effective procedures. Fortunately, as the toilet training research continues, more sophisticated efforts are being reported (e.g., Bettison, 1986), and the science of toilet training mentally retarded persons has continued to expand.

As Bettison (1978, 1986) has illustrated, toileting is a rather complex skill dependent not only on learning but also on maturational factors. Further, though many of the behaviors in the toileting chain are easily observed (e.g., approaching the toilet, handling clothes, voiding in the toilet), other essential skills in the chain are not so easily observed (e.g., inhibition of voiding as the bladder begins to fill). The several skills involved in successful independent toileting must also be linked in the correct sequence, and, during portions of the chain, multiple skills have to be performed simultaneously (e.g., inhibiting voiding while approaching the toilet). It is not surprising that the acquisition of independent toileting may often require special emphasis with the mentally retarded individual.

The objective of the present chapter is to provide a general update of the toilet training research with mentally retarded persons. To begin, the subskills of successful independent toileting will be described briefly followed by a discussion of some of the common training procedures. The two major training programs will then be summarized and compared, followed by a detailed review of the research published since 1980. The final sections of the chapter will contain discussions of some new developments from the recent research and the areas in which research may still be needed, as well as some suggestions for choosing toilet training programs.

THE BASIC SUBSKILLS OF TOILETING

A comprehensive understanding of successful toileting requires a breakdown of the skills that must be mastered to achieve fully independent toileting. This becomes particularly important with the severely and profoundly mentally retarded who may not readily respond to a simple reward for successful voiding and punishment for accidents approach. Such programs may be successful in increasing the number of voidings in the toilet and reducing toileting accidents. However, fully independent toileting, in which the client recognizes internal cues and then carries out the entire toileting sequence independently, often requires attention to the acquisition of specific subskills in this lengthy chain of behaviors.

A complete listing of the major subskills of fully independent toileting, in sequence, includes at least the following: (1) the inhibition of reflex voiding as the bowel or bladder fills, (2) approaching the toilet, (3) lowering clothing, (4) sitting on the toilet or standing facing the toilet, (5) voiding in the toilet, (6) using tissue as appropriate, (7) standing up, (8) flushing the toilet, and (9) raising clothing. This list may be intimidating for the trainer of profoundly mentally retarded individuals. Even in the case where the majority of these skills are already in the individual's behavioral repertoire, they must be performed in the correct sequence and in response to the appropriate cues. Many individuals may also need special assistance in attending to cues that occur at various points throughout this sequence of behaviors. Sensitivity to these issues will help the trainer identify weak links in the toileting sequence that may interfere with the successful acquisition of fully independent toileting (Bettison, 1986).

TOILET TRAINING PROCEDURES

Toilet training programs can be very simple or complex, depending upon the goals of training and the behavioral repertoire of the trainee(s). One of the simpler approaches involves prompting the client to go to the toilet and providing rewards for elimination in the toilet. Some type of punishment is often applied for toileting accidents (i.e., voiding in some place other than in the toilet). Prompts to void in the toilet may be given on a regular schedule (e.g., every 2 hours), or on an individually determined schedule, based upon an assessment of when reflex voiding responses tend to occur. This simple procedure for toilet training may be successful and cost effective for the client who already performs the majority of the skills in the toileting sequence and simply needs practice in performing the sequence in response to bowel and/or bladder cues. In addition, if the goal of training is simply to improve bowel or bladder continence but not independent toileting, these procedures may be all that is needed.

Additional techniques may be added to remediate weaknesses in various subskills. For example, if dressing skills are lacking, a graduated guidance procedure can be added to train them. The same is true for the skills of approaching the toilet and flushing, if the client has difficulty with those parts of the toileting sequence.

Many trainers use electronic signaling devices to enable the rapid detection of voiding responses. These devices are activated by a stream of urine either in the clothing (pants alarm) or in the toilet (toilet alarm). They allow the trainer to respond rapidly to accidents, either with punishment or the initiation of the toileting sequence in the case of the pants alarm, or the reliable administration of reward in the case of the toilet alarm.

Encouraging clients to consume extra liquids is another common procedure in toileting programs. This procedure is intended to increase the number of training opportunities during the program, since voiding is not naturally a high-rate response. Thompson and Hanson (1983) reported that a large percentage of the published work concerned with toilet training involves some sort of hydration technique. They also reported that precautions should be taken to avoid overhydration.

Smith (1979) categorized the basic types of toileting programs into "timing" and "potting" methods. In his view, programs that attempt to predict the occurrence of a voiding response and prompt the trainee to the toilet at those times (timing method) are theoretically different from programs that toilet the trainee at arbitrary intervals (potting method). He suggests that the potting method may be the procedure of choice, because the timing method tends to train the client to perform the toileting sequence at the time of a reflex voiding, which is dangerously close to an accident, rather than at times when the bladder is not necessarily full (Smith, 1979). A formal comparison of the two methods will be discussed later.

MAJOR CONTEMPORARY TRAINING PROGRAMS

Two intense training programs have had a significant influence on current procedures for training toileting skills to mentally retarded persons: Azrin and Foxx's (1971) "rapid" program and Van Wagenen's "forward-moving" approach (Mahoney, Van Wagenen, & Meyerson, 1971; Van Wagenen, Meyerson, Kerr, & Mahoney, 1969). Both programs will be described in some detail in the following sections.

The Van Wagenen et al. (1969) Method

In the forward-moving procedure training does not involve a rigid potting schedule, but trials are carried out when a reflex voiding response occurs. Smith (1979) would describe this approach as a timing method. The subject is fitted with a pants alarm to allow immediate detection of a voiding response. With the onset of the pants alarm the trainer yells "No!" to startle the trainee and inhibit voiding. The trainee is then rapidly assisted to the toilet, positioned appropriately for voiding, and finally encouraged to reinitiate voiding in the toilet. When the trainee begins to perform those steps independently (prompts are faded as the trainee takes more initiative), the removal and replacement of clothing is added to the sequence using a graduated guidance procedure. The trainee is encouraged to consume extra liquids throughout training to increase training trials. In the original test of this method, eight profoundly mentally retarded children were trained to be fully independent in urinating in a relatively short time period (Van Wagenen et al., 1969).

Mahoney et al. (1971) introduced a modification of the basic forward-moving procedure. Prior to beginning training as detailed above, trainees received practice in approaching the toilet and lowering their clothing in response to an auditory signal produced by the trainer using a remote-control device. This pretraining procedure was intended to give the trainee extra practice on the approach/clothes removal behaviors so that training time could be saved when the original forward-moving procedure began. Any appreciable improvement over the original procedure is not obvious from the results presented.

The Azrin and Foxx (1971) Method

The rapid program approach (Azrin & Foxx, 1971; Foxx & Azrin, 1973) has generated a considerable amount of attention, with at least eight studies directed at testing the method or some variation of it with mentally retarded persons (e.g., Bettison, Davison, Taylor, & Fox, 1976; Luiselli, Reisman, Helfen, & Pemberton, 1979; Sadler & Merkert, 1977; Smith, Britton, Johnson, & Thomas, 1975; A. Song, R. Song, & Grant, 1976). This approach is an intense potting procedure in terms of Smith's (1979) terminology. The trainee, fitted with a pants alarm, sits in close proximity to the toilet and consumes extra fluids. If the trainee's pants are dry during checks at 5-minute intervals, social and edible rewards are administered. At 30-minute intervals, the trainee is seated on the toilet until elimination occurs, or for a maximum of 20 minutes. Reward is provided for appropriately eliminating in the toilet. If an accident is discovered during pants checks, an overcorrection procedure ("Full Cleanliness Training") is implemented. During this procedure, the trainee is reprimanded, required to remove clothes and shower, and forced to wash and hang up dirty clothes. The trainee must also clean the soiled area with a mop. At the end of Full Cleanliness Training, a time-out procedure is implemented during which rewards are withheld but toileting sessions are continued. The program also utilizes pants and toilet alarms for the detection of voiding, and a graduated guidance technique to teach dressing during potting trials. Prompts for approaching the toilet are gradually faded until the trainee approaches independently. Following this, prompts for approach are no longer given.

Comparison of the Two Training Programs

Both the Azrin and Foxx (1971) and the Van Wagenen et al. (1969) programs have been successful in developing fully independent toileting in some severely and profoundly mentally retarded clients. However, the programs are quite different procedurally and in their theoretical underpinnings. The Van Wagenen et al. (1969) program takes advantage of reflex voiding episodes to practice a forward-moving toileting sequence that is very similar to the final desired behavior (i.e., fully independent toileting). The pants alarm is used to help signal the onset of a reflex voiding episode, and the trainee receives practice in inhibiting the voiding response under one set of stimulus conditions and initiating the response under another set of stimulus conditions. To repeat, it is a timing procedure using Smith's (1979) terminology, and a particular precise one (i.e., training trials are not initiated until a reflex voiding response occurs). A primary advantage seems to be the specific training to inhibit voiding. The procedure is a classical conditioning one, in which the bladder cues are the conditioned stimulus, the loud "No!" from the trainer the unconditioned stimulus, and the inhibition of voiding the unconditioned response that, as a result of training, occurs in response to the bladder cues. The Azrin and Foxx (1971) program emphasizes relatively intense social learning and reinforcement principles. High-density reinforcement and a strong punishment procedure are the principle components. The pants alarm is used as an aid in detecting accidents so that punishment procedures can be implemented immediately, and not as a signal to start the toileting sequence.

The Van Wagenen et al. (1969) procedure is theoretically appealing, particularly with its direct focus on the inhibition of voiding under stimulus conditions in which voiding would result in an accident, and the encouragement of voiding under stimulus conditions that lead to an appropriate elimination. The Azrin and Foxx (1971) procedures do not directly address this seemingly crucial skill. In the first edition of this chapter, we recognized the popularity and success of the Azrin and Foxx (1971) procedure, but we suggested that the Van Wagenen *et al.* (1969) procedure should be considered a viable alternative because it appears to require less time and little punishment.

Smith (1979) performed a comparison of three different toilet training approaches that provides some valuable empirical data addressing the question of the relative effectiveness of the Van Wagenen *et al.* (1979) and the Azrin and Foxx (1971) programs. Two of the methods were intensive, individual approaches, one modeled after the Azrin and Foxx (1971) method and the other having some similarities to the Mahoney *et al.* (1971) version of the Van Wagenen *et al.* (1969) program. The third procedure was a group approach using a traditional institutional potting procedure. Both intensive training approaches were found to be better than the traditional group method. The Azrin and Foxx (1971) procedure produced five of five independent toileters, whereas the Mahoney *et al.* (1971) procedure produced four of five independent toileters. According to the author the fifth subject in the latter group was a particularly resistant client who may not have responded to either program. In spite of the similarity in results, Smith (1979) recommended the Azrin and Foxx (1971) procedure over the Mahoney *et al.* (1971) method. The special remote-control pants alarm of Mahoney *et al.* (1971) was more expensive than the pants alarm of the Azrin and Foxx (1971) procedure, and the trainers apparently preferred the Azrin and Foxx (1971) technique. It should be noted, however, that Smith modified both training approaches, especially the Mahoney *et al.* (1971) approach, so that the comparison is not a direct one. In addition, as stated above, the Mahoney *et al.* (1971) modification is not necessarily an improvement over the Van Wagenen *et al.* (1969) procedure, which does not require the expensive remote-control alarm system.

REVIEW OF RECENT LITERATURE

As mentioned in the introduction, toilet training research with mentally retarded persons has been published consistently over the past two and one-half decades. In this section, some of the research published since 1980 will be reviewed. Combining this review with the literature review section of the McCartney and Holden (1981) chapter will give the applied researcher or clinician a reasonably complete, although not totally comprehensive, coverage of toilet training research with mentally retarded persons.

Most of the research in recent years continues to utilize some variation of the Azrin and Foxx (1971) procedure. Demonstration or pilot projects continue to be common, and the generality of these procedures has been demonstrated with various groups. The robustness of the basic technique has also been demonstrated; that is, a variety of procedural modifications have been investigated with generally positive results. The isolated demonstration or pilot projects that were published since 1980 will first be briefly reviewed. Then the work of Bettison (1986), who has carried out a rather systematic analysis of toilet training procedures, will be discussed in more detail.

Lancioni (1980) applied a variation of the Azrin and Foxx (1971) program to the training of deaf-blind profoundly mentally retarded children who exhibited high rates of self-stimulatory behavior. These children had acquired basic dressing skills prior to the initiation of the toilet training program, so it was not necessary to intensively train these skills as part of the toileting program.

Subjects were trained for 4 hours daily. Prior to each training session, they were given a smaller breakfast than usual to make edible rewards more effective. Extra fluids were given at 5-minute intervals, beginning before training and continuing into the training session. In the first phase of training, the children were seated just outside the toilet stall and wore a pants alarm. They were checked for dryness at approximately 5-minute intervals and were rewarded with back rubs if dry. Prompts to go to the toilet were given every 20 minutes on the first training day only, and each of the following behaviors was reinforced with edibles if the toileting sequence was self-initiated: voiding in the toilet, raising pants, and returning to the chair. This process continued until independent toileting was occurring, after which the reward was discontinued for voiding and raising pants and was given only after the client returned to the chair.

Punishment was administered when the pants alarm signaled an accident. The children were required to walk on a series of raised blocks, which apparently was an aversive consequence. They were then allowed to change clothes.

As independent toileting began to occur consistently with the child seated just outside the toilet stall, a second phase of training was initiated. In this phase, the subjects were stationed in a hallway outside the bathroom, and the same training contingencies were used. Independent toileting from the hallway led to the third phase, which involved using the same procedures with the subject located back in the classroom. As independent toileting began to occur from the classroom, the extra fluids were gradually removed, and the frequency of dry pants checks was reduced.

After the intense training phases were ended, a maintenance phase was instituted that included edible reinforcement after fully independent toileting, back rubs after only three widely spaced dry pants checks, and the omission of dry pants checks for the remainder of the day after an accident.

A multiple-baseline procedure (three groups of three children each) was used to evaluate treatment effects. Training produced a rapid increase in independent toileting and a decrease in accidents for all groups. It also generalized to other portions of the day when the only procedures in effect were assisted toileting and simple reward for voiding in the toilet (i.e., baseline conditions for this study). Eight of nine subjects maintained their newly acquired skills for 44 days.

This study demonstrates the effectiveness of the Azrin and Foxx (1971) program with deaf-blind children. The multiple-baseline design illustrated that treatment was effective, and the generalization phase, though it was relatively short and contained some fairly powerful treatment procedures in itself, gave some indication of the longevity of the treatment effects.

In attempting to show that positive results could be obtained with a less intense toileting program included as part of the client's daily routine, Lancioni and Ceccarani (1981) introduced a new innovation into their training procedure: the use of plastic "potties." The general procedure involved the increased consumption of liquids, more frequent sessions of assisted toileting (i.e., toileting behavior after an initial prompt from the trainer), and punishment. Two different interventions (A and B) were used. In the initial phase of both interventions, the profoundly mentally retarded subjects were maintained in their normal daily activities and were prompted to toilet themselves at 55-minute intervals. They were rewarded for three behaviors: voiding in the toilet, walking out of the bathroom after voiding, and returning to the classroom. They were punished after accidents by being required to walk on their knees and bending to their knees and rising repeatedly for approximately 1½ minutes. The only difference in the two interventions was the use of an extra discriminative stimulus for toileting. Intervention A required the subject to carry a red plastic "potty" to the bathroom and insert it in the toilet before voiding. Potties were placed all around the classroom area as reminders to use the toilet. In Intervention B, the potties were not used. In the latter phases of both interventions the number of assisted toileting sessions was reduced and then finally discontinued (subjects using Intervention B did not progress beyond this point). As the subjects progressed further in Intervention A, reinforcement was reduced to the point where it was given only upon the client's return to the classroom after successful independent toileting. The use of the potties was also faded out, and the consumption of liquids was reduced to near normal levels.

Using a multiple-baseline across subjects analysis, the authors demonstrated that Intervention A was effective. Each subject's accident rate was reduced to zero, and all toileting was fully independent after 7 to 10 days of training. Intervention B produced some reduction in accidents in its initial phases, but no increase in independent toileting. However, when these subjects were switched to Intervention A, they showed the same rapid progress as the original subjects using that procedure.

In a second experiment, Lancioni and Ceccarani (1981) investigated whether punishment was a necessary procedure for clients who were accident free but did not exhibit independent toileting. They used the same interventions as were used in the first experiment, except that punishment was omitted. The effect of the potty devices on the development of independent toileting using this less intense training approach was evident. When potties were used, progress was rapid in spite of the omission of punishment for accidents. The positive training effects found during training in both experiments generalized well to other portions of the clients' day. Follow-up results showed maintenance of the skills for 60 days.

These studies illustrate that a less intense procedure that does not involve the disruption of the daily routine can be effective in developing independent toileting in some clients. The use of the potties was an interesting innovation that probably functions as a reminder to use the toilet, and as a discriminative stimulus for the initial steps in the toileting sequence. Lancioni and Ceccarani's (1981) hypothesis that punishment acts primarily to reduce toileting accidents, and is not a critical procedure in increasing the rate of independent toileting, received some support from the second experiment.

Both Lancioni (1980) and Lancioni and Ceccarani (1981) continued to provide reward at the end of a successful toileting action during the follow-up phase, and this apparently was a permanent procedure in the setting where these clients lived. Although the improvement in the independence of these clients is unquestionable, it seems that in most applied settings it would be possible and desirable to reduce excessive dependence on artificial contingencies, such as the provision of edibles for the performance of toileting skills.

The clients in Lancioni and Ceccarani's (1981) study also appeared to have a number of prerequisite toileting subskills. They all had basic dressing skills, and apparently required little prompting to initiate the toileting sequence. Also, since their accident rate prior to training was fairly low, they apparently had some ability to inhibit voiding prior to training. A low-intensity procedure such as this may not be effective with clients that have fewer prerequisite skills.

Richmond (1983) trained toileting skills to four young (2–3 years) developmentally retarded children who appeared, according to the author, to be profoundly mentally retarded. Subjects were trained to have fewer toileting accidents in an experiment designed to show how a simplified potting procedure could have beneficial effects with much less time and effort than an intense training program. The training procedures were simple. Potting intervals were reduced from once an hour during baseline to once every 15 minutes during treatment. Social praise was provided for being dry just prior to toileting, and liquid reward and social praise were provided for voiding in the toilet. Accidents were punished with a reprimand and a simple correction procedure (i.e., changing clothes, washing, disposing of dirty clothes, and dressing). The potting interval was kept at 15 minutes the first week, but was gradually increased to 2 hours over a period of 4 weeks.

Using a multiple-baseline design across children, the experimenter was able to show the beneficial effects of this treatment on accident rate for each child. Further, the effect was maintained for 7 to 8 weeks when baseline conditions were in effect. No attempt was made to train or even systematically evaluate further improvements in toileting beyond a decreased accident rate, though some improvement in prevoiding behaviors (e.g., approaching the toilet, lowering pants, etc.) was reported.

This study achieved its objective of demonstrating that a limited, yet desirable improvement could be obtained with a simple program that was easy to administer. The impression given is that this level of improvement was all that the situation would allow, given the age of the children and the environmental conditions.

Hobbs and Peck (1985) provided a simple reward for toilet eliminations and/or punishment for accidents program to 12 profoundly mentally retarded females residing in an institution. No attempt to attain self-initiated toileting was reported. Clients were rewarded for eliminating in the toilet during assisted toileting sessions every 2 hours, and were punished after accidents with decreased social contact, removal from desirable activities, and the delay of meals. Mean percentage of correct eliminations (obtained by dividing the number of voidings in the toilet by the total number of voidings) for the training group improved from 50% to 83% over a 12-week period. There was no improvement over the same period for a no-training control group. The positive results in the training group were maintained for 1 year, as illustrated by a 2-day follow-up observation.

Hobbs and Peck (1985) demonstrated once again that the application of simple operant procedures has a positive effect on accident rate with institutionalized mentally retarded persons. This finding has been demonstrated by others (e.g., Dayan, 1964; Waye & Melnyr, 1973), but this study included a comparison group and a long-term follow-up probe.

Bettison (1986) has reported on a series of studies that have begun to answer some of the more difficult questions in regard to the toilet training of mentally retarded persons: What is the effectiveness of various procedures used in complex training programs? and What program modifications can improve training results for the more difficult-to-train client? Her adept comparisons and choice of techniques reveal a thorough knowledge of operant principles and toilet training problems.

In her dissertation (reported in Bettison, 1986), Bettison compared the effectiveness of three of the major components of the Azrin and Foxx (1971) program. The first major training strategy evaluated was the application of contingent consequences (i.e., reward for toilet voiding and punishment for accidents). A control group for this condition received noncontingent consequences in about the same number and pattern as the training group. The second major training strategy was the use of shaping procedures to train nonvoiding toileting skills. Trainers performed these skills for the subjects in the control condition for this strategy. The use of alarms was the third major Azrin and Foxx (1971) training strategy tested. In the control condition for this strategy, alarms were activated in about the same pattern and frequency as they would occur if used in training; however, they were not associated with voiding.

The results were disappointing. The three training strategies were not significantly more effective than control conditions, and they did not produce differential effects. Most of the subjects did improve, however, and almost half of them achieved self-initiated toileting.

These results are certainly not as impressive as those normally reported when the Azrin and Foxx (1971) program is used. Bettison (1986) suggested that her trainees did not have as many preexisting skills as the trainees in some other studies. Thus, the subjects in those studies were better prospects for successful training. She also suggested that the Azrin and Foxx (1971) program does not specifically train all of the skills in the toileting sequence. Because of the "potting" nature of the procedure, some crucial skills are not directly taught, such as the inhibition of the voiding response to increasing bowel or bladder pressure. Also, the nature of the procedure allows a number of toilet-sitting trials during which voiding does not occur, in spite of the hydration procedures used. Finally, Bettison (1982) noted that her trainees had particular difficulty discriminating when to pull pants down as opposed to when to pull them up.

Bettison (1982) developed a detailed chaining program that includes several existing strategies as well as some new ones. The program also emphasizes the training or monitoring of all of the subskills in the self-toileting sequence. As described in Bettison (1986), the basic procedure is a backward-chaining procedure. Each skill in the chain is trained to a predetermined criterion level of performance so that nothing is left to chance, and bowel and bladder tension are treated as essential discriminative stimuli.

The program begins (Bettison, 1986) with training the last two responses in the toileting chain (i.e., standing from the toilet and pulling pants up). After the criterion is reached on these two steps, the rest of the chain is added to the sequence, but only the specific step next in line for strengthening is trained on any given trial. On each trial, the trainer quickly moves the trainee through the earlier skills in the sequence, uses a graduated guidance procedure with the training step, and allows independent performance of the skills after the training step. Early in the training program, trials are always initiated by bowel and/or bladder tension cues to ensure that these cues become essential discriminative stimuli in the toileting chain. To accomplish this, a pants alarm is used to detect the onset of voiding, and, as in the Van Wagenen et al. (1969) procedure, the trainer shouts "No!" to produce an inhibition of the voiding response, which serves as direct practice of that important skill. Next, as described above, the trainer takes the trainee quickly through the toileting chain, and the inevitable reward at the end of each trial serves to strengthen the entire chain of behavior. At the end of training subjects are gradually moved further from the toilet, and the use of alarms and extra fluids is eliminated.

Bettison (1982) increased the durations of the pants alarm and the toilet signal (in this case, a light rather than an auditory alarm) to further emphasize the presence of bowel and bladder tension prior to voiding in the toilet and the lack of tension after voiding in the toilet as discriminative stimuli. The pants alarm is allowed to sound from onset until voiding begins in the toilet. The toilet light remains on from the initiation of voiding in the toilet until the end of the toileting chain. The intent of these modifications is to strengthen the awareness of bladder or bowel tension as a discriminative cue for the behaviors prior to voiding in the toilet, and to strengthen the awareness of bowel or bladder relaxation as a discriminative cue for the postvoiding skills in the chain. This procedure should be especially beneficial in overcoming the problem of discriminating when to pull pants down or when to pull them up (Bettison, 1986), because additional stimuli are added to facilitate this discrimination.

In comparing her chaining approach to the Azrin and Foxx (1971) program, Bettison (1986) found that the chaining method was superior on three measures, by (1) increasing the rate of toilet voiding, (2) increasing self-initiated uses of the toilet, and (3) reducing accidents, although this latter finding was not statistically significant.

Bettison's (1986) analysis of toileting behavior and procedures is important. The toileting program she proposed (Bettison, 1982, 1986) holds great promise for the training of clients with severe learning deficiencies, though she recognizes that additional modifications in the procedure may be needed. The treatment has many similarities to the Van Wagenen et al. (1969) approach, but it goes further in placing great emphasis on the importance of each subskill within the toileting sequence, which is certainly a requirement for the client who does not respond to less comprehensive programs.

NEW DEVELOPMENTS

As stated in the introduction to this chapter, because toilet training research utilizing operant principles with mentally retarded persons was still in its early developmental phases in 1981, the knowledge base at the time of the first edition of this chapter was encouraging but somewhat limited. The research to that time had demonstrated that operant procedures worked, that some form of improvement was possible with all clients, and that more intense approaches produced more independent toileters. What has been learned since that time? The following sections will discuss some new findings from Bettison's (1986) work, as well as some impressions from the literature as a whole.

An initial and very basic impression is that further refinements are needed in toilet training programs to achieve success with the more difficult-to-train client, at least in terms of full toileting independence. Although the literature review in the 1981 chapter did not emphasize it, some studies were already showing less than a 100% success rate (e.g., Bettison et al., 1976). Other studies were reporting total success with clients who were described as profoundly mentally retarded when other evidence, such as the IQ scores reported, suggested that higher ability subjects were included in the sample. Other studies gave little or no evidence to substantiate the diagnostic level, so doubts remain concerning the actual capabilities of the subjects trained. In more recent work, Bettison (reported in Bettison, 1986) found several clients who improved in some aspects of toileting but failed to achieve full independence. The impression given in the 1970s of guaranteed success with the new toilet training programs was prematurely optimistic when more recent data are considered.

Bettison's work (1986) also demonstrated that a more detailed and comprehensive approach to evaluating and training all of the subskills of fully independent toileting is needed to improve the success rate of training efforts. A primary skill neglected in the major potting procedures (e.g., Azrin & Foxx, 1971) is the ability to inhibit voiding as the bladder and/or bowel begins to fill. If this skill is not directly trained, the effectiveness of the program may be limited, particularly when it comes to the reduction of accidents.

Bettison (1986) found a preliminary trend suggesting that her chaining procedure, which directly trains this skill, is more effective in reducing accidents than a potting procedure.

Another important factor often neglected in toilet training programs, and one that creates problems for profoundly mentally retarded persons, is discriminating the appropriate stimuli that signal "pants down" as opposed to "pants up" (Bettison, 1986). Strategies designed to enhance this discrimination may be needed for the successful training of these clients.

When comparing intense training programs and various major training strategies within such programs, the results have not been particularly revealing. As reported above, when Smith (1979) compared versions of the Azrin and Foxx (1971) and the Van Wagenen et al. (1969) programs, little difference in the success rate was found. Bettison (1986) has also found little reason to prefer any major training component of the Azrin and Foxx procedure over others. Therefore, until further research is performed in this area, it might be concluded, as did both Smith (1979) and Bettison (1986), that the crucial aspect of the intense toilet training programs is their structured framework, rather than any particular training procedures.

The advance in our knowledge of toilet training procedures with mentally retarded persons has been slow in the last few years. However, researchers are just now beginning to venture beyond a period of demonstration and pilot projects into a period of component analyses and the closer examination of critical variables. They are discovering the many complexities involved in training toileting skills. Continued pursuit of this new phase of research, which is well illustrated by the work of Bettison (1986), may lead to further advances in the next few years.

SUGGESTIONS FOR FUTURE RESEARCH

This section will begin by suggesting what type of research is not needed. Projects that simply demonstrate that operant procedures improve the toileting skills of mentally retarded persons are now of limited usefulness. Operant principles have been shown to have a positive effect in virtually every published report. Also, research showing the effect of variations in Azrin and Foxx's (1971) training program are not beneficial unless they involve a reexamination of the theory supporting the program. The basic program has already been adequately replicated.

There are some procedural replications that might expand the knowledge base. Replication with some distinct subgroups might be helpful, for example, in demonstrating that an intense training program is successful with subjects having no prerequisite toileting skills. The standard approaches have not achieved total success in developing fully independent toileting with these clients.

Studies that evaluate the interaction of the client's level of prerequisite toileting skills with various training procedures would also provide useful information for applied researchers and clinicians. Preferably, such studies would do more than just demonstrate that less intense procedures are sufficient for training clients with several prerequisite skills, whereas more intense procedures are needed for less capable clients. Instead, they would demonstrate the effectiveness of tailoring a toileting program to match the individual's prerequisite toileting skills. For example, individuals who seem to have particular difficulty in inhibiting reflex voidings might benefit more from the use of a pants alarm to signal the occurrence of reflex voidings and a startle procedure (i.e., the trainer immediately shouts "No!" to elicit directly the appropriate muscular response), than from a more traditional potting approach.

Clear component analyses of the more influential training packages are also needed. For example, subjects who are trained with the full Azrin and Foxx (1971) procedure could be compared to other groups of clients who receive the full procedure minus one of the major components. The more critical components of the total program would be identified by comparing each group's performance with the group receiving the full program. The more beneficial the procedure, the more its absence from the total program would disrupt acquisition of toileting skills relative to the full program. Although not necessarily using this particular approach, some analysis of procedural components has already been done (Bettison, 1986), but more is needed.

Bettison's (1982) new chaining procedure also warrants further research, particularly with the client who is resistant to other intensive techniques. As discussed above, the special emphasis on providing additional stimuli to improve the discrimination of bowel or bladder cues, as well as the revival of the Van Wagenen et al. (1969) procedure to directly train the inhibition of voiding are theoretically appealing procedures. There is evidence that the chaining program is more effective than the Azrin and Foxx (1971) program for the client with few prerequisite skills (Bettison, 1986), but this finding requires further replication.

CHOOSING A TREATMENT PROGRAM

The terminal behavior desired is a primary factor to be considered in choosing a toilet training program. It has been repeatedly shown that a reduction of accidents can be obtained with the majority of clients, assuming there are no physiological contraindications. In most cases, simply adding contingent consequences for accidents and toilet voidings is effective in achieving some reduction, if not the total elimination, of accidents. This reduction may be fragile, however, in that environmental disruptions or schedule changes may lead to a reoccurrence of accidents, since the client's behavior may continue to be dependent upon staff vigilance, assistance, and a constant environment.

If fully independent toileting is the goal of training, a more intense procedure may be needed for the rapid development of such skills with the severely or profoundly mentally retarded individual. Such a program as the

Azrin and Foxx (1971) rapid method of toilet training may be effective in this case, particularly if there are preexisting toileting skills, such as the ability to inhibit voiding inappropriately. The procedure may even be modified significantly with good success if the situation demands it. For example, less intense punishment procedures have been used successfully (e.g., Smith, 1979). In some cases, particularly if the client is not having frequent accidents, punishment might not be necessary (e.g., Lancioni & Ceccarani, 1981), or it can be quite different in nature from the "Full Cleanliness Procedure" originally prescribed.

If the potential trainee does not exhibit fully independent toileting, but has most of the toileting subskills in his or her behavioral repertoire, and the normal daily environment allows full and easy access to toileting facilities, a procedure less intense than that of Azrin and Foxx (1971) may allow the trainee to remain in a normal training routine and still learn to be independent in toileting. Such a procedure may meet with less resistance from administrators and parents, and be less stressful for trainees and trainers than staying in or near the bathroom for long intervals and being excluded from normal activities (Lancioni & Ceccarani, 1981). The criterion behavior will probably not be attained as rapidly, however.

In the case where the client to be trained has limited or nonexistent toileting subskills, a comprehensive procedure such as Bettison's chaining method (Bettison, 1982) may be the program of choice. The extra emphasis on training each subskill, as well as the unique use of pants and toilet alarms as discriminative stimuli, may be particularly beneficial in such cases. However, further demonstrations of the effectiveness of this procedure are necessary before it can be strongly recommended.

The above discussion should serve to remind the clinician that the toilet training program chosen should be tailored to the trainee's needs, which can be closely determined after extensive observation of the trainee and interviews with the family and/or staff providing daily care (Bettison, 1978). The clinician should also keep in mind that it may be useless to train more independence than the trainee's normal environment can support. For example, if staff or family members will not allow free access to the toilet, then it is useless to train a client to independently initiate the toileting sequence. This behavior will be quickly extinguished after the training program is completed.

CONCLUSIONS

The research emphasizing the use of operant learning principles to train toileting skills has succeeded in providing a technology that effectively remediates one of the most basic and degrading skill deficits of mentally retarded persons. The large majority of these individuals can now achieve some degree of improvement in toileting skills that will allow greater independence and more exposure to a normal environment. Fully independent toileting is also possible, as demonstrated by the significant number of profoundly mentally retarded individuals who have attained this level of ability. This advancement is remarkable for a relatively short period of time. Just 25 years ago there was little to offer severely and profoundly mentally retarded individuals in regard to toilet training. Ellis's (1963) theoretical description of the stimulus–response principles that might be useful in training toileting skills to mentally retarded persons stimulated a very important and fruitful area of research.

Now that some fairly effective training programs have been tested, the applied researcher must further develop and refine the toilet training technology. Some individuals do not attain fully independent toileting even with the use of very intense, up-to-date programs. Further analyses comparing some of the major training strategies used in toileting programs should also be performed to determine the most effective components.

As further progress is made in the coming years, it should become possible to perform a detailed evaluation of prerequisite toileting skills and then prescribe the right "mix" of procedures in order to allow the fastest rate of improvement and the highest level of toileting independence possible for each trainee.

REFERENCES

Azrin, N., & Foxx, R. (1971). A rapid method of toilet training the institutionalized retarded. *Journal of Applied Behavioral Analysis, 4,* 89–99.

Bettison, S. (1978). Toilet training the retarded: Analysis of the stages of development and procedures for designing programs. *Australian Journal of Mental Retardation, 5,* 95–100.

Bettison, S. (1982). *Toilet training to independence for the handicapped. A manual for trainers.* Springfield, IL: Charles C Thomas.

Bettison, S. (1986). Behavioral approaches to toilet training for retarded persons. In N. R. Ellis & N. W. Bray (Eds.), *International review of research in mental retardation* (Vol. 14, pp. 319–350). Orlando, FL: Academic Press.

Bettison, S., Davison, D., Taylor, P., & Fox, B. (1976). The long-term effects of a toilet training program for the mentally retarded: A pilot study. *Australian Journal of Mental Retardation, 4,* 18–35.

Dayan, M. (1964). Toilet training retarded children in a state residential institution. *Mental Retardation, 2,* 116–117.

Ellis, N. (1963). Toilet training the severely defective patient: An S-R reinforcement analysis. *American Journal of Mental Deficiency, 68,* 99–103.

Foxx, R., & Azrin, N. (1973). *Toilet training the retarded: A rapid program for day and nightime independent toileting.* Champaign, IL: Research Press.

Hobbs, T., & Peck, C. (1985). Toilet training people with profound mental retardation: A cost effective procedure for large residential settings. *Behavioral Engineering, 9,* 50–57.

Konarski, E., & Diorio, M. (1985). A quantitative review of self-help research with the severely and profoundly mentally retarded. *Applied Research in Mental Retardation, 6,* 229–245.

Lancioni, G. (1980). Teaching independent toileting to profoundly retarded deaf-blind children. *Behavior Therapy, 11,* 234–244.

Lancioni, G., & Ceccarani, P. (1981). Teaching independent toileting within the normal daily program. *Behavior Research of Severe Developmental Disabilities, 2,* 79–96.

Luiselli, J. L., Reisman, J., Helfen, C. S., & Pemberton, B. W. (1979). Toilet training in the classroom: An adaptation of Azrin and Foxx's rapid toilet training procedure. *Behavioral Engineering, 1979, 5,* 89–93.

Mahoney, K., Van Wagenen, R., & Meyerson, L. (1971). Toilet training of normal and retarded children. *Journal of Applied Behavioral Analysis, 4,* 173–181.

McCartney, J. R., & Holden, J. C. (1981). Toilet training for the mentally retarded. In J. L. Matson & J. R. McCartney (Eds.), *Handbook of behavior modification with the mentally retarded* (pp. 29–60). New York: Plenum Press.

Richmond, G. (1983). Shaping bowel and bladder continence in developmentally retarded pre-school children. *Journal of Autism and Developmental Disorders, 13,* 197–204.

Sadler, W., & Merkert, F. (1977). Evaluating the Foxx & Azrin toilet training procedure for retarded children in a day training center. *Behavior Therapy, 8,* 499–500.

Smith, P. (1979). A comparison of different methods of toilet training the mentally handicapped. *Behaviour Research and Therapy, 17,* 33–43.

Smith, R., Britton, P., Johnson, M., & Thomas, D. (1975). Problems involved in toilet training of institutionalized mentally retarded individuals. *Behaviour Research and Therapy, 3,* 301–302.

Song, A., Song, R., & Grant, P. (1976). Toilet training in school and its transfer in the living unit. *Journal of Behavior Therapy and Experimental Psychiatry, 1976, 7,* 281–284.

Thompson, T., & Hanson, R. (1983). Overhydration: Precautions when treating urinary incontinence. *Mental Retardation, 21,* 139–143.

Van Wagenen, R., Meyerson, L., Kerr, N., & Mahoney, K. (1969). Field trials of a new procedure for toilet training. *Journal of Experimental Child Psychology, 8,* 147–159.

Waye, M., & Melnyr, W. (1973). Toilet training of a blind retarded boy by operant conditioning. *Journal of Behavior Therapy and Experimental Psychology, 4,* 267–268.

10

Acquisition of Self-Help Skills

MARIE E. TARAS AND MARY MATESE

Self-help skills, or daily living skills, may be defined as those behaviors that allow individuals to care independently for their own bodily needs. The mentally retarded person needs to be able to eat, use the toilet, dress, and perform personal hygiene to meet basic requirements for independence and normalcy. Once these skills are acquired, caregivers could redirect time and effort previously devoted to basic care to education and training of residents, thus facilitating a more productive environment.

In recognition of the importance of self-help skills, an abundance of behaviorally oriented research evaluating and developing new techniques of teaching these skills has been conducted over the last 25 years. The first practical application of behavior modification methods to teach daily living skills to mentally retarded people appeared around 1963 from the Pinecrest State School in Louisiana, in the work of Ellis (1963), Dayan (1964), and Bensberg, Colwell, and Cassel (1965). Since that time, three approaches to behavior modification have been described in the literature as the primary techniques that are used to teach self-help skills to mentally retarded persons in residential facilities, and in special educational and parent training programs. These three methods are graduated guidance, backward chaining, and forward chaining. The purpose of this chapter is to describe and assess these techniques and to discuss their application to specific areas of self-help skills.

PROCEDURES UTILIZED IN TEACHING SELF-HELP SKILLS

General strategies for teaching self-help skills will be reviewed, including response chaining, graduated guidance, prompting, fading, and independence training. The chapter has been organized in this fashion to facilitate understanding of the basic methods employed in the research conducted to date. Specific and detailed programs of applying these procedures will be described in our review of the various topics, such as feeding, toilet training, and personal hygiene. These techniques are relevant for many problems of

MARIE E. TARAS AND MARY MATESE • Department of Psychology, Louisiana State University, Baton Rouge, Louisiana 70803.

persons with mental retardation. However, they are discussed most frequently with respect to self-help skills.

Prompts and Fading Techniques

Prompts are stimuli that increase the probability of a target behavior. They are used singularly, in combination, or as part of a hierarchy. There are four primary types of prompts: verbal, gestural, modeling, and physical. Research in this area seems to indicate that no prompt functions well by itself. For example, gestural prompts are much more successful when some verbalization precedes it, whereas verbal prompts by themselves have a very low rate of self-initiation and lead to a longer acquisition time (Glendenning, Adams, & Sternberg, 1983). In a study conducted by Glendenning et al. (1983), comparing sequences of verbal, gestural, and physical prompts, they found that a combination of verbal prompts and physical assistance led to a significantly higher rate of self-initiated responses.

Fading, a second related technique, is the transition of stimulus control from prompts to task-related stimuli. Timing is crucial in the process of fading; premature removal of a prompt can result in a high error rate, which precludes acquisition of the target behavior (Touchette, 1968). Unnecessarily prolonging the prompting process, however, could nurture dependence on stimuli provided by the trainer (Touchette & Howard, 1984). Two commonly used methods of fading described by Billingsley and Romer (1983) are the "least-to-most" intrusive prompt order and the "most-to-least" intrusive prompt order (cited in Godby, Gast, & Wolery, 1987; Snell, 1987). Instructors have indicated a preference for the least-to-most prompt hierarchy (Walls, Crist, Sienicki, & Grant, 1981), which consists of a general instruction, then successively more restrictive prompts (i.e., specific verbal direction, modeling, and physical guidance) if the client is still in need of more assistance (Marholin, O'Toole, Touchette, Berger, & Doyle, 1979). The most-to-least prompt hierarchy merely follows this sequence in reverse, and there is very little difference in the effectiveness of either technique (Walls, Crist, Sienicki, & Grant, 1981).

A fading procedure that has received widespread attention over the past decade in the self-help literature is the prompt delay procedure which functions by inserting an interval of time between the presentation of the task and the response prompt, thus shifting control to stimuli inherent in the task (Walls, Dowler, Haught, & Zawlocki, 1984). Research on this topic conducted by Touchette and Howard (1984) found that implementing a delay prior to prompting increased stimulus control transfer, and this rate could be accelerated by consequences favoring self-initiated responses. There are two primary types of prompt delay procedures: constant time delay and progressive time delay. The first block of trials is typically presented at zero-second delay. Constant time delay places a fixed interval of time between the novel stimulus and the response prompt, whereas the progressive time delay method places increasing increments of time intervals between presentation of the initial stimulus and the controlling prompt. The progressive delay procedure has been found to be more efficient than the least restrictive prompt sequence in terms of amount of instructional time, fewer trials to criterion, and lower error rates (Godby *et al.*, 1987). However, studies comparing these two instructional methods caution that further examination is needed in looking at the relative efficiency of these two techniques for discrete and chained responses (e.g., Bennett, Gast, Wolery, & Schuster, 1986; Godby *et al.*, 1987). Finally, Handen and Zane (1987) reviewed 26 studies that used the delayed prompt procedure and stated that "the paucity of literature contrasting the efficacy of delayed prompting with other training procedures precludes the drawing of any valid conclusions regarding the relative advantages of the various training methods" (p. 328). Nonetheless, we do know that such methods are effective and warrant attention by the reader.

Graduated Guidance

Graduated guidance utilizes the whole task method of teaching in which the person attempts every step in the sequence during each learning trial. The initial program of this type was developed by Azrin and his associates with self-feeding (Azrin & Armstrong, 1973) and dressing (Azrin, Schaeffer, & Wesolowski, 1976). The three types of prompts typically used to assist in task performance are gestural, verbal, and physical. The latter two methods are used primarily in the early training period. The trainer fades prompts intuitively, always giving the client the minimal physical assistance necessary to perform the targeted task. Any attempts at self-initiation are verbally reinforced, and the trainer maintains a shadowing position, keeping his or her hands 2 to 3 inches away from the client's in order to correct any errors or hesitations. This approach works extremely well with severely and profoundly mentally retarded clients, especially those who tend to become dependent on physical prompts. However, the subtleties of this technique are difficult to teach to some paraprofessional staff. Its unstructured, general approach sometimes makes it difficult for staff members to know when and how much physical guidance is needed in a specific instance; therefore, it is not well suited to apply to a variety of self-help skills (Watson & Uzzell, 1980).

More frequently used is the "constant contact" physical assistance technique. The teacher first puts his or her hand on the student's hand, then the student's wrist, then the forearm, the elbow, and finally the shoulder (Snell, 1987). As with Azrin's procedure, only as much physical assistance required for task completion is used, but the trainer begins with the most restrictive physical prompt as opposed to the least restrictive hierarchy. Both programs recommend high density reinforcement. Verbal and physical reinforcement for each completed step of a task-analyzed behavior and an edible or activity reinforcer at the end of the chain are not uncommon. Given the necessity of overt assistance, graduated guidance has become a common form of treatment.

Response Chaining

A second major instructional method for training self-help skills is response chaining (e.g., Azrin & Foxx, 1971; Watson & Uzzell, 1980). Typically, the response is broken down into separate teachable components usually through task analysis (Snell, 1987). These tasks are then trained via a forward or backward chaining procedure.

Forward Chaining

In forward chaining, the first step of the task-analyzed sequence is learned using a predetermined criterion. For example, if an instructor wanted to teach shoe-tying using forward chaining, he or she would first have the resident learn how to grasp both shoelaces and pull them tightly. Once the client could do this five times in succession, without the assistance of prompts, the next step, crossing the laces over, could be approached. Subsequent steps are then added one at a time in a forward sequence beginning with step 1, then step 2, and so on. The instructor typically begins with a verbal prompt and then moves to a gestural prompt or models for the client, whichever seems most appropriate. If the client still needs assistance, a physical prompt is used (Watson & Uzzell, 1980). Forward chaining is ideally suited to severely, moderately, and mildly mentally retarded clients with receptive language skills in which extensive physical prompting is not required (Watson & Uzzell, 1980). The advantages of this technique includes its low error rate on the part of the learner (Walls, Zane, & Ellis, 1981; Walls et al., 1984) and its adaptation to a large number of self-help programs (Watson & Uzzell, 1980). However, because the structure of forward chaining allows only for a maximum of one additional step per trial, it requires more time for training than whole task presentation (Walls et al., 1984).

Backward Chaining

Backward chaining is similar to forward chaining in that tasks are broken down into functional units. However, the task-analyzed steps are taught in reverse sequence in comparison to forward chaining, starting with the last step first. There is very little difference in the relative effectiveness of forward and backward chaining (Walls, Zane, & Ellis, 1981). The typical prompt hierarchy for this technique is verbal, gestural, and physical, with the more restrictive prompts being faded first (Watson & Uzzell, 1980). This instructional method works well with the severely and profoundly mentally retarded, but it is not recommended for clients who become dependent on physical prompts because it lacks a gradual fading procedure (Watson & Uzzell, 1980). Backward chaining is relatively easy to teach to paraprofessional staff, and, like forward chaining, it has been adapted to a large number of daily living skills programs (Watson & Uzzell, 1980).

Whole Training and Chaining

There has been some investigation into the relative merits of whole task presentation and chaining techniques, where specific incremental steps are trained. These studies (e.g., Nettlebeck & Kirby, 1976; Walls, Zane, & Ellis, 1981) tend to be homogeneous in nature as they generally involve teaching mildly to moderately mentally retarded individuals vocational assembly tasks. Both Nettlebeck and Kirby (1976) and Walls, Zane, and Ellis (1981) found chaining techniques to be a better instructional tool than the whole task teaching method. Also, chaining results in lower error rates, compared to the whole task presentation, which may result in fewer maladaptive responses during instructional sessions (Bennett *et al.*, 1986; Weeks & Gaylord-Ross, 1981). However, chaining techniques are not very efficient in that they require much more of a trainer's time and attention, since he or she must ensure that each additional step is mastered as well as all combinations of steps (Nettlebeck & Kirby, 1976).

A literature review conducted by Spooner and Spooner (1984) found no conclusive advantage to whole task training and chaining. They concluded:

> In the final analysis, it may be that different learners do better with different procedures, and that when different tasks are used (e.g., dressing v. vocational) different results are obtainable. (p. 123)

The advantages, if indeed they are present, may be idiosyncratic. Thus, varying methods may need to be tried before optimal results can be established.

Independence Training

Independence training is a packet of treatment procedures that can be used in conjunction with standard classroom training and has been used in teaching a wide variety of self-help skills (Matson, 1982). These methods differ somewhat from those mentioned earlier in the chapter in that operant and social learning principles are considered. Techniques utilized in independence training consist of peer and self-reinforcement, self-monitoring, and evaluation, *in vivo* modeling by the trainer, and trainer-assisted performance of the target skills by the resident (Matson & Marchetti, 1980). The primary goal of this procedure is to increase independent functioning in a typically dependent population (Matson & Marchetti, 1980). Advantages of independence training are numerous. First, it has been proven to be more effective than a number of conventional behavioral treatments for training some self-help and social skills (Matson, 1980, 1982; Matson, DiLorenzo, & Esveldt-Dawson, 1981; Matson & Marchetti, 1980; Matson, Marchetti, & Adkins, 1980). Also, it requires less one-to-one supervision and requires about as much time as traditional treatment programs (Matson *et al.*, 1981). Additionally, it enhances consent to treatment by increasing feedback and responsibility of clients in their treatment programs. Finally, both staff members and clients have positively reacted to independence training and seem to enjoy the increased interaction this method provides (Matson, 1980). To date the research indicates that supplementing traditional classroom training with self-regulating techniques can facilitate acquisition of self-help skills. However, it should be cautioned that although this technique is applicable to mildly and moderately mentally retarded persons, it may have less applicability with severely and profoundly mentally retarded persons.

In the following section, we will examine how each of the above described procedures are incorporated into teaching specific self-help skills to mentally retarded persons. Where applicable, each topic section will be divided in two main sections: one section will address acquisition of self-help skills, and a second section will deal with decelerative techniques that are utilized to ameliorate inappropriate or socially unacceptable behaviors that interfere with appropriate self-help skills acquisition.

TEACHING SPECIFIC SELF-HELP SKILLS

Self-Feeding

Techniques and programs aimed at increasing appropriate self-feeding skills of mentally retarded persons encompass a large body of research. Critical reviews of training self-feeding skills are provided by Reid (1982), Reid, Wilson, and Faw (1983), and Snell (1987). One reason for this great emphasis is that it is the first basic self-help skill in the normal developmental sequence to be acquired (Reid, 1982). Thus, self-feeding is logically a basic and necessary set of skills to acquire before other independent self-help skills are targeted for intervention (Reid, 1982; Reid et al., 1983). Another reason for the large number of self-feeding studies is that lack of appropriate self-feeding skills constitutes a major area of frustration for and demand on caregivers, be they parents or staff. If these clients are left to feed themselves, the resulting situation is messy, hectic, and aversive to the caregiver. Handicapped persons often eat with their hands, off the floor, and may throw or spill food (Redd, Porterfield, & Anderson, 1979). Any attempts to prevent spillage usually requires interruption of the feeding response and/or restraint, which sets up an ensuing battle between the client and caregiver. On the other hand, caregivers may decide to bypass the disruptive self-feeding scenes and to feed the child themselves. Although this avoids the mess and struggle, it consumes a great deal of one person's time, three times a day, which is often impractical, if not impossible, in placements where staff to student ratios are low. Additionally, this later approach fosters increased dependence on the adult. Clients who have not learned to feed themselves, especially as they become older, severely limit opportunities for positive interpersonal interactions and productive work (Bender & Valletutti, 1985). Also, this may limit the opportunity for their placement in less restrictive settings.

Acquisition of Self-Feeding Skills

Operant procedures are especially well-suited to training self-feeding skills because food, which is a powerful and primary reinforcer, is built into the feeding program (O'Brien, Bugle, & Azrin, 1972). Ideally, once a client has learned to eat appropriately, the consumption of food should provide continued, natural reinforcement to maintain correct eating skills (Redd *et al.*, 1979). However, this has not occurred (Groves & Carroccio, 1971; O'Brien *et al.*, 1972; Whitney & Barnard, 1966). Although food is an inherently powerful reinforcer, it can be obtained more easily and faster through incorrect eating behaviors, such as eating with one's hands, than correct eating skills (Redd *et al.*, 1979).

Graduated Guidance

Albin (1977) employed the whole task method of graduated guidance in teaching three profoundly mentally retarded children to eat with a spoon. Graduated guidance went from least restrictive (verbal prompt) to the most restrictive (physical prompt). For example, with the food in front of the child, he or she was given one verbal instruction to pick up the spoon. If the child did not respond appropriately in two seconds, the staff physically placed their hands around the child's and the spoon, and guided the child to use the spoon to place food in the mouth. Praise and physical reinforcement were contingent upon food entering the mouth.

Backward Chaining

Backward chaining entails teaching the particular skill's task-analyzed steps in reverse; that is, the last step is trained to criterion, then the second from last step is taught, and so on until all the steps comprising the behavior are trained. Backward chaining combined with prompting, such as physical guidance, was used in several studies to teach basic self-feeding skills to mentally retarded persons (Bensberg *et al.*, 1965; Berkowitz, Sherry, & Davis, 1971; Gorton & Hollis, 1965; Murphy & Zahm, 1978; O'Brien *et al.*, 1972; Ross & Oliver, 1969; Song & Gandhi, 1974). In particular, O'Brien *et al.* (1972), via five meals a day and with these techniques, increased spoon usage in a profoundly retarded 6-year-old girl. The eating response was broken down into the following six steps: (1) the spoon was placed in the child's hand, which was held by the teacher's hand; (2) the child's hand was guided and the spoon was dipped into the food and held about 1 inch above the bowl once loaded with food; (3) the spoon was brought to within 2 inches of the child's mouth; (4) the child's mouth was gently opened by the teacher's hand on the child's chin; (5) the spoon was guided into the child's mouth; and (6) the child's hand was guided through an upward and outward motion to ensure that the food was removed from the spoon.

After the sequence was correctly performed for three successive guided trials, the teacher manually guided the child through one less step of the sequence. In other words, by releasing the child's hand further from her mouth, she was required to finish more of the responses independently. The amount of guidance was gradually decreased as the child's self-feeding skills increased.

Prompts

Low-functioning mentally retarded persons who do not have any self-feeding skills may initially require a high level of physical prompts (Banderdt & Bricker, 1978; Richman, Sonderby, & Kahn, 1980). Procedures require the caretaker to hold the client's hand around the utensil and physically guide him or her through the steps to self-feeding (e.g., loading food onto the utensil, lifting it toward the mouth, etc.). As the client becomes more adept, the amount of physical guidance can be gradually faded. For example, instead of grasping the client's hand, the caretaker may move the prompt to the wrist, forearm, elbow, and eventually the shoulder. However, in training multiple utensil use in 24 institutionalized mentally retarded clients, Nelson, Cone, and Hanson (1975) found that physical guidance was more effective than modeling. Therefore, physical prompts are not just reserved for the lower functioning clients.

For the mentally retarded person who has minimal self-feeding skills, training can be conducted by combining verbal prompts with modeling of appropriate self-feeding behaviors (Butterfield & Parson, 1973; O'Brien & Azrin, 1972). In doing so, the teacher would instruct the client, while at the same time demonstrating the desired behavior. For example, as the teacher instructs the resident to lift a utensil, the teacher is simultaneously lifting a utensil. O'Brien and Azrin (1972) compared the appropriate eating behaviors of a training and a control group. The training group received verbal prompts, modeling, and physical guidance (i.e., the least-to-most approach), whereas the control group received no special training. At posttest and at a 2-week follow-up, the training group emitted fewer eating errors than the control group. In addition, O'Brien and Azrin (1972) included a social validity measure in their study and found that their mentally retarded clients ate with less errors in the institution's dining area than did a group of normals in a public restaurant.

For the mentally retarded with advanced feeding skills, verbal prompts alone may be sufficient to correct inappropriate eating behaviors (Redd *et al.*, 1979). This situation may consist of observing the client eating and providing instructions and feedback.

Independence Training

Matson, Ollendick, and Adkins (1980), in an attempt to approximate normal mealtime behaviors with 40 severely and profoundly mentally retarded residents, utilized independence training and targeted 26 behaviors (e.g., stays seated during meals; chews food before swallowing; uses fork appropriately; uses napkin; elbows off the table) for intervention. The 26 behaviors were grouped into five levels of eating behaviors: (1) orderliness, (2) eating behavior, (3) utensil usage, (4) neatness, and (5) table manners, which were arranged hierarchically from the most basic (i.e., orderliness) to advanced self-feeding (i.e., table manners). At the beginning of the 3-month training period, residents were placed into groups corresponding to one of the above five levels, based upon pretaining eating skills. Special eating-related privileges (e.g., sitting at a preferred table or helping in meal preparation and clean-up) were contingent upon progression through each group of skills. A least-to-most restrictive prompting approach was used to correct performance, beginning with a verbal prompt, then modeling, and, if needed, manual guidance. The specific and unique training techniques included *in vivo* modeling by peers, peer social reinforcement, self-evaluation, and monitoring. Residents were responsible for evaluating their performance and that of their peers. This resulted in repeated exposure to training procedures, and increased discrimination, in oneself and others, of appropriate eating behaviors. At posttest and 4 months later, the training group consistently completed more appropriate feeding behaviors than a matched control group.

Combination of Procedures

Perhaps the most widely cited feeding program is the work of Azrin and Armstrong (1973). These clinicians developed an intensive feeding program that incorporated several procedures, and was designed for remediating severe feeding deficits and to be more effective and achieve faster improvements than traditional programs (Reid, 1982). The program was field tested with 11 profoundly mentally retarded, institutionalized persons, whose target behaviors were eating with various utensils and performing different eating behaviors, such as cutting and buttering. The specifics of the program entailed mini-meals (i.e., small meals served hourly throughout the day), graduated guidance going from most-to-least restrictive prompts to guide the utensil to the student's mouth, different training procedures for each utensil to prevent confusion and distractions, physically interrupting inappropriate behaviors (e.g., eating with hands), positive practice and restitutional overcorrection for spilling (i.e., child cleaned up his or her own spills and/or practiced appropriate handling of the utensil), and multiple trainers. All of the students in Azrin and Armstrong's (1973) study acquired the targeted skills. These results suggest a greater and quicker response to treatment than traditional procedures. Similar intensive feeding programs have been modeled after Azrin and Armstrong (1973), but results have not been achieved as quickly (Stimbert, Minor, & McCoy, 1977).

Deceleration of Inappropriate Mealtime Behaviors

Several operant techniques have been used to decrease inappropriate mealtime behavior. For example, brief time-out from food by removing the resident from the table (Albin, 1977; Berkowitz *et al.*, 1971; Martin, McDonald, & Omichinski, 1971) or removing the resident's food (Barton, Guess, Garcia, & Baer, 1970; Christian, Hollomon, & Lanier, 1973; Cipani, 1981; Groves & Carroccio, 1971; O'Brien & Azrin, 1972; Whitney & Barnard, 1966) could be utilized as natural punishers for inappropriate behavior (Redd *et al.*, 1979). Inappropriate mealtime behaviors punished with time-out included throwing utensils or food, spilling food, stealing food, eating with one's hands, screaming, or inappropriate use of utensils. Another common decelerative technique was brief, contingent restraint of hand(s) and reprimand for inappropriate use of hands (e.g., eating with hands, throwing food, stealing food, eating too quickly) (Favell, McGimsey, & Jones, 1980; Henriksen & Doughty, 1967; O'Brien & Azrin, 1972). Some studies, such as the intensive feeding programs of Azrin and Armstrong (1973) and of Stimbert *et al.* (1977), and the Richman *et al.* (1980) study, have decelerative techniques (e.g., overcorrection) built into the program.

Thompson, Iwata, and Poynter (1979) decreased the pathological tongue thrusting (reverse swallowing) of a 10-year-old cerebral palsy, mentally retarded boy through the combination of a differential reinforcement of other behavior (DRO) (presenting food when his tongue was in) and a punishment procedure (gently pushing the tongue back in with a spoon). Most studies have included reinforcement contingent upon appropriate eating behaviors with a punishment procedure contingent upon inappropriate eating behaviors to decrease mealtime behavior problems (Reid, 1982).

Another inappropriate eating behavior that is often seen in mentally retarded persons and that has been extensively documented in the literature is chronic rumination/vomiting. A complete review of the topic is beyond the scope of this chapter; however, the more common decelerative techniques used to treat the behavior will be presented. Interested readers who desire more extensive programs are directed to a review of rumination and vomiting treatment research by Starin and Fuqua (1987). Behavioral techniques that have successfully treated rumination and/or vomiting in mentally retarded individuals include: contingent exercise (Daniel, 1982); differential reinforcement procedures (Conrin, Pennybacker, Johnston, & Rast, 1982; McKeegan, Estill, & Campbell, 1987; Mulick, Schroeder, & Rojahn, 1980); electric shock (Kohlenberg, 1970; Luckey, Watson, & Musick, 1968; Watkins, 1972); food satiation (Borreson & Anderson, 1982; Foxx, Snyder, & Schroeder, 1979; Libby & Phillips, 1979; Rast & Johnston, 1986); lemon juice (Becker, Turner, & Sajwaj, 1978; Glasscock, Friman, O'Brien, & Christophersen, 1986; Marholin, Luiselli, Robinson, & Lott, 1980); and overcorrection (Duker & Seys, 1977; Foxx *et al.*, 1979; Simpson & Sasso, 1978).

Toilet Training

Toilet training, along with self-feeding, is perhaps the most commonly trained self-help skill with the developmentally disabled/mentally retarded individual, because bladder and bowel incontinence is a common problem.

The lack of appropriate toileting behaviors can be extremely problematic for a client. It can result in restriction from normal daytime activities and certain training programs, and can cause certain health-related problems, such as skin irritation and urinary tract infections (Barmann, Katz, O'Brien, & Beauchamp, 1981). Administrative concerns with the problem of incontinence include the severe drain on staff resources as paraprofessionals prefer not to work with incontinent residents (Levine & Elliott, 1970) and the heavy load on supportive services, such as hospital laundry (Dayan, 1964). From a more humane perspective, appropriate toileting is a fundamental, yet important skill that can prevent social ostracism, and is an essential component for the mentally retarded person's self-dignity (Baumeister & Klosowski, 1965; Butler, 1976). In addition, clients who are physically capable of being toilet trained, but are not, are likely to be excluded from social interactions (Bender & Valletutti, 1985). Thus, effective toilet training techniques, which can be implemented within typical institutions' limited resources, are a necessity. Fortunately, behaviorally based techniques fit neatly within the framework, and this approach has the most to offer (Smith, Britton, Johnson, & Thomas, 1975).

Acquisition of Toileting Skills

There are two basic goals in training appropriate toileting. First, to teach simple continence in order for the individual to remain clean and dry. Secondly, and most important, the individual must master the complex chain of behaviors necessary for independent toileting. Certain groups of mentally retarded persons are more amenable to behavioral interventions in toileting skills than others. Clients who are young at the time of treatment initiation, have an IQ score of 20 or more (Lohmann, Eyman, & Lask, 1967), and a relatively high level of pretraining toileting skills are more likely to master successfully appropriate toileting (Osarchuk, 1973). However, success with operant techniques, which have been applied to a broad range of clientele, has occurred (Osarchuk, 1973). These procedures will be discussed in detail in the following sections.

Diurnal Enuresis and Encopresis

The bulk of research on incontinence deals mainly with daytime training programs. There are three main classifications of toilet training procedures: graduated guidance, shaping, and a combination of the two.

Graduated Guidance

Perhaps the most important study featuring this behavior-shaping technique was conducted by Azrin and Foxx (1971). Graduated guidance was used to facilitate the entire behavior chain necessary for independent toileting: approaching the toilet, pulling one's pants down before eliminating, pulling them back up, and flushing the toilet bowl after eliminating. The minimal prompt necessary to induce the client to exhibit the target behavior was used. For example, if the trainer wanted the student to undress, he or she would start with no prompt at all, then point at the student's pants. If this still failed to elicit the desired response, the trainer would give a verbal instruction and, finally, would give increasing amounts of physical assistance to guide the student through the entire act. Studies that also used graduated guidance include Azrin, Bugle, and O'Brien (1971), Barmann *et al.* (1981), Jason (1977), Mahoney, Van Wagenen, and Meyerson (1971), Van Wagenen, Meyerson, Kerr, and Mahoney (1969), and Williams and Sloop (1978).

Shaping

A second procedure used to train toileting skills is shaping by successive approximations. Unfortunately, studies that use this procedure give very little detail about how this was actually implemented. For example, Baumeister and Klosowski (1965) gave a description of shaping typical to this literature: attendants "were instructed to attend to specific behaviors associated with the eliminative process and to reinforce immediately those which were adaptive in nature" (p. 25). In general, these studies have not had favorable results when compared with those using graduated guidance (i.e., Levine & Elliott, 1970).

Prompts

All four types of prompts (verbal, gestural, modeling, and physical) have been used in training independent toileting behavior. Doleys and Arnold (1975) trained toilet-sitting behavior in an 8-year-old mentally retarded boy by using a peer as a model for which their client was reinforced for imitating. Mahoney *et al.* (1971) and Van Wagenen *et al.* (1969) used a combination of verbal commands and physical guidance to teach prerequisite toileting behavior. If a student began to urinate inappropriately, they approached him or her calling "Stop!" in a loud voice, rapidly walked the student to the toilet, and physically placed him or her in the sex-appropriate position for elimination. None of the previously mentioned reports gave much detail about fading of prompts. Azrin and Foxx (1971), however, gave a very comprehensive account of their prompt and fading procedures. They used a least restrictive hierarchy of prompts (which include verbal, gestural, and physical) along with a group training procedure that encouraged modeling of toileting behavior by other residents. Although Azrin and Foxx (1971) recommended that prompts be faded at the very start of training, Smith (1979) warned that if prompts are faded too abruptly, the initial independent toiletings are not stable enough to maintain, as they may be responses to inappropriate external stimuli.

Combination of Procedures

Very few studies that teach independent toileting skills use more than one method. Richmond (1983) used verbal reinforcement to shape adaptive toileting skills and resorted to graduated guidance only if necessary. Additionally, Smith *et al.* (1975) reported using shaping and chaining procedures, although they did not go into specific detail about how this was implemented into their program. It is interesting to note that although chaining techniques have proven to be effective for training social skills, there is a paucity of data on its use in toilet training.

Until this point, only methods of training prerequisite behaviors necessary for independent toileting have been discussed. In the following sections, procedures that train a client to attend to proprioceptive stimuli and eliminate correctly into the commode will be reviewed. These techniques include the use of mechanical devices, the timed plotting method, and the regular potting method.

Mechanical Devices

Two apparatuses that may be used to aid in remediating the problem of daytime incontinence are the portable pants alarm, which is used to detect inappropriate micturation in clothing, and the toilet bowl alarm, which detects appropriate eliminations into the commode. Basically, these automated devices have an electrical circuit that is completed by moisture from voiding, which, in turn, activates an auditory signal. Details concerning construction and operating these devices can be found in studies conducted by Azrin and Foxx (1971), Azrin *et al.* (1971), Herreshoff (1973), and Hobbs and Peck (1985). Hanson, Doughty, and Lunneborg (1985) described a plan for an automated reward toilet bowl alarm that automatically reinforces appropriate eliminations with edibles. This device eliminates a potential difficulty of current methods that reinforce appropriate elimination into the toilet. In other words, procedures that do not use an automatic alarm may inadvertently reinforce retention of bodily wastes while the resident is sitting on the toilet, because trainers must wait nearby to dispense immediately reinforcers for appropriate elimination. Since the resident's departure from the bathroom marks the end of constant attention from the teacher, the resident may actually be punished for proper elimination (Passman, 1975). Pants alarms facilitate transfer of stimulus control from external, artificial cues, such as a trainer's command, to bladder-tension cues, as inappropriate eliminations can be immediately detected and consequated. Mechanical training devices are useful in that they allow the trainer freedom to carry out other duties rather than constantly attending to residents for signs of incontinence, and because they permit the immediate delivery of consequences. Furthermore, mechanically trained clients have less of a regression problem because they are taught to respond to proprioceptive stimuli (Osarchuk, 1973).

Timed Potting and Regular Potting

A second method, often used in conjunction with mechanical devices for training appropriate elimination in mentally retarded individuals, is to simply place the person on the toilet and reinforce them when they urinate and/or defecate into the toilet. This goal can be approached in two ways. The first method, regular potting, entails toileting the client at arbitrarily set time intervals. The second approach, timed potting, schedules toileting around predicted times of incontinent episodes. These predicted times can be derived statistically or clinically (i.e., identifying behaviors which precede elimination) (Baumeister & Klosowski, 1965). Smith (1979) compared timed and regular toileting methods and found that both obtained similar results, but that regular toileting was simpler in terms of instrumentation and procedure.

Intensive Individual and Group Training

A final factor to be considered in selecting a toilet training program for mentally retarded persons is whether an intensive individual or a group training approach should be used. Although effective group training procedures, which can be carried out within the economical and staffing limitations of the typical institution, have been developed (i.e., Hobbs & Peck, 1985), individual training methods have been demonstrated to be more effective in terms of results and cost (Smith, 1979).

Nocturnal Enuresis

Nocturnal enuresis is a major problem in the mentally retarded population as illustrated in a survey conducted by Smith (1981), which found that 43% of 1,330 predominantly adult patients in an institution for the mentally handicapped were nocturnally enuretic. Despite the scope of this problem and the fact that operant conditioning techniques have been proven to be more effective than traditional potting methods (Sloop & Kennedy, 1973), there is a paucity of published reports in this area (Smith, 1981).

Mechanical Devices

Behaviorally based approaches typically use an automated device, based on the same principle as the pants and toilet bowl alarm, known as the *bell and pad* to remediate nighttime incontinence. For a complete description, see Foxx and Azrin (1974). The bell and pad causes an alarm to sound when the resident urinates in bed, enabling staff to immediately require the client to complete elimination in the toilet rather than toileting him or her at arbitrarily determined times. Although the training method described above has a limited amount of efficacy (Williams & Sloop, 1978), a more comprehensive behavioral program developed by Azrin, Sneed, and Foxx (1973) generally obtains more significant results within a shorter time span.

General Considerations in Toilet Training

Other components, such as overhydration and punishment, can be added to any day or nighttime toilet training program. The relative advantages and disadvantages are described in the following section.

Deceleration of Inappropriate Toileting Behaviors

The most commonly used aversive consequence used in toilet training is restitution overcorrection, which simply requires that the client restore the environment to its former state. An example of this procedure would be having clients clean themselves, their clothing, and any furniture they may have soiled following each inappropriate elimination. There are many advantages in using restitution. First, the individual assumes responsibility for his or her own inappropriate behavior. A second advantage is that it involves the client's own clothing, which may exert discriminative control over soiling, rather than external stimuli (i.e., a time-out room) (Doleys & Arnold, 1975). Furthermore, restitution is relatively easy to implement, and staff cooperation is high since it emphasizes individual responsibility (Matson, 1977). Overall, this procedure has many useful implications for toilet training mentally retarded persons as it replaces disruptive behaviors with more adaptive behaviors (Freeman & Pribble, 1974).

A potential disadvantage of this simple overcorrection technique is that it can result in a confrontation between a student and a caregiver, who does not have substantial prior training (Doleys & Arnold, 1975; Matson, 1975). Moreover, physical injury may result from further attempts to implement these procedures.

A second punishment procedure commonly used is time-out. The client is removed from a more reinforcing environment to a less reinforcing one for a predetermined time period. Azrin and Foxx (1971) used a 1-hour time-out period, in which the resident did not receive edibles or social rewards in conjunction with restitution. The effectiveness of the time-out period as a punisher may be determined by its length. For example, Smith (1979) compared a training program with a brief (10 minutes) time-out period to a similar program in which a time-out period was not implemented, and found no significant difference in outcome. Other aversive consequences described in the literature include administration of a cold bath after bed-wetting (Tough, Hawkins, McArthur, & Van Ravenswaay, 1971) and one spank after each episode of daytime incontinence (Azrin et al., 1971). These latter methods are likely to be deemed inappropriate in the present climate with respect to the intrusiveness of various treatments.

Hydration

Yet another component of many toilet training programs is hydration (e.g., Azrin & Foxx, 1971; Richmond, 1983; Van Wagenen et al., 1969). Clients are given large volumes of liquids, thus facilitating more frequent opportunities to teach appropriate toileting through increased number of voiding episodes. Although this method, used as part of a behavioral treatment for enuresis, has shown a good deal of success, researchers should be aware of several precautions. Excessive intake of free water (appropriate amounts are dictated by body weight) can lead to an electrolyte imbalance known as *hyponatremia*, which can be fatal. Symptoms of hyponatremia include nausea, emesis, grand mal seizures, muscular twitching, and coma. Programs using hydration should screen clients' medical histories for conditions that make them more susceptible to water intoxications. Persons having a seizure disorder, hydrocephaly, spinal injury or who are being treated with medications that increase urinary retention should never be overhydrated. For a complete discussion of these concerns, interested readers should refer to Thompson and Hanson (1983).

In conclusion, it seems that the biggest difficulty in analyzing the efficacy of different toilet training regimes is a lack of agreed upon standards by which to evaluate the plethora of programs currently available. Similarly, few comparative studies have been conducted to date in which direct tests of various treatment procedures are made. The extreme seriousness of this problem, given the fact that people are likely to be restricted from a community placement because of toileting problems, strongly argues for more research on this topic. The reader is also referred in this book to Chapter 9, on toilet training, which describes treatments for this problem in more detail.

INDEPENDENT DRESSING

The ability to dress oneself is another basic skill that many severely or profoundly mentally retarded persons may not have in their repertoires. Although the training of independent dressing skills is as important to mentally retarded persons as is self-feeding and toilet training, there is considerably less research conducted on this important topic. Nevertheless, several investigators have published critical reviews on the teaching of independent dressing skills (Reid, 1982; Reid et al., 1983; Snell, 1987). Whitman, Scibak, and Reid (1983) emphasized several reasons why it was important for mentally retarded individuals to acquire this skill. First, acquisition of self-sufficient dressing skills gives mentally retarded persons greater control over their lives, rather than depending on caregivers to dress and undress them (Reid, 1982). This additional control may also aid any possible transition to a less restrictive setting. Moreover, such dependence on caregivers requires much of their time, which could be spent teaching more advanced skills to the residents, such as communication (Bender & Valletutti, 1985; Reid, 1982). Lastly, self-dressing is socially important for mentally retarded persons, because dressing skills affect appearance, which plays a large role in interpersonal interactions with nonretarded persons (Reid, 1982). In fact, clothing is a very powerful means of nonverbal communication (Newton, 1976).

Acquisition of Independent Dressing

Unlike the self-feeding strategies, independent dressing procedures do not involve an inherent reinforcer (e.g., food), unless the environment is extremely cold and clothing provides immediate warmth (Reid, 1982). Nor, in contrast to toilet training, is there immediate, built-in consequence (e.g., wet pants) to maintain independent dressing (Reid, 1982). Therefore, reinforcement must be provided externally. Another important factor to consider in training independent dressing skills is generalization across different settings and times, given the location where and time when dressing usually occurs (Reid *et al.*, 1983). Typically, dressing skills are required in the morning and evening in the privacy of the person's bedroom or bathroom. In contrast, most training and research are conducted at set times during the day at the convenience of the teacher. This may be necessary to ensure that a sufficient amount of time can be spent on training of this sort. However, whenever possible, generalization across settings and times should be incorporated into programs aimed at training independent dressing skills.

Forward Chaining

Forward chaining was the main technique used by Martin, Kehoe, Bird, Jensen, and Darbyshire (1971) to teach a whole series of independent dressing skills, both basic and complex. Targeted dressing behaviors, such as putting on underpants, undershirt, bra, sweater, socks, and lacing and tying shoes, were taught to 11 severely mentally retarded female students. The same basic procedure was utilized for training putting on a sweater, socks, underpants, and undershirt. First of all, the skill was task analyzed into five basic steps; each step had to be completed successfully on three successive trials before the next step was trained. For example, in training the first step of putting on a sweater, it was placed inside out in front of the student and she was to identify the inside and outside. The second step involved turning the sweater right side out. The student's hands were guided into the sweater from the bottom. She was then physically prompted to grab the sleeves and pull them back through the bottom of the sweater. Physical guidance by the experimenter in this step and the following three steps was gradually faded until the student could perform each step unassisted. In step three, the student pulled the sweater over her head. Finding the tag, and placing it at the back of the neck comprised step four. The final step of the sequence consisted of placing the student's arms in the sleeves. During training, the student earned a reinforcer by performing all previously learned steps. In other words, in the beginning phases of treatment the student earned a reinforcer for minimal performance, whereas at the end of training, she was only reinforced upon correct completion of the entire task. In a similar fashion (i.e., through forward chaining), the students were taught how to lace and tie shoes and how to put on a bra. After treatment most of the students were able to perform correctly the tasks in less than half the initial time. However, not all students were taught each task.

Backward Chaining

Backward chaining has been used to teach basic dressing and undressing skills to mentally retarded persons (Azrin *et al.*, 1976; Bensberg *et al.*, 1965; Ross & Oliver, 1969). A specific case in point is the study conducted by Minge and Ball (1967). In this early study, six profoundly mentally retarded persons were trained, through the use of physical and verbal prompts and gestures in a backward chaining sequence, to put on and take off a shirt (or dress), pants, and socks. For example, elastic-banded pants were utilized to teach taking pants off. The first step consisted of having the student, who was seated with pants nearly off, remove the pants from one foot only. The next step, while still seated, entailed having the student remove the pants which were at his or her knees. Finally, the student removed the pants completely. The students stayed at each step until they could perform the step correctly in response to four of the first five directions given per session. The trainer began with physical guidance, then gestures, and, finally, verbal directions only. Reinforcement consisted of praise and food, in which each student was required to earn a breakfast and a lunch during training sessions to increase attention and motivation. At posttraining, the students differentially improved their dressing and undressing skills; that is, they correctly completed more undressing than dressing responses. In particular, the mean number of correct responses for putting on pants remained at zero for posttraining.

Backward chaining was also used in a program to teach exceptional children three different clothes-fastening skills (i.e., zipping, snapping, and buttoning) (Edgar, Maser, & Haring, 1977). The criterion for moving from one step to the next was correct performance of the current step at least three consecutive times without assistance. The task of zipping was task-analyzed into the following seven sequences of behavior, in which the amount of zipping required of the student increased with each step: (1) The teacher engages the zipper, while the student pinches the zipper handle, zips up, and locks the zipper; (2) the teacher engages the zipper, while the student holds the edge of the vest near the bottom left side of the zipper, zips up, and locks the zipper; (3) the student pinches and holds the zipper mechanism, while the teacher inserts the slider, and the student zips it up; (4) the student pinches the slider and engages the zipper with assistance; (5) the student engages the zipper independently; (6) the student positions, engages, and zips up the zipper with no prompts; and (7) the student learns to unzip. Similarly, the skill of snapping was broken down into the following five behavioral sequences: (1) The teacher positions both halves of the snap and holds the bottom half, while the student uses his or her fingers to push the top half down until it fastens; (2) the teacher positions and holds the bottom half of the snap, while the student holds the top half of the snap and uses his or her thumb to push the top of the snap down until it fastens; (3) the teacher holds the bottom half of the snap, while the student pinches the top half, lines it up with the bottom half, and fastens; (4) the student pinches the bottom half of the snap and fastens it independently; and (5) the student learns to unsnap. Finally, buttoning behavior was task-analyzed into the following six incremental sequences: (1) The teacher inserts the button half-way into the buttonhole and holds the edge of the vest below the buttonhole, while the student pinches the button and pulls it through the buttonhole. (2) The teacher inserts the button halfway into the buttonhole, while the student pinches the edge of the vest below the buttonhole and pulls the button through the buttonhole. (3) The teacher turns the buttonhole out so that, from the back side of the buttonhole, the student can see the teacher's thumb as it covers the buttonhole. The student pinches the edge of the button and holds the button next to the teacher's buttonhole thumb. Then the teacher pulls the buttonhole over the button, and the student finishes buttoning. (4) The student pinches the buttonhole and holds the button next to his or her buttonhole thumb, while the teacher pulls the buttonhole over the button and the student finishes buttoning. (5) The student holds the button next to his or her buttonhole thumb and lifts up the index finger of the buttonhole hand and pinches the button. The student then releases his or her button hand and uses this hand to pull the buttonhole over the button while pulling the button through. Lastly, (6) the student learns to unbutton. These steps are followed in the sequence presented, and the training strategies described above are used. Although success has been reported with this program in field testing, no controlled empirical testing of the effectiveness of the program was reported.

Forward and Backward Chaining

One unique study task analyzed and described in detail the steps for teaching buttoning to severely/profoundly mentally retarded children, yet the sequence of steps was a combination of forward and backward chaining (Adelson-Bernstein & Sandow, 1978). This training utilized manual guidance and verbal prompts, and a special button vest with one button (1–2 inches in diameter) and one buttonhole. The first step, in which the child finds and grasps the button, is a forward chaining step. However, in the second step (backward chaining), the child is performing the last step in the sequence, that is, pulling the button through the buttonhole, which was put into position by the teacher. Finding the buttonhole is the third step in this training regimen. Fourth, the child puts the button in the buttonhole. The third and fourth steps are taught according to a forward chaining sequence. In the last step of the sequence, the child wears a button vest with three buttons sewn on, and is taught through backward chaining to align the buttons and put them through the buttonholes; that is, initially, only the top button is left undone. After the child can successfully button the top button, the top two buttons are left undone, until the vest is completely open and the child is required to align and button all three buttons. Each step of the sequence is broken down further into substeps, giving detailed instructions for teachers on how to hold the child's hand. Then the teacher gradually fades manual guidance until the child is able to perform the step successfully. Unfortunately, no field data were presented to support the effectiveness of the procedure.

Prompts

Prompting is often used to train independent dressing behaviors utilizing the whole task method (Karen & Maxwell, 1967; King & Turner, 1975). King and Turner (1975) targeted several dressing skills, including undressing, putting clothes (i.e., socks, shoes, shirt, and pants) away, getting a new article of clothing and putting it on (including snapping and zipping), with a profoundly mentally retarded young adult. Each independent dressing skill was trained with the whole task method, and instruction began with modeling by the trainer if the client did not correctly perform the task on his own. If the behavior was not imitated, physical prompts were utilized to achieve task completion. Further task analysis of the steps was not provided. As training progressed, the client required fewer physical and verbal prompts, and dressed and undressed quicker than at pretraining. At the end of training, all dressing skills had been mastered, except the putting on of shirts and socks. The authors speculated that if larger shirts and socks were used, then the client would probably have achieved success with those articles of clothing.

Combination of Procedures

Just as in teaching self-feeding skills, Azrin and his colleagues have developed an intensive training program for the teaching of independent dressing skills to profoundly mentally retarded persons (Azrin et al., 1976). Lengthy and intensive training sessions were conducted with seven profoundly mentally retarded adults to teach dressing and undressing skills. Specifically, the program included the following 12 steps: (1) There was a forward sequence whole task presentation (i.e., the resident participated in each step of the task in the normal sequence, from first to last, at one presentation). (2) Each trial consisted of the entire dressing sequence, utilizing five types of slip-on clothing (i.e., underpants, shoes, socks, pants, and shirt with no laces, buttons, zippers, belts, or snaps), not just one article of clothing. (3) Initially, oversized (two sizes too big) garments were utilized for training, and when the student no longer required manual guidance on a particular size, the next smaller size was used. (4) Reinforcers intrinsic to dressing and undressing (i.e., the student's appearance was praised while standing in front of a mirror) were used in addition to individually identified reinforcers; also, edibles, praise, and physical stroking were used on a near-continuous basis contingent upon the responding or the lack of resistance, instead of reinforcing only response completion. (5) Initially, verbal instructions were given throughout a trial, rather than only at the beginning, and proceeded from the most general (i.e., "get dressed") to more structured and specific (i.e., "pull up your pants"). (6) A major component was manual guidance, which went from least to most restrictive (i.e., first a verbal prompt was given, then gesture, physical prompting, and, if necessary, physical prompting along with verbal instructions). (7) Fading procedures, such as prompt delay (i.e., instructions and gesturing were repeated every 10 seconds for 1 minute before a physical prompt was used), graduated guidance (i.e., easing of the trainer's physical guidance when the student began to respond on his or her own), and intermittent guidance (i.e., light and momentary physical contact initiated only when the student was not responding independently or when the student had difficulty), were incorporated into the program. (8) The length of the training sessions was intensified to 2 to 3 hours, twice per day. (9) To minimize confusion, undressing was taught separately from dressing. (10) To guarantee initial success, the easier skill of undressing (first removing shoes, then socks, pants, underpants, and, lastly, shirt) was taught before dressing (with the trainer dressing the student for the next undressing trial). (11) Multiple trainers (i.e., two) were used until the student could be easily managed by one. Lastly, (12) the goal of the intensive program was to teach independent dressing skills to profoundly mentally retarded persons within a few days, and have it be an enjoyable experience.

During training sessions, residents were seated in a chair to eliminate the unsteadiness of standing. Students were trained to use both hands to dress and undress. In an average of 12 hours, over the course of 3 or 4 training days, all 7 residents learned to dress and undress themselves in response to instructions. However, attempts at replicating these results have failed (Diorio & Konarski, 1984). Of the three profoundly mentally retarded clients used by Diorio and Konarski (1984), only two reached the criteria for undressing, while none of the three reached the criteria for dressing, despite 108.2 hours of training.

Deceleration of Inappropriate Dressing Behaviors

Inappropriate dressing behaviors exhibited by mentally retarded clients can include (1) incorrect responses, (2) severely disruptive behaviors related to the training of independent dressing skills, or (3) an inappropriate dressing-related behavior, such as public disrobing. Martin, McDonald, and Omichinski (1971) utilized decelerative techniques for both incorrect responses and disruptive behavior occurring during training sessions. For example, incorrect responses were consequated with a reprimand and time-out (i.e., ignoring the child) for approximately 10 seconds, whereas severely disruptive behavior was followed by a reprimand and a slap across the client's fingers.

Another type of inappropriate dressing-related behavior often exhibited by mentally retarded clients, which is socially undesirable and potentially health hazardous, is public disrobing (Durana & Cuvo, 1980). Durana and Cuvo (1980) reported on the inconsistencies in the effectiveness produced by DRO, so they proposed the use of two other procedures in conjunction with DRO with a profoundly mentally retarded female. One procedure was restitutional overcorrection, which required the client to restore the disturbed situation to a greatly improved state, and the second procedure was negative practice, whereby the client was required to dress and undress repeatedly either 10 times or for a half hour. Similarly, Foxx (1976) utilized restitutional and positive practice overcorrection to treat public disrobing in two profoundly mentally retarded females. Specifically, restitutional overcorrection entailed having the clients, who usually only wore a dress, dress in panties, bra, slip, and panty hose and tie their shoes. The positive practice overcorrection component made the women attend to the clothing needs and personal appearance of the other residents on the ward by buttoning or zipping their unfastened clothing, straightening disarrayed clothing, placing footwear on those with bare feet, and combing tousled hair. Hamilton, Stephens, and Allen (1967) treated public disrobing and clothes ripping by utilizing time-out with physical restraint.

PERSONAL HYGIENE

Personal hygiene/grooming skills include all self-care behaviors excluding toileting, feeding, and dressing (Reid et al., 1983). Examples of different personal hygiene behaviors include showering/bathing (with hand and face washing), toothbrushing, shaving, and hair care. Although these basic personal hygiene skills are critical if individuals are to attempt to take minimal care of themselves, behavioral research of the training of these skills with the severely and profoundly mentally retarded is very sparse (Whitman et al., 1983). Acquisition of such skills is important in that it enables the mentally retarded person to move toward independent living (Reid et al., 1983). Moreover, lack of appropriate personal hygiene skills in mentally retarded persons will invariably lead to decreased interpersonal and social experiences (Bender & Valletutti, 1985).

Toothbrushing

Of all the basic personal hygiene skills, toothbrushing has received the most attention from researchers. This situation may be because basic dental hygiene is important for medical/health reasons (e.g., gum disease, cavities, etc.), as well as interpersonal interactions (e.g., bad breath, appearance). Further, this skill may be easier to teach than some others, and it would be appealing to caregivers to be in a position whereby they do not have to frequently stick their hands into clients' mouths.

Acquisition of Toothbrushing Skills

Prompts

Verbal instructions, modeling (Bensberg et al., 1965; Wolber, Carne, Collins-Montgomery, & Nelson, 1987), physical guidance (Fowler, Johnson,

Whitman, & Zukotynski, 1978), and praise and tokens have been used in several toothbrushing skills training programs (Abramson & Wunderlich, 1972; Horner & Keilitz, 1975). Specifically, Horner and Keilitz (1975) taught eight mildly and moderately retarded persons how to brush their teeth via the whole task method. However, since the residents did not know how to perform the entire sequence of the behavior, task analysis was used first, whereby the desired behavior was broken down into 15 component steps (e.g., Step 1, pick up and hold the toothbrush; Step 4, apply toothpaste to brush; Step 7, brush the biting surfaces of the teeth; Step 10, rinse the mouth; Step 14, put equipment away, etc.). Each component step was trained using the least restrictive procedure (i.e., verbal instructions) first, then, if necessary, using verbal instructions with more restrictive procedures (i.e., modeling, then physical prompts) to ensure correct responding. Praise and tokens were given for correct performance of each step.

Maintenance of Toothbrushing Skills

Once independent toothbrushing has been established, several reinforcement techniques have been utilized to maintain this self-help behavior. Wehman (1974) utilized a star chart within a token economy to encourage continued independent toothbrushing among moderately and severely mentally retarded geriatric women. Similarly, Swain, Allard, and Holborn (1982) used stickers as incentives in a "Good Toothbrushing Game" to increase the cleanliness of teeth of nonhandicapped first and second graders.

These data clearly show the importance and utility of some treatment procedures for this important subgroup of hygiene skills. Given this promise, more research of this type is definitely needed.

Washing

There are other hygiene problems that have been treated as well. Washing is obviously an important hygiene skill and will now be discussed.

Acquisition of Washing Skills

As described here, washing skills include showering, washing of the hands and face, and shaving (males).

Forward Chaining

The skill of washing and drying of hands and face was task analyzed into 12 steps and trained, via forward chaining, to 11 severely mentally retarded girls at a training school (Treffry, Martin, Samels, & Watson, 1970). The 12 washing steps were: (1) pointing to the hot water tap on command; (2) pointing to the cold water tap on command; (3) placing the plug in the sink; (4) placing water in the sink; (5) wetting hands with the facecloth; (6) washing hands with the facecloth and soap; (7) wetting face with the facecloth; (8) washing face with the facecloth and soap; (9) rinsing soap from hands; (10) rinsing soap from face; (11) drying hands; and (12) drying face. Later, Steps 4 to 12 had to be broken down into smaller components. For example, Step 4 (placing water in the sink) was further task-analyzed into (a) turning on the hot water tap, (b) turning off the hot water tap, (c) turning on the cold water tap, and (d) turning off the cold water tap. Training began with Step 1, using edible and social reinforcement for correct responses. The criterion for mastery was 10 correct responses to the verbal prompt. Once Step 1 was trained to mastery, then Step 2 was trained, and so on. During training sessions, after 5 to 15 minutes was spent training the current step, the resident would be guided through the rest of the sequence. Training consisted of verbal prompts and the least amount of physical guidance as needed to complete the step.

Prompts

Bensberg et al. (1965) used verbal instructions and gestures to train hand-washing, among other skills, to severely and profoundly mentally retarded clients. Visual prompts, that is, sequential pictorial cues, were utilized by Thinesen and Bryan (1981) to train face washing, shaving, and other self-help skills (e.g., making the bed, cleaning glasses, dressing, etc.) to three mildly to moderately mentally retarded male residents in a group home. The men were provided with a photo album, each page of which concentrated on one behavior and contained three photographs of the skill to be performed, arranged in a pictorial sequence, and one photo of the reinforcer to be received contingent upon successful performance of the skill. After being instructed to perform the behavior, the trainer would determine if the resident had successfully completed it and would rate the performance as pass or fail. If the resident passed, then he received praise and the reinforcer which was depicted in the photo album for that particular skill. If he failed, he was instructed to repeat the behavior, and no other consequences were administered.

Independence Training

Matson, Marchetti, and Adkins (1980) trained 25 moderately to profoundly mentally retarded adults to complete more showering steps using independence training, as compared to 25 residents receiving standard training, and 25 controls. The target behavior, showering, was operationally defined and task analyzed into the following 29 steps (asterisked steps had to be completed in the order listed): (1) place towel and washcloth on stand beside the shower; *(2) turn on the water faucet; *(3) adjust the temperature; *(4) step under the water until the body is wet; *(5) lather cloth with soap and place soap in tray; *(6) wash face with cloth; (7) wash left arm with cloth; *(8) wash under left arm with cloth; (9) wash right arm with cloth; *(10) wash under right arm with cloth; (11) wash chest and stomach with cloth; *(12) wash genital area with cloth; *(13) wash buttocks with cloth; (14) wash left leg with cloth; (15) wash right leg with cloth; (16) rinse off and wring out washcloth; *(17) rinse off soap and turn off water; (18) get towel; (19) dry face; (20) dry arms; (21) dry remainder of body; (22) dry chest and stomach; (23) dry genital area; (24) dry back; (25) dry buttocks; (26) dry right leg; (27) dry left leg; (28) put towel and cloth in dirty clothes hamper; and (29) apply deodorant to underarms. Criterion for successful completion was passing at least 18 steps, including all asterisked items (in the correct order). Training for the standard treatment group consisted of verbal prompts, modeling, manual guidance, social reinforcement, shaping, fading, and chaining, as determined by their frequency of citation in the self-help literature. The procedures utilized for the independence training group were those also used in the standard training group, with the addition of self-evaluation and monitoring. The self-evaluation and monitoring phase took place at week's end, when the residents were asked to evaluate their performance throughout the week. Social reinforcement was given for accurate and honest answers, regardless of performance. If no progress was made during the week, the resident was prompted to supply possible reasons why and suggest alternative ways in which to improve future performance. If the resident completed more steps than on the previous week, social reinforcement was given, along with a small star to place on the progress chart, as a form of public recognition and self-monitoring. As measured by pre- and posttreatment measures, independence training was superior to standard training procedures and no treatment, and it was the preferred method of the residential staff. In a similar study by Matson et al. (1981), independence training was effective in group training showering behavior to 36 moderately to severely mentally retarded adults. Independence consisted of first having the trainer model, while providing verbal instructions, the task-analyzed steps to groups of three residents. Then the residents began their showers. When an error was detected, the trainer asked another resident in the triad to verbalize the cues necessary for correct performance. At the end of showering, residents were asked to evaluate their own performance, and were given feedback from the trainer. Residents who received independence training performed significantly better than controls on posttest measures.

Deceleration of Inappropriate Washing Behaviors

While training hands and face washing, Treffry et al. (1970) incorporated a 15-second time-out procedure (the child was ignored) contingent upon inappropriate responses to the verbal prompts, or resistance to the physical guidance. While in time-out, if the child continued to behave inappropriately, such as throwing soap or abusing other children, the child received a slap to the fingers.

Conclusion

The objective of this chapter was to present the techniques and practical applications necessary in order to train successfully a variety of basic self-help skills to mentally retarded persons. Such techniques included backward and forward chaining, graduated guidance, prompting, and independence training. These techniques have been utilized to train such self-help skills as independent feeding, toileting, dressing, and personal hygiene. Evidently, operant procedures are effective in helping mentally retarded persons acquire various independent daily living skills. Numerous task-analyzed steps are presented, with detailed instructions, to aid the reader/caregiver in direct, practical application of the operant procedures for use in educational and treatment planning. In addition, operant techniques are presented that are often required to decrease inappropriate behavior that would otherwise interfere with the acquisition of more appropriate independent self-help skills.

Much has been done in the area of self-help skills with mentally retarded persons. Interestingly, however, there is not anywhere near the research activity one would expect, given the great deal of practical application of these principles and procedures in clinical settings. With the recent federal mandated hours of programming daily, there are virtually no mentally retarded persons who are not impacted with treatments for the problem behaviors that are outlined in this chapter. Perhaps more than any other area, we need to know what can be trained, with whom, most efficiently. Although some promising data are available, much is yet to be done in this area.

Self-feeding and toilet training have received perhaps the most research in this area of study, and rightly so. The hierarchy of skills trained should be based on which skills are likely to lead to the greatest independence for the client. The relationship of skill building to aggression and self-injury and other problem behavior areas is most certainly a topic deserving study. Furthermore, prerequisite skills, such as compliance and being able to follow simple instructions, while rarely discussed, are of extreme importance in the overall development of a comprehensive treatment approach.

Although most of these procedures and their practical applications have been empirically researched and validated, additional research is needed in the areas of comparative studies of the effectiveness of various procedures, and in the skill areas of independent dressing and personal hygiene.

References

Abramson, E. E., & Wunderlich, R. A. (1972). Dental hygiene training for retardates: An application of behavioral techniques. *Mental Retardation, 10,* 6–8.

Adelson-Bernstein, N., & Sandow, L. (1978). Teaching buttoning to severely/profoundly retarded multihandicapped children. *Education and Training of the Mentally Retarded, 13,* 178–183.

Albin, J. B. (1977). Some variables influencing the maintenance of acquired self-feeding behavior in profoundly retarded children. *Mental Retardation, 15,* 49–52.

Azrin, N. H., & Armstrong, P. M. (1973). The "mini-meal": A method for teaching eating skills to the profoundly retarded. *Mental Retardation, 11,* 9–11.

Azrin, N. H., & Foxx, R. M. (1971). A rapid method of toilet training the institutionalized retarded. *Journal of Applied Behavior Analysis, 4,* 89–99.

Azrin, N. H., Bugle, C., & O'Brien, F. (1971). Behavioral engineering: Two apparatuses for toilet training retarded children. *Journal of Applied Behavior Analysis, 4,* 249–253.

Azrin, N. H., Sneed, T. J., & Foxx, R. M. (1973). Dry bed: A rapid method of eliminating bedwetting (enuresis) of the retarded. *Behaviour Research and Therapy, 11,* 427–434.

Azrin, N. H., Schaeffer, R. M., & Wesolowski, M. D. (1976). A rapid method of teaching profoundly retarded persons to dress by a reinforcement-guidance method. *Mental Retardation, 14,* 29–33.

Banerdt, B., & Bricker, D. (1978). A training program for selected self-feeding skills for the motorically impaired. *AAESPH Review, 3,* 222–229.

Barmann, B. C., Katz, R. C., O'Brien, F., & Beauchamp, K. L. (1981). Treating irregular enuresis in developmentally disabled persons. *Behavior Modification, 5,* 336–346.

Barton, E. S., Guess, D., Garcia, E., & Baer, D. M. (1970). Improvement of retardates' mealtime behaviors by timeout procedures using multiple baseline techniques. *Journal of Applied Behavior Analysis, 3,* 77–84.

Baumeister, A., & Klosowski, R. (1965). An attempt to group toilet train severely retarded patients. *Mental Retardation, 3,* 24–26.

Becker, J. V., Turner, S. M., & Sajwaj, T. E. (1978). Multiple behavioral effects of the use of lemon juice with a ruminating toddler-age child. *Behavior Modification, 2,* 267–278.

Bender, M., & Valletutti, P. J. (1985). *Teaching the moderately and severely handicapped: A functional curriculum for self-care, motor skills, and household management* (Vol. 1, 2nd ed.). Austin, TX: Pro-Ed.

Bennett, D. L., Gast, D. L., Wolery, M., & Schuster, J. (1986). Time delay and system of least prompts: A comparison in teaching manual sign production. *Education and Training of the Mentally Retarded, 21,* 117–129.

Bensberg, G. J., Colwell, C. N., & Cassel, R. H. (1965). Teaching the profoundly retarded self-help activities by behavior shaping techniques. *American Journal of Mental Deficiency, 69,* 674–679.

Berkowitz, S., Sherry, P. J., & Davis, B. A. (1971). Teaching self-feeding skills to profound retardates using reinforcement and fading procedures. *Behavior Therapy, 2,* 62–67.

Billingsley, F. F., & Romer, L. T. (1983). Response prompting and the transfer of stimulus control: Methods, research, and conceptual framework. *Journal of the Association for the Severely Handicapped, 8,* 3–12.

Borreson, P. M., & Anderson, J. L. (1982). The elimination of chronic rumination through a combination of procedures. *Mental Retardation, 20,* 34–38.

Butler, J. F. (1976). Toilet training a child with spina bifida. *Journal of Behavior Therapy and Experimental Psychiatry, 7,* 63–65.

Butterfield, W. H., & Parson, R. (1973). Modeling and shaping by parents to develop chewing behavior in their retarded child. *Journal of Behavior Therapy and Experimental Psychiatry, 4,* 285–287.

Christian, W. P., Hollomon, S. W., & Lanier, C. L. (1973). An attendant operated feeding program for severely and profoundly retarded females. *Mental Retardation, 11,* 35–37.

Cipani, E. (1981). Modifying food spillage behavior in an institutionalized retarded client. *Journal of Behavior Therapy and Experimental Psychiatry, 12,* 261–265.

Conrin, J., Pennypacker, H. S., Johnston, J., & Rast, J. (1982). Differential reinforcement of other behaviors to treat chronic rumination of mental retardates. *Journal of Behavior Therapy and Experimental Psychiatry, 13,* 325–329.

Daniel, W. H. (1982). Management of chronic rumination with a contingent exercise procedure employing topographically dissimilar behavior. *Journal of Behavior Therapy and Experimental Psychiatry, 13,* 149–152.

Dayan, M. (1964). Toilet training retarded children in a state residential institution. *Mental Retardation, 2,* 116–117.

Diorio, M. S., & Konarski, E. A., Jr. (1984). Evaluation of a method for teaching dressing skills to profoundly mentally retarded persons. *American Journal of Mental Deficiency, 89,* 307–309.

Doleys, D. M., & Arnold, S. (1975). Treatment of childhood encopresis: Full cleanliness training. *Mental Retardation, 13,* 14–16.

Duker, P. C., & Seys, D. M. (1977). Elimination of vomiting in a retarded female using restitutional overcorrection. *Behavior Therapy, 8,* 255–257.

Durana, I. L., & Cuvo, A. J. (1980). A comparison of procedures for decreasing public disrobing of an institutionalized profoundly mentally retarded woman. *Mental Retardation, 18,* 185–188.

Edgar, E., Maser, J. T., & Haring, N. G. (1977). Button up!: A systematic approach for teaching children to fasten. *Teaching Exceptional Children, 9,* 104–105.

Ellis, N. R. (1963). Toilet training the severely defective patient: An S-R reinforcement analysis. *American Journal of Mental Deficiency, 68,* 98–103.

Favell, J. E., McGimsey, J. F., & Jones, M. L. (1980). Rapid eating in the retarded: Reduction by nonaversive procedures. *Behavior Modification, 4,* 481–492.

Fowler, S. A., Johnson, M. R., Whitman, T. L., & Zukotynski, G. (1978). Teaching a parent in the home to train self-help skills and increase compliance in her profoundly retarded adult daughter. *AAESPH Review, 3,* 151–161.

Foxx, R. M. (1976). The use of overcorrection to eliminate the public disrobing (stripping) of retarded women. *Behaviour Research and Therapy, 14,* 53–61.

Foxx, R. M., & Azrin, N. H. (1974). *Toilet training the retarded: A rapid program for day and nighttime independent toileting.* Champaign, IL: Research Press.

Foxx, R. M., Snyder, M. S., & Schroeder, F. (1979). A food satiation and oral hygiene punishment program to suppress chronic rumination by retarded persons. *Journal of Autism and Developmental Disorders, 9,* 399–412.

Freeman, B. J., & Pribble, W. (1974). Elimination of inappropriate toileting behavior by overcorrection. *Psychological Reports, 35,* 802.

Glasscock, S. G., Friman, P. C., O'Brien, S., & Christophersen, E. R. (1986). Varied citrus treatment of ruminant gagging in a teenager with Batten's disease. *Journal of Behavior Therapy and Experimental Psychiatry, 17,* 129–133.

Glendenning, N. J., Adams, G. L., & Sternberg, L. (1983). Comparison of prompt sequences. *American Journal of Mental Deficiency, 88,* 321–325.

Godby, S., Gast, D. L., & Wolery, M. (1987). A comparison of time delay and system of least prompts in teaching object identification. *Research in Developmental Disabilities, 8,* 283–306.

Gorton, C. E., & Hollis, J. H. (1965). Redesigning a cottage unit for better programming and research for the severely retarded. *Mental Retardation, 3,* 16–21.

Groves, I. D., & Carroccio, D. F. (1971). A self-feeding program for the severely and profoundly retarded. *Mental Retardation, 9,* 10–12.

Hamilton, J., Stephens, L., & Allen, P. (1967). Controlling aggressive and destructive behavior in severely retarded institutionalized residents. *American Journal of Mental Deficiency, 71,* 852–856.

Handen, B. L., & Zane, T. (1987). Delayed prompting: A review of procedural variations and results. *Research in Developmental Disabilities, 8,* 307–330.

Hanson, R. H., Doughty, N. R., & Lunneborg, D. (1985). A portable automated reward potty chair. *Behavioral Engineering, 9,* 76–78.

Henriksen, K., & Doughty, R. (1967). Decelerating undesired mealtime behavior in a group of profoundly retarded boys. *American Journal of Mental Deficiency, 72,* 40–44.

Herreshoff, J. K. (1973). Two electronic devices for toilet training. *Mental Retardation, 11,* 54–55.

Hobbs, T., & Peck, C. A. (1985). Toilet training people with profound mental retardation: A cost effective procedure for large residential settings. *Behavioral Engineering, 9,* 50–57.

Horner, R. D., & Keilitz, I. (1975). Training mentally retarded adolescents to brush their teeth. *Journal of Applied Behavior Analysis, 8,* 301–309.

Jason, L. A. (1977). Evaluating the Foxx and Azrin toilet training procedure for retarded children in a day training center. *Behavior Therapy, 8,* 499–500.

Karen, R. L., & Maxwell, S. J. (1967). Strengthening self-help behavior in the retardate. *American Journal of Mental Deficiency, 71,* 546–550.

King, L. W., & Turner, R. D. (1975). Teaching a profoundly retarded adult at home by nonprofessionals. *Journal of Behavior Therapy and Experimental Psychiatry, 6,* 117–121.

Kohlenberg, R. J. (1970). The punishment of persistent vomiting: A case study. *Journal of Applied Behavior Analysis, 3,* 241–245.

Levine, M. N., & Elliott, C. B. (1970). Toilet training for profoundly retarded with a limited staff. *Mental Retardation, 8,* 48–50.

Libby, D. G., & Phillips, E. (1979). Eliminating rumination behavior in a profoundly retarded adolescent: An exploratory study. *Mental Retardation, 17,* 94–95.

Lohmann, W., Eyman, R. K., & Lask, E. (1967). Toilet training. *American Journal of Mental Deficiency, 71,* 551–557.

Luckey, R. E., Watson, C. M., & Musick, J. K. (1968). Aversive conditioning as a means of inhibiting vomiting and rumination. *American Journal of Mental Deficiency, 73,* 139–142.

Mahoney, K., Van Wagenen, R. K., & Meyerson, L. (1971). Toilet training of normal and retarded children. *Journal of Applied Behavior Analysis, 4,* 173–181.

Marholin, D., Luiselli, J. K., Robinson, M., & Lott, I. T. (1980). Response-contingent taste-aversion in treating chronic ruminative vomiting of institutionalised profoundly retarded children. *Journal of Mental Deficiency Research, 24,* 47–56.

Marholin, D., O'Toole, K. M., Touchette, P. E., Berger, P. L., & Doyle, D. A. (1979). "I'll have a Big Mac, large fries, large Coke, and apple pie," . . . or teaching adaptive community skills. *Behavior Therapy, 10,* 236–248.

Martin, G. L., Kehoe, B., Bird, E., Jensen, V., & Darbyshire, M. (1971). Operant conditioning in dressing behavior of severely retarded girls. *Mental Retardation, 9,* 27–31.

Martin, G. L., McDonald, S., & Omichinski, M. (1971). An operant analysis of response interactions during meals with severely retarded girls. *American Journal of Mental Deficiency, 76,* 68–75.

Matson, J. L. (1975). Some practical considerations for using the Foxx and Azrin rapid method of toilet training. *Psychological Reports, 37,* 350.

Matson, J. L. (1977). Simple correction for treating an autistic boy's encopresis. *Psychological Reports, 41,* 802.

Matson, J. L. (1980). A controlled group study of pedestrian-skill training for the mentally retarded. *Behaviour Research and Therapy, 18,* 99–106.

Matson, J. L. (1982). Independence training vs. modeling procedures for teaching phone conversation skills to the mentally retarded. *Behaviour Research and Therapy, 20,* 505–511.

Matson, J. L., & Marchetti, A. (1980). A comparison of leisure skills training procedures for the mentally retarded. *Applied Research in Mental Retardation, 1,* 113–122.

Matson, J. L., Marchetti, A., & Adkins, J. A. (1980). Comparison of operant- and independence-training procedures for mentally retarded adults. *American Journal of Mental Deficiency, 84,* 487–494.

Matson, J. L., Ollendick, T. H., & Adkins, J. A. (1980). A comprehensive dining program for mentally retarded adults. *Behaviour Research and Therapy, 18,* 107–112.

Matson, J. L., DiLorenzo, T. M., & Esveldt-Dawson, K. (1981). Independence training as a method of enhancing self-help skills acquisition of the mentally retarded. *Behaviour Research and Therapy, 19,* 399–405.

McKeegan, G. F., Estill, K., & Campbell, B. (1987). Elimination of rumination by controlled eating and differential reinforcement. *Journal of Behavior Therapy and Experimental Psychiatry, 18,* 143–148.

Minge, M. R., & Ball, T. S. (1967). Teaching of self-help skills to profoundly retarded patients. *American Journal of Mental Deficiency, 71,* 864–868.

Mulick, J. A., Schroeder, S. R., & Rojahn, J. (1980). Chronic ruminative vomiting: A comparison of four treatment procedures. *Journal of Autism and Developmental Disorders, 10,* 203–213.

Murphy, M. J., & Zahm, D. (1978). Effect of improved physical and social environment on self-help and problem behaviors of institutionalized retarded males. *Behavior Modification, 2,* 193–210.

Nelson, G. L., Cone, J. D., & Hanson, C. R. (1975). Training correct utensil use in retarded children: Modeling vs. physical guidance. *American Journal of Mental Deficiency, 80,* 114–122.

Nettlebeck, T., & Kirby, N. H. (1976). A comparison of part and whole training methods with mildly mentally retarded workers. *Journal of Occupational Psychology, 49,* 115–120.

Newton, A. (1976). Clothing: A positive part of the rehabilitation process. *Journal of Rehabilitation*, 42, 18–22.

O'Brien, F., & Azrin, N. H. (1972). Developing proper mealtime behaviors of the institutionalized retarded. *Journal of Applied Behavior Analysis, 5*, 389–399.

O'Brien, F., Bugle, C., & Azrin, N. H. (1972). Training and maintaining a retarded child's proper eating. *Journal of Applied Behavior Analysis, 5*, 67–72.

Osarchuk, M. (1973). Operant methods of toilet behavior training of the severely and profoundly retarded: A review. *Journal of Special Education, 7*, 423–437.

Passman, R. H. (1975). An automatic device for toilet training. *Behaviour Research and Therapy, 13*, 215–220.

Rast, J., & Johnston, J. M. (1986). Social versus dietary control of ruminating by mentally retarded persons. *American Journal of Mental Deficiency, 90*, 464–467.

Redd, W. H., Porterfield, A. L., & Andersen, B. L. (1979). *Behavior Modification: Behavioral approaches to human problems*. New York: Random House.

Reid, D. H. (1982). Trends and issues in behavioral research on training feeding and dressing skills. In J. L. Matson & F. Andrasik (Eds.), *Treatment issues and innovations in mental retardation* (pp. 213–240). New York: Plenum Press.

Reid, D. H., Wilson, P. G., & Faw, G. D. (1983). Teaching self-help skills. In J. L. Matson & J. A. Mulick (Eds.), *Handbook of mental retardation* (pp. 429–442). New York: Pergamon Press.

Richman, J. S., Sonderby, T., & Kahn, J. V. (1980). Prerequisite vs. in vivo acquisition of self-feeding skill. *Behaviour Research and Therapy, 18*, 327–332.

Richmond, G. (1983). Shaping bladder and bowel continence in developmentally retarded preschool children. *Journal of Autism and Developmental Disorders, 13*, 197–204.

Ross, P., & Oliver, M. (1969). Evaluation of operant conditioning with institutionalized retarded children. *American Journal of Mental Deficiency, 74*, 325–330.

Simpson, R. L., & Sasso, G. M. (1978). The modification of rumination in a severely emotionally disturbed child through an overcorrection procedure. *AAESPH Review, 3*, 145–150.

Sloop, E. W., & Kennedy, W. A. (1973). Institutionalized retarded nocturnal enuretics treated by a conditioning technique. *American Journal of Mental Deficiency, 77*, 717–721.

Smith, L. J. (1981). Training severely and profoundly mentally handicapped nocturnal enuretics. *Behaviour Research and Therapy, 19*, 67–74.

Smith, P. S. (1979). A comparison of different methods to toilet training the mentally handicapped. *Behaviour Research and Therapy, 17*, 33–34.

Smith, P. S., Britton, P. G., Johnson, M., & Thomas, D. A. (1975). Problems involved in toilet-training profoundly and mentally handicapped adults. *Behaviour Research and Therapy, 13*, 301–307.

Snell, M. E. (1987). *Systematic instruction of persons with severe handicaps*. Columbus, OH: Merrill Publishing.

Song, A. Y., & Gandhi, R. (1974). An analysis of behavior during the acquisition and maintenance phases of self-spoon feeding skills of profound retardates. *Mental Retardation, 12*, 25–28.

Spooner, F., & Spooner, D. (1984). A review of chaining techniques: Implications for future research and practice. *Education and Training of the Mentally Retarded, 10*, 114–124.

Starin, S. P., & Fuqua, R. W. (1987). Rumination and vomiting in the developmentally disabled: A critical review of the behavioral, medical, and psychiatric treatment research. *Research in Developmental Disabilities, 8*, 575–605.

Stimbert, V. E., Minor, J. W., & McCoy, J. F. (1977). Intensive feeding training with retarded children. *Behavior Modification, 1*, 517–529.

Swain, J. J., Allard, G. B., & Holborn, S. W. (1982). The good toothbrushing game: A school-based dental hygiene program for increasing the toothbrushing effectiveness of children. *Journal of Applied Behavior Analysis, 15*, 171–176.

Thinesen, P. J., & Bryan, A. J. (1981). The use of sequential pictorial cues in the initiation and maintenance of grooming behaviors with mentally retarded adults. *Mental Retardation, 19*, 247–250.

Thompson, G. A., Jr., Iwata, B. A., & Poynter, H. (1979). Operant control of pathological tongue thrust in spastic cerebral palsy. *Journal of Applied Behavior Analysis, 12*, 325–333.

Thompson, T., & Hanson, R. (1983). Overhydration: Precautions when treating urinary inconti-nence. *Mental Retardation, 21,* 139–143.

Touchette, P. (1968). The effects of graduated stimulus change on the acquisition of a simple discrimination in severely retarded boys. *Journal of the Experimental Analysis of Behavior, 11,* 39–48.

Touchette, P. E., & Howard, J. S. (1984). Errorless learning: Reinforcement contingencies and stimulus control transfer in delayed prompting. *Journal of Applied Behavior Analysis, 17,* 175–188.

Tough, J. H., Hawkins, R. P., McArthur, M. M., & Van Ravenswaay, S. (1971). Modification of enuretic behavior by punishment: A new use for an old device. *Behavior Therapy, 2,* 567–574.

Treffry, D., Martin, G., Samels, J., & Watson, C. (1970). Operant conditioning of grooming behavior of severely retarded girls. *Mental Retardation, 8,* 29–33.

Van Wagenen, K., Meyerson, L., Kerr, N. J., & Mahoney, K. (1969). Field trials of a new procedure for toilet training. *Journal of Experimental Child Psychology, 8,* 147–159.

Walls, R. T., Crist, K., Sienicki, D. A., & Grant, C. (1981). Prompting sequences in teaching independent living skills. *Mental Retardation, 19,* 243–246.

Walls, R. T., Zane, T., & Ellis, W. D. (1981). Forward and backward chaining, and whole task methods. *Behavior Modification, 5,* 61–74.

Walls, R. T., Dowler, D. L., Haught, P. A., & Zawlocki, R. J. (1984). Progress delay and unlimited delay of prompts in forward chaining and whole task training strategies. *Education and Training of the Mentally Retarded, 19,* 276–284.

Watkins, J. T. (1972). Treatment of chronic vomiting and extreme emaciation by an aversive stimulus: Case study. *Psychological Reports, 31,* 803–805.

Watson, L. S., Jr., & Uzzell, R. (1980). Teaching self-help skills to the mentally retarded. In J. L. Matson & J. R. McCartney (Eds.), *Handbook of behavior modification with the mentally retarded* (pp. 151–175). New York: Plenum Press.

Weeks, M., & Gaylord-Ross, R. (1981). Task difficulty and aberrant behavior in severely handi-capped. *Journal of Applied Behavior Analysis, 14,* 449–463.

Wehman, P. (1974). Maintaining oral hygiene skills in geriatric retarded women. *Mental Retarda-tion, 12,* 20.

Whitman, T. L., Sciback, J. W., & Reid, D. H. (1983). *Behavior modification with the severely and profoundly retarded: Research and applications.* New York: Academic Press.

Whitney, L. R., & Barnard, K. E. (1966). Implications of operant learning theory for nursing care of the retarded child. *Mental Retardation, 4,* 26–29.

Williams, F. E., & Sloop, E. W. (1978). Success with a shortened Foxx-Azrin toilet training program. *Education and Training of the Mentally Retarded, 4,* 399–402.

Wolber, G., Carne, W., Collins-Montgomery, P., & Nelson, A. (1987). Tangible reinforcement plus social reinforcement versus social reinforcement alone in acquisition of toothbrushing skills. *Mental Retardation, 25,* 275–279.

11

Community Living Skills

JEFFREY S. DANFORTH AND RONALD S. DRABMAN

In 1986, a United States District Court in Alabama approved the consent settlement of the *Wyatt v. Stickney* litigation (Marchetti, 1987) thus bringing to a close the most significant court-related event prompting community placement of mentally retarded people. It is important to note that the court enjoined Alabama "to continue to make substantial progress in placing members of the plaintiff class in community facilities and programs" (Marchetti, 1987, p. 252).

Wyatt v. Stickney, in conjunction with efforts of those who espouse the philosophy of "normalization," has resulted in the community placement of a significant number of mentally retarded (and mentally ill) people. Normalization, as it has been defined by such proponents as Nirje (1969) and Wolfensberger (1972), espouses that mentally retarded individuals be accorded the same basic educational, social, and habitation privileges as those maintained by the rest of society in which that individual lives. The result, in this country, was a decline in population of the institutionalized mentally retarded of over 70,000 from 1971 to 1982 (Scheerenberger, 1982). Yet most of the individuals who have entered the community are still, in effect, separated from mainstream society. As Sarason (1974) noted,

> Few things are as destructive of the psychological sense of community . . . as the tendency to segregate the atypical person, to place him in a special geographical area where he will be with his "own kind" and receive "special handling." (p. 161)

In spite of the trend toward community placement, it is clear that exposing mentally retarded individuals to the community is only a beginning step to achieving normalization. In order for mentally retarded citizens to merge into community settings, both in a social and practical independent living sense, many skill deficits need to be overcome through explicit training in community living skills. Educators, acknowledging this need, are now incorporating community living skills into the curriculum of special needs students (Brown *et al.*, 1983; Snell, 1983; Wilcox & Bellamy, 1982; Wuerch & Voeltz, 1982).

JEFFREY S. DANFORTH • Department of Psychiatry, University of Massachusetts Medical School, 55 Lake Avenue North, Worcester, Massachusetts 01655.   RONALD S. DRABMAN • Department of Psychiatry and Human Behavior, University of Mississippi Medical Center, 2500 North State Street, Jackson, Mississippi 39216.

In their 1981 review of community living skills, Marchetti and Matson noted limited behavioral research on training independent living skills, but they predicted an expansion of this training in the next few years. The purpose of this chapter was to review the experimental research on community living skills since that time. Three categories of skills were covered: food-related skills, leisure skills, and pragmatic domestic skills. Following this, generalization and methodological research issues were discussed.

FOOD-RELATED SKILLS

An area that has received increased attention recently is food-related skills. These skills consist of self-help behaviors that allow individuals to plan meals independently, as well as acquire and cook nutritious food. Institutionalized people are usually not responsible for selecting or preparing their own food; therefore, clients placed in the community often need to acquire these behaviors. Skills to be examined under this rubric include shopping, menu planning, cooking, and eating out.

Shopping

Shopping for their own food allows individuals to function more independently in community-based domestic environments, and is an essential survival skill for independent living. Although descriptive studies suggested that the technology was available to teach handicapped children and adolescents nutrition education (Stapley, Smith, Bittle, Andrews, & Nuckolls, 1984) and supermarket shopping skills (Wheeler, Ford, Nietupski, Loomis, & Brown, 1980), the test-teach design employed in these studies failed to provide experimental evidence that the teaching programs were responsible for the skill acquisition.

A controlled study by Nietupski, Welch, and Wacker (1983) attempted to determine if picture prompts and calculators facilitated grocery item purchasing by four moderately to severely retarded young adult males (mean IQ of 39, and age of 20). Given one paper money denomination, a money card displaying pictures of bills, a calculator, and a 10-item grocery list, students were taught an 8-step task that included deducting the cost of the grocery items from the money available. A multiple probe design across students was used to assess the effectiveness of the teaching program, which included modeling, praising correct performance, and verbally prompting, modeling, or physically guiding the student after incorrect performance. The multiple probe design called for periodic rather than continuous probes of student behavior in order to attenuate extinction problems associated with prolonged baseline conditions. Students achieved the skill as a result of the training procedure, and they maintained their skills as assessed by a generalization probe conducted in a local supermarket. However, as pointed out by these researchers, the program did not address basic shopping skills, such as obtaining and maneuvering a cart and searching for items.

In a subsequent study (Gaule, Nietupski, & Certo, 1985), a multiple probe design across skill clusters was used to assess the effectiveness of the same training format to teach three clusters of behavior: preparing a shopping list for one meal, locating and obtaining the items in the supermarket, and purchasing the items. Three moderately/severely handicapped young adult males (mean IQ of 35, and age of 18) were taught in classrooms and at the supermarket. The skills were acquired, but unreinforced probe trials 2 and 4 weeks after termination showed only partial skill maintenance. This may have been the result of relatively low accuracy criterions (80%, 67%, and 100%) that were required of the students on each of the three skill clusters. Positive aspects of this research included a more detailed task analysis of shopping skills.

A second line of shopping research was initiated by Matson (1981) who taught shopping skills to mentally retarded adults using "independence training," a treatment package first described in Matson (1980a). An important component of this research was the degree to which shopping skills generalized over time and to novel settings. Twenty mildly retarded adults (10 males and 10 females, mean age of 34) were matched and divided into a treatment group and a no-treatment control group. The 14-component chain of skills taught ranged inclusively from selecting the correct grocery store to lifting the groceries from the checkout counter and carrying them out. Treatment included alternating classroom and *in vivo* sessions with instructions, feedback, modeling, behavioral rehearsal, social reinforcement, and self-evaluation. The independence training model encourages clients to evaluate their own as well as other clients' performance. A one-way ANCOVA showed that, in the treatment group, the number of shopping skills completed correctly increased significantly after the posttest, the 2-month follow-up test, and in the generalization store where no training had occurred.

A second study (Matson & Long, 1986) replicated and extended these findings to include adaptive use of hand-held calculators while shopping. A question raised by Matson's studies concerned classroom versus *in vivo* training with respect to generalization to novel settings.

McDonnell and Horner (1985) compared *in vivo* training with *in vivo* combined with simulation training. Simulation training was defined by them as "an approach in which relevant stimuli (or approximations of relevant stimuli) are presented outside their normal stimulus context (i.e., in the classroom)" (p. 324). *In vivo* training involved training in a single supermarket. Four males and four females (mean IQ of 43, and age of 19) were taught to select groceries off of store shelves from a list of 15 items. A two-level multiple baseline across students was used, and probes were conducted in markets frequented by each student's family. *In vivo* training alone resulted in immediate but moderate improvements in the percentage of target items selected correctly. Subjects showed greater improvement when they received *in vivo* plus simulation training, and the results maintained in the students' family supermarkets. McDonnell and Horner made an important point when they distinguished comparing classroom and *in vivo* settings from teaching in the presence of relevant stimulus dimensions likely to be encountered. *In vivo* instruction does not ensure that all relevant stimulus conditions that are encountered in the natural environment are also encountered in one live training site, but sometimes this can be arranged in a classroom environment.

Haring, Kennedy, Adams, and Pitts-Conway (1987) investigated the effectiveness of videotaped modeling as a procedure to promote generalization across settings. Three 20-year-old autistic individuals (2 males, 1 female, with Vineland Adaptive Behavior Scale Levels of 4–5 years old) were taught purchasing skills in a store via praise and graduated prompt levels. Generalization probes were conducted in three other community stores. The percentage of correct responses in probe stores did not increase until after classroom training, with videotapes showing peers modeling purchases in the generalization stores.

Generalization to novel stores is a theme common to shopping skills research. This essential aspect of shopping behavior was taught in the classroom by simulated stimulus conditions portrayed either on chalkboards (Matson, 1981; Matson & Long, 1986), in slides (McDonnell & Horner, 1985), or in film (Haring *et al.*, 1987). The critical feature has been simulating conditions as they will be found in community store settings. In any case, there is no research at this time that indicates that mentally retarded clients can be taught generalized shopping skills without some *in vivo* training experience, suggesting that the ambiance of a natural store setting is difficult to replicate in a classroom.

Menu Planning

Another area of importance is nutritional meal planning. In conjunction with shopping skills, training in this area should facilitate independent community living. The ability to prepare nutritionally adequate menus is one predictor of successful independent housing among mentally retarded persons (Schalock, Harper, & Carver, 1981). Diets poor in nutrition can adversely affect almost all forms of mental and physical handicaps (Brown, Davis, & Flemming, 1979), and it has been suggested that excess weight may be a particular problem for mentally retarded people (Emery, Watson, Watson, Thompson, & Biderman, 1985; Fox, Burkhart, & Rotatori, 1983). Baseline shopping patterns of mentally retarded adults consist of impulsive, rather random selections (Williams & Ewing, 1981). They often chose from only one food group, for example, meat, ignoring vegetables and fruits, grain, and dairy products (Reitz, 1984; Sarber & Cuvo, 1983). Thus, teaching nutritional menu planning is a logical extension of shopping research.

Sarber, Halasz, Messmer, Bickett, and Lutzker (1983) showed in a single case study that menu planning and grocery shopping skills could be taught to a 34-year-old mildly mentally retarded woman (IQ of 57). Shortly thereafter,

Sarber and Cuvo (1983) conducted a follow-up with four mentally retarded adults (2 males and 2 females, mean IQ of 72, and age of 29). A multiple probe design across subjects assessed the effectiveness of a program to teach them to plan 1 week of nutritious meals, devise a grocery list, and find the food from the grocery list in the supermarket. Training was conducted in the classroom and in a supermarket. Each task was described in detail, broken down into component parts, and rehearsed. For incorrect responses, instructions were repeated, the response was verbally or manually modeled, verbal and physical prompts were provided if necessary, and then practice followed. The results showed that subjects performed each task poorly in baseline, but strong improvement was shown after training, in a different probe supermarket, and in follow-up maintenance tests 1 week and 1 month later. Pre- and posttraining results also indicated that the three subtasks could be successfully chained together. Additional data were provided on time spent shopping and on nutritional ratings of the menus and their variety.

An even more comprehensive program included teaching five mildly mentally retarded adults (3 females, 2 males, mean IQ of 76, and age 22) to plan nutritious meals within a $25 weekly budget (Wilson, Cuvo, & Davis, 1986). The authors pointed out that budgeting is an integral part of meal planning because many handicapped people live on fixed incomes. A multiple-baseline design across skill clusters showed that training skills in planning healthy meals and writing a grocery list resulted in a weekly food bill averaging $56.25. After direct training, budgets approached the $25 criterion. The success of this program was in part a function of the prerequisite monetary and community skills the subjects already had. This fact points out that the range of skills trained should be determined on the basis of the client's disability and the manner of living (independent, group home, etc.) that is desired. Thus, research on all levels of shopping skill function is appropriate.

Cooking

A related line of research includes teaching clients to cook the food purchased. In an early report of this training, Matson (1979) described how moderately to severely mentally retarded adults (12 males and 12 females) learned basic cooking methods common to the preparation of a number of meals. Later, Johnson and Cuvo (1981) used a multiple baseline across subjects and responses to evaluate a procedure to train boiling, baking, and broiling skills to four retarded adults (3 males and 1 female, mean IQ of 59, and age of 32). Training consisted of pictorial recipes, graduated prompt levels, praise, and a histogram to provide visual feedback on the accuracy of each client's daily performance. Results showed the success of the training program with idiosyncratic generalization between similar cooking tasks. Follow-up tests 7 to 11 days after training revealed reasonable maintenance. The authors of both cooking studies wisely pointed out the benefits of teaching responses that covary across skill dimensions.

Eating Out

Normalized eating skills that provide independence and mobility to mentally retarded individuals include skills that allow them to eat out. These skills allow independence by giving a person the option of eating elsewhere rather than returning home for each meal. In addition, eating in restaurants is a potential source of socialization.

Most restaurant training research is aimed at performance in fast-food restaurants. In one study (Marholin, O'Toole, Touchette, Berger, & Doyle, 1979), four adult males (mean Peabody Picture Vocabulary Test score of 34, and age of 52) were taught to ride a bus to a McDonald's Restaurant, purchase a meal, and pay for it. A multiple-baseline design across subjects showed that the training procedures resulted in increased correct responding by each subject.

This research was extended in a study looking at classroom-based instruction for locating, ordering, paying, eating, and exiting from McDonald's (van den Pol *et al.*, 1981). Subjects were three young adult males, ages ranging from 17 to 22, with IQ scores ranging from 46 to 75. Slides depicting scenes from McDonald's and a simulated restaurant counter served as apparatus. Students responded to questions about slides and role-played restaurant interactions. Correct responses received social and descriptive praise. Incorrect responses produced feedback, modeling, and a remedial trial. Importantly, response definitions and descriptions of training procedures for each skill were provided in a detailed table format. Probe assessments were conducted in a McDonald's Restaurant. A multiple baseline across subjects and skill components showed that the percentage of correct responses within each skill component increased after training, and was maintained in a similar fast-food restaurant (Burger King), and in a 1-year follow-up. The follow-ups were conducted without the subjects' knowledge to ensure that the skills were generalized to settings that did not include known trainers.

A more recent study compared the effects of simulated classroom training that was provided immediately prior, and $1\frac{1}{2}$ hours prior to the *in vivo* training that is often necessary with severely handicapped persons (Nietupski, Clancy, Wehrmacher, & Parmer, 1985). Two mentally retarded boys (ages 8 and 13) who were considered untestable on the Stanford Binet, learned to walk to the counter at a fast-food restaurant and buy french fries and a Coke. A combination multiple probe design across students/alternating treatments design suggested the timing of the simulation training, relative to *in vivo* training, was not a factor in skill acquisition.

Research on food-related skills illustrated that complex skill clusters can be taught to mentally retarded people, and that prosthetics often aid in such skill acquisition. More extensive research needs to be conducted on cooking skills and on programs to teach appropriate skills for more formal restaurant dining.

LEISURE ACTIVITIES

Scientific and public policy advances in the field of mental retardation have allowed more emphasis to be placed on basic leisure skills (Fain, 1986). Leisure activities by mentally retarded individuals often do not develop unless specific program direction is given. Previous research indicated that, compared to nonretarded people, noninstitutionalized mentally retarded persons spent the majority of their leisure time in passive isolated activities, such as watching TV and listening to the radio (Birenbaum & Re, 1979; Reiter & Levi, 1981). This finding suggests that many mentally retarded people are actually functionally institutionalized in community settings (Crapps, Langone, & Swaim, 1985; Salzberg & Langford, 1981). The seriousness of this issue can be better understood when one considers that lack of friendship and social interaction are associated with a person's failure to perform adequate leisure activities. Thus, we agree with Frith, Mitchell, and Roswal's (1980) recommendation that recreation and leisure activities should be included in Individualized Education Plans (IEP) for all mentally retarded students. Skills examined under this rubric include recreation, free time, and cooperative activities.

Recreation

A modeling technique designed to teach diving into a swimming pool to a 12-year-old boy with an IQ of 54 is an example of research on recreational skills (Feltz, 1980). Diving could be considered representative of recreational skills that retarded people avoid because of perceived risk; yet they often report a desire to participate. Diving skills were broken down into 18 units, with the teacher using explanation, modeling, a peer model, student description of the task, and practice with physical guidance. An unaided follow-up after 3 weeks illustrated skill maintenance.

Schleien, Certo, and Muccino (1984) used a multiple baseline across skill components to demonstrate the effectiveness of a program to teach independent bowling skills to a 16-year-old boy with an IQ of 32. Instruction took place at a bowling alley, and adaptive picture cards were used to assist with such aspects as informing the attendant of shoe size. Verbal and physical prompts, praise, and modeling were used to teach the boy to bowl one string, order a soft drink from the concession stand, and make a purchase from the vending machine. An impressive aspect of this study was the follow-up probes conducted at three different bowling alleys showing that the skills generalized across settings. It was speculated that the functional nature of the skills accounted for the generalization.

In another study on recreational skills (Luyben, Funk, Morgan, Clark, & Delulio, 1986) three mentally retarded adult males (mean IQ of 32, with ages ranging from 24–52) were taught to use a soccer pass. The pass was analyzed into nine components, with the men receiving descriptive praise for correct performance. Incorrect responses were followed by descriptive correction and a maximum-to-minimum prompt reduction procedure ranging from full physical prompts to less guided prompts. Most research reviewed here used prompts ranging from least to most intrusive as the need arose. However, Luyben *et al.* (1986) indicated that pilot work showed that strategy resulted in higher error rates, lower acquisition rates, and subsequently negative emotional responses. A multiple-baseline design across subjects provided evidence that the skill acquisition was due to the training procedures, and generalization probes in another gym 57 and 276 days after training indicated a well-established skill.

A second line of recreation research has focused on the relation between physical fitness and exercise. As indicated earlier, mentally retarded individuals tend to be less active than nonretarded individuals, and this factor can result in lower exercise performance levels (Coleman, Ayoub, & Friedrich, 1976; Maksud & Hamilton, 1974). Physical training programs can lead to decreased weight and improved maximal oxygen consumption (Schurrer, Weltman, & Brammell, 1985). A second reason that mentally retarded individuals show poor physical fitness is the failure of physical fitness programs to incorporate motivational or generalization strategies.

In response to this finding, Allen and Iwata (1980) compared the baseline levels of participation by 10 retarded adults (6 males and 4 females, mean age of 42) in exercise versus game-like physical education activities. Participation in games was the higher frequency behavior. Access to games was then made contingent upon completion of exercise to determine if the former might reinforce the latter, according to principles established by Premack (1959). Exercise did indeed increase after the implementation of the group Premack contingency, illustrating that access to games can reinforce exercise behavior. The utility of this finding was that no tangible reinforcers were used, and most phys ed programs would have the equipment necessary to implement similar activities.

Coleman and Whitman (1984) extended this research by programming maintenance by including a component whereby 17 mentally retarded individuals (10 females and 7 males, mean IQ of 55, ages ranging from 40–68) were to self-monitor and self-reinforce their exercise behavior. In baseline, subjects were simply told to exercise, whereas in treatment, prompts and modeling were used to teach the clients to record their exercise behavior and provide themselves with praise and access to backup reinforcers, such as records and magazines. A multiple-baseline design across groups showed a general increase in exercise frequency that was maintained when program supervision was transferred to workshop staff.

Free Time

Fain (1986) distinguished between recreation and leisure, noting that the former involves engagement in activities, such as bowling, swimming, or exercise, whereas the latter is not specific to any activity but instead implies free expression in which persons simply do what they want in their free time.

The paradox is that whereas leisure is not associated with structured activities, in many cases structured education is necessary so that mentally retarded people will have free-time skills other than TV viewing.

This point was made clear in a study by Adkins and Matson (1980) that demonstrated that prompts to use an activity room and a discussion about leisure activities had little impact on the use of leisure time by six institutionalized mentally retarded women (mean age of 32). A multiple baseline across subjects, with a return to baseline between interventions, showed that only after a specific leisure skill was trained did frequency of participation in leisure time increase. Teachers modeled potholder making, gave minimal prompts and verbal praise, and taught the women to evaluate their own performance. A 6-week follow-up showed continued interest in leisure-time activity.

In another study, Schleien, Wehman, and Kiernan (1981) taught three severely mentally retarded adults (2 males and 1 female, mean IQ of 22, and age of 39), whose only leisure activity was TV watching, to throw darts. A combination of multiple-baseline design across subjects, and changing criterion design with increased height and distance from the dart board was used. Instructional sessions consisted of verbal cues and prompts, modeling, physical prompts, and praise. As a result of training, each adult was able to master a 7-step dart-throwing sequence. Generalization probes showed that the skill transferred to three other settings and was maintained after 4 months. Most importantly, two of the adults were observed to throw darts spontaneously on several occasions over 4 months, illustrating use of their free time in an enjoyable manner.

Other research has looked at the more general use of free time. For example, Schleien, Kiernan, and Wehman (1981) provided six moderately retarded adults (3 males and 3 females, ages ranging from 27–52) with leisure counseling sessions, introduced recreational materials, and trained these adults in their use. An ABAB design demonstrated an increased rate of high-quality leisure time when the program was introduced.

In an interesting study on the general use of free time, Jones, Favell, Lattimore, and Risley (1984) examined the rate of engagement with toys emitted by wheelchair bound, multiply handicapped people (10 females and 3 males, mean Bayley developmental levels of 4.1 months, mean age of 17). In baseline, average engagement with toys occurred less than 20% of the time. Treatment consisted of presenting the subjects with toys of varying stimulus dimensions and determining individual preferences. Based on this analysis, preferred toys were attached to a holder that was part of the wheelchair apparatus. A multiple-baseline design across two groups showed an increase in toy engagement for 11 of the 13 subjects, with 90-day follow-ups indicating maintenance.

Subsequent studies on use of free time have focused on promoting generalization and maintenance of skills. This type of research is essential because the use of free-time skills denotes choice and involvement without external help. Haring (1985) assessed the effects of training play behavior on response generalization to related and novel toys. Four moderate to severely handicapped children (3 males and 1 female, mean IQ of 40, and age of 6) were taught to play with detailed training toys via praise, modeling, instruction, and physical prompts. Assessment with a multiple probe design showed that training with subsequent toys required fewer trials, and training with similar less detailed (more abstract) toys was facilitated. This generalization was accounted for by noting the functional similarity of the play responses and the related stimulus features of the toys.

In an examination of free-time use, Nietupski *et al.* (1986) trained three students (2 males and 1 female, mean IQ of 40, and age of 17) to select and initiate play with age-appropriate leisure materials. A multiple probe design across subjects showed that in baseline all three students had low levels of engagement in leisure activity. Through the use of praise and verbal and physical prompts, rates of selecting an activity and in participating rose substantially for each subject. An interesting aspect of this study was an explicit schedule of praise during training that was faded from fixed internal 30-second schedule, to a fixed internal 2-minute schedule, to no praise during probes and follow-up. This may explain the rapid acquisition and maintenance of the leisure activity 4 months later. Leisure-time research often assumes that appropriate behavior will be naturally reinforced by the consequences of the leisure activity (see Baer & Wolf, 1970). The nature of these natural consequences is an area greatly in need of more research.

Cooperative Activities

The importance of cooperative play activity to the social and emotional development of children has long been recognized (Eriksen, 1977; Piaget, 1951). Cooperative play activities provide a setting to learn rule-following, to form friendships, and to improve motor functioning. Baseline observations of the play behavior of mentally retarded people often indicated self-directed independent play with few attempts to engage the environment. This finding is consistent with research indicating that play behavior does not develop naturally for most retarded people (Li, 1981; Wehman, 1975).

In spite of the importance attributed to social play behavior, research in this area often presents serious methodological difficulties. Marchant and Wehman (1979) taught severely mentally retarded children (mental ages ranging from 21–46 months, ages 8–9) to play the Picture Lotto Game together, and Donder and Nietupski (1981) had nonhandicapped adolescents teach playground activities to mentally retarded male peers (mean IQ of 49, and age of 14). Descriptions of the treatment procedures were vague, however, and would be difficult to replicate. The same was true of a study that programmed indoor cooperative table games for severely mentally retarded adolescents (7 males and 3 females, mean age of 16) (Jeffree & Cheseldine, 1984). A dance program for educable mentally retarded teenagers described by Crain, McLaughlin, and Eisenhart (1983) and another program describing severe and profound adults who learned to play Lotto together (Nietupski & Svoboda, 1982), had no experimental control.

Fajardo and McGourty (1983) operationalized developmental play milestones for three groups of 15-year-old male adolescents with retardation ranging from mild to severe. Subjects in each group had matched controls. Modeling, prompting, and an increasing schedule of fixed interval (FI) food and token reinforcement (ranging from FI 3 minutes to FI 30 minutes) for specific play behaviors resulted in improved interactional play ratings. Unfortunately, these gains declined again on a 7-day posttest suggesting that the approximately 4 hours of training was not sufficient to result in persistent change.

Some research on cooperative play has focused on severely mentally retarded people. In one study, Wacker, Berg, and Moore (1984) showed that formally pairing teenagers together to play with board games they were already competent in resulted in increased rates of participation in on-task cooperative play behavior (target students were 1 male and 1 female, mean IQ of 31, and age of 19). This research was compared in an alternating treatment design to a condition wherein a group of teenagers were simply shown the games and told to play together. Thus, a minor change in staff interaction resulted in significant changes, suggesting pragmatic applications to the classroom.

In another study, Keogh, Faw, Whitman, and Reid (1984) used a multiple probe design across subjects to assess the effectiveness of a program to teach board games to two severely retarded adolescent boys (mean age of 17). Trainers used verbal instructions, modeling of play behavior, and self-instruction, prompting, and praise. The program included individual training, dyad training, and free-play intervention. Interestingly, none of the skills acquired generalized to subsequent conditions without training, and additional training was necessary to ensure maintenance.

Lagomarcino, Reid, Ivancic, and Faw (1984) used the dance behavior of higher functioning retarded people as the standard for dance training to institutionalized severe and profound retardates ranging in age from 14 to 19. A multiple-baseline design across subjects assessed a training program that consisted of praise, verbal feedback, modeling, and physical guidance. Three of four subjects acquired dance skills, but, as in a number of studies with severely mentally retarded individuals, some minor staff intervention was necessary to maintain generalization over time and settings.

The pursuit of leisure is a broad skill area in need of substantial research. As indicated by these studies, teaching leisure skills provides the opportunity for social interaction, but training in social skills is often necessary to ensure that such interactions are not limited because of skill deficits (see Marchetti & Campbell, Chapter 12, in this volume). Broadly speaking, the target response for leisure pursuits includes initiation of activity, performance, and sustained activity. Wehman and Schleien (1980) have also suggested that variables, such as leisure preference, age appropriateness, and access to desired activities, need to be studied. To date, the only variable that has been researched in depth is skill proficiency, although initial work on preference has begun.

PRAGMATIC DOMESTIC SKILLS

Pragmatic domestic skills for mentally retarded individuals include a wide range of useful behaviors that increase the likelihood of independent functioning and social acceptance within the community. Included in this domain are laundry skills, monetary skills, traveling skills, fire safety training, and telephone skills.

Laundry Skills

Appropriate laundering skills contribute to the normalization process by allowing mentally retarded persons more independence and also contribute to community acceptance by improving appearance. In addition, compared to paying a commercial laundry, economic advantages are apparent.

Cuvo, Jacobi, and Sipko (1981) used a home economics room as a setting to teach sorting, washing, and drying clothes to five moderately and mildly retarded students (4 males and 1 female, mean age of 20, and IQ of 46). Each task was analyzed into component steps, and a multiple baseline across these steps and students was used to evaluate the effectiveness of the teaching program. The details of the training procedures provided in this report might serve as an exemplar for any research on community living skills. Three levels of training procedures were used with prompt levels ordered from less to more, or more to less if a great deal of assistance was required. Such procedures as verbal instruction, correction, and praise, ranging from continuous to a fixed-ratio 8 schedule, were used in addition to a histogram, which provided performance feedback to the students. The proportion of target steps performed correctly improved to near mastery as a result of the training, and additional data were provided on the proportion of prompt types used.

This research was extended in a study that assessed generalization over settings and time (Thompson, Braam, & Fuqua, 1982). Three trainable/educable male mentally retarded students (mean age of 18) were taught laundering skills in a simulated apartment. A multiple probe design across skill components indicated that the instruction, modeling, and graduated guidance training program package was effective. In addition, an assessment in a public laundromat and a follow-up 10 months later indicated generalization of skills for 2 of 3 students.

A subsequent study by Morrow and Bates (1987) accentuated the importance of generalization across settings. Three types of school-based instructional materials were compared relative to their impact on generalization to community laundromats: pictured materials, a cardboard replication, and a home washing machine. The stimulus dimensions of each were carefully detailed. Subjects were nine residents of a state institution (5 males and 4 females, mean IQ of 33, and age of 18). Although the cardboard replication and washing machine functioned as effective stimuli within the training settings, demonstration of laundry skills in the community was limited until training in the natural environment occurred.

Monetary Skills

Relative to research on other community-living skills, work conducted on monetary skills has been rigorous and extensive (Marchetti & Matson, 1981). Money management is an important skill for the mentally retarded individual, especially in light of the competitive employment situations into which well-trained retarded people can enter (see Martin & Mithaug, Chapter 13, in this volume).

Prerequisite skills for money management are coin identification and math. Frank and McFarland (1980) developed such a program for 43 elementary-aged educable mentally retarded children (23 males and 20 females, mean IQ of 71, and age of 9). Instructional procedures taken from a previous study (Borakove & Cuvo, 1977) consisted of modeling, imitation, and corrective feedback in the use of a number line consisting of cardboard strips with coins glued on. Responses to a coin skills acquisition test and a generalization test showed improved scores for students in both one-to-one conditions and small group instruction, whereas a control group showed no improvement.

This investigation was extended by Frank and Wacker (1986) in a program designed to utilize coin skills by having four elementary school students (IQs ranging from 58 to 70, ages ranging from 11–13) purchase items from their school store. The coin skills transferred to items the students were not trained to buy, but removal of the coin number line resulted in a substantial skill decrement. Thus, the practicality of the number line was questionable. Frank and Wacker noted that its size made it too cumbersome for use in a supermarket, but it was useful for teaching entry level monetary values, and it may be helpful in structured home and workshop settings.

A second line of monetary skills research has focused on higher level banking skills and the question of simulation versus *in vivo* training. Bourbeau, Sowers, and Close (1986) used a multiple baseline across subjects to assess a classroom-based program designed to teach four secondary level educable mentally retarded (EMR) students (IQs ranging from 53 to 66, ages ranging from 17–21) depositing and withdrawal skills. Because classroom training was not efficient, additional *in vivo* training was required to achieve appropriate performance in a novel bank.

Shafer, Inge, and Hill (1986) used simulated conditions to teach a moderately mentally retarded 25-year-old man with an IQ of 46 how to use an automated bank machine. A multiple probe design across target behaviors, a clear task analysis of the dependent variable, and explicit descriptions of the training design add to the importance of this study. An inexpensive replica of an automatic banking machine was used so that the trainer could describe and model the task in the subject's home. The subject practiced while receiving descriptive praise and prompts when necessary. The program resulted in appropriate depositing skills. As in most simulation research, additional training was required for improved *in vivo* performance, but when the skill was achieved, a 6-month follow-up illustrated near perfect maintenance. This study provided good balance with respect to the positive and negative aspects of simulation training. *In vivo* practice was not feasible because the bank machine was frequently used by customers and repeated errors would have caused the machine to confiscate the bank card. On the other hand, the automatic bank machine was slightly modified during training, and this minor stimulus change resulted in training conditions that no longer corresponded to *in vivo* conditions. The difficulties illustrated that *in vivo* versus simulation training probably should not be considered an either/or question.

Traveling Skills

Training in independent travel skills is important for mentally retarded people both in institutional and community settings. This training facilitates opportunities for a variety of educational experiences, employment, shopping, eating out, leisure activities, and social engagements in the community. However, these opportunities are secondary to the improved levels of safety that skills can provide, both with respect to automobile accidents involving pedestrians, and the ability to escape from danger. Recent traveling skills research has included both pedestrian skills and use of public transportation.

Most of the research on pedestrian skills has been directly influenced by Page, Iwata, and Neef (1976), Matson (1980a), and Neef, Iwata, and Page (1978); (see also Marchetti & Matson, 1981, for a review).

Gruber, Reeser, and Reid (1979) used a multiple baseline across subjects to evaluate a program to teach four profoundly mentally retarded young adult males (mean IQ of 11, and age of 22) in a state facility to walk 1,000 feet from their living area to school. Training procedures included verbal instructions and resident practice with contingent praise and edible treats. Incorrect responses resulted in verbal reprimands and/or physical prompts. A backward chaining format was implemented so that whenever a subject reached performance criterion for a prescribed distance, training procedures were initiated an additional 50 feet away from the school. Posttraining sessions followed wherein trainers were gradually faded from view. Follow-up observations 1 to 8 weeks after training revealed 100% maintenance. Interestingly, residents were also walking from school back to their residences without training.

Another study that facilitated educational services was conducted by Colozzi and Pollow (1984) who taught five moderate and severely mentally retarded students (3 males and 2 females, mental ages ranging from 3–6, chronological ages ranging from 7–12) to walk from the point where their taxi left them at school into their classroom. Walking was presented as a total task rather than broken into units, and teachers gradually faded physical prompts and instructions as students' performance improved. Experimental control was demonstrated by a multiple baseline across subjects. Follow-up data showed 100% skill maintenance from 7 weeks to 2 years later. The subjects in this study and in the Gruber *et al.* (1979) research had walked their respective routes on previous occasions, so it might be most accurate to describe the programs' functions as establishing stimulus control by other environmental variables rather than skill acquisition *per se*, but this does not detract from the programs' contribution.

Another study that involved a backward chaining format was conducted by Cipani, Augustine, and Blomgren (1982) who taught two profoundly mentally retarded female residents (Fairview Self-Help quotients of 7 and 10, ages 53 and 31) of a state institution to ascend stairs quickly and safely. Physical guidance and edible reinforcers were gradually faded, and incorrect responses (e.g., taking three steps at a time) resulted in a 30-second time-out during which the clients were held still at the starting point. A multiple-baseline design illustrated substantial gains by both subjects, and most treatment gains were maintained on three different sets of stairs and 8 months later.

In a study designed to assess classroom versus community training procedures, 18 members of a residential facility (mean IQ of 49, and age of 41) were assigned to two groups and taught to cross intersections (Marchetti, McCartney, Drain, Hooper, & Dix, 1983). A model of city blocks was used in the classroom group, and the community group received training on community streets. The community training approach was much more effective.

A second line of traveling skills research focused on use of public transportation, specifically bus riding. Robinson, Griffith, McComish, and Swasbrook (1984) indicated that a combined classroom/community training program might effectively teach such skills to workshop trainees (mean IQ of 53, and age of 27). In a controlled study, 27 people (mean age of 35) with mild to severe mental retardation were assigned to one of three groups and taught to locate a bus stop, to signal, to board, and then to exit the bus (Marchetti, Cecil, Graves, & Marchetti, 1984). This detailed report compared three types of training: classroom training involved a simulated model of the city, a simulated bus, and slide presentations of relevant stimuli; community training was conducted in town; and facility-grounds training was performed on the grounds with appropriate props. The training procedures were similar in all three locales and consisted of verbal and physical prompts that were gradually faded out. All three training procedures resulted in significant gain from pre- to posttest, but the facility-grounds group showed the greatest improvement, with the fewest sessions required to complete the program at approximately half the cost and time relative to the other programs. Community training was the next best approach, indicating once again that stimulus dimensions comparative to real-life situations are imperative.

Welch, Nietupski, and Hamre-Nietupski (1985) used a multiple probe design to validate a procedure to teach six moderately retarded young adults (4 females and 2 males, mean IQ of 44, and age of 19) to evaluate whether they had missed the bus and to problem solve if they did. A prosthetic card with two clockfaces assisted the students. One clock indicated "late," the other "on time," and the students compared this card to their watches to determine if they were late. Simulated instruction was conducted at a mock bus stop. Three students performed adequately on community probes, the others required additional *in vivo* training.

Research in traveling skills consisted of generally well controlled, detailed studies. The report by Welch *et al.* (1985) suggested the importance of research on ways mentally retarded individuals can cope with the unexpected when traveling. It is inevitable that buses will be late, and people will get lost. A truly independent person must respond appropriately, yet such skills may be difficult to maintain given their relatively infrequent use.

Fire Safety Training

Fire safety training is another research area where people are trained to respond to unexpected problems. In a previous review on emergency skills, Marchetti and Matson (1981) reported only one fire safety study (Matson, 1980b). It is disconcerting that, in the years since, only one experimentally controlled study has been reported, especially in light of data suggesting the poor fire self-preservation abilities of mentally retarded people who live in community-based residences (MacEachron & Janicki, 1983; MacEachron & Krauss, 1985).

Rae and Roll (1985) anecdotally described a program in which profoundly mentally retarded people (6 females and 4 males, ages 22–42) were taught to escape from a fire. Haney and Jones (1982) established a design to program maintenance and generalization of skills needed to exit from a burning house at night. Subjects were three mentally retarded children (2 male and 1 female, mean IQ of 33, and age of 15). Training sessions consisted of verbal instruction, practice, social praise for correct responses, and candy when the entire response sequence was completed. Errors were followed by modeling and continued practice. During maintenance training, prompts, feedback, and social praise were faded, and children were taught to acquire candy on their own when they responded appropriately. Generalization training sessions were conducted in separate rooms. A multiple baseline across subjects established that children acquired 80% of the required emergency responses during training. Maintenance scores 2 to 4 months later declined slightly, and there were further declines in generalization probes in different rooms.

Like most studies that represent one of the first in an area, this experiment provoked more questions than it answered. For example: Is training subjects to respond to pictures of fire and smoke functionally appropriate considering other simulation research reported? What should be done about accuracy rates less than 100%? How do we train a response that might occur both infrequently and in the absence of adult trainers? Might it be best to train in the location the client is most likely to escape from? Fire and other safety skills training is a community living skill in need of much empirical research.

Telephone Skills

A community skill that has sometimes been trained as part of emergency skills is appropriate use of telephones (Risley & Cuvo, 1980). Telephone skills can also provide some parsimony to everyday life and the opportunity for social contact.

Smith and Meyers (1979) compared modeling with verbal instructions and modeling alone as means of teaching telephone skills to people with moderate to profound retardation (42 males and 18 females, mean age of 46). Subjects were assigned to groups, and results generally showed that verbal instruction added little to the modeling procedure.

In a systematic follow-up, Matson (1982) compared modeling and independence training as means to teach telephone conversation skills. Assessment consisted of trainers individually asking nine open-ended questions over the telephone to mildly mentally retarded adults (25 females and 20 males, mean IQ of 61, and age of 38). The modeling procedure was based on that described by Smith and Meyers (1979), and independence training was based on Matson (1980a). Results showed that independence training was significantly more effective than modeling alone in teaching appropriate phone skills.

Karen, Astin-Smith, and Creasy (1985) used a multiple-baseline design across subjects and skills to assess a program to teach phone-answering skills to six female high school students (mean IQ of 59, and age of 25). The skills consisted of calling someone to the phone, referring the caller to another number, dealing with a wrong number, and taking a message. Training procedures, consisting of verbal and physical prompts and social reinforcement, were described in exacting detail. The results showed the procedures to be generally effective during posttraining assessments and monthly follow-ups.

Recently Horner, Williams, and Stevely (1987) focused on generalized telephone use by special education high school students (2 males and 2 females, mean IQ of 45, and age of 19). Horner and his colleagues focused on simulation training that assessed the key stimulus/response relations in a given situation, and provided those relations in a training setting. A multiple baseline across subjects and behavior was used to evaluate the selection of stimulus dimensions and the training program, which consisted of verbal instructions, prompts, praise, and modeling. Behaviors taught included receiving and making telephone calls. Assessment showed a substantial increase in the number of correct responses from a set of telephone calls "systematically constructed to present subjects with the range of different situations they might encounter" (p. 233) in both home and school. Support was provided for the efficacy of training in simulation settings with materials representing the broad range of stimulus conditions likely to be encountered.

GENERALIZATION

Although it has been noted previously (Cuvo & Davis, 1983; Martin, Rusch, & Heal, 1982), this review once again indicates that generalization to the community environment encountered by the mentally retarded individual is the fundamental component of a community-living skill. A skill that does not generalize to a person's environment cannot be considered a community-living skill. Too much research has continued to use the "train and hope" (Stokes & Baer, 1977) method of achieving generalization. In this approach, generalization was assessed but not programmed. This strategy contradicts most behavior analytic research on stimulus control, which suggests that subjects tend to discriminate settings, not generalize across them.

Another less than desirable method frequently used to program generalization is called "sequential modification" (Stokes & Baer, 1977). In these cases, researchers trained subject behavior, assessed for generalization, failed to find any, so training simply continued in the community setting. It was unlikely that responses trained in this fashion would generalize to other community settings.

Fortunately, two treatment programs that produce generalization across settings have been designed: general case procedures and independence training. Each of these will be discussed in turn.

Arising from the concerns about generalization across settings, a debate emerged regarding training in schools versus *in vivo* training. Research that has focused on arranging stimulus training conditions as they would appear in the real-life environment showed that the school-based versus *in vivo* question was the wrong issue. Rather, the key question was: Are the stimulus relations that controlled the desired response in the training setting the same stimulus relations likely to be encountered in the natural environment? If so, then generalization to that environment was more likely to occur.

The training program that grew from such speculation is referred to as *general case programming*. This program emerged from educational research by Engelmann and his colleagues (Becker, Engelmann, & Thomas, 1975; Engelmann & Carnine, 1982). The first step in these training programs required the teacher to survey and operationalize the stimulus conditions under which the desired response was likely to be performed. The goal was to target the entire range of relevant stimulus events that controlled the desired behavior in the natural environment. Then, the teacher programmed this range of stimulus conditions to occur in the training settings. This methodology could be employed in either simulated or *in vivo* settings because the important ingredient was the stimuli that control behavior, not the location of training.

The type of problem that good general case programming can overcome was well illustrated by a minor problem encountered by Morrow and Bates (1987). Subjects were trained to perform laundry skills, but before the community follow-up could be completed, the price of doing a wash in the laundromat rose from 75 cents to 85 cents. The skill cluster trained included putting 75 cents into the washing machine, but this response was not consistent with the new response required by the price change, so a new skill component (putting in 85 cents) had to be trained. Of course, all research is limited by the cognitive capacities of the subjects, but ideally successful general case programming would have had the subjects learn to match the price listed in the laundromat with the appropriate coins. Changing the price of a load of laundry may seem trivial at first glance, but this exemplifies the type of dilemma likely to be encountered by mentally retarded persons living in the community, and the problem is not trivial if the appropriate generalized skill is not available.

A second program with elements designed to enhance generalization is *independence training*, first described by Matson (1980a). Generally, the first phase of this program was conducted in a classroom setting where subjects learned to verbalize appropriate responses to relevant stimuli, and a second phase was conducted either at a simulated or *in vivo* setting where the responses were practiced. Training was usually conducted in small groups. Verbal and physical prompts were used to evoke the behavior in training and to cue other group members to attend to the trainee currently practicing. The trainer evaluated subject performance, then the target subjects evaluated their own performance, followed by positive evaluations from other members of the training group, with the trainer consequating the accuracy of the evaluations. Trainees took turns functioning as the target subject. Generalization was enhanced by training subjects to evaluate their performance. This behavior served functionally to (1) reinforce skill performance in the absence of the trainer and (2) provide a solid cognitive conceptualization of the desired response. Also, training settings resembled those likely to be actually encountered.

A related concern is the assessment of generalization. Research consistently included observations in other settings and follow-up assessments. In a number of cases, training trials were included in these assessments, but researchers mislabeled the data as representing generalization. These types of data do not constitute generalization as defined by Stokes and Baer (1977),

> the occurrence of relevant behavior under different, non-training conditions (i.e., across subjects, settings, people, behaviors, and/or time) without the scheduling of the same events in those conditions as had been scheduled in training conditions. (p. 350)

The scientific validity of many studies would be enhanced by excluding training from generalization settings.

Most of the community skills research adequately examined acquisition of target behavior. Future research needs to continue to address generalization over subject's settings and time (Drabman, Hammer, & Rosenbaum, 1979), both in the form of programming for generalization and of assessing the degree to which it occurs.

METHODOLOGY

A majority of the articles reviewed in this chapter indicated experimental control through either group designs or within-subject comparisons, usually controlled by either multiple baselines or multiple probe designs. A common problem observed in the within-subject designs was multiple baselines across only two subjects or two behaviors. The integrity of the logic behind the multiple-baseline design involving multiplicative probabilities is decreased when there are less than three variables. Many of the studies could have been substantially improved by the addition of a third measured variable.

Teach/test designs of an AB format were still used in some studies, but this was less prevalent than previous reviews had indicated, and it is hoped that the use of this design will decline precipitously.

A methodological problem that could hinder replication and applicability of community skills research was the many vague and/or incomplete descriptions of the subjects, training procedures, and target responses. Replicability is a basic characteristic of sound research, and if an applied mental retardation worker cannot replicate a training procedure, then the significance of the research is limited. Additionally, studies that demonstrated the effectiveness of a treatment procedure, but failed to provide adequate descriptions of training procedures, made it difficult to specify which element(s) of the procedure (e.g., consequences, prompts, task analysis) were responsible for the positive outcome. Detailed training procedures and operational definitions for each target behavior would have enhanced the replicability of many of the studies.

Most of the research reported IQ, age, and sex of the subjects. These demographics are important for replication and application. Other subject characteristics that need to be reported more often include number of years institutionalized, current living arrangements and family support, prerequisite behaviors, language ability, disruptive behaviors, compliance, and physical handicaps. The inclusion of these factors would augment comparison of studies in efforts to define what population has been taught what skills.

SOCIAL VALIDITY

Some of the studies reported attempts to establish the importance of the skill taught in real life. In this regard, most of the skills had face validity, but a significant contribution could be made if the behaviors that account for most of the variance in successful community living were established and the definitions operationalized.

Very few of the studies gave any indication that the skills were subsequently used by the individuals after the research project terminated. The danger of excluding such information is that researchers are left open to the criticism that the study was done simply to prove that the technology exists, thus making it possible to teach certain skills to certain handicapped populations. This is an admirable goal, but what about the subjects in the research? Do they find their new skills useful or enjoyable? Reporting such information would add just as much social validity as reports from "experts" do, and it would establish the significance of the research question.

CONCLUSION

Empirical behavioral research on programs to teach community living skills to mentally retarded people has been reviewed. Research demonstrated that many complex community skills could be analyzed into component parts and taught via common techniques, such as instructions, modeling, behavioral rehearsal, graduated prompt levels, contingent descriptive praise, and the subsequent fading of such procedures. Indeed, it is remarkable how much progress has been made in teaching community skills to mentally retarded individuals. However, a lack of programmed generalization strategies often leads to poor maintenance or generalization across settings. On the positive side, treatment designs, such as general case programming and independence training, have established the feasibility of teaching behavior that may generalize. Methodological problems, such as a lack of experimental control, multiple baselines across only two components, and incomplete descriptions of treatment procedures, limited the possibilities for replication and applicability of many studies.

REFERENCES

Adkins, J., & Matson, J. L. (1980). Teaching institutionalized mentally retarded adults socially appropriate leisure skills. *Mental Retardation, 18,* 249–252.

Allen, L. D., & Iwata, B. A. (1980). Reinforcing exercise maintenance using existing high-rate activities. *Behavior Modification, 4,* 337–354.

Baer, D. M., & Wolf, M. M. (1970). The entry into natural communities of reinforcement. In R. Ulrich, T. Stachnik, & J. Mabry (Eds.), *Control of human behavior: Volume II* (pp. 319–324). Glenview, IL: Scott, Foresman.

Becker, W., Engelmann, S., & Thomas, D. (1975). *Teaching 2: Cognitive learning and instruction.* Chicago: Science Research Associate.

Birenbaum, A., & Re, M. A. (1979). Resettling mentally retarded adults in the community—Almost 4 years later. *American Journal of Mental Deficiency, 83,* 323–329.

Borakove, L. S., & Cuvo, A. J. (1977). Facilitative effects of coin displacement on teaching coin summation to mentally retarded adolescents. *American Journal of Mental Deficiency, 81,* 350–356.

Bourbeau, P. E., Sowers, J., & Close, D. W. (1986). An experimental analysis of generalization of banking skills from classroom to bank settings in the community. *Education and Training of the Mentally Retarded, 21,* 98–107.

Brown, J. E., Davis, E., & Flemming, P. L. (1979). Nutritional assessment of children with handicapping conditions. *Mental Retardation, 17,* 129–132.

Brown, L., Nisbet, J., Ford, A., Sweet, M., Shiraga, B., York, J., & Loomis, R. (1983). The critical need for nonschool instruction in educational programs for severely handicapped students. *Journal of the Association for the Severely Handicapped, 8,* 71–77.

Cipani, E., Augustine, A., & Blomgren, E. (1982). Teaching profoundly retarded adults to ascend stairs safely. *Education and Training of the Mentally Retarded, 17,* 51–54.

Coleman, A. E., Ayoub, M. M., & Friedrich, D. W. (1976). Assessment of the physical work capacity of institutionalized mentally retarded males. *American Journal of Mental Deficiency, 80,* 629–635.

Coleman, R. J., & Whitman, T. L. (1984). Developing, generalizing, and maintaining physical fitness in mentally retarded adults: Toward a self-directed program. *Analysis and Intervention in Developmental Disabilities, 4,* 109–127.

Colozzi, G. A., & Pollow, R. S. (1984). Teaching independent walking to mentally retarded children in a public school. *Education and Training of the Mentally Retarded, 19,* 97–101.

Crain, C., McLaughlin, J., & Eisenhart, M. (1983). The social and physical effects of a 10-week dance program on educable mentally retarded adolescents. *Education and Training of the Mentally Retarded, 18,* 308–312.

Crapps, J. M., Langone, J., & Swaim, S. (1985). Quantity and quality of participation in community environments by mentally retarded adults. *Education and Training of the Mentally Retarded, 20,* 123–129.

Cuvo, A. J., Jacobi, L., & Sipko, R. (1981). Teaching laundry skills to mentally retarded students. *Education and Training of the Mentally Retarded, 16,* 54–64.

Cuvo, A. J., & Davis, P. K. (1983). Behavior therapy and community living skills. In M. Hersen, R. Eisler, & P. Miller (Eds.), *Progress in behavior modification* (Vol. 14, pp. 132–156). New York: Academic Press.

Donder, D., & Nietupski, J. (1981). Nonhandicapped adolescents teaching playground skills to their mentally retarded peers: Toward a less restrictive middle school environment. *Education and Training of the Mentally Retarded, 16,* 270–276.

Drabman, R. S., Hammer, D., & Rosenbaum, M. J. (1979). Assessing generalization in behavior modification with children: The generalization map. *Behavioral Assessment, 1,* 203–219.

Emery, C. L., Watson, J. L., Watson, P. J., Thompson, D. M., & Biderman, M. D. (1985). Variables related to body weight status of mentally retarded adults. *American Journal of Mental Deficiency, 90,* 34–39.

Engelmann, S., & Carnine, D. (1982). *Theory of instruction: Principles and applications.* New York: Irvington.

Eriksen, E. (1977). *Toys and reasons.* New York: Norton.

Fain, G. S. (1986). Leisure: A moral imperative. *Mental Retardation, 24,* 261–263.

Fajardo, D. M., & McGourty, D. G. (1983). Promoting social play in small groups of retarded adolescents. *Education and Training of the Mentally Retarded, 18,* 300–307.

Feltz, D. L. (1980). Teaching a high-avoidance motor task to a retarded child through participant modeling. *Education and Training of the Mentally Retarded, 15,* 152–155.

Fox, R., Burkhart, J. E., & Rotatori, A. F. (1983). Eating behavior of obese and nonobese mentally retarded adults. *American Journal of Mental Deficiency, 87,* 570–573.

Frank, A. R., & McFarland, T. D. (1980). Teaching coin skills to EMR children: A curriculum study. *Education and Training of the Mentally Retarded, 15,* 270–278.

Frank, A. R., & Wacker, D. P. (1986). Analysis of a visual prompting procedure on acquisition and generalization of coin skills by mentally retarded children. *American Journal of Mental Deficiency, 90,* 468–472.

Frith, G. H., Mitchell, J. W., & Roswal, G. (1980). Recreation for mildly retarded students: An important component of individualized education plans. *Education and Training of the Mentally Retarded, 15,* 199–203.

Gaule, K., Nietupski, J., & Certo, N. (1985). Teaching supermarket shopping skills using an adaptive shopping list. *Education and Training of the Mentally Retarded, 20,* 53–59.

Gruber, B., Reeser, R., & Reid, D. H. (1979). Providing a less restrictive environment for profoundly retarded persons by teaching independent walking skills. *Journal of Applied Behavior Analysis, 12,* 285–297.

Haney, J. I., & Jones, R. T. (1982). Programming maintenance as a major component of a community-centered preventive effort: Escape from fire. *Behavior Therapy, 13,* 47–62.

Haring, T. G. (1985). Teaching between class generalization of toy play behavior to handicapped children. *Journal of Applied Behavior Analysis, 18,* 127–139.

Haring, T. G., Kennedy, C. H., Adams, M. J., & Pitts-Conway, V. (1987). Teaching generalization of purchasing skills across community settings to autistic youth using videotape modeling. *Journal of Applied Behavior Analysis, 20,* 89–96.

Horner, R. H., Williams, J. A., & Stevely, J. D. (1987). Acquisition of generalized telephone use by students with moderate and severe mental retardation. *Research in Developmental Disabilities, 8,* 229–247.

Jeffree, D. M., & Cheseldine, S. E. (1984). Programmed leisure intervention and the interaction patterns of severely mentally retarded adolescent: A pilot study. *American Journal of Mental Deficiency, 88,* 619–624.

Johnson, B. F., & Cuvo, A. J. (1981). Teaching mentally retarded adults to cook. *Behavior Modification, 5,* 187–202.

Jones, M. L., Favell, J. E., Lattimore, J., & Risley, T. R. (1984). Improving independent engagement of nonambulatory multihandicapped persons through the systematic analysis of leisure materials. *Analysis and Intervention in Developmental Disabilities, 4,* 313–332.

Karen, R. L., Astin-Smith, S., & Creasy, D. (1985). Teaching telephone-answering skills to mentally retarded adults. *American Journal of Mental Deficiency, 89,* 595–609.

Keogh, D. A., Faw, G. D., Whitman, T. L., & Reid, D. H. (1984). Enhancing leisure skills in severely retarded adolescents through a self-instructional treatment package. *Analysis and Intervention in Developmental Disabilities, 4,* 333–351.

Lagomarcino, A., Reid, D. H., Ivanvic, M. T., & Faw, G. D. (1984). Leisure-dance instruction for severely and profoundly retarded persons: Teaching an intermediate community living skill. *Journal of Applied Behavior Analysis, 17,* 71–84.

Li, A. K. F. (1981). Play and the mentally retarded child. *Mental Retardation, 19,* 121–126.

Luyben, P. D., Funk, D. M., Morgan, J. K., Clark, K. A., & Delulio, D. W. (1986). Team sports for the severely retarded: Training a side-of-the-foot soccer pass using a maximum to minimum prompt reduction strategy. *Journal of Applied Behavior Analysis, 19,* 431–436.

MacEachron, A. E., & Janicki, M. P. (1983). Self-preservation ability and residential fire emergencies. *American Journal of Mental Deficiency, 88,* 157–163.

MacEachron, A. E., & Krauss, M. W. (1985). Self-preservation ability and residential fire emergencies: Replication and criterion-validity study. *American Journal of Mental Deficiency, 90,* 107–110.

Maksud, M. G., & Hamilton, L. H. (1974). Physiological responses of EMR children to strenuous exercise. *American Journal of Mental Deficiency, 79,* 32–38.

Marchant, J., & Wehman, P. (1979). Teaching table games to severely retarded children. *Mental Retardation, 17,* 150–152.

Marchetti, A., & Matson, J. L. (1981). Training skills for community adjustment. In J. L. Matson & J. R. McCartney (Eds.), *Handbook of behavior modification with the mentally retarded* (pp. 211–246). New York: Plenum Press.

Marchetti, A. G. (1987). *Wyatt v. Stickney:* A consent decree. *Research in Developmental Disabilities, 8,* 249–259.

Marchetti, A. G., McCartney, J. R., Drain, S., Hooper, M., & Dix, J. (1983). Pedestrian skills training for mentally retarded adults: Comparison of training in two settings. *Mental Retardation, 21,* 107–110.

Marchetti, A. G., Cecil, C. E., Graves, J., & Marchetti, D. C. (1984). Public transportation instruction: Comparison of classroom instruction, community instruction, and facility-grounds instruction. *Mental Retardation, 22,* 128–136.

Marholin, D., II, O'Toole, K. M., Touchette, P. E., Berger, P. L., & Doyle, D. A. (1979). "I'll have a Big Mac, large fries, large coke, and apple pie," . . . or teaching adaptive community skills. *Behavior Therapy, 10,* 236–248.

Martin, J. E., Rusch, F. R., & Heal, L. W. (1982). Teaching community survival skills to mentally retarded adults: A review and analysis. *Journal of Special Education, 16,* 243–267.

Matson, J. L. (1979). A field tested system of training meal preparation skills to the mentally retarded. *British Journal of Mental Subnormality, 25,* 14–18.

Matson, J. L. (1980a). A controlled group study of pedestrian-skill training for the mentally retarded. *Behaviour Research and Therapy, 18,* 99–106.

Matson, J. L. (1980b). Preventing home accidents: A training program for the retarded. *Behavior Modification, 4,* 397–410.

Matson, J. L. (1981). Use of independence training to teach shopping skills to mildly mentally retarded adults. *American Journal of Mental Deficiency, 86,* 178–183.

Matson, J. L. (1982). Independence training vs modeling procedures for teaching phone conversation skills to the mentally retarded. *Behaviour Research and Therapy, 20,* 505–511.

Matson, J. L., & Long, S. (1986). Teaching computation/shopping skills to mentally retarded adults. *American Journal of Mental Deficiency, 91,* 98–101.

McDonnell, J. J., & Horner, R. H. (1985). Effects of in vivo versus simulation-plus in vivo training on the acquisition and generalization of grocery item selection by high school students with severe handicaps. *Analysis and Intervention in Developmental Disabilities, 5,* 323–343.

Morrow, S. A., & Bates, P. E. (1987). The effectiveness of three sets of school based instructional materials and community training on the acquisition and generalization of community laundry skills by students with severe handicaps. *Research in Developmental Disabilities, 8,* 113–136.

Neef, N. A., Iwata, B., & Page, T. (1978). Public transportation training: In vivo versus classroom instruction. *Journal of Applied Behavior Analysis, 11,* 331–344.

Nietupski, J., & Svoboda, R. (1982). Teaching a cooperative leisure skill to severely handicapped adults. *Education and Training of the Mentally Retarded, 17,* 38–43.

Nietupski, J., Welch, J., & Wacker, D. (1983). Acquisition, maintenance, and transfer of grocery item purchasing skills by moderately and severely handicapped students. *Education and Training of the Mentally Retarded, 18,* 279–286.

Nietupski, J., Clancy, P., Wehrmacher, L., & Parmer, C. (1985). Effects of minimal versus lengthy delay between simulated and in vivo instruction on community performance. *Education and Training of the Mentally Retarded, 20,* 190–195.

Nietupski, J., Hamre-Nietupski, S., Green, K., Varnum-Teeter, K., Twedt, B., LePera, D., Scebold, K., & Hanrahan, M. (1986). Self-initiated and sustained leisure activity participation by students with moderate/severe handicaps. *Education and Training of the Mentally Retarded, 21,* 259–264.

Nirje, B. (1969). The normalization principle and its human management implications. In R. Kugel & W. Wolfensberger (Eds.), *Changing patterns in residential services for the mentally retarded.* Washington, DC: President's Committee on Mental Retardation.

Page, T. J., Iwata, B. A., & Neef, N. A. (1976). Teaching pedestrian skills to retarded persons: Generalization from the classroom to the natural environment. *Journal of Applied Behavior Analysis, 9,* 433–444.

Piaget, J. (1951). *Play, dreams, and imitation in childhood.* London: Heineman.

Premack, D. (1959). Toward empirical behavior laws: 1. Positive reinforcement. *Psychological Review, 66,* 219–233.

Rae, R., & Roll, D. (1985). Fire safety training with adults who are profoundly mentally retarded. *Mental Retardation, 23,* 26–30.

Reiter, S., & Levi, A. M. (1981). Leisure activities of mentally retarded adults. *American Journal of Mental Deficiency, 86,* 201–203.

Reitz, A. L. (1984). Teaching community skills to formally institutionalized adults: Eating nutritionally balanced diets. *Analysis and Intervention in Developmental Disabilities, 4,* 299–312.

Risley, R., & Cuvo, A. J. (1980). Training mentally retarded adults to make emergency telephone calls. *Behavior Modification, 4,* 513–526.

Robinson, D., Griffith, J., McComish, K., & Swasbrook, K. (1984). Bus training for developmentally disabled adults. *American Journal of Mental Deficiency, 89,* 37–43.

Salzberg, C. L., & Langford, C. A. (1981). Community integration of mentally retarded adults through leisure activity. *Mental Retardation, 19,* 127–131.

Sarason, S. B. (1974). *The psychological sense of community: Prospects for a community psychology.* San Francisco: Jossey-Bass.

Sarber, R. E., & Cuvo, A. J. (1983). Teaching nutritional meal planning to developmentally disabled clients. *Behavior Modification, 7,* 503–530.

Sarber, R. E., Halasz, M. M., Messmer, M. C., Bickett, A. D., & Lutzker, J. R. (1983). Teaching menu planning and grocery shopping skills to a mentally retarded mother. *Mental Retardation, 21,* 101–106.

Schalock, R. L., Harper, R. S., & Carver, G. (1981). Independent living placement: Five years later. *American Journal of Mental Deficiency, 86,* 170–177.

Scheerenberger, R. C. (1982). *Public residential facilities for the mentally retarded.* National Association of Superintendents of Public Residential Facilities for the Mentally Retarded. Madison, WI.

Schleien, S. J., Kiernan, J., & Wehman, P. (1981). Evaluation of an age-appropriate leisure skills program for moderately retarded adults. *Education and Training of the Mentally Retarded, 16,* 13–19.

Schleien, S. J., Wehman, P., & Kiernan, J. (1981). Teaching leisure skills to severely handicapped adults: An age appropriate darts game. *Journal of Applied Behavior Analysis, 14,* 513–519.

Schleien, S. J., Certo, N. J., & Muccino, A. (1984). Acquisition of leisure skills by a severely handicapped adolescent: A data based instructional program. *Education and Training of the Mentally Retarded, 19,* 297–305.

Schurrer, R., Weltman, A., & Brammell, H. (1985). Effects of physical training on cardiovascular fitness and behavior patterns of mentally retarded adults. *American Journal of Mental Deficiency, 90,* 167–169.

Shafer, M. S., Inge, K. J., & Hill, J. (1986). Acquisition, generalization, and maintenance of automated banking skills. *Education and Training of the Mentally Retarded, 21,* 265–272.

Smith, M., & Meyers, A. (1979). Telephone-skills training for retarded adults: Group and individual demonstrations with and without verbal instruction. *American Journal of Mental Deficiency, 83,* 581–587.

Snell, M. (1983). *Systematic instruction of the moderately and severely handicapped.* Columbus, OH: Charles E. Merrill.

Stapley, V. J., Smith, M. A. H., Bittle, J. B., Andrews, F. E., & Nuckolls, L. J. (1984). Food and nutrition education for children who are mentally retarded. *Mental Retardation, 22,* 289–293.

Stokes, T. F., & Baer, D. M. (1977). An implicit technology of generalization. *Journal of Applied Behavior Analysis, 10,* 349–367.

Thompson, T. J., Braam, S. J., & Fuqua, R. W. (1982). Training and generalization of laundry skills: A multiple probe evaluation with handicapped persons. *Journal of Applied Behavior Analysis, 15,* 177–182.

van Den Pol, R. A., Iwata, B. A., Ivanvcic, M. T., Page, T. J., Neef, N. A., & Whitley, F. P. (1981). Teaching the handicapped to eat in public places: Acquisition, generalization, and maintenance of restaurant skills. *Journal of Applied Behavior Analysis, 14,* 61–69.

Wacker, D. P., Berg, W. K., & Moore, S. J. (1984). Increasing on-task performance of students with severe handicaps on cooperative games. *Education and Training of the Mentally Retarded, 19,* 183–190.

Wehman, P. (1975). Establishing play behaviors in mentally retarded youth. *Rehabilitation Literature, 38,* 98–105.

Wehman, P., & Schleien, S. (1980). Assessment and selection of leisure skills for severely handicapped individuals. *Education and Training of the Mentally Retarded, 15,* 50–57.

Welch, J., Nietupski, J., & Hamre-Nietupski, S. (1985). Teaching public transportation problem solving skills to young adults with moderate handicaps. *Education and Training of the Mentally Retarded, 20,* 287–295.

Wheeler, J., Ford, A., Nietupski, J., Loomis, R., & Brown, L. (1980). Teaching moderately and severely handicapped adolescents to shop in supermarkets using pocket calculators. *Education and Training of the Mentally Retarded, 15,* 105–112.

Wilcox, B., & Bellamy, G. T. (Eds.). (1982). *Design of high school programs for severely handicapped students.* Baltimore: Brookes.

Williams, R. D., & Ewing, S. (1981). Consumer roulette: The shopping patterns of mentally retarded persons. *Mental Retardation, 19,* 145–149.

Wilson, P. G., Cuvo, A. J., & Davis, P. K. (1986). Training a functional skill cluster: Nutritious meal planning within a budget, grocery list writing, and shopping. *Analysis and Intervention in Developmental Disabilities, 6,* 179–201.

Wolfensberger, W. (1972). *The principle of normalization in human services.* Washington, DC: National Institute on Mental Retardation.

Wuerch, B. B., & Voeltz, L. M. (1982). *Longitudinal leisure skills for severely handicapped learners: The Ho'onanea Curriculum Component.* Baltimore: Brookes.

V

Treating Social and Emotional Problems

12

Social Skills

ALLEN G. MARCHETTI AND VINCENT A. CAMPBELL

INTRODUCTION

The most striking aspect of the literature pertaining to social skills theory, training, and evaluation is the lack of a clear and generally accepted definition of social skills. Major conceptual and definitional differences exist between behavioristic and trait theorists and practitioners regarding the molecular versus molar focus of study and treatment (McFall, 1982). These differences bear directly on definitional matters and the psychological processes involved in social skills. Curran (1979a) indicated his inclination is to "limit the construct of social skill to motoric behavior" (p. 323), but admits to ambivalence regarding the inclusion of cognition as a factor in social skills. On the other hand, Trower (1979) suggested that social skill has perceptual, cognitive, and performance components. Likewise, McFall (1982) favored a multiprocess conception of social skills, suggesting a model consisting of decoding (perceptual), decision (cognitive), and encoding (performance) skills. The tendency toward including more processes and behaviors within the scope of social skills led Curran (1979a) to state,

> If we do not restrain ourselves and put some limits on the construct of social skill, it will expand to include all human behavior, and social skills training will soon come to mean any process which is capable of producing changes in human behavior. (p. 323)

Distinctions have been made between social performance and social skills (McFall, 1982), the former being a "general evaluative term referring to the quality or adequacy of a person's overall performance in a particular task," whereas social skills refer to "the specific abilities required to perform competently at a task" (pp. 12, 13). In this context, social performance can be viewed as a molar evaluation of a person's overall behavior in a social situation, whereas skills can be seen as the constituent behaviors that contribute to the overall performance.

Bernstein (1981) discussed the difficulties that result from the lack of a consistent definition of social skills. Unfortunately, her solution, as is the case

ALLEN G. MARCHETTI • Georgia Retardation Center, 4770 Peachtree Road N.E., Atlanta, Georgia 30338.   VINCENT A. CAMPBELL • Department of Mental Health and Mental Retardation, 135 South Union Street, Montgomery, Alabama 36130.

with a number of authors, is to coin yet another term, "interpersonal skills," that relates to the general area of social skills and to define it. Such an approach does little to clarify a situation already rife with terms and definitions. Because of the wide variety of psychological processes, behaviors, theories, and applications that relate directly or tangentially to contacts between people, we will attempt, in this chapter, to address the topic very broadly and will present reports of studies that are described by their authors as addressing the development of interpersonal behavior in mentally retarded people. In this chapter, no new definition or innovative terms will be proposed.

In general, social skills training is an area of applied behavior analysis that is noteworthy, in part, because of the wide range of populations identified as displaying deficiencies. Clinical and nonclinical applications of social skills training procedures have been employed with regard to schizophrenia (Bellack, Hersen, & Turner, 1976; Hersen & Bellack, 1976; Hersen, Eisler, & Miller, 1973; Shephard, 1986), social anxiety (Trower, 1986), depression (Libet & Lewinsohn, 1973; Williams, 1986), substance abuse (Monti, Abrams, Binkoff, & Zwick, 1986), alcoholism (Miller & Eisler, 1977), dating skills in college students (Hedquist & Weinhold, 1970), delinquency (Henderson & Hollin, 1986), criminal and antisocial behavior (Howells, 1986), and mental retardation (Matson & DiLorenzo, 1986).

Curran (1979a) commented that social skills training is a heterogeneous treatment approach that may vary in structure, content, theoretical orientation, and other dimensions. For our purposes, social skills training refers to a broad category of applied behavior analysis and intervention techniques. They are applied to assist clients acquire responses, which when displayed during interpersonal interactions, will be deemed appropriate for the situation.

The issue of social behavior is central for mentally retarded people. The current definition of mental retardation requires that a person display impairments in adaptive behavior concurrent with significantly subaverage intelligence (Grossman, 1983). Adaptive behavior scales typically contain items or dimensions that measure social functioning (Meyers, Nihira, & Zetlin, 1979). Studies of the factor structure of adaptive behavior scales have yielded dimensions of positive behavior that have been described as social. Lambert and Nicoll (1976) identified "social responsibility" as a dimension of adaptive behavior using the American Association on Mental Deficiency (AAMD) Adaptive Behavior Scale (ABS)—Public School Version. Factor analysis of Part 1 of the ABS by Nihira (1976) yielded a Personal-Social Responsibility factor.

The social skills training approaches that are covered in this chapter are limited to response acquisition programs. Programs designed to decrease or eliminate maladaptive behaviors are not included. Consideration is also limited to social behavior as distinct from other adaptive behavior domains, such as work or leisure, that are affected by social performance. Further, programs designed to develop more basic self-help skills, such as dining and toileting, are not included, although deficiencies in these areas are likely to elicit strong social responses from other people.

The material that follows is organized to highlight evaluation and training procedures that have been employed with mentally retarded people. A comprehensive review of the literature bearing on social skills training of mentally retarded people is beyond the scope of this chapter. Within this context, studies are cited that exemplify the evaluation and training procedures. More comprehensive reviews of this literature may be found in Andrasik and Matson (1985), Matson and DiLorenzo (1986), Matson, DiLorenzo, and Andrasik (1983), and Robertson, Richardson, and Youngson (1984).

EVALUATION OF SOCIAL SKILLS AND SOCIAL SKILLS TRAINING

A sizable body of literature has developed on the evaluation of social skills. However, problems continue to exist with regard to the methods used to assess social skills, the level of assessment (i.e., molar or molecular), and the scales or other measures used in evaluation (Bellack, 1983). A more fundamental problem relating to the evaluation of social skills has to do with the continuing absence of a suitable and generally agreed upon definition (Zigler, Balla, & Hoddap, 1984). Another problem of considerable proportions is that few, if any, of the procedures used to assess social skills are valid, reliable, and practical (Gresham & Elliott, 1987).

This general literature bears indirectly on issues confronted by the evaluator of social skills of mentally retarded people. By definition, mentally retarded people demonstrate impairments in adaptive behavior, a major component of which is social behavior (Grossman, 1983). The cognitive limitations characteristic of mental retardation add to the concerns regarding client-based sources of information, such as self-reports and role-playing, that are widely used in social skills evaluation. Issues of considerable importance with a mentally retarded population, such as the cognitive ability to acquire skills and to generalize across situations, may be of lesser concern with a nonretarded group.

Although controversy regarding such conceptual issues as molar and molecular models of social skills (McFall, 1982) have parallels in evaluation, there is somewhat less overall disagreement regarding the objectives of social skills assessment. The following material deals with social skills assessment from the point of view of the purpose of evaluation, that is, global assessment of social skills, identification of specific deficits, and evaluation of training outcomes, particularly as related to mentally retarded people. For broader and more detailed presentations of material related to evaluation of social skills, the reader is encouraged to refer to Bellack (1979a,b), Curran (1979b), Curran and Wessberg (1981), and Conger and Conger (1986).

OBJECTIVES OF SOCIAL SKILLS EVALUATION

Social skills may be assessed at several levels depending on the objective of the evaluation. At a molar level, evaluation is directed at identifying individuals with an overall deficiency in social performance. Such overall evaluations generally focus on typical performance of the individual and indicate whether or not a social deficiency exists in comparison to some norm group. The evaluations typically do not focus on etiological factors. At a somewhat lower level of evaluation, domains or dimensions of social performance are examined to identify those that result in poor social performance. For instance, a person may be found deficient in greeting behaviors. At a molecular level, deficiencies in specific component behavior of a particular social dimension are identified for remediation through training.

Bellack (1979b) provided guidelines for the behavioral evaluation of social skills. They include determining whether a person displays general social skills deficiencies, identifying the circumstances under which these deficiencies are displayed, identifying the etiology of the deficiency in social performance, and specifying the behavioral components of the overall skill that the clients lacks and that result in deficient performance. To this list may be added evaluating the outcomes of social skills training programs (Kazdin, 1977) and consideration of the social environment in which the client is expected to respond appropriately in social situations. In the following section, social skills evaluation is discussed in light of three evaluative purposes: (1) evaluating overall social performance, (2) identifying specific social deficiencies, and (3) assessing the outcome of social skills training. Within each section relating to the purpose of social skills evaluation, the sources of data and problems are discussed.

Evaluation of Overall Social Skills

Unlike nonretarded individuals who present for treatment of social skills deficits in a relatively circumscribed area, mentally retarded people are generally deficient across a broad spectrum of social behavior (Affleck, 1977). Zigler, Balla, and Hoddap (1984) have raised questions regarding the use of social adaptation (i.e., adaptive behavior) as a diagnostic criterion for mental retardation, primarily because of a lack of precision as to the nature of the construct and, as a result, the lack of validity of the scales. Measures of social skills of mentally retarded people generally consist of items that bear on social awareness, greeting behaviors, and interpersonal manners. However, in many cases, the social nature of the skills subsumed under the label *social skills* is remote. For instance, the Fairview Social Skills Scale for Mildly and Moderately Retarded (Ross & Giampiccolo, 1972) includes items related to toileting, dining, dressing and other self-help behaviors. In other instances, the area of social skills is tapped by relatively few items. The American Association on Mental Deficiency (AAMD) Adaptive Behavior Scale includes seven items for evaluating global social skills: Cooperation, consideration for others, awareness of others, interaction with others, participation in group activities, selfishness, and social maturity. An improvement in this test appears to have been made with the Vineland Adaptive Behavior Scales (Sparrow, Balla, & Cicchetti, 1984), which includes 37 items within three domains of socialization—interpersonal relationships, play and leisure time, and coping skills. These two widely used scales provide detailed norms for interpreting social performance of mentally retarded people (McCarver & Campbell, 1987). The Social Performance Survey Schedule (Matson, Helsel, Bellack, & Senatore, 1983), is a social behavior inventory developed specifically for use with a mentally retarded population. It provides a multidimensional assessment of social skills but does not provide norms for comparative evaluation of a particular client's performance.

Interference mechanisms have been cited by Curran (1979b, 1985; Curran & Wessberg, 1981; Affleck, 1977) as affecting social skills performance. The cognitive limitations inherent in mental retardation impose a ceiling effect both on the acquisition of specific social skills and on the ultimate level of social performance that may be realized by mentally retarded people. As cognitive impairment increases, the ultimate level of social behavior development can be expected to decrease.

A second class of interference mechanisms that have an adverse potential for the social performance of mentally retarded people is concerned with motivational and personality factors. Zigler has written extensively on the effect of differential motivational factors that affect the behavior of mentally retarded people (Zigler, 1966, 1969; Zigler & Balla, 1982; Zigler et al., 1984). Although the focus of much of Zigler's work has centered on the effect of noncognitive factors on cognitive performance, the experiential and developmental histories of many mentally retarded people can be seen to have manifestations in social performance. Such factors, as identified by Zigler and his associates, include wariness, expectation of failure, differential reinforcement hierarchies, anxiety, outerdirectedness, effects of institutions, and imitative behavior (Balla & Zigler, 1979). Consideration must be given to these variables, which may result in poor social performance, and it must not be assumed that overall deficiencies in social performance are due to a lack of learning of the component behaviors.

The four most commonly employed sources of information for social skills evaluation are self-report methods, *in vivo* observations of behavior, observations of behavior during simulated situations, and observation of behavior during role-play situations (Bellack, 1979a). Although these sources have been characterized as lacking in psychometric foundation (Bellack, 1979b), the most commonly used source of information regarding the social skills of mentally retarded people is an informant who is familiar with the client's typical behavior (Meyers et al., 1979). Informant-based evaluations have been criticized for lack of interrater reliability, emotional involvement of the informant, and lack of precision in terminology (e.g., "always," "usually," "sometimes," "never") (Meyers et al., 1979). Widely used scales such as the AAMD Adaptive Behavior Scale (Nihira, Foster, Shellhaas, & Leland, 1974) and the Vineland Adaptive Behavior Scales (Sparrow et al., 1984) typically rely on informants.

Several inventories and standardized observation approaches have been developed for use with mentally retarded populations. A major problem with such instruments has to do with the situational specificity of social behavior (Powers & Handleman, 1984). Relying as they do on informant reports or observations in highly specific situations, these scales make use of only a small sample of social behavior as the basis for evaluation. A version of the Social Performance Survey Schedule (Lowe & Cautela, 1978) has been adapted for use with mentally retarded people. The resulting instrument contains 57 items in 4 dimensions that were obtained through factor analysis (Matson, Helsel, Bellack, & Senatore, 1983). Although the instrument has promise for use with this population, no norms are provided that indicate age- and sex-related profiles of social performance. The Behavioral Interpersonal Problem Solving Test (Vaughn, Ridley, & Cox, 1983) involves the scoring by a trained examiner of subject responses to interpersonal problem situations. Again, this instrument provides no norms for evaluating the relative performance of the mentally retarded subject.

Identification of Specific Social Deficiencies

The majority of social skills training studies do not address the issue of identifying target deficiencies for remediation. Typically, skills are selected *a priori*, and comparisons are made between skill acquisition techniques or between subject groups. However, the social skills trainer of mentally retarded people must identify social deficiencies that are particularly problematic, or must establish a training hierarchy related to the subject's particular developmental level. Evaluation scales of overall behavior, such as the AAMD Adaptive Behavior Scale and the Vineland Adaptive Behavior Scales, generally contain some items that relate to the social performance of mentally retarded people. However, such scales typically provide a unitary score for social functioning, which does little to inform the evaluator of specific deficiencies (Bellack, 1979a). These scales typically do not evaluate the skills along a continuum of performance, but assess in an all-or-none fashion. As noted above, these scales provide little information regarding factors that may contribute to the deficiency. Once it has been determined that the client is deficient in social skills, a much more specific evaluation is needed to identify the specific component behaviors in which the client is deficient. The primary approaches to this task include social validation, sociometric methods, informant reports, and task analysis.

Social validation techniques (Wolf, 1978) have been employed to identify specific social deficiencies of mentally retarded people (Kazdin & Matson, 1981). Within this evaluation approach, behavioral inventories may be used to identify specific components of behaviors that contribute to acceptable behavior within circumscribed situations that are vital to overall training objectives, such as living in more normalized residential settings. Once a scale or inventory of behavior is developed, individual clients may be rated by employing subjective evaluation to determine the specific deficiencies that inhibit successful performance.

A procedure employed by Strain (1983), in a study involving developmentally disabled 3- to 5-year-old children in mainstream classes, appears to have promise with regard to identifying behavioral goals. In this study, social skills were included or excluded for consideration in a preschool social skills curriculum based on the social status of nonhandicapped classmates of handicapped children. This approach appears to deal quite effectively with the lack of empirical basis for social validation, which relies on professional judgment regarding the types of social skills that contribute to effective social interactions.

Task analysis of the specific behavioral interaction may be employed to break it down into the specific component motor behaviors. Within the task analysis, the component behaviors are identified and arranged hierarchically in such a manner that a particular client's performance may be evaluated in terms of component skills that are or are not in his or her behavioral repertoire (Powers & Handleman, 1984). Task analysis of social interactions are complicated by the situational specificity of social behavior (Kazdin, 1977). As noted by Bijou (1981), task analysis must be tailored to the learning and behavioral repertoire of the individual child. In this regard, social validation may be used to provide a basis for an initial task analysis. However, the learning progress of the individual must be monitored periodically to promote effective learning.

As is true when evaluating the overall social performance of a mentally retarded person, the social skills evaluator and trainer must take factors other than skill deficiencies into account when identifying social skills deficiencies for training. It is important to bring cognitive factors into consideration when setting training goals. For instance, the differential social expectations within institutions, sheltered community residential settings, and independent living must be factors when setting the overall goals of a particular social skills training program. Evaluation of social skills, and the setting of training goals, should consider the developmental level of the client (Harris & Ferrari, 1983; Powers & Handleman, 1984). As noted by Greenspan (1979), developmental level has a direct bearing on such related issues as role taking, social inference, social comprehension, insight, moral judgment, referential communication, and social problem solving. These processes are developmental in nature, are strongly related to cognitive understanding of social situations, and have a direct impact on the production of competent display of social behavior.

Evaluation of Outcome of Training

There are two broad issues related to the assessment of social skills training outcomes: determining whether there has been a change in the target behavior and evaluating the practical significance of the behavioral change in terms of the client's day-to-day performance (Kazdin, 1977). In a research context, the first issue usually is approached experimentally by comparing the results of a treatment group with groups receiving no treatment or other treatments. The second issue relates to the significance of the behavior change in the light of some standard of behavior or reference group, and the extent to which the behavior change is maintained over time and generalizes across social situations. Although both areas are of concern to the social skills trainer, determining the practical significance of a behavior change probably presents greater difficulty to the practitioner. In general, it may be stated that experimentally significant behavioral change does not necessarily mean that a practical change has occurred in the client's behavior.

Social validation (Kazdin, 1977; Kazdin & Matson, 1981; Wolf, 1978) has been proposed for evaluating the practical significance of training programs. This approach employs two components: social comparison and subjective evaluation (Kazdin & Matson, 1981). The social comparison component, as the term implies, involves the comparison of a client's social behavior after treatment with that of some appropriate peer group. As is true with the use of the social validation approach in identifying target behaviors for training, a problem exists with regard to identification of an appropriate criterion group with which to compare the client's posttreatment behavior (Curran, 1979a; Kazdin, 1977). Considering the attainment ceiling imposed on many mentally retarded people by cognitive interference, it may be unrealistic to use a non-retarded criterion group. Subjective evaluation, the second component of social validation, relies on the judgment of informants regarding the overall performance of the client. Kazdin (1977) has commented on problems that may be associated with the use of subjective evaluation, including the face validity of instruments used to evaluate global social performance, lack of reliability between raters, and bias of the evaluator toward the client. One recommendation with regard to the last concern involves the use of evaluators with no prior experience with the client.

The issue of criterion groups is especially difficult with more severely mentally retarded clients (Kazdin, 1977). For these persons, it is not realistic to use a nonretarded criterion group. A more useful approach to this problem may be to identify mentally retarded people whose social skills are not viewed as problematic as a criterion group and to assess the client's posttreatment behavior in light of their performance. Again, the approach taken by Strain (1983) for developing curriculum goals may be of use in evaluating treatment outcomes. Using some means, such as sociometric analysis, to identify people who demonstrate high- and low-performance levels, and comparing post-treatment behavior of the client against that of the high-performance group would provide a more objective criterion of training success.

As noted above, assessment of the practical aspects of behavior change involves evaluation of the extent to which the desired change is maintained over time and has generalized beyond the immediate training situation. Follow-up observations of target behaviors have been employed in a number of studies to determine the extent to which it has been maintained over time (e.g., Bramston & Spence, 1985; Matson & Senatore, 1981; Senatore, Matson, & Kazdin, 1982; Turner, Hersen, & Bellack, 1978; Wildman, Wildman, & Kelly, 1986). Unfortunately, follow-up probes for maintenance of target skills has not become a routine procedure in training studies (Mash & Terdal, 1977).

Few studies have assessed the issue of generalization of social skills. Stainback, Stainback, and Strathe, in a review of generalization of social skills (1983) identified four categories of generalization: "(a) generalization across settings, (b) generalization across individuals, (c) generalization across settings and individuals, and (d) generalization across settings, individuals, and behaviors" (p. 293). Although a number of studies reviewed in this chapter attempted to assess generalization over individuals and settings by employing role-playing, subject/confederates interactions, and so forth, few evaluated the target behaviors in actual community settings during natural social events. Because of the situational specificity of social skills, and the difficulty encountered by mentally retarded people in generalizing learned responses (Campione & Brown, 1977), it is important that assessment of training programs include generalization probes.

TRAINING APPROACHES: THEORY TO PRACTICE

Social skills training involving mentally retarded people has taken various forms in applied and in research settings. An array of treatment procedures has been used to target interpersonal and/or personal skills through both molar and/or molecular approaches. Procedures have been validated in individual case experimental designs (Deutsch & Parks, 1978; Geller, Wildman, Kelly, & Laughlin, 1980; Matson & Adkins, 1980; Matson & Stephens, 1978) and in group comparison studies (Senatore et al., 1982). In recent years, social skills training procedures have been extended in their application across the entire lifespan to enhance social competence. Social skills training procedures have been applied in educational settings (Brown & Shaw, 1986; Odom & Strain, 1984), institutions (Bates, 1980; Foxx, McMorrow, & Mennemeir, 1984; Matson, 1978; Matson & Earnhart, 1981), and community and natural environments (Senatore et al., 1982; Stacy, Doleys, & Malcolm, 1979; Wildman et al., 1986).

Application of social skills training procedures to enhance the social competence of persons with mental retardation is a relatively recent development, with the majority of applied research reports appearing in the literature in the last two decades. The origins of these procedures can be traced, however, to the work of such early researchers as Thorndike, Pavlov, and Watson, who formulated their theories at the turn of the century (Phillips, 1985; Shaw & Costanzo, 1970).

Postulates regarding the role of social imitation learning have been traced to early theorists, such as Watson and Rayner (1920) and Mary Carver Jones (1924). Other researchers, such as Bellack and Hersen (1977), attribute the development of social skills training techniques to the work of psychotherapists, such as Salter (1949), Wolpe (1958), and Lazarus (1971), and to the work on social competence by Zigler and Phillips (1960, 1961).

The work of these theorists laid the foundation for more recent research on development of social behavior (Bandura, 1965, 1969). Bandura (1969) provided a comprehensive framework for a social-learning interpretation of the mechanisms regulating behavior. Bandura indicated that "the type of behavior that a person exhibits partly determines his environmental contingencies which, in turn, influence his behavior" (p. 63). Bandura wrote extensively about the role of imitation, modeling, and vicarious processes in response acquisition or change.

Within the field of mental retardation, a broad array of studies have been published that report the use of behaviorally based social skills training procedures. These range from studies employing simple contingencies (Brodsky, 1967) to complex social skills packages that include instruction, modeling, role-playing, performance feedback, social reinforcement, and *in vivo* demonstration (Bates, 1980; Bornstein, Bach, McFall, Friman, & Lyons, 1980; Matson, 1980, 1984). The specific training approaches employed have varied depending on the social skills dimensions or specific behaviors that have been targeted. These procedures will be reviewed in the next section of this chapter.

Although some theorists have taken a molecular approach to social skills, emphasizing such behaviors as eye contact, facial expression, smiling, gesturing, voice loudness, hand-shaking, attentiveness, and so forth, others have chosen to focus on molar skill areas, such as assertiveness, conversational skills, cooperative behavior, or generalized interpersonal interaction (Robertson et al., 1984). Although the literature reflects applications of both molar and molecular training approaches, practical outcomes of training efforts must be viewed within the context of the performance of functional skills that are displayed appropriately across time, persons, places, and circumstances. For example, a number of molecular social skills may be taught which, when displayed in context and the correct sequence, comprise a molar skill, such as greeting. The component molecular skills may include approach, extension of the hand, grip, and hand-shaking. However, if the individual engages in inappropriate conversation while performing these component behaviors, the interaction would not be considered to be an adequate greeting. Likewise, greeting neighborhood adults in such a manner may be considered appropriate, whereas the same behavior may not be considered to be appropriate if employed with young children.

In many cases, the method used to train social skills has been determined by the nature of the target behaviors. A molecular view of behaviors that comprise social skills includes "verbal and non-verbal behaviors by which (individuals) affect the responses of other persons in the interpersonal context" (Van Hasselt, Hersen, Whitehill, & Bellack, 1979, p. 415), and an operant approach to developing these specific observable skills may be appropriate. On the other hand, a more molar orientation holds that social behavior involves the proper application of motoric, cognitive, and affective skills (Davies & Rogers, 1985), and an approach that includes a cognitive component, such as role taking, may be indicated.

Trower, Bryant, and Argyle (1978) indicated that effective social behavior consists of the following skills and behaviors:

1. Nonverbal motoric behaviors: facial expressions, gestures, body contact, and appearance

2. Verbal behaviors: asking questions, making small talk, and performing social rituals (e.g., greetings)
3. Affective behaviors: expressing attitudes and feelings, recognizing internal emotional cues, referential communication, and empathic responding
4. Social cognitive skills: interpersonal problem solving, role taking, thinking empathically, discrimination of social cues, understanding social norms, and linking together a sequence of thoughts and behaviors (cited in Davies & Rogers, 1985, p. 187)

To teach this range of social behaviors, various social skills training approaches have been employed. The treatment approaches that are reviewed in the following section include operant, psychotherapeutic, cognitive, and social-learning methods. Representative studies will be cited to demonstrate the application of each approach. The categorization of these approaches is somewhat arbitrary because many studies employ several training methods. For example, the social skills training package (Matson & Stephens, 1978) includes many varied treatment approaches applied in combination.

Operant Approaches

Operant conditioning, often referred to as *respondent* or *Type R conditioning*, was originally postulated by Thorndike (1898, 1932, 1935, 1949). Based on his work with animals, Thorndike formulated the law of effect, which basically indicated that the probability of the reoccurence of a response is increased if it is followed by a satisfying state of affairs or a reinforcing stimulus, and that nonreinforced responses tend to be discontinued.

The strength of the response or the adequacy of performance is influenced by (1) how immediate the reinforcement is applied following the behavior, (2) how frequent the reinforcement is provided, and (3) the amount and number of reinforcers administered (DeCecco & Crawford, 1974). B. F. Skinner, who is most closely associated with the recent application of operant techniques, wrote extensively about the control of behavior which he saw as clearly outside the control of the organism. Skinner indicated that

> It is now clear that we must take into account what the environment does to an organism not only before but after it responds. Behavior is shaped and maintained by its own consequences. Once this fact is recognized, we can formulate the interaction between organism and environment in a much more comprehensive way. (cited in DeCecco & Crawford, 1974, p. 187)

Operant techniques have been used to develop molecular social skills, primarily motoric and simple verbal behaviors. They also have been used as a component of other treatment approaches. The most common application of operant techniques involves the selection of a target behavior, task analysis, and reinforcement for successive approximations of the target behavior.

Brodsky (1967) studied the application of operant techniques with two institutionalized mentally retarded females who rarely initiated social contact. He differentially reinforced one subject for initiating verbal interaction on the ward and in the natural environment, whereas the other subject received reinforcement for appropriate social statements on the ward. Training did not occur in the natural environment. Brodsky found increased appropriate verbal responding for both subjects, but the behavior change did not generalize for the subject who did not receive programming in the natural environment.

Stokes, Baer, and Jackson (1974) found that rudimentary greeting responses, such as hand waving, could be taught to a severely handicapped person through the use of operant procedures, which utilized edible reinforcers and contingent praise upon response.

Hopkins (1968) targeted smiling behavior in two children who were mentally retarded. Using edible reinforcers, social reinforcement, and reinforcement scheduling, he demonstrated that he could positively effect the target behavior.

Other researchers have used operant techniques in conjunction with instruction and feedback to increase socially appropriate behavior. Whitman, Mercurio, and Caponigri (1970) were able to increase ball playing in two boys who were mentally retarded through operant techniques that included the use of physical prompts, verbal instruction, and verbal and edible reinforcers. Adaptive conversational speech was successfully taught by Whitman, Burish, and Collins (1972) to four mentally retarded adolescents, using tangible reinforcers paired with information feedback.

Although numerous studies have shown that operant techniques can positively enhance rudimentary social behavior, results have not demonstrated that their application alone is effective for generalizing learning across settings or individuals.

Psychotherapy

Psychotherapeutic techniques have been applied in a limited number of studies to enhance adjustment of persons with mental retardation. In its strictest sense, the term *psychotherapy* includes methods, such as psychoanalysis, nondirective or directive counseling, and psychodrama. The term has also been loosely applied to informal verbal therapies with counselors, ministers, and the like (Chaplin, 1968).

Because of its reliance on verbal communication, traditional psychotherapy has been applied in only a limited number of cases with persons who are mentally retarded. In these instances, it has been with those individuals who are higher functioning and who demonstrate relatively high cognitive development.

Matson and Senatore (1981) compared traditional psychotherapy, social skills training, and no treatment. First, they established a social validation criterion as it related to socially appropriate behavior in a workshop setting in order to select target behaviors. Subjects were 35 adults in the mild-to-moderate range of mental retardation who resided in the community with their parents or in a group home setting. Therapy groups included three to five clients who attended 1-hour sessions, twice weekly, for 5 weeks. Target behaviors included appropriate statements of one word, appropriate statements of more than one word, and inappropriate statements. Traditional psychotherapy included discussions related to the subjects' activities in the sheltered workshop, and, if necessary, the subjects were encouraged and prompted to discuss their interests and concerns. The researchers placed emphasis on empathy, genuineness, respect, and concreteness. Additionally, attention was given to establishing behaviors that enhance "group norms which promote trust, cohesiveness, universality, security, hope, and interpersonal learning" (Matson & Senatore, 1981, p. 376), with the objective of increasing appropriate social interaction in the workshop setting. The social skills training procedures (described in more detail later in this chapter), which were aimed specifically at the target behaviors, proved more effective than the traditional psychotherapy and no-treatment conditions. The authors concluded that "traditional psychotherapy had no marked positive effects, despite previous research suggesting that this treatment may be useful for enhancing interpersonal skills of the mentally retarded" (p. 380).

Other studies have employed traditional psychotherapy to remediate social and other deficits of persons with mental retardation (Argyle, Bryant, & Trower, 1974; Bialer, 1967; Sternlicht, 1966). However, few studies have been methodologically rigorous, and the majority do not provide a sufficient description of methodology to permit replication. In only a few cases has psychotherapy been compared to other treatment procedures, and generalization of learning has not been carefully assessed. Additionally, it is unclear from a review of the literature specifically which portion of the population of persons with mental retardation might benefit from this approach.

Cognitive Therapy

In its broadest sense, cognitive therapy applies to a wide range of treatment approaches. The bases for application of this approach are the

> hypotheses that: (a) cognitive factors (thoughts, images, memories, etc.) are intimately related to dysfunctional behavior, and (b) modification of such factors is an important mechanism for producing behavior change. (Thase, 1986, p. 60)

Application of cognitive therapies has not been reported extensively in the research literature. Lindsey (1986) indicated that this limited attention to assessment of cognitions and attitudes toward social interaction is a critical omission because it has been demonstrated with other populations that social cognitions are important for interpersonal interaction. Additionally, it has been demonstrated that simply having adequate social skills does not result in social interaction. Social interaction may be affected by avoidance of social contact because of a lack of confidence, poor self-image, attitudes attributed toward others, and a fear of failure in social situations.

Greenspan (1979) proposed a model of social intelligence that includes seven constructs subsumed under three major categories: (1) social sensitivity, (2) social insight, and (3) social communication. These include role taking, social inference, social comprehension, psychological insight, moral judgment, referential communication, and social problem solving. Many of these abilities have been targeted in research applying cognitive approaches.

Lindsey (1986), in a report on three case studies with persons who were mildly mentally retarded, concentrated on attitudes and beliefs about social interaction. He demonstrated that significant cognitive change could be effected, which resulted in positive change in the amount and nature of social interactions. Through the application of therapies that focus directly on behaviors, such as negative social self-statements and predetermined expectations of social failure, Lindsey demonstrated that concurrent cognitive changes can occur regardless of changes in social skill proficiency.

Smith (1986) and Castles and Glass (1986) focused on the ability of persons with mental retardation to apply interpersonal problem-solving strategies. These authors cited the inability of persons with mental retardation to resolve interpersonal conflicts and persuade others to cooperate in achieving interpersonal goals as reasons for poor social status. Problem-solving techniques enable persons who have adequate social skills to decide what response is appropriate in a given situation. The procedures used in studies of social problem solving typically present a social situation and focus on

> (a) generation of alternate solutions, (b) evaluation of probable consequences, (c) selection of the best alternatives, and (d) enumeration of specific means to implement the solutions chosen. (Castles & Glass, 1986, p. 37)

Smith (1986) found similarities in the type and number of strategies produced by persons with mental retardation and mental age-matched nonretarded subjects presented with interpersonal problem situations. However, he found that the nonretarded subjects used a broader range of problem-solving strategies than their mentally retarded counterparts.

Castles and Glass (1986) compared interpersonal problem–skill training, social skills training, and a combination of these two procedures in an attempt to increase problem-solving ability of 33 moderately and mildly mentally retarded adults. Using the 4-step procedure described above with role playing to determine the probable consequence of each solution, the authors found differential effects with the treatment procedures and between mildly and moderately mentally retarded subjects. Subjects who were trained using only problem-solving strategies showed no significant improvement in role-playing performance of social behaviors, but mildly mentally retarded subjects improved in problem-solving performance. Results of the study did not generalize to untrained situations.

Bramston and Spence (1985) compared "cognitive social-problem solving," social skills training, an attention placebo control, and no-treatment to enhance social competence. Like Castles and Glass (1986), they found that social skills training enhanced performance of basic social skills. However, the cognitive social-problem solving procedure resulted in greater improvement in the generation of alternate solutions. After 3 months, treatment gains were not maintained for either condition. Researchers have also targeted other cognitive skill areas, such as role-taking ability (Affleck, 1975; Blacher-Dixon & Simeonsson, 1978), cooperative behavior (Turner *et al.*, 1978), and other cognitively based skill areas.

Social Learning Techniques

Social learning theory has evolved largely from the work of Miller and Dollard (1941) and Bandura and Walters (1963), who postulated comprehensive theories of imitative behavior. These techniques have been applied in numerous studies to target a multitude of behaviors, including conversational skills (Wildman *et al.*, 1986), appropriate and inappropriate verbal interaction (Matson, 1980), prosocial behavior (Turner *et al.*, 1978), assertiveness (Stacy *et al.*, 1979), cooperative behavior (Gibson, Lawrence, & Nelson, 1976), giving and receiving compliments (King, Marcattilio, & Hanson, 1981), inappropriate gestures, posture, and hand movements (Bornstein *et al.*, 1980), handling criticism and differing with others (Bates, 1980)—just to mention a few.

Social learning techniques refer to a broad array of treatment strategies that include instruction, modeling, role playing, behavioral rehearsal, performance feedback, social praise, and *in vivo* demonstration. By far, most of the research involving the training of social skills has applied these treatment strategies either individually or in combination. *Instruction* provides the subject with detailed information as to the behavior he or she should display during a social interaction. *Modeling* provides a demonstration of how a particular skill should be performed, and may be demonstrated by the trainer (Matson & Senatore, 1981), a confederate (Senatore *et al.*, 1982), or a peer/assistant trainer (Matson, 1980). Such procedures may also be applied "live" or through video applications (Gibson *et al.*, 1976), whereas others have used these techniques in combination (Wildman *et al.*, 1986). Matson (1986) indicated that the term *modeling* is actually a generic term which encompasses both imitation and observational learning. "Imitation is the observation and displaying of a series of responses," whereas observation learning "refers to learning that occurs from the observation of others, and often the behaviors learned are not precisely imitated" (p. 150). *Role playing* incorperates performance of the targeted behavior with application of reinforcement techniques for approximation to the desired target behaviors. Role-playing situations may involve the use of models, simulated settings, or *in vivo* demonstration (Marchetti, Cecil, Graves, & Marchetti, 1984). Typically, a confederate or therapist interacts with the client to enhance performance. *Behavioral rehearsal* may be used in conjunction with modeling and requires that the client practice or repeat the desired response while receiving prompting from the trainer or while performing the desired behaviors independently (Senatore *et al.*, 1982). *Performance feedback* provides an evaluation of the quality of the response with instruction regarding ways to improve the resulting response. Feedback has included verbal guidance following skill performance, demonstration, as well as video applications in which clients study their performance on tape immediately after role playing and/or behavioral rehearsal (Meredith, Saxon, Doleys, & Kyzer, 1980). *Social praise* involves the application of an array of reinforcement strategies, including verbal praise, smiles, gestures, and/or application of other interpersonal reinforcers. Finally, *in vivo demonstration* involves the performance of the target behavior to demonstrate generalization and to ensure skill maintenance.

As previously indicated, these techniques have been applied independently or in combination. Application of the full spectrum of these techniques is often referred to in the literature as a social skills training package (Matson & Stephens, 1978). The reader is cautioned that similar terminology is often applied in social skills studies for procedurally dissimilar techniques. For example, modeling may include the trainer as the model, or a confederate, or a peer, and may involve live or taped modeling sequences.

Nelson, Gibson, and Cutting (1973), in one of the first studies comparing the differential effectiveness of (1) modeling, (2) instruction and feedback, and (3) a combination of these approaches, found that the combination of procedures was more effective in increasing the social behavior of a mildly retarded child than the individual applications. However, they cautioned that, in this single case study, treatment effects were confounded with sequence effects.

Gibson *et al.* (1976) also compared the efficacy of these three approaches. The target skill was peer interaction that included verbalizations, recreation, and cooperation. Three mentally retarded adults served as subjects. Modeling was presented using videotaped sequences. Results indicated that although the three treatment groups improved on the target behaviors from baseline levels, these procedures were differentially effective. The most effective procedure was the combination of modeling and instruction and feedback, followed by instruction and feedback, with the least effective procedure being the application of modeling alone.

Turner *et al.* (1978) targeted prosocial behaviors (i.e., eye contact, number of words spoken, smiles, appropriate intonation, overall assertiveness) in one of the first applications of a package of social skills techniques, including instruction, modeling, role playing, behavioral rehearsal, feedback, and reinforcement. They demonstrated the effectiveness of these procedures in this single case study. Results were maintained at a 6-month follow-up for the majority of the skills targeted.

Matson and Stephens (1978) were the first to refer to the combination of these procedures as a "social skills training package." In a study that employed these procedures, these researchers targeted negative social behaviors, such as arguing and fighting. Four adult females who were diagnosed with mental retardation and psychosis served as subjects. It was found that the frequency of fighting and arguing decreased significantly, and appropriate use of target behaviors, such as posture, speech content, affect, and so forth, increased significantly through the application of these procedures.

Stacy *et al.* (1979) successfully employed the social skills training package described above to target assertiveness in previously institutionalized mentally retarded persons. They demonstrated the efficacy of these procedures for individuals who reside in community settings, such as group homes.

Senatore *et al.* (1982) compared the standard social skills training package with an identical condition, which included active rehearsal, and a no-treatment control condition. Clients who received active rehearsal were to act out responses by rehearsing the target behaviors. Desired behaviors were gradually shaped through application of prompts by the trainer. The inclusion of the active rehearsal component proved more effective than the standard package alone.

Several studies have also employed video technologies in combination with the treatment approaches detailed above. These techniques have proved effective when used to provide immediate feedback showing subjects the adequacy of their responses (King *et al.*, 1981; Meredith *et al.*, 1980).

Another unique training strategy has been the application of a modified table game to teach six skill areas, including compliments, social interaction, politeness, criticism, social confrontation, and questions and answers (Foxx *et al.*, 1984). The researchers made the movement of playing pieces on a "Sorry" game board contingent upon responding correctly to a game card, which was related to the target behavior. Results showed that the game was effective in increasing social/vocational skills.

The research literature continues to grow with regard to the application of social learning techniques to social deficiencies of persons with mental retardation. It is apparent from a review of the literature that these techniques are effective in increasing the social competence of these persons. However, further research is needed to compare the differential effectiveness of these procedures and to evaluate more carefully maintenance and generalization of learned skills.

SUMMARY

Despite the significant body of research related to the conceptualization of social skills and the specific application of social skills training procedures with mentally retarded people, problems persist with regard to definitions, assessment approaches, and training methods. It is unclear from the literature specifically what psychological processes and behaviors are included under the rubric of social skills. Several investigators have interpreted the term *social skills* broadly to include only the motoric behaviors involved in social interactions, whereas others have argued to include perceptual, cognitive, and behavioral components in the concept. Adding to the conceptual confusion is the tendency for investigators to opt for new terms that relate to social skills. At this time, there is very little need for additional terminology in this area.

Research is needed for the development of standardized evaluation methodology and normative data. Social validation techniques may serve as a preliminary source of information concerning the components of social interactions and evaluations of social performance. However, such information requires empirical validation as well as social validation. It is strongly recommended that social skills investigators include maintenance and generalization probes as routine components of training outcome measures.

The social skills literature is replete with studies in which baseline measures of performance are compared with posttreatment performance of some specific social behavior. Generally, these studies have targeted a behavior that was selected *a priori*. The outcome of these studies invariably demonstrates that mentally retarded subjects, most commonly moderately and mildly retarded subjects, can learn specific social skills (perhaps this is an artifact of nonsignificant studies rarely being published). What is needed are studies that view training outcomes within the context of some specific social environment in which meaningful behavior change results in more functional social performance. A technology for training specific skills has been developed; further research is needed to conceptualize and evaluate adequate social performance and its overall development in mentally retarded people.

REFERENCES

Affleck, G. G. (1975). Role-taking ability and the interpersonal competencies of retarded children. *American Journal of Mental Deficiency, 80,* 312–316.

Affleck, G. G. (1977). Interpersonal competencies of the mentally retarded. In P. Mittler (Ed.), *Research to practice in mental retardation: Vol. II. Education and training* (pp. 85–91). Baltimore: University Park Press.

Andrasik, F. S., & Matson, J. (1985). Social skills training for the mentally retarded. In L. L'Abate & M. Milan (Eds.), *Handbook of social skills training and research* (pp. 418–454). New York: Wiley.

Argyle, M., Bryant, B., & Trower, P. (1974). Social skills training and psychotherapy: A comparative study. *Psychological Medicine, 4,* 435–443.

Balla, D., & Zigler, E. (1979). Personality development in retarded persons. In N. R. Ellis (Ed.), *Handbook of mental deficiency, psychological theory and research* (2nd ed., pp. 143–168). Hillsdale, NJ: Lawrence Erlbaum.

Bandura, A. (1965). Vicarious processes: A case of no-trial learning. In L. Berkowetz (Ed.), *Advances in experimental social psychology,* (Vol. 2, pp. 1–55). New York: Academic Press.

Bandura, A. (1969). *Principles of behavior change.* New York: Holt, Rinehart & Winston.

Bandura, A., & Walters, R. H. (1963). *Social learning and personality development.* New York: Holt, Rinehart & Winston.

Bates, P. (1980). The effectiveness of interpersonal skills training on the social skill acquisition of moderately and mildly retarded adults. *Journal of Applied Behavior Analysis, 13,* 237–248.

Bellack, A. S. (1979a). A critical appraisal of strategies for assessing social skill. *Behavioral Assessment, 1,* 157–176.

Bellack, A. S. (1979b). Behavioral assessment of social skills. In A. S. Bellack & M. Hersen (Eds.), *Research and practice in social skills training* (pp. 75–104). New York: Plenum Press.

Bellack, A. S. (1983). Recurrent problems in the behavioral assessment of social skill. *Behaviour Research and Therapy, 21,* 29–41.

Bellack, A. S., & Hersen, M. (1977). *Behavior modification: An introductory textbook.* Baltimore: Williams & Wilkins.

Bellack, A. S., Hersen, M., & Turner, S. M. (1976). Generalized effects of social skills training in chronic schizophrenics: An experimental analysis. *Behaviour Research and Therapy, 14,* 391–398.

Bernstein, G. (1981). Research issues in training interpersonal skills for the mentally retarded. *Education and Training of the Mentally Retarded, 16,* 70–74.

Bialer, I. (1967). Psychotherapy and other adjustment techniques with the mentally retarded. In

A. A. Baumeister (Ed.), *Mental retardation: Appraisal, education, and rehabilitation* (pp. 138–180). Chicago: Aldine.

Bijou, S. W. (1981). Behavioral teaching of young handicapped children: Problems of application and implementation. In S. W. Bijou & R. Ruiz (Eds.), *Behavior modification: Contributions to education* (pp. 97–110). Hillsdale, NJ: Lawrence Erlbaum.

Blacher-Dixon, J., & Simeonsson, R. J. (1978). Effect of shared experience on role-taking performance of retarded children. *American Journal of Mental Deficiency, 83,* 21–28.

Bornstein, P., Bach, P., McFall, M., Friman, P., & Lyons, P. (1980). Application of a social skills training program in the modification of interpersonal deficits among mentally retarded adults: A clinical replication. *Journal of Applied Behavior Analysis, 13,* 171–176.

Bramston, P., & Spence, S. H. (1985). Behavioral versus cognitive social-skills training with intellectually-handicapped adults. *Behaviour Research and Therapy, 23,* 239–246.

Brodsky, C. (1967). The relation between verbal and nonverbal behavior change. *Behaviour Research and Therapy, 5,* 182–191.

Brown, G. S., & Shaw, M. (1986). Social skills training in education. In C. Hollin & P. Trower (Eds.), *Handbook of social skills training* (Vol. 1, pp. 59–78). New York: Pergamon Press.

Campione, J. C., & Brown, A. L. (1977). Memory and metamemory development in educable retarded children. In R. V. Kail, Jr., & J. W. Hagen (Eds.), *Perspectives on the development of memory and cognition* (pp. 367–406). Hillsdale, NJ: Lawrence Erlbaum.

Castles, E., & Glass, C. (1986). Training in social and interpersonal problem-solving skills for mildly retarded and moderately retarded adults. *American Journal of Mental Deficiency, 91,* 35–42.

Chaplin, J. P. (1968). *Dictionary of psychology.* New York: Dell Publishing Co.

Conger, J. C., & Conger, A. J. (1986). Assessment of social skills. In A. R. Ciminero, K. S. Calhoun, & H. E. Adams (Eds.), *Handbook of behavioral assessment* (2nd ed., pp. 526–560). New York: Wiley.

Curran, J. P. (1979a). Social skills: Methodological issues and future directions. In A. S. Bellack & M. Hersen (Eds.), *Research and practice in social skills training* (pp. 319–354). New York: Plenum Press.

Curran, J. P. (1979b). Pandora's box reopened? The assessment of social skills. *Journal of Behavioral Assessment, 1,* 55–71.

Curran, J. P. (1985). Social competency training. In H. A. Marlowe, Jr., & R. B. Weinberg (Eds.), *Competence development* (pp. 146–176). Springfield, IL: Charles C Thomas.

Curran, J. P., & Wessberg, H. W. (1981). Assessment of social inadequacy. In D. H. Barlow (Ed.), *Behavioral assessment of adult disorders* (pp. 405–438). New York: Guilford Press.

Davies, R., & Rogers, E. (1985). Social skills training with persons who are mentally retarded. *Mental Retardation, 23,* 186–196.

DeCecco, J., & Crawford, W. (1974). *The psychology of learning and instruction.* Englewood Cliffs: NJ: Prentice-Hall.

Deutsch, M., & Parks, A. L. (1978). The use of contingent music to increase appropriate conversational speech. *Mental Retardation, 16,* 33–36.

Foxx, R., McMorrow, M., & Mennemeir, M. (1984). Teaching social/vocational skills to retarded adults with a modified table game: An analysis of generalization. *Journal of Applied Behavior Analysis, 17,* 343–352.

Geller, M. I., Wildman, H. E., Kelly, J. A., & Laughlin, C. S. (1980). Teaching assertive and commendatory social skills to an interpersonally deficient retarded adolescent. *Journal of Clinical Child Psychology, 9,* 17–21.

Gibson, F., Lawrence, P., & Nelson, R. (1976). Comparison of three training procedures for teaching social responses to developmentally disabled adults. *American Journal of Mental Deficiency, 81,* 379–387.

Greenspan, S. (1979). Social intelligence in the retarded. In N. R. Ellis (Ed.), *Handbook of mental deficiency, psychological therapy and research* (2nd ed., pp. 483–531). Hillsdale, NJ: Lawrence Erlbaum.

Gresham, F. M., & Elliott, S. N. (1987). The relationship between adaptive behavior and social skills: Issues in definition and assessment. *Journal of Special Education, 21,* 167–181.

Grossman, H. J. (1983). *Classification in mental retardation.* Washington, DC: American Association on Mental Deficiency.

Harris, S. L., & Ferrari, M. (1983). Developmental factors in child behavior therapy. *Behavior Therapy, 14,* 54–72.

Hedquist, F., & Weinhold, B. K. (1970). Behavioral group counseling with socially anxious and unassertive college students. *Journal of Counseling Psychology, 17,* 237–242.

Henderson, M., & Hollin, C. (1986). Social skills training and delinquency. In C. Hollin & P. Trower (Eds.), *Handbook of social skill training* (Vol. 1, pp. 79–101). New York: Pergamon Press.

Hersen, M., & Bellack, A. S. (1976). Social skills training for chronic psychiatric patients: Rational, research findings and future directions. *Comprehensive Psychiatry, 17,* 559–580.

Hersen, M., Eisler, R. M., & Miller, P. M. (1973). Development of assertive responses: Clinical measurement and research considerations. *Behaviour Research and Therapy, 11,* 505–521.

Hollin, C., & Trower, P. (1986a). *International series in experimental social psychology* (Vol. 1). New York: Pergamon Press.

Hollin, C., & Trower, P. (1986b). *International series in experimental social psychology* (Vol. 2). New York: Pergamon Press.

Hopkins, B. L. (1968). Effects of candy and social reinforcement, instruction, and reinforcement schedule learning on the modification and maintenance of smiling. *Journal of Applied Behavior Analysis, 2,* 121–129.

Howells, K. (1986). Social skills training and criminal and antisocial behavior in adults. In C. Hollin & P. Trower (Eds.), *Handbook of social skills training* (Vol. 1, pp. 185–210). New York: Pergamon Press.

Jones, M. C. (1924). The elimination of children's fears. *Journal of Experimental Psychology, 7,* 383–390.

Kazdin, A. E. (1977). Assessing the clinical or applied importance of behavior change through social validation. *Behavior Modification, 1,* 427–451.

Kazdin, A. E., & Matson, J. L. (1981). Social validation in mental retardation. *Applied Research in Mental Retardation, 2,* 39–53.

King, R., Marcattilio, A. J., & Hanson, R. (1981). Some functions of videotape equipment in training social skills to institutionalized mentally retarded adults. *Behavioral Engineering, 6,* 159–167.

Lambert, N., & Nicoll, R. (1976). Dimensions of adaptive behavior of retarded and nonretarded public school children. *American Journal of Mental Deficiency, 81,* 135–146.

Lazarus, A. A. (1971). *Behavior therapy and beyond.* New York: McGraw-Hill.

Libet, J., & Lewinsohn, P. (1973). The concept of social skill with special reference to the behavior of depressed persons. *Journal of Consulting and Clinical Psychology, 40,* 304–312.

Lindsey, W. (1986). Cognitive changes after social skills training with young mildly mentally handicapped adults. *Treatment Deficiency Research, 30,* 81–88.

Lowe, M. R., & Cautela, J. R. (1978). A self-report measure of social skill. *Behavior Therapy, 9,* 535–544.

Marchetti, A., Cecil, C., Graves, J., & Marchetti, D. (1984). Public transportation instruction: Comparison of classroom instruction, community instruction, and facility grounds instruction. *Mental Retardation, 22,* 128–136.

Mash, E. J., & Terdal, L. G. (1977). After the dance is over: Some issues and suggestions for follow-up assessment in behavior therapy. *Psychological Reports, 41,* 1287–1308.

Matson, J., DiLorenzo, T., & Andrasik, F. (1983). A review of behavior modification procedures for treating social skills deficits and psychiatric disorders of the mentally retarded. In J. Matson & S. F. Andrasik (Ed.), *Treatment issues and innovations in mental retardation* (pp. 415–543). New York: Plenum Press.

Matson, J. L. (1978). Training socially appropriate behaviors to moderately retarded adults: A social learning approach. *Scandinavian Journal of Behavior Therapy, 7,* 167–175.

Matson, J. L. (1980). Acquisition of social skills by mentally retarded adult training assistants. *Journal of Mental Deficiency Research, 24,* 129–135.

Matson, J. L. (1984). Social skills training. *Psychiatric Aspects of Mental Retardation Reviews, 3,* 1–4.

Matson, J. L. (1986). Modeling. In A. S. Bellack & M. Hersen (Eds.), *Dictionary of behavior therapy techniques* (pp. 150–151). New York: Pergamon Press.

Matson, J. L., & Adkins, J. (1980). A self-instructional social skills training program for mentally retarded persons. *Mental Retardation, 18,* 245–248.

Matson, J. L., & DiLorenzo, T. (1986). Social skills training and mental handicap and organic impairment. In C. Hollin & P. Trower (Eds.), *Handbook of social skills training* (Vol. 2, pp. 67–90). New York: Pergamon Press.

Matson, J. L., & Earnhart, T. (1981). Programming treatment effects to the natural environment: A procedure for training institutionalized retarded adults. *Behavior Modification, 5,* 27–37.

Matson, J. L., & Senatore, V. (1981). A comparison of traditional psychotherapy and social skills training for improving interpersonal functioning of mentally retarded adults. *Behavior Therapy, 12,* 369–382.

Matson, J. L., & Stephens, R. M. (1978). Increasing appropriate behavior of explosive chronic psychiatric patients with social skills training package. *Behavior Modification, 2,* 61–76.

Matson, J. L., Helsel, W. J., Bellack, A. S., & Senatore, V. (1983). Development of a rating scale to assess social skills deficits in mentally retarded adults. *Applied Research in Mental Retardation, 4,* 399–407.

McCarver, R. B., & Campbell, V. A. (1987). Future developments in the concept and application of adaptive behavior. *Journal of Special Education, 21,* 197–207.

McFall, R. M. (1982). A review and reformulation of the concept of social skills. *Behavioral Assessment, 4,* 1–33.

Meredith, R., Saxon, S., Doleys, D., & Kyzer, B. (1980). Social skills training with mildly retarded young adults. *Journal of Clinical Psychology, 36,* 1000–1009.

Meyers, C. E., Nihira, K., & Zetlin, A. (1979). The measurement of adaptive behavior. In N. R. Ellis (Ed.), *Handbook of mental deficiency, psychological theory and research* (2nd ed., pp. 431–481). Hillsdale, NJ: Lawrence Erlbaum.

Miller, N. E., & Dollard, J. (1941). *Social learning and imitation.* New Haven, CT: Yale University Press.

Miller, P. M., & Eisler, R. M. (1977). Assertive behavior of alcoholics: A descriptive analysis. *Behavior Therapy, 8,* 146–149.

Monti, P., Abrams, D., Binkoff, J., & Zwick, W. (1986). Social skills training and substance abuse. In C. Hollin & P. Trower (Eds.), *Handbook of social skills training* (Vol. 2, pp. 111–142). New York: Pergamon Press.

Nelson, R., Gibson, F., & Cutting, D. S. (1973). Videotaped modeling: The development of three appropriate social responses in a mildly retarded child. *Mental Retardation, 11,* 22–28.

Nihira, K. (1976). Dimensions of adaptive behavior in institutionalized mentally retarded children and adults: Developmental perspective. *American Journal of Mental Deficiency, 81,* 215–226.

Nihira, K., Foster, R., Shellhaas, M., & Leland, H. (1974). *AAMD adaptive behavior scale.* Washington, DC: American Association on Mental Deficiency.

Odom, S. L., & Strain, P. S. (1984). Classroom-based social skills instructions for severely handicapped preschool children. *Topics in Early Childhood Special Education, 4,* 97–116.

Phillips, E. L. (1985). Social skills: History and prospect. In L. L'Abate & M. Milan (Ed.), *Handbook of social skills training and research* (pp. 3–21). New York: Wiley.

Powers, M. D., & Handleman, J. S. (1984). *Behavioral assessment of severe behavioral developmental disabilities.* Rockville, MD: Aspen Systems.

Robertson, I., Richardson, A., & Youngson, S. (1984). Social skills with mentally handicapped people: A review. *British Journal of Clinical Psychology, 23,* 241–264.

Ross, R. T., & Giampiccolo, J. S. (1972). *Fairview social skills scale for mildly and moderately retarded.* Costa Mesa, CA: Fairview State Hospital.

Salter, A. (1949). *Conditional reflex therapy.* New York: Farrar, Straus & Giroux.

Senatore, V., Matson, J. L., & Kazdin, A. E. (1982). A comparison of behavioral methods to train social skills to mentally retarded adults. *Behavior Therapy, 13,* 313–324.

Shaw, M., & Costanzo, P. (1970). *Theories of social psychology.* New York: McGraw-Hill.

Shepherd, G. (1986). Social skills training and schizophrenia. In C. Hollin & P. Trower (Eds.), *Handbook of social skills training* (Vol. 2, pp. 9–37). New York: Pergamon Press.

Smith, D. (1986). Interpersonal problem-solving skills of retarded and nonretarded children. *Applied Research in Mental Retardation, 7,* 431–442.

Sparrow, S. S., Balla, D. A., & Cicchetti, D. V. (1984). *Vineland adaptive behavior scales.* Circle Pines, MN: American Guidance Service.

Stacy, D., Doleys, D., & Malcolm, R. (1979). Effects of social skills training in a community based program. *American Journal of Mental Deficiency, 84,* 152–158.

Stainback, W., Stainback, S., & Strathe, M. (1983). Generalization of positive social behavior by severely handicapped students: A review and analysis of research. *Education and Training of the Retarded, 18,* 293–299.

Sternlicht, M. (1966). Psychotherapeutic procedures with the retarded. In N. R. Ellis (Ed.), *International review of research in mental retardation* (Vol. 2, pp. 279–354). New York: Academic Press.

Stokes, T., Baer, D., & Jackson, R. (1974). Programming the generalization of a greeting response in four retarded children. *Journal of Applied Behavioral Analysis, 7,* 599–610.

Strain, P. S. (1983). Identification of social skill curriculum targets for severely handicapped children in mainstream preschools. *Applied Research in Mental Retardation, 4,* 369–382.

Thase, M. E. (1986). Cognitive therapy: In A. Bellack & M. Hersen (Eds.), *Dictionary of behavior therapy techniques.* New York: Pergamon Press.

Thorndike, E. L. (1898). *Animal intelligence.* New York: Macmillan.

Thorndike, E. L. (1932). *Educational psychology.* New York: Teachers College, Columbia University.

Thorndike, E. L. (1935). *The psychology of wants, interests, and attitudes.* New York: Appleton-Century-Crofts.

Thorndike, E. L. (1949). *Selected writings from a connectionist's psychology.* New York: Appleton-Century-Crafts.

Trower, P. (1979). Fundamentals of interpersonal behavior: A social-psychological perspective. In A. Bellack & M. Hersen (Eds.), *Research and practice in social skills training* (pp. 3–40). New York: Plenum Press.

Trower, P. (1986). Social skills training and social anxiety. In C. Hollin & P. Trower (Eds.), *Handbook of social skills training* (Vol. 2, pp. 39–65). New York: Pergamon Press.

Trower, P., Bryant, B., & Argyle, M. (1978). *Social skills and mental health.* Pittsburg, PA: University of Pittsburg Press.

Turner, S. M., Hersen, M., & Bellack, A. S. (1978). Social skills training to teach prosocial behaviors in an organically impaired and retarded patient. *Journal of Behavior Therapy and Experimental Psychiatry, 9,* 253–258.

Van Hasselt, V., Hersen, M., Whitehill, M. B., & Bellack, A. S. (1979). Social skills assessment and training for children: An evaluative review. *Behaviour Research and Therapy, 17,* 413–417.

Vaughn, S. R., Ridley, C. A., & Cox, J. (1983). Evaluating the efficacy of an interpersonal skills training program with children who are mentally retarded. *Education and Training of the Mentally Retarded, 18,* 191–196.

Watson, J. B., & Rayner, P. (1920). Conditional emotional reactions. *Journal of Experimental Psychology, 3,* 1–14.

Whitman, T. L., Mercurio, J. R., & Caponigri, V. (1970). Development of social responses in two severely retarded children. *Journal of Applied Behavior Analysis, 3,* 133–138.

Whitman, T. L., Burish, T., & Collins, C. (1972). Development of interpersonal language responses in two moderately retarded children. *Mental Retardation, 10,* 40–45.

Wildman, B. G., Wildman, H. E., & Kelly, W. J. (1986). Group conversational-skills training and social validation with mentally retarded adults. *Applied Research in Mental Retardation, 7,* 443–458.

Williams, J. M. G. (1986). Social skills training and depression. in C. Hollin & P. Trower (Eds.), *Handbook of social skills training* (Vol. 2, pp. 91–110). New York: Pergamon Press.

Wolf, M. M. (1978). Social validity: The case for subjective measurement of how applied behavior analysis is finding its heart. *Journal of Applied Behavior Analysis, 11,* 203–214.

Wolpe, J. (1958). *Psychotherapy by reciprocal inhibition.* Stanford, CA: Stanford University Press.

Zigler, E. (1966). Mental retardation: Current issues and approaches. In M. L. Hoffman & L. W.

Hoffman (Eds.), *Review of child development research* (Vol. 2, pp. 107–168). New York: Russell Sage.

Zigler, E. (1969). Developmental versus difference theories of mental retardation and the problem of motivation. *American Journal of Mental Deficiency, 73,* 536–555.

Zigler, E., & Balla, D. (1982). Motivation and personality factors in the performance of the retarded. In E. Zigler & D. Balla (Eds.), *Mental retardation: The developmental-difference controversy* (pp. 9–26). Hillsdale, NJ: Lawrence Erlbaum.

Zigler, E., & Phillips, L. (1960). Social effectiveness and symptomatic behaviors. *Journal of Abnormal and Social Psychology, 61,* 231–238.

Zigler, E., & Phillips, L. (1961). Social competence and outcome in psychiatric disorder. *Journal of Abnormal and Social Psychology, 63,* 264–271.

Zigler, E., Balla, D., & Hoddap, R. (1984). On the definition and classification of mental retardation. *American Journal of Mental Deficiency, 89,* 215–230.

13

Consumer-Centered Transition and Supported Employment

JAMES E. MARTIN, DENNIS E. MITHAUG, MARTIN AGRAN, AND JAMES V. HUSCH

Upon leaving school, the majority of young adults with learning and behavior problems experience unemployment, social isolation, and economic dependence. Recent follow-up studies of special education graduates suggest that little more than one third are employed full-time, live independently, and are self-supporting. The consistency of this pattern across several statewide studies leaves little doubt about the magnitude of the problem (Fardig, Algozzine, Schwartz, Hensel, & Westling, 1985; Hasazi, Gordon, & Roe, 1985; Mithaug, Horiuchi, & Fanning, 1985; Mithaug, Horiuchi, & McNulty, 1987).

The situation is even worse for graduates who are mentally retarded. Hasazi, Gordon, Roe, Hull, *et al.* (1985) reported that 43% of their sample of special education graduates in Vermont were employed in nonsubsidized or nonsheltered workshop jobs. Of those working, only 23% were employed full-time. Wehman, Kregel, and Seyfarth (1985) reported more disheartening findings. In a sample of special education graduates from Virginia, 36% of the former students with mental retardation were working in nonsheltered jobs—almost all of whom were mildly mentally retarded. Only 12% of the workers with moderate and severe mental retardation were employed in community jobs. In other words, "a total of *43%* of those individuals labeled *mildly mentally retarded* were *unemployed,* compared with *78%* of those labeled *moderately or severely mentally retarded*" (Wehman, Kregel, & Seyfarth, 1985, p. 97). Schalock *et al.* (1986) reported that in a rural Nebraska sample, 58% of the mildly handicapped and 25% of the moderately and severely mentally retarded were employed. Most recently, Edgar and Levine (1988) found that 38% of former Washington students in the moderate/severe category and 45% in the mild category were employed, but less than 10% of these former students were working full-time at minimum wage or better. Most telling, almost 50% of the former mentally retarded students (almost equally split between

JAMES E. MARTIN, DENNIS E. MITHAUG, AND JAMES V. HUSCH • Department of Special Education, University of Colorado at Colorado Springs, Colorado Springs, Colorado 80933. MARTIN AGRAN • Department of Special Education, Utah State University, Logan, Utah 84322.

the mild and the moderate/severe categories) were not involved in any work activity outside the home.

In this chapter, we will review briefly the present vocational training system and the attitudes of parents regarding the employment of their handicapped children. The transition and supported employment initiatives will be examined as a means to improve postschool success. The remainder of this chapter introduces the Adaptability Instruction Model, an instructional approach whereby consumers play a central role in the job-match, placement, and maintenance procedures.

POSTSCHOOL SHELTERED WORKSHOPS

Many young adults with mental retardation who leave school receive services from sheltered workshops. Unfortunately, there is little consumer movement from the sheltered programs to integrated employment. In fact, for persons who fail to leave a sheltered workshop within 6 months of entry, it is likely they will remain permanently (Rusch & Mithaug, 1980). Nationwide, fewer than 12% of all sheltered workshop employees who are mentally retarded advance to nonsheltered employment (Bellamy, Rhodes, & Albin, 1986).

PARENTAL ATTITUDE TOWARD EMPLOYMENT

Many parents of adult children with mental retardation, especially those who may have a child with a severe disability, are reluctant to have their son or daughter involved in community-based vocational programming until the last year of high school, or to be employed outside of sheltered workshops following graduation (Hill, Seyfarth, Banks, Wehman, & Orelove, 1987; Seyfarth, Hill, Orelove, McMillan, & Wehman, 1987). This attitude is important because parental support and employment preparation during the school years appear to be related to employment success (Brickey, Campbell, & Browning, 1985; McLoughlin, Garner, & Callahan, 1987). Kernan and Koegel (1980; cited in Schutz, 1986) examined the impact of family support upon the employment status of a group of mentally retarded workers. Their results indicated that parental support correlated with successful employment. Schutz (1986), Goodall, Wehman, and Cleveland (1983), and Kochany and Keller (1981) reported that, when family support is not present, individuals were more likely to be in sheltered employment, to lose their community jobs if they were employed outside of sheltered employment, or not to seek employment at all. Hill et al. (1987) concluded that

> much more parent/professional communication is needed to improve parental expectations for the vocational potential of their children who are mentally retarded. . . . at present, parents' expectations do not concur with the . . . professional expectations which hold that most persons who are mentally retarded can effect transition into the mainstream of employment. (p. 22)

TRANSITION INITIATIVE

In response to the inability of current education and habilitation practices to assure reasonable transitions, several educators and postschool service providers have initiated a nation-wide movement to develop more effective service delivery models (Bellamy, Rhodes, Mank, & Albin, 1988; Krause & MacEachron, 1982; McLoughlin et al., 1987; Wehman & Kregel, 1985). These initiatives include: (1) cooperative transition agreements between education and adult service agencies (Hardman & McDonnell, 1987; Stodden & Boone, 1987); (2) transition services that use community-based training, functional curriculum, opportunities for integrated social interaction, and job-matching procedures to achieve supported employment placements (Rusch, 1986; Wehman, Moon, Everson, Wood, & Barcus, 1988); (3) individualized transition plans (Hardman & McDonnell, 1987); and (4) parent/professional partnerships (Bellamy et al., 1988; Bronicki & Turnbull, 1987; Close & Keating, 1988; Schutz, 1986).

Missing Links

Parents of former special education graduates suggest that transition efforts "should assist the student to become more independent in understanding what he or she needs and wants, how to set personal goals . . . and to select action plans that will lead to desired outcomes" (Mithaug, Horiuchi, & McNulty, 1987, p. 59). Instead the transition initiative's focusing upon "cooperative interagency agreements," "community-based programming," and "individualized transition plans" *ignore* the student—the primary consumer of services. Student choice and meaningful involvement in the planning process are given little consideration. For example, McDonnell and Hardman (1985) recommended that "the formal transition plan should be developed in a cooperative meeting between parents, the high school teacher, a case management service representative, and relevant adult service providers" (p. 277). Where is the student? Mithaug, Martin, Frazier, and Allen (1988) ask how can students be expected to assume responsibility for their long-term employment success if they are systematically excluded from decision making—from the choices that will impact them in important ways? This current state of affairs is contrary to the intent of the transition initiative put forward by the U.S. Department of Special Education and Rehabilitative Services:

> Transitions are an important part of normal life. As roles, locations, and relationships change, all of us must *adapt* [italics added], and we do so with more or less disruption or stress. The transition . . . to working life calls for a range of choices about career options, living arrangements, social life, and economic goals that have lifelong consequences. For individuals with disabilities, this transition often is made more difficult by limitations that can be imposed by others' perceptions of disability and by the complex array of services that are intended to assist adult adjustment. (Will, 1984, p. 2)

LONG-TERM CONSUMER IMPACT

We believe that school-based and postschool vocational programs established as a result of the transition initiative must have a structure that includes consumer input. Vocational instruction and placement programs should empower people by addressing such questions as: Are consumers' input and decision making emphasized? Do consumers learn to make informed choices, and do these choices affect placement decisions? Does the program establish dependent relationships or does it promote independence? What instructional activities encourage consumers to make their own choices, decisions, to participate in the development of their own individualized education or rehabilitation plan, and to manage their own environment? Are they happy with changes they make in their lives?

In the remaining sections of this chapter, we address these questions. We will examine consumer empowerment, review current instructional approaches, and describe how adaptability instruction improves the long-term employment of workers with mental retardation.

Consumer Empowerment

Consumer empowerment is the ability and opportunity to choose, to set goals, and to make decisions. Consumers cannot become more independent by participating only in socially integrated settings and increasing their task independence. As Mithaug, Martin, Husch, Agran, and Rusch (1988) indicate, "consumers can experience social integration without being productive or independent; they can be independent but not productive or socially integrated" (p. 90). Independence is making choices and decisions on one's own and then being responsible for the consequences. In the following example, Murphy, in contrast to Steve who remained in a sheltered job, became personally independent when he became employed in a community job and decided for himself what to do, when to do it, and with whom:

> Three years ago, Steve and Murphy, who were diagnosed as being mildly to moderately mentally retarded, were working in a typical sheltered workshop and living in a nursing home for mentally retarded adults. Their morning routine consisted of being awakened by service attendants, waiting in line to use the rest room, eating cafeteria-style in a large dining hall, and traveling to the sheltered workshop with other residents in a yellow agency school bus. After being directed to their work stations by supervisory aides, Steve and Murphy assembled and later disassembled objects, menial tasks that lacked correspondence with jobs found in competitive employment. For their efforts, Steve and Murphy were paid well below minimum wage, approximately $0.76 per hour. During their workday, they talked with other retarded individuals or the few staff members present.
>
> After the day's work, Steve and Murphy returned to the nursing home to watch television in the day room with other residents. Usually after dinner they once again watched television, talked with other residents, or were entertained by local community volunteer groups. About once a week they went on a planned social outing to a nearby discount store to buy miscellaneous and needed personal care items. On returning to the home, Steve and Murphy found little privacy. Even

after they retired for the evening, staff entered their room for bed checks throughout the night.

Today there is a dramatic difference in the quality of one of their lives. Unfortunately, Steve's life is not different. His daily routine has changed little, if any. . . .

Murphy, on the other hand, is experiencing a new and exciting life. For the
past 3 years, he has been employed as a kitchen laborer in the food service division
of a local university and lives in his own apartment. During Murphy's recent visit to
Steve in the nursing home, they discussed Murphy's job, some new items he
bought for the apartment with the money he made, and the girl he met at work.
Murphy told Steve about his new assignment—operating the new dishwasher.
Next, he invited Steve over for dinner to show off his new toaster oven and coffee
maker. Finally, he talked to Steve about going to the movies with his new girlfriend.
As Murphy said good-by, Steve commented that he, too, would like to become
involved in a similar training program so that he could have money to spend at the
movies and live in his own apartment. (Martin, Schneider, Rusch, & Geske, 1982,
p. 59)

Two young adults involved with People First of Colorado Springs made
the same point in a recent newsletter of the Colorado Association for Retarded Citizens. Dennis Schwed stated: "I want to better myself and be a
better person. . . . I think that people ought to listen to us" ("Playing the
waiting game," 1988, p. 1). Debbie Allen agreed: "We need to show . . . that
we are people with ideas and we can make good decisions, too" (p. 1).

Current Instructional Approach

The dominant instructional approach in use today is one in which teachers and vocational supervisors make the decisions and students respond pas-
sively throughout the day. Guess, Benson, and Siegel-Causey (1985) suggested that all too often program staff members determine what students should
learn, how they will be taught, and where the instruction will take place.
Instead of being considered self-directing, persons with mental retardation
are all too often perceived as "mere objects of external manipulation" (p. 234).
Young adults with mental retardation learn to react to and depend on the
cues and consequences of others. They learn to be dependent—not independent (Rusch, Martin, & White, 1985).

As a result, young adults with mental retardation do not have the opportunity to express preferences and make choices. Seldom do school or vocational programs ask students what jobs they like the best or what work
conditions they prefer. Guess and Siegel-Causey (1985) suggested that students should become more self-directed, not less. Adaptability instruction is
an approach to help students become more self-directed and more in control
of the environment in which they live.

Adaptability Instruction Model

The Supported Employment Partnership at the University of Colorado at
Colorado Springs and the Self-Instructional Research Project at Utah State

University use the Adaptability Instruction Model to empower consumers. Implicit in this model is the notion that individuals who are mentally retarded can learn to make choices and be less dependent on others (Agran & Moore, 1987).

The Adaptability Instruction Model consists of four components: (1) decision making, (2) independent performance, (3) self-evaluation, and (4) adjustment (Mithaug, Martin, & Agran, 1987). During decision making, students make choices regarding the type of work they want to do and then develop a plan for the amount of work they will accomplish and time-lines or schedules for completing that work. During independent performance, they learn to follow their own plans by beginning their work as scheduled, completing the amount they specified, and ending work on time. During self-evaluation, they learn to monitor their own performance and behaviors by self-recording work outcomes, such as the time they begin and end work, the amount of work they complete, the accuracy of their work, and the times they end work. By comparing these outcomes with their own expectations, they are able to conclude if they met their own goals and objectives. This allows them to determine an appropriate adjustment for their next work period.

Need to Adapt

Workers need to adapt to on-the-job changes in order to maintain a satisfactory level of performance. The Colorado Employability Skills Survey reported that differences between school and work accuracy and problem-solving skills produced entry-level adjustment problems (Colorado Department of Education, 1983). Goal setting, independent performance, self-evaluation, and adjustment are the essential skills students and young adults need to learn to solve on-the-job problems. These skills enable persons to self-manage their own environment.

Self-Management

The Adaptability Instruction Model is based upon self-management, an approach that encourages the control of one's behavior through self-regulation of antecedent or consequent stimuli (Bandura, 1969; Kurtz & Neisworth, 1976; Martin, Burger, Elias-Burger, & Mithaug, 1988; Skinner, 1974). The three classes of self-management are: (1) antecedent cue regulation, (2) self-monitoring/self-evaluation, and (3) self-consequation (Gifford, Rusch, Martin, & White, 1984). Antecedent cue regulation is the use of prompts and cues that lead the consumer to the needed response. It alters the stimulus conditions that precede target behaviors (Martin, 1982). Antecedent cue regulation "limits the range of discriminative stimuli controlling the desired behavior, and might incorporate procedures such as the use of picture cues" (Gifford et al., 1984, p. 293) or self-instructions (Agran & Martin, 1987). Self-monitoring is the initial step in establishing self-control (Rosenbaum & Drabman, 1979). It is a two-stage process whereby the consumer must first become aware of his or her own behavior "by discriminating the occurrence or nonoccurrence of a specific behavior; second, the person usually records or reports the observation" (Martin, 1982, p. 18). Self-consequation is the use of self-reinforcement or self-recruited feedback to increase or decrease behavior (Buckley & Mank, 1988; Mank & Horner, 1987).

An analysis of 280 scholarly reviews and 808 research reports on self-management from 1957 to 1986 strongly supports the use of goal setting, planning, self-monitoring, self-evaluations, and adjustment procedures for both nonhandicapped and handicapped populations (Mithaug, Martin, Agran, & Rusch, 1988). Conclusions reached in reviews of the use of self-management procedures by individuals who are mentally retarded further demonstrate their use to facilitate the acquisition, maintenance, and generalization of behavior (Agran & Martin, 1987; Martin et al., 1988; Shapiro, 1981).

From 1973 to early 1987, 77 studies were published that investigated the use of self-management procedures with individuals who were mentally retarded. An analysis of these studies enabled Martin et al. (1988) to conclude that

> self-control (self-management) procedures enable individuals who are mentally retarded to become more independent. . . . About half of these studies included maintenance and generalization checks . . . and in almost all of these cases the self-control strategy helped achieve maintenance and/or generalization. Interestingly, in the few studies that compared self-control strategies to traditional intervention, the self-control strategies were more successful than trainer-based approaches. (p. 48)

The VITAL Checklist and Curriculum Guide (VCCG)

Mithaug, Martin, and Burger (1987a) operationalized the four adaptability concepts into the VITAL Checklist and Curriculum Guide (VCCG). The VCCG is a criterion-referenced mastery assessment that "evaluates the essential problem solving and adaptability skills all students need to become independent at school, at home, and at work" (Mithaug, Martin, & Burger, 1987a, p. 1). It includes 43 skills that enable students to set goals, determine action plans to meet the goal, take that action and monitor their performance, evaluate their actions, and then determine any need for adjustments the next time the task has to be completed.

Agran, Martin, and Mithaug (1987) administered the VCCG to 428 students from 37 schools in 21 districts across 10 Colorado cities. Figure 1 presents student profiles from those assessments. Note the similarity between profiles of all groups: Decision Making and Independence were highest, whereas Self-Evaluation and Adjustment were the lowest. The performance of the primary-aged normal elementary students was higher than any special education group. Students who were mentally retarded scored the lowest of all. These data also suggest the limited degree to which students' educational programs emphasized adaptability skills.

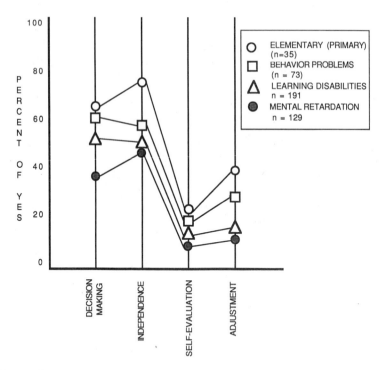

FIGURE 1. VITAL Checklist Adaptability profiles across different categorical groups.

Adaptability Demonstration and Research

The Transition Research and Demonstration Project at the University of Colorado at Colorado Springs has produced considerable information on how to teach adaptability skills to students with mental retardation. Three examples of these demonstration studies follow.

In one demonstration study, four secondary-level students with moderate mental retardation who worked in a grocery store used picture forms and schedules to (1) select the jobs they liked the best, (2) set goals, (3) independently schedule and follow their task schedules, (4) evaluate performance, (5) compare their performance to standards of performance, and (6) make necessary adjustments. Figure 2 depicts one of the forms they used to evaluate their performance when bringing carts in from the parking lot and whether they needed help or completed the task independently. The second study demonstrated that four students who were moderately mentally retarded could use picture-based forms to determine if their abilities and interests matched the job requirements and conditions. After selecting their own on-the-job try-out sites, the students scheduled tasks and independently completed them in the proper sequence. Then, they self-evaluated their performance, compared it to supervisor evaluations, and decided what to adjust the next time. The third study demonstrated that a class of secondary students with moderate to severe mental retardation could learn crucial adaptability

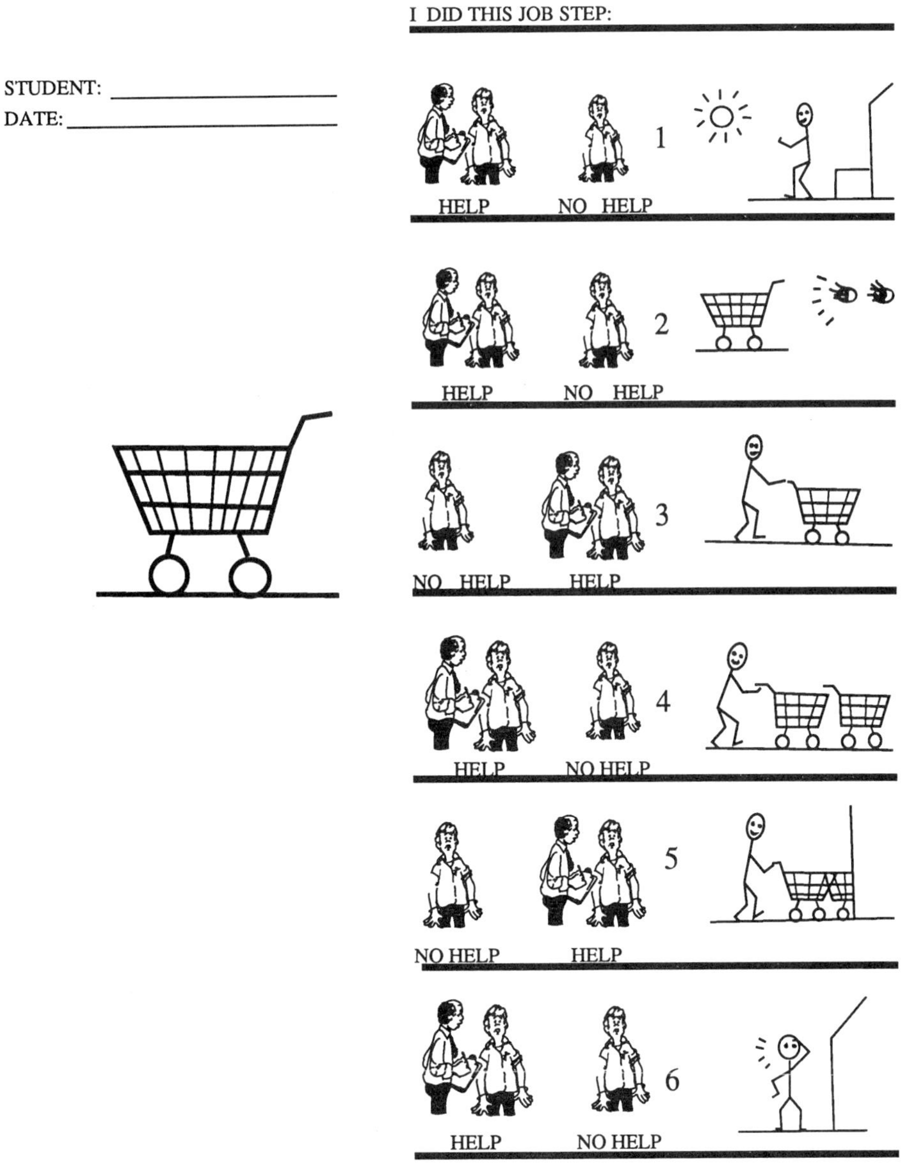

I DID THIS JOB STEP:

STUDENT: _____

DATE: _____

FIGURE 2. Example of self-evaluation form used at a grocery store job.

skills through completion of in-class activities. Each student completed a classroom-based sequence of self-directed picture-cued lessons. After about 5 months of systematic in-class intervention, students learned many adaptability skills, which generalized across nontrained tasks and settings.

Agran and his associates at Utah State University have investigated the effects of antecedent self-management control procedures on the problem-solving skills of students with mild through severe mental retardation. For example, four students with mental retardation who were employed as housekeeping trainees in a hospital were having difficulty completing job tasks in a specified order (Agran, Fodor-Davis, & Moore, in press). To enhance their performance, they learned to emit task-specific self-instructions prior to each task. As depicted in Figure 3, following training, job-task se-

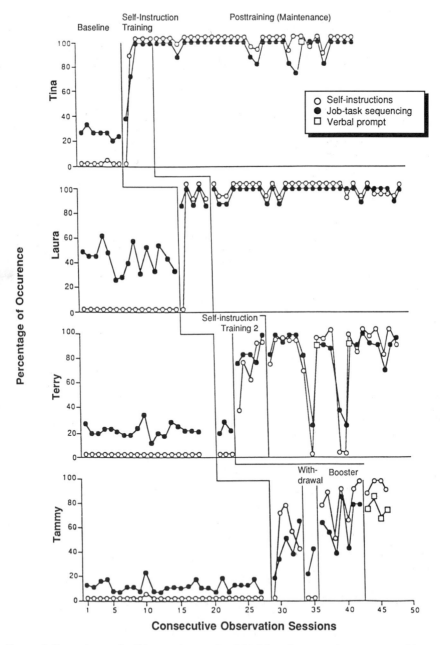

FIGURE 3. Percentages of self-instructions emitted for job task-sequencing across participants.

quencing for all students increased dramatically and maintained for up to 3 months; concomitant increases in task completion were also observed.

In another investigation, five adolescents with severe handicaps who were being trained to acquire a variety of janitorial skills were instructed to use self-generated verbal prompts and/or picture cues prior to their performance (Agran, Fodor-Davis, Moore, & Deer, 1988). Results indicated that training improved the work performance of all participants. Last, Moore, Agran, and Fodor-Davis (in press) trained four employees with severe handicaps to use a number of antecedent self-management strategies (i.e., self-instructions, goal setting, picture cues) to enhance decision making and productivity. The training produced marked increases in productivity.

Summary

Clearly, adaptability instruction can enhance students' self-management and empower their ability to become more independent. Most importantly, adaptability instruction will provide participants with the skills they need to be their own change agents rather than passive recipients of the decisions of teachers, job coordinators, and coaches.

VOCATIONAL INSTRUCTION AND PLACEMENT

Besides empowering consumer decision making, school-based instructional programs and postschool supported employment operations need to teach their consumers to take advantage of the fundamental opportunity integrated placements offer to learn to adapt to changing circumstances. Rather than assume that on-going supervision is sufficient for success, we must consider goals and strategies that encourage consumers to become independent. This will require partnership between schools, community agencies, parents, and consumers.

School-Based Instruction

We believe educational programs that serve students who are mentally retarded need to combine functional skill training and in-school integrated social skill experiences with community-based instructional activities (Sailor *et al.*, 1986). As shown in Figure 4, during the early school years, the focus of activity is within the regular classroom, supplemented by needed individual or group functional skill training activity. Integration into regular school activities during these years promotes social interaction skills. Specific skill training activities and adaptability instruction can occur through individual or group instruction in specialized or mainstreamed settings. Most of the activity that occurs during the middle and high school years takes place in the community, outside the school building (see Mithaug, Martin, Agran, & Rusch, 1988, and Mithaug, Martin, & Husch, 1988, for detailed information about school-based adaptability instruction).

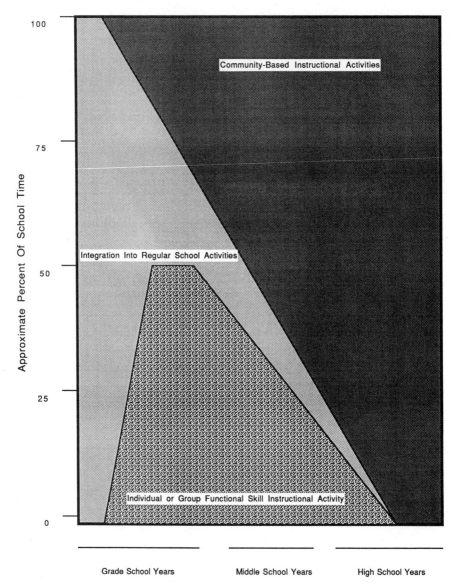

FIGURE 4. Recommended distribution of school-day time by type of activities across elementary, middle school, and secondary school years.

Results from the many recent follow-up studies strongly suggest needed change in secondary-level programming. As Edgar (1987) points out:

Few mildly handicapped students (and virtually no severely involved students) move from school to community jobs that allow for independent living. The truth is that the secondary curriculum for special education students appears to have very little, if any, impact on their eventual adjustment to community life. . . . A logical conclusion is that a major change in secondary programs for special education is

> urgently required. . . . The only solution is radical (no namby-pamby modification
> or cosmetic addition to existing programs) shift in focus of secondary curriculum
> away from academic to functional vocational, independent living tasks. (p. 560)

Employment preparation and experiences are the most important factors related to employment success (McLoughlin *et al.*, 1987). During middle school through high school, the percentage of time spent in community-based vocational training should increase, from less than 10% of the school day in the early grades to all day during the last 3 or 4 years of high school. Beginning by the age of 12, students who are mentally retarded should participate more often in community-based vocational programs (Rusch & Chadsey-Rusch, 1985; Wehman, Kregel, & Barcus, 1985). These programs should sample a range of entry-level occupations rather than focus upon one job (Pumpian, West, & Shepard, 1988). During the later school years, students should rotate every month or so through different job try-out sites, until they are placed into a paid job. At this time, a level of support should be provided that replicates postschool supported employment programs. Once the student is stabilized, transfer is made to the postschool supported work program. School- and community-based vocational programs need to follow federal and state labor laws to ensure safety and fair payment of wages. (See Martin & Husch, 1987, for a review of how to establish school vocational programs in accordance with labor laws and regulations.) Finally, transition plans for services provided by a postschool-supported employment program should be established no later than the last year of school (Wehman, Wood, Everson, & Parent, 1985).

Postschool-Supported Employment Programs

The 1986 amendments of the U. S. Rehabilitation Act established supported employment as a goal for individuals for whom competitive employment has not traditionally occurred. Supported employment includes (1) paid work, (2) work in an integrated nonsheltered setting, (3) instruction to learn needed behaviors, and (4) on-going support to maintain a job. In contrast with traditional employment programs, which do not meet the needs of many workers who require on-going support to maintain a job, the central feature of supported employment programs is long-term follow-up and support. Supported employment is for workers who need permanent support to be successful in competitive employment (Mithaug *et al.*, 1988). It is "inappropriate for persons who would be better served in time-limited preparation programs leading to independent employment" (Wehman & Kregel, 1985, p. 220).

Various supported employment alternatives include (1) individual-supported jobs in community businesses (Bellamy *et al.*, 1988; Rusch, 1986; Wehman *et al.*, 1988), (2) mobile work crews (Mank, Rhodes, & Bellamy, 1986), (3) enclaves (Valenta & Rhodes, 1985), and (4) entrepreneurial (Bellamy *et al.*, 1988). Each of these employment models is described briefly in Table 1.

There are model-supported employment programs in Illinois (Lagomar-

TABLE 1
Supported Employment Models

Individual-supported jobs in community businesses

One person with severe disabilities is employed by a community firm. After intensive on-the-job training, a job coach provides long-term follow-up.

Mobile Work Crews

Small group of workers who typically complete service industry jobs (e.g., janitorial or groundskeeping work) at community businesses. As with an individual placement, a job coach provides long-term follow-up.

Enclaves

A small group of persons with severe disabilities who work at a community business. As with an individual placement, a job coach provides long-term follow-up.

Entrepreneurial

A small group of workers, helped by consultants and nonhandicapped workers, establish and operate their own business. The workers own the business and share the profits. Employment can occur through individual-supported jobs, mobile crews, or enclaves.

---

cino, 1986), Virginia (Wehman, 1986b), Vermont (Vogelsberg, 1986), Oregon (Bellamy *et al.*, 1988), and other states. They are cost effective in relation to the placement of mentally retarded individuals in sheltered workshops and provide more opportunities for social integration (Martin *et al.*, 1982; Wehman & Kregel, 1985). However, the interactions that typically occur between job coaches, supervisors, and the consumer all too often promote dependence rather than independence (Mithaug, Martin, Agran, & Rusch, 1988). Perhaps, this is why the average duration of employment per individual in the nation's longest running supported employment program ranges from 13.5 to 19 months ("Supported employment: What the data tell us," 1988).

Purpose of Supported Employment

One primary purpose of supported employment is for consumers to be as autonomous and adaptable as possible (Buckley & Mank, 1988). Unfortunately, most interactions between job coaches, supervisors, and consumers promotes the need for supervision while inhibiting adaptive responding (Gifford *et al.*, 1984). Self-management approaches "demonstrate an important, and exciting, new approach to teaching and supporting vocational skills" (Mank & Horner, 1988, p. 169). We believe adaptability instruction, which is based upon self-management approaches, empowers consumers at their employment sites.

CONSUMER-CENTERED SUPPORTED EMPLOYMENT MODEL

Secondary-aged students and unemployed adults or those working in sheltered workshops need to make the transition to employment. Figure 5 depicts a model suggesting how this can be undertaken. Consumer-centered ongoing assessment is central to this process. We use the Job Match Assess-

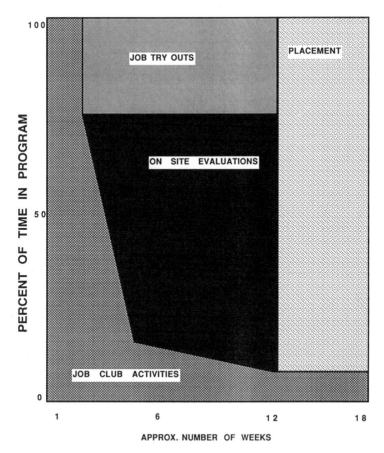

FIGURE 5. Recommended distribution of time across job tryouts, on-site evaluations, and job-club activities prior to and after a supported employment placement.

ment process described later. Prior to a paid job placement, each consumer experiences three activities: (1) processing self-assessment information and planning options in a job-club format, (2) on-site evaluations where job preferences and abilities are compared to the demands of different work sites, and (3) job tryouts where on-the-job adaptability skills are learned. Students complete job tryouts and self-administer on-site evaluations from the middle school years on. Students obtain a paid job at least two years prior to leaving school. Following a paid placement, support responsibilities are gradually transferred from the schools to adult providers. When students graduate from school, they are working in a paid job that they enjoy and receive support and follow-up services from a postschool supported employment program.

VOCATIONAL ASSESSMENT

Functional assessment determines and then matches a worker's abilities, interests, and needs to the requirements of a community job (Martin, 1986).

To facilitate placement, contemporary assessments measure performance in relation to specific on-the-job demands (Agran *et al.*, 1989; Menchetti & Rusch, in press; Menchetti, Rusch, & Owens, 1982). The job match assessment is an informal approach designed for use with supported employment programs. It suggests a supported employment option in relation to the level of assistance needed at various work sites for each worker.

Job Match Assessment Process

The Job Match Assessment process (Martin, Mithaug, & Husch, 1988) compares consumers' skills to the demands expected across different targeted work environments. It assesses the entry-level, vocational, social/personal, and adaptability skills employers expect workers to possess (Mithaug, Martin, & Agran, 1987; Rusch, Schutz, & Agran, 1982; Salzberg, Agran, & Lignugaris-Kraft, 1986; Salzberg, Likins, McConaughy, Lignugaris-Kraft, & Stowitschek, 1989). A teacher, counselor, or vocational supervisor determines what skills are required for each job by interviewing supervisors and workers. Direct observation is used to verify interview data and add any skills not already identified. Next, a situational assessment is used to evaluate the person's skills and abilities. This assessment specifies the level of cue the person will need to complete each task in relation to various job expectations. A profile is generated from the results, indicating the most appropriate type of supported employment program for each targeted job.

The Job Match Assessment assumes that each person is able to complete all required tasks. Rather than assessing the ability or inability to perform a skill, the Job Match Assessment identifies the cue that enables the person to complete the task. The three cue levels are: (1) teacher- or supervisor-delivered cues, (2) permanent cues, and (3) self-generated cues. Level 3 self-generated cues mean that the person can perform the task with self-delivered verbal prompts or instructions. The next highest level indicates that the person can read and follow printed instructions, photographs, or drawings to complete a task. Finally, when a teacher, supervisor, or job coach prompts a student, the lowest level is marked. Thus, a person's support level and subsequent type of supported employment placement can be determined for each job.

Levels of Consumer-Centered Independence

Mithaug, Martin, Husch, Agran, and Rusch (1988) detail 10 levels of consumer-centered independence, which range from making a single independent response to setting goals, making plans, and adjusting performance in relation to self-assessed feedback information. The levels define the range of independent performance possible—from completion of a single-step task to a detailed analysis of a person's own activities and desires. Table 2 explains these 10 levels.

The various types of supported employment placements can be matched to independence levels. A person whose independence levels range from 1 to 4 would function best with the degree of support provided by an enclave. A person whose independence levels range from 5 to 6 would receive the best degree of support from a mobile crew. Workers who function with independence levels of 7 to 9 can function well in individual placement with periodic follow-up by the job coach. Finally, a person who is at independence level 10 is a candidate for competitive employment. (See Mithaug, Martin, Husch, Agran, & Rusch, 1988, for a detailed discussion of independence levels and corresponding supported employment placements.)

CONSUMER-CENTERED VOCATIONAL ASSESSMENT

Consumer-centered assessments allow individuals with mental retardation to evaluate their own needs. They use this information to match placements to their own needs, interests, and abilities. This is a radical shift from current practices, because most secondary students do not attend their own staffings, let alone participate in the decision-making process that directly affects them (Mithaug, Martin, Agran, & Rusch, 1988). The Supported Employment Partnership at the University of Colorado at Colorado Springs has developed and field-tested a two-part consumer-centered vocational assessment process (Martin, Mithaug, & Husch, 1988). The first assessment establishes a job match; the second secures a successful placement. Table 3 outlines the process.

TABLE 2
Levels of Consumer-Centered Independence

1. A single response
2. Completion of a single-step task
3. Completion of a multiple-step task
4. Completion of a routine single-step task[a]
5. Completion of a routine multiple-step task[a]
6. Completion of a variable multiple-task sequence
7. Action sequence and self-evaluation
8. Plans, action sequence, and self-evaluation
9. Goals, plans, action sequence, and self-evaluation
10. Goals, plans, action sequence, self-evaluation, and adjustment

[a]Required to get material needed to do task and return/delivery material and product.

TABLE 3
Two-Part Consumer-Centered Vocational Assessment

I. Job-match assessment
  A. Self-assessment of strengths (completed during job-club activities)
    1. Social/personal
    2. Occupational
    3. Community functioning
  B. Self-assessment of preferred jobs (completed during job-club activities)
    1. General
    2. Paired comparisons
  C. Self-assessment of preferred job characteristics (completed during job-club activities and on-site)
    1. Environmental traits
    2. Shift and time traits
    3. Job traits
  D. Self-evaluation of job tasks (completed on-the-job and discussed during job-club activities)
    1. Task requirements
    2. Schedule requirements
II. Placement assessments
  A. Long-term contracts (completed during job-club activities and at on-the-job tryouts)
    1. Goals (including job and work condition preferences)
    2. Skills and behaviors
    3. Self-evaluation
    4. Adjustment
  B. Short-term contracts (completed during job-club activities and on-the-job)
    1. Goals
    2. Skills and behaviors
    3. Self-evaluation
    4. Adjustment

Format

Individuals with mild to severe mental retardation complete the job-match and maintenance assessments themselves. They work on paper-and-pencil tasks during job-club activities and situational assessments. Each assessment form consists of line drawings that are paired with printed words presented in a left-to-right, top-to-bottom sequence. Prerequisite skills require looking at a drawing and responding to what it means. The situational assessment uses similar forms to direct consumer observations and self-evaluations. Each assessment is individualized to meet the needs and abilities of different consumers. A form can consist of one drawing or many.

Administration and Response Consistency

Consumers complete the placement assessments several times over a period of weeks. Their response consistency helps to determine the amount of assistance consumers need to make decisions. When response consistency reaches a minimum of 80% across at least three administrations, the consumer is making reliable choices. Lower levels require that the individuals receive support and guidance in decision making. Consumers use their self-assessments to develop their IEP (Individual Education Plan) or their IWRP (Individual Written Rehabilitation Plan).

Job-Match Assessment

The job-match assessment consists of a four-step process. First, consumers determine their strengths and weaknesses in social/personal, occupational, community functioning, and work-related leisure domains. Second, they determine the jobs they like. Third, they assess preferred job characteristics and then confirm them through on-site observations. Last, they observe the tasks at preferred jobs and compare them with their preferences and their own strengths and weaknesses. The job match occurs through situational assessments and job-club activities. Each of the four steps in the process is discussed below.

Self-Assessment of Strengths

The self-assessment of strengths is the first consumers complete. Its purpose is twofold. It provides a structured opportunity for the vocational staff to become acquainted with the consumer, and consumers with the other members of their job-club group. Second, it provides consumers with an opportunity to learn to evaluate themselves in terms of their own strengths and weaknesses. Consumers answer questions about vocationally important skills and abilities, including social/personal, occupational, community functioning, and work-related leisure preferences and habits. They complete assessments at least three times over several days. Parents, former teachers, and others familiar with the consumer also use the forms to evaluate the consumer's behavior. Consumers compare their evaluations with those completed by significant others. Each consumer then uses the results to compare his or her abilities to specific job requirements. Figure 6 provides an example of part of the assessment form used by the Supported Employment Partnership.

Self-Assessment of Job Preferences

First, consumers complete a general job-preference assessment, which consists of 12 to 15 line drawings representing locally available entry-level jobs. Each consumer simply circles or checks the drawings representing the jobs he or she likes. Each individual completes the assessment at least three times or until three or four jobs are consistently marked. This procedure provides initial preference data that are needed for the more detailed paired-comparison assessment.

Next, the consumers complete a paired-comparison assessment of pre-

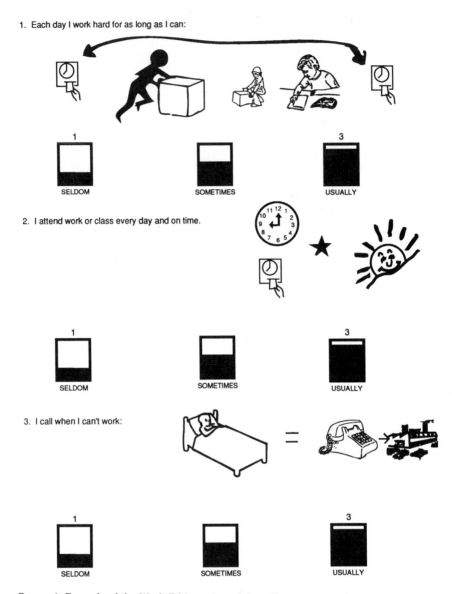

FIGURE 6. Example of the Work Ethic section of the self-assessment of strengths form.

ferred and nonpreferred jobs to determine their initial job preferences. Each consumer evaluates at least 10 line drawings of different jobs two at a time (see examples of two jobs in Figure 7). A teacher, counselor, or another consumer can present the drawings. The presenter controls the order so that the consumer can compare each drawing (see example of the job pairs in Table 4). The pool of jobs includes the preferred jobs identified in the general assessment, one or two jobs that are too difficult for the person to complete,

LAUNDRY/DRY CLEANERS

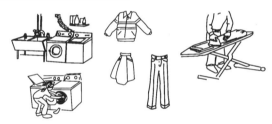

OUTDOOR MAINTENANCE/LAWN SERVICE

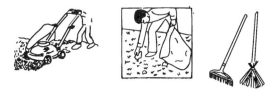

FIGURE 7. Two drawings used with the paired-comparison job preference assessment.

and others likely to be available in the community. Most individuals with mental retardation need five or six administrations of the paired comparisons to rank their preferred jobs reliably.

Self-Assessment of Preferred Job Characteristics

This assessment determines the consumer's preferences for specific job characteristics that are associated with the work site, worker role, and work schedule. Consumers assess three categories of job characteristics: (1) en-

TABLE 4
*Occupational Preferences Determined
through Paired-Comparison Testing*

1. Janitorial/housecleaning	Social activities
2. Laundry/dry cleaners	Outdoor maintenance
3. Cashier	Janitorial/housecleaning
4. Social activities	Laundry/dry cleaners
5. Outdoor maintenance	Cashier
6. Janitorial/housecleaning	Laundry/dry cleaners
7. Social activities	Outdoor maintenance
8. Cashier	Social activities
9. Janitorial/housecleaning	Outdoor maintenance
10. Cashier	Laundry/dry cleaners

Procedures

Consumer is presented all possible combinations of jobs and the choices are recorded. This is repeated at least three times or until a pattern of consistent choices is obtained.

vironmental (inside vs. outside); (2) worker (sitting vs. standing); and (3) shift and time (day vs. evenings). Figure 8 depicts several items from this assessment. Most questions present contrasting characteristics (i.e., work alone or with other people). As before, consumers circle or mark the line drawing representing preferred characteristics and complete the assessment at least three times over as many days or until they reach a 70% consistency level.

Self-Assessment of Job Tasks

Prior to the initial job tryout, consumers complete structured on-site assessments to learn task and schedule requirements. They observe several jobs, including preferred, nonpreferred, and novel jobs, and then self-assess the tasks and schedules associated with each. Figure 9 provides an example of

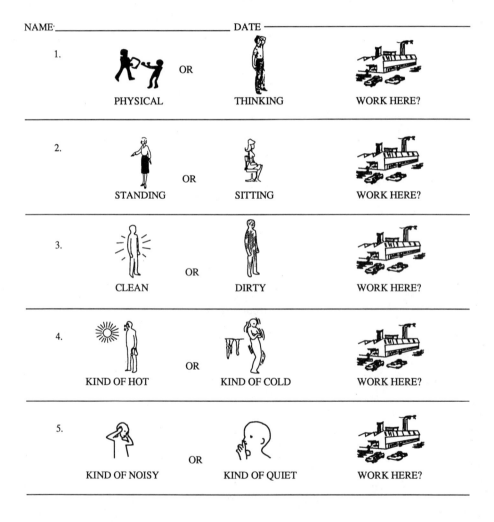

1.	PHYSICAL	OR	THINKING	WORK HERE?
2.	STANDING	OR	SITTING	WORK HERE?
3.	CLEAN	OR	DIRTY	WORK HERE?
4.	KIND OF HOT	OR	KIND OF COLD	WORK HERE?
5.	KIND OF NOISY	OR	KIND OF QUIET	WORK HERE?

FIGURE 8. Sample page to determine on-site job characteristics.

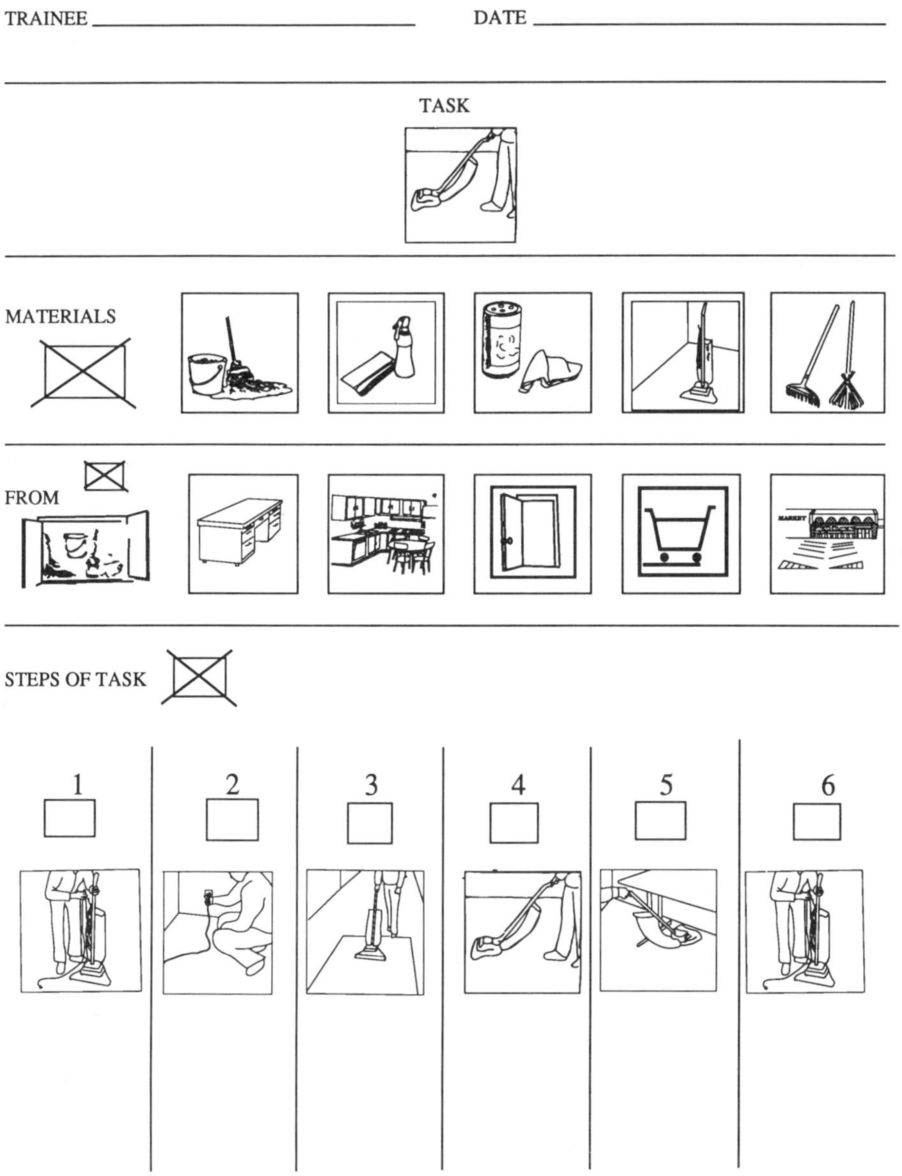

TRAINEE _____   DATE _____

FIGURE 9. Example of a self-assessment job task form for a maid's position.

the self-assessment form for a maid's vacuuming task. While observing a maid working, consumers check the boxes indicating the work materials required and where they are located. As the maid completes each step of the task, consumers check the corresponding step on the form. They repeat this process for all tasks in a job. After completing the on-site task self-assessment, the assessment of job characteristics is administered during job-club activities. After several jobs have been observed, the paired-comparison job preference assessment is repeated.

Obtaining a Job Match

During the four-step job match, consumers observe several jobs and match work characteristics to their own strengths, weaknesses, and preferences. After they compare their observations with their preferences, they decide on a job tryout location where they complete their placement assessments.

Placement Assessments

During job placements, a job coach provides support to enable consumers to learn skills necessary to maintain employment. Many workers who are mentally retarded need this systematic instruction (Test, Grossi, & Keul, 1988). Typically, job coaches provide prompts, instructions, or even do the work themselves to maintain the job, learn new tasks, move from one job to another job, or adapt to a change in the shift. Seldom do consumers adjust on their own. We believe the worker does not need to depend upon a job coach so much. Many workers who are mentally retarded can learn to manage their own work. The job coach should orchestrate and encourage this self-management and advocate issues beyond the worker's control. The job coach develops and supplies the worker with needed forms and organizes the information so that the worker can review it during job-club discussions.

Adaptability Contracts

Adaptability contracts are self-management forms that consumers use to (1) set goals and performance objectives, (2) develop work schedules, (3) monitor their own progress, (4) evaluate their results, and (5) decide what adjustment to make the next time. There are two contracts: (1) the long-term contract for setting goals and plans for several weeks, months, or even years, and (2) the short-term contract for day-to-day planning and evaluation on-the-job. Consumers use the short-term contract to monitor their progress on their long-term plan.

The long-term contract contains goals, choice options, plan, results, evaluation, and adjustment sections. The focus for the long-term contract during job try-outs is to validate the job match. Figure 10 presents the first page of a long-term adaptability contract used by our Supported Employment Partnership. The sections for goals and choices present job characteristics and job-choice options, respectively. The consumer completes these sections after being at a job tryout site for several days. In the remaining sections, the consumer examines other aspects of the work site, including time and days worked and money earned. Consumers record their observations on the contract forms. Then, consumers use information from their daily contracts to

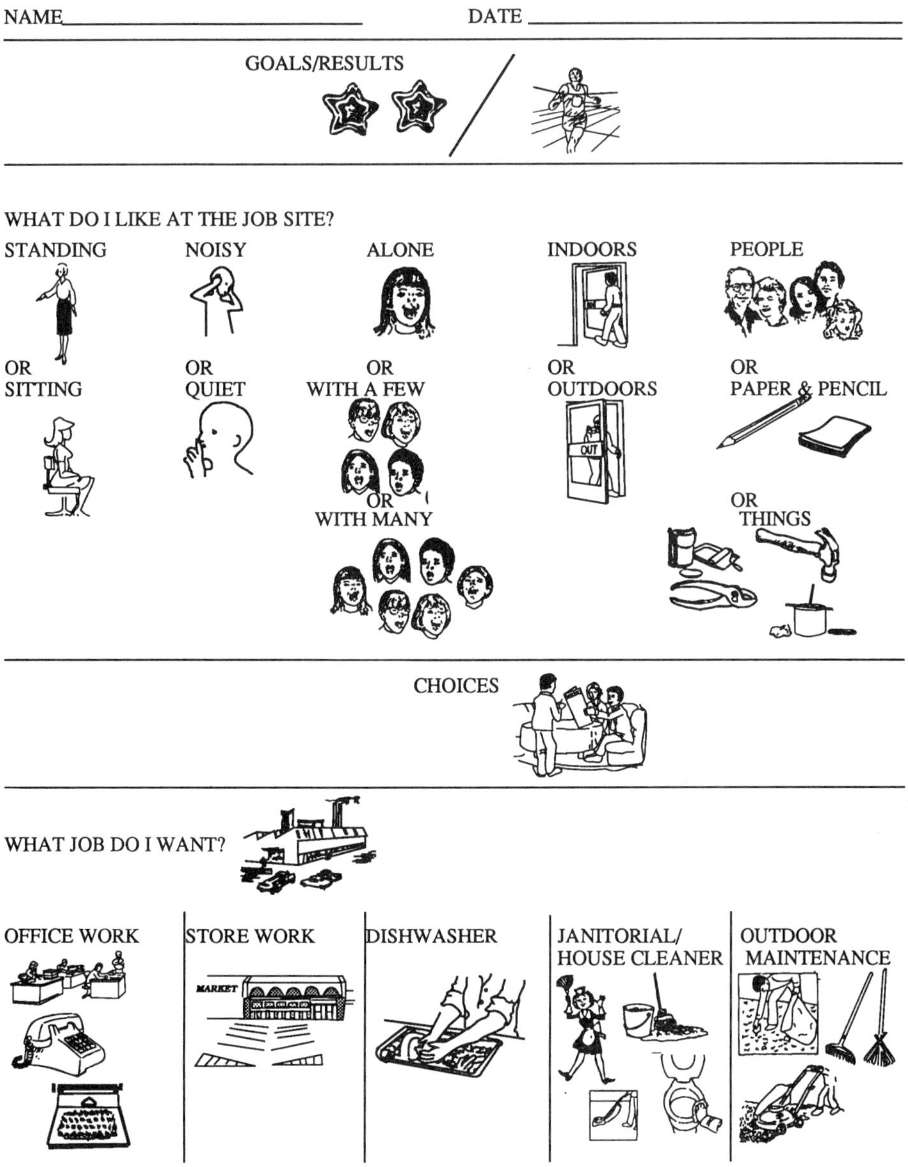

NAME_____   DATE _____

GOALS/RESULTS

WHAT DO I LIKE AT THE JOB SITE?

| STANDING | NOISY | ALONE | INDOORS | PEOPLE |

| OR SITTING | OR QUIET | OR WITH A FEW | OR OUTDOORS | OR PAPER & PENCIL |

OR WITH MANY

OR THINGS

CHOICES

WHAT JOB DO I WANT?

| OFFICE WORK | STORE WORK | DISHWASHER | JANITORIAL/ HOUSE CLEANER | OUTDOOR MAINTENANCE |

FIGURE 10. Example of a page taken from a long-term adaptability contract.

evaluate their progress and determine appropriate adjustments for their long-term contract.

The short-term contract reflects day-to-day changes on-the-job. This requires workers to monitor their performance each day, to make short-term decisions, and to determine on-the-job performance adjustments. The contract includes plan, work, evaluation, and adjust sections. The plan section details the day's responsibilities, and the work section allows consumers to self-monitor their performance. In the evaluation section, they compare actual performance with expectations. The plan can be expanded to include unique issues. Figure 11 presents a contract for a fast-food restaurant, which focuses upon the consumer's appearance and work attitude.

The immediate supervisor evaluates consumers' performance each day by using a similar form. Then the workers compare their evaluations with those of the job supervisor. Discrepancies between the two evaluations require new decisions in the adjust section, which the workers express by marking directly on the contract. Many on-the-job supervisors do not provide honest feedback, preferring always to rate the "handicapped worker" higher than his or her performance deserves. A crucial job coach role is to facilitate honest evaluation.

Task Sequence Cards

If the task sequence in the daily contract is insufficient to cue performance for each step of each task, the job coach develops job cards, such as the one presented in Figure 12. It provides step-by-step drawings of what needs to be done. The workers simply follow the instructions depicted by each drawing. After completing a step, they check it to monitor their progress through the sequence. Several job cards can be sequenced together to facilitate independent completion of all the tasks. The job coach can vary the complexity of visual cues depending on the needs of the work site and the abilities of the workers. For instance, in lobby clean-up, the workers must do one set of tasks if the restaurant is busy, and another if it is slow. The job coach can build this decision-tree into the daily contract so that consumers can make this important discrimination and then make the correct decision *independently*.

Job Maintenance

Adaptability contracts assist consumers to make the adjustments necessary for long-term placements. They reflect changes in consumer needs and interests as well as changes in job requirements. The long-term contract can also include recreational or residential goals as it evolves into a "life plan" accompanied by short-term contracts that assist in the management of day-to-day activities. It is this dynamic interplay between contract plans, performance, evaluations, and adjustments that will assure long-term success for consumers as they learn to adjust on their own.

SUMMARY

We must help consumers think and act on their own. To do this, we need to change our collective intervention orientation. For too long, we have viewed consumers as passive recipients of our actions. The Adaptability In-

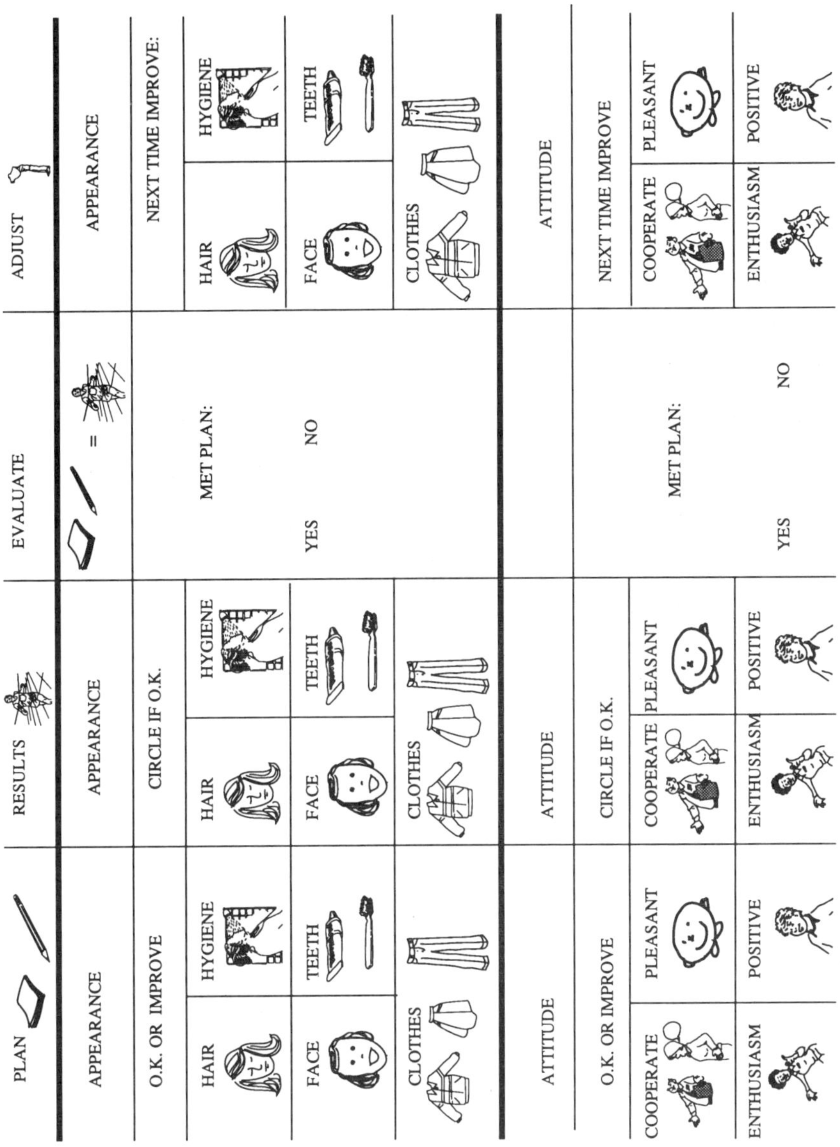

FIGURE 11. Example of a page taken from a daily adaptability contract focusing upon appearance and work attitude.

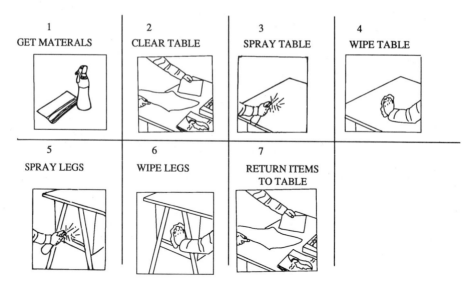

FIGURE 12. Sample job card.

struction Model, based upon sound self-management research, is an intervention approach that includes the consumer. Through the use of pictures and drawings, individuals who are mildly, moderately, and severely mentally retarded can learn to plan, to complete tasks independently, to evaluate their performance, to compare their performance to a standard, and to make adjustments. These skills will enable many workers to be successful at their community jobs and make more choices for themselves.

Supported employment programs provide a means for adults who are mentally retarded to become productive members of society. By working in partnership with consumers, parents, educators, and agency representatives, we can alter existing practices to improve consumers' independence and adaptability. These efforts will produce positive long-term consequences for consumers as they learn how to make decisions, perform work schedules independently, evaluate their own performance and their work expectations, and change their behavior accordingly—not only for today, but for their future as well.

ACKNOWLEDGMENTS. We express appreciation to Mike Allen, past president of Parents Encouraging Parents for his help in expanding our thoughts. This parent organization is based in Colorado Springs. We also express our sincere appreciation to Arlene Waters-Karlan, teacher in the Harrison School District in Colorado Springs, for her inspiring teaching ability. Support for the preparation of this chapter was provided in part from grants from the U.S. Office of Special Education and Rehabilitative Services, Colorado Division of Rehabilitation, Colorado Department of Education, and the Mid-Colorado Regional Commission for the Developmentally Disabled of Colorado Springs.

REFERENCES

Agran, M., & Martin, J. E. (1987). Applying a technology of self-control in community environments for mentally retarded individuals. In M. Hersen, R. M. Eisler, & P. M. Miller (Eds.), *Progress in behavior modification* (Vol. 21, pp. 108–151). Newbury Park, CA: Sage Publications.

Agran, M., & Moore, S. (1987). Transitional programming: Suggesting an adaptability model. In J. L. Matson & R. P. Barrett (Eds.), *Advances in mental retardation and developmental disabilities* (Vol. 3, pp. 179–208). Greenwich, CT: JAI Press.

Agran, M., Fodor-Davis, J., & Moore, S. C. (1986). The effects of self-instructional training on job task-sequencing: Suggesting a problem-solving strategy. *Education and Training of the Mentally Retarded, 21,* 273–281.

Agran, M., Fodor-Davis, J., Moore, S. C., & Deer, M. (1988). *The effects of self-generated prompting procedures on the instruction-following skills of students with severe handicaps.* Manuscript submitted for publication.

Agran, M., Martin, J. E., & Mithaug, D. E. (1987). Transitional assessment for students with mental retardation. *Diagnostique, 12,* 173–184.

Bandura, A. (1969). *Principles of behavior modification.* New York: Holt, Rinehart & Winston.

Bellamy, G. T., Rhodes, L. E., & Albin, J. M. (1986). Supported employment. In W. E. Kiernan & J. A. Stark (Eds.), *Pathways to employment for adults with developmental disabilities* (pp. 129–138). Baltimore: Brookes.

Bellamy, G. T., Rhodes, L. E., Mank, D. M., & Albin, J. M. (1988). *Supported employment.* Baltimore: Brookes.

Brickey, M. P., Campbell, K. M., & Browning, L. J. (1985). A five-year follow-up of sheltered workshop employees placed in competitive jobs. *Mental Retardation, 23,* 67–83.

Bronicki, G. J., & Turnbull, A. P. (1987). Family-professional interactions. In M. Snell (Ed.), *Systematic instruction of persons with severe handicaps* (3rd ed., pp. 9–35). Columbus, OH: Charles E. Merrill.

Buckley, J., & Mank, D. M. (1988). Self-management programming for supported employment. In D. O. Olsen & P. Ferguson (Eds.), *Disability research: Issues in policy and practice* (pp. 63–90). Eugene, OR: University of Oregon Specialized Training Program.

Close, D. W., & Keating, T. J. (1988). Community living and work. In R. Gaylord-Ross (Ed.), *Vocational education for persons with handicaps* (pp. 87–108). Mountain View, CA: Mayfield.

Colorado Department of Education. (1983). *Colorado employability skills survey.* Denver: Author.

Edgar, D. (1987). Secondary programs in special education: Are many of them justifiable? *Exceptional Children, 53,* 555–561.

Edgar, E., & Levine, P. (1988). A longitudinal study of graduates of special education. *Interchange, 8*(2), 3–5. (Newsletter from the University of Illinois Transition Institute).

Fardig, D. B., Algozzine, R. F., Schwartz, S. E., Hensel, J. W., & Westling, D. L. (1985). Postsecondary vocational adjustment of rural mildly handicapped students. *Exceptional Children, 52,* 115–121.

Gifford, J., Rusch, F. R., Martin, J. E., & White, D. M. (1984). Autonomy and adaptability: A proposed technology for maintaining work behavior. In N. Ellis & N. Bray (Eds.), *International review of research in mental retardation* (Vol. 12, pp. 285–314). New York: Academic Press.

Goodall, P. A., Wehman, P., Cleveland, P. (1983). Job placement for mentally retarded individuals. *Education and Training of the Mentally Retarded, 18,* 271–278.

Guess, D., & Siegel-Causey, E. (1985). Behavioral control and education of severely handicapped students: Who's doing what to whom and why? In D. Bricker & J. Filler (Eds.), *Severe mental retardation: From theory to practice* (pp. 230–243). Reston, VA: Council for Exceptional Children.

Guess, D., Benson, H. A., & Siegel-Causey, E. (1985). Concepts and issues related to choice making and autonomy among persons with severe disabilities. *Journal of the Association for Persons with Severe Handicaps, 10,* 79–86.

Hardman, M., & McDonnell, J. (1987). Implementing federal transition initiatives for youths with severe handicaps: The Utah community-based transition project. *Exceptional Children, 53,* 493–498.

Hasazi, S. B., Gordon, L. R., & Roe, C. A. (1985). Factors associated with employment status of handicapped youth exiting high school from 1979–1983. *Exceptional Children, 51,* 493–469.

Hasazi, S. B., Gordon, L. R., Roe, C. A., Hull, M., Finck, D., & Salembier, G. (1985). A statewide follow-up on post-high school employment and residential status of students labelled, "mentally retarded". *Education and Training of the Mentally Retarded, 20,* 222–234.

Hill, M. L., Banks, D., Handrich, R. R., Wehman, P. H., Hill, J. W., & Shafer, M. S. (1987). Benefit-cost analysis of supported competitive employment for persons with mental retardation. *Research in Developmental Disabilities, 8,* 71–89.

Hill, J., Seyfarth, J., Banks, P. D., Wehman, P., & Orelove, F. (1987). Parent attitudes about working conditions of their adult mentally retarded sons and daughters. *Exceptional Children, 54,* 9–23.

Johnson, D. R., Bruininks, R. H., & Thurlow, M. L. (1987). Meeting the challenge of transition service planning through improved interagency cooperation. *Exceptional Children, 53,* 522–530.

Kernan, K., & Koegel, R. (1980). *Employment experiences of community-based mildly retarded adults.* Working paper No. 14, Socio-Behavioral Group, Mental Retardation Research Center, School of Medicine, University of California, Los Angeles.

Kochany, L., & Keller, J. (1981). An analysis and evaluation of the failure of severely disabled individuals in competitive employment. In P. Wehman (Ed.), *Competitive employment: New horizons for severely disabled individuals* (pp. 181–198). Baltimore: Brookes.

Krause, M. W., & MacEachron, A. E. (1982). Competitive employment training for mentally retarded adults: The supported work model. *American Journal of Mental Deficiency, 86,* 650–653.

Kregel, J., Wehman, P., Seyfarth, J., & Marshall, K. (1986). Community integration of young adults with mental retardation: Transition from school to adulthood. *Education and Training of the Mentally Retarded, 21,* 35–42.

Kurtz, P. D., & Neisworth, J. T. (1976). Self-control possibilities for exceptional children. *Exceptional Children, 42,* 212–217.

Lagomarcino, T. R. (1986). Community services: Using the supported work model within an adult service agency. In F. R. Rusch (Ed.), *Competitive employment issues and strategies* (pp. 65–75). Baltimore: Brookes.

Mank, D., & Horner, R. H. (1987). Self-recruited feedback: A cost-effective procedure for maintaining behavior. *Research in Developmental Disabilities, 8,* 91–112.

Mank, D., & Horner, R. H. (1988). Instructional programming in vocational education. in R. Gaylord-Ross (Ed.), *Vocational education for persons with handicaps* (pp. 142–173). Mountain View, CA: Mayfield.

Mank, D., Rhodes, L., & Bellamy, G. T. (1986). Four supported employment models. In W. Kiernan and J. Stark (Eds.), *Pathways to employment for adults with developmental disabilities* (pp. 139–153). Baltimore: Brookes.

Martin, J. E. (1982). *Time-setting generalization assessment of mentally retarded adults acquired self-control in the preparation of complex meals after withdrawal of training components and trainers.* Unpublished doctoral dissertation, Department of Special Education, University of Illinois at Urbana-Champaign.

Martin, J. E. (1986). Identifying potential jobs. In F. R. Rusch (Ed.), *Competitive employment issues and strategies* (pp. 165–186). Baltimore: Brookes.

Martin, J. E. & Husch, J. V. (1987). School-based vocational training and labor laws. *Journal of the Association for Persons with Severe Handicaps, 12,* 140–144.

Martin, J. E., Schneider, K. E., Rusch, F. R., & Geske, T. G. (1982). Training mentally retarded individuals for competitive employment: Benefits of transitional employment. *Exceptional Education Quarterly, 3,* 58–66.

Martin, J. E., Mithaug, D. E., & Husch, J. V. (1988). *How to teach adaptability in community training and supported employment.* Colorado Springs, CO: Ascent Publications.

Martin, J. E., Burger, D. L., Elias-Burger, S., & Mithaug, D. E. (1988). Application of self-control strategies to facilitate independence. In N. Bray (Ed.), *International review of research in mental retardation* (Vol. 15, pp. 155–193). New York: Academic Press.

McDonnell, J., & Hardman, M. (1985). Planning the transition of severely handicapped youth from school to adult services: A framework for high school programs. *Education and Training of the Mentally Retarded, 20,* 275–286.

McLoughlin, C. S., Garner, J. B., & Callahan, M. (1987). *Getting employed, staying employed.* Baltimore: Brookes.

Menchetti, B. M., & Rusch, F. R. (in press). Vocational evaluation and eligibility for rehabilitation services. In P. Wehman & S. Moon (Eds.), *Vocational rehabilitation and supported employment.* Baltimore: Brookes.

Menchetti, B. M., Rusch, F. R., & Owens, D. (1982). Assessing the vocational needs of mentally retarded adolescents and adults. In J. L. Matson & S. E. Bruening (Eds.), *Assessing the mentally retarded* (pp. 247–284). New York: Grunne & Stratton.

Mithaug, D. E., Horiuchi, C. N., & Fanning, P. N. (1985). A report on the Colorado statewide follow-up survey of special education students. *Exceptional Children, 51,* 397–404.

Mithaug, D. E., Horiuchi, C. N., & McNulty, B. A. (1987). *Parent report on the transition of students graduating from Colorado special education programs in 1978 and 1979.* Denver: Colorado Dept. of Education.

Mithaug, D. E., Martin, J. E., & Agran, M. (1987). Adaptability instruction: The goal of transitional programming. *Exceptional Children, 53,* 500–505.

Mithaug, D. E., Martin, J. E., & Burger, D. L. (1987a). *VITAL independence training and adaptability learning.* Colorado Springs, CO: Ascent Publications.

Mithaug, D. E., Martin, J. E., & Burger, D. L. (1987b). *VITAL checklist and curriculum guide.* Colorado Springs, CO: Ascent Publications.

Mithaug, D. E., Martin, J. E., Agran, M., & Rusch, F. R. (1988). *Why special education students fail: How to teach them to succeed.* Colorado Springs, CO: Ascent Publications.

Mithaug, D. E., Martin, J. E., Frazier, E., & Allen, M. (1988). *What special education teenagers must learn at home.* Colorado Springs, CO: Ascent Publications.

Mithaug, D. E., Martin, J. E., & Husch, J. V. (1988). *How to teach success strategies to students with special needs.* Colorado Springs, CO: Ascent Publications.

Mithaug, D. E., Martin, J. E., Husch, J. V., Agran, M., & Rusch, F. R. (1988). *When will persons in supported employment need less support?* Colorado Springs, CO: Ascent Publications.

Moore, S. C., Agran, M., & Fodor-Davis, J. (in press). Using self-management strategies to increase the production rates of workers with severe handicaps. *Education and training of the mentally retarded.*

Nietupski, J., Hamre-Nietupski, S., Welch, J., & Anderson, R. (1983). Establishing and maintaining vocational training sites for moderately and severely handicapped students: Strategies for community/vocational trainers. *Education and Training of the Mentally Retarded, 18,* 169–175.

Pancsofar, E. L. (1986). Assessing work behavior. In F. R. Rusch (Ed.), *Competitive employment issues and strategies* (pp. 93–102). Baltimore: Brookes.

Playing the waiting game. (1988, March). *Association for Retarded Citizens News for Colorado,* p. 1.

Pumpian, I., West, E., & Shepard, H. (1988). Vocational evaluation of persons with severe handicaps. In R. Gaylord-Ross (Ed.), *Vocational education for persons with handicaps* (pp. 355–386). Mountain View, CA: Mayfield.

Revell G., Wehman, P., & Arnold, S. (1985). Supported work model of competitive employment for mentally retarded persons: Implications for rehabilitative services. In P. Wehman & J. Hill (Eds.), *Competitive employment for persons with mental retardation: From research to practice* (pp. 46–64). Richmond, VA: Virginia Commonwealth University.

Rosenbaum, M. S., & Drabman, R. S. (1979). Self-control training in the classroom: A review and critique. *Journal of Applied Behavior Analysis, 12,* 467–485.

Rusch, F. R. (1986). Introduction to supported work. In J. Chadsey-Rusch, C. H. Hanley-Maxwell, L. A. Phelps, & F. Rusch (Eds.), *School-to-work transition issues and models* (pp. 36–57). Champaign, IL: Transition Institute, College of Education, University of Illinois.

Rusch, F. R., & Chadsey-Rusch, J. (1985). Employment for persons with severe handicaps: Curriculum development and coordination of services. *Focus on Exceptional Children, 17*(9), 1–8.

Rusch, F. R., & Mithaug, D. E. (1980). *Vocational training for mentally retarded adults.* Champaign, IL: Research Press.

Rusch, F. R., Schutz, R. P., & Agran, M. (1982). Validating entry-level survival skills for service occupations: Implications for curriculum development. *Journal of the Association for the Severely Handicapped, 7*, 32–41.

Rusch, F. R., Martin, J. E., & White, D. M. (1985). Competitive employment: Teaching mentally retarded employees to maintain their work behavior. *Education and Training of the Mentally Retarded, 20*(3), 182–189.

Rusch, F. R., Mithaug, D. E., & Flexor, R. W. (1986). Obstacles to competitive employment and traditional program options for overcoming them. In F. R. Rusch (Ed.), *Competitive employment issues and strategies* (pp. 7–21). Baltimore: Brookes.

Rusch, F. R., Chadsey-Rusch, J., & Lagomarcino, T. (1987). Preparing students for employment. In M. Snell (Ed.), *Systematic instruction of persons with severe handicaps* (pp. 471–490). Columbus, OH: Charles E. Merrill.

Sailor, W., Halvorsen, A., Anderson, J., Goetz, L., Gee, K., Doering, K., & Hunt, P. (1986). Community intensive instruction. In R. H. Horner, L. H. Meyer, & H. D. Fredericks (Eds.), *Education of learners with severe handicaps* (pp. 251–288). Baltimore: Brookes.

Salzberg, C. L., Agran, M., & Lignugaris-Kraft, B. (1986). Behaviors that contribute to entry-level employment: A profile of five jobs. *Applied Research in Mental Retardation, 7*, 299–314.

Salzberg, C. L., Likins, M., McConaughy, E. K., Lignugaris-Kraft, B., & Stowitschek, J. J. (1986). Social competence and employment of retarded persons. In N. Bray (Ed.), *International review of research in mental retardation*. (Vol. 14, pp. 225–257). Orlando, FL: Academic Press.

Schalock, R. L., Wolzen, B., Ross, I., Elliott, B., Werbel, G., & Peterson, K. (1986). Post-secondary community placement of handicapped students: A five-year follow-up. *Learning Disability Quarterly, 9*, 295–303.

Schutz, R. P. (1986). Establishing a parent-professional partnership to facilitate competitive employment. In F. Rusch (Ed.), *Competitive employment issues and strategies* (pp. 289–302). Baltimore: Brookes.

Seyfarth, J., Hill, J. W., Orelove, F., McMillan, J., & Wehman, P. (1987). Factors influencing parents' vocational aspirations for their children with mental retardation. *Mental Retardation, 25*(6), 357–362.

Shapiro, E. S. (1981). Self-control procedures with the mentally retarded. In M. Hersen, R. M. Eisler, & P. M. Miller (Eds.), *Progress in behavior modification* (Vol. 12, pp. 265–297). New York: Academic Press.

Skinner, B. F. (1974). *About behaviorism*. New York: Alfred A. Knopf.

Stodden, R. A., & Boone, R. (1987). Assessing transition services for handicapped youth: A cooperative interagency approach. *Exceptional Children, 53*, 537–545.

Supported employment: What the data tell us. (Spring, 1988). *Employment News*. Eugene, OR: Specialized Training Program, University of Oregon.

Test, D. W., Grossi, T., & Keul, P. (1988). A functional analysis of the acquisition and maintenance of janitorial skills in a competitive work setting. *Journal of the Association for Persons with Severe Handicaps, 13*(1), 1–7.

Valenta, L., & Rhodes, L. (1985). Industry-based supported competitive employment for persons with severe handicaps. *Journal of the Association for Persons with Severe Handicaps, 10*, 12–21.

Vogelsberg, R. T. (1986). Competitive employment in Vermont. In F. R. Rusch (Ed.), *Competitive employment issues and strategies* (pp. 35–49). Baltimore: Brookes.

Wacker, D. P., & Berg, W. K. (1987). Generalizing and maintaining work behavior. In F. R. Rusch (Ed.), *Competitive employment issues and strategies* (pp. 129–140). Baltimore: Brookes.

Wehman, P. (1986a). Supported competitive employment for persons with severe disabilities. *Journal of Applied Rehabilitation Counseling, 17*(4), 24–29.

Wehman, P. (1986b). Competitive employment in Virginia. In F. R. Rusch (Ed.), *Competitive employment issues and strategies* (pp. 23–33). Baltimore: Brookes.

Wehman, P., & Kregel, J. (1985). A supported work approach to competitive employment of individuals with moderate and severe handicaps. *Journal of the Association for Persons with Severe Handicaps, 10*, 3–11.

Wehman, P., Kregel, J, & Barcus, J. M. (1985). From school to work: A vocational transition model for handicapped students. *Exceptional Children, 52*, 25–37.

Wehman, P., Kregel, J., & Seyfarth, J. (1985, December). Employment outlook for young adults with mental retardation. *Rehabilitation Counseling Bulletin*, pp. 90–98.

Wehman, P., Wood, W., Everson, J. M., & Parent, W. (1985). A supported employment approach to transition. *American Rehabilitation, 11*(3), 12–16.

Wehman, P., Moon, M. S., Everson, J. M., Wood, W., & Barcus, J. M. (1988). *Transition from school to work.* Baltimore: Brookes.

Wehman, P. H., Kregel, J., Barcus, J. M., & Schalock, R. L. (1986). Vocational transition for students with developmental disabilities. In W. E. Kiernan & J. A. Stark (Eds.), *Pathways to employment for adults with developmental disabilities* (pp. 113–128). Baltimore: Brookes.

Will, M. (1984). *OSERS programming for the transition of youth with disabilities: Bridges from school to working life.* Washington, DC: Office of Special Education and Rehabilitative Services (OSERS), U. S. Department of Education.

14

Emotional Problems I
Anxiety Disorders and Depression

BETSEY A. BENSON

INTRODUCTION

Anxiety disorders and depression in mentally retarded persons have received less attention than other behavior disorders. The inattention is not because anxiety and depression are rare among mentally retarded individuals; survey data indicate that these problems are relatively common. Rather, anxiety disorders and depression may be overlooked because individuals experiencing these problems are less difficult for caretakers to deal with than individuals who are aggressive or noncompliant. Thus, mentally retarded persons with anxiety disorders or depression may be less readily identified and referred for treatment.

A second factor that may have contributed to a lack of attention to anxiety disorders and depression was the belief that mentally retarded persons were *not* subject to the same types of emotional problems as nonretarded persons. This situation was especially true in the area of depression, where mentally retarded persons were said to be too psychologically immature to develop depressive disorders (Gardner, 1967). Consequently, there was a tendency to overlook anxiety disorders and depression in mentally retarded persons or to attribute maladaptive behaviors to the individual's cognitive limitations.

In recent years, it has become generally accepted that mentally retarded persons experience the full range of emotional disorders (Philips, 1967). However, it will become apparent that where anxiety disorders and depression are concerned, much of the research has focused on a few specific disorders whereas others have not been studied.

Following a brief review of the survey research on anxiety disorders and depression in mentally retarded individuals, the two groups of disorders will be dealt with separately in the discussion of assessment and treatment.

BETSEY A. BENSON • Department of Psychology, University of Illinois at Chicago, Chicago, Illinois 60680.

FREQUENCY OF ANXIETY DISORDERS AND DEPRESSION

The survey data have been fairly consistent regarding the frequency of occurrence of anxiety disorders and depression among mentally retarded individuals, surprisingly so, considering the wide geographic dispersion of the surveys and the varied methods of obtaining information. Three outpatient clinic surveys found similar rates of occurrence. Philips and Williams (1975) reported the three major problems noted by parents of 100 mentally retarded children referred to a psychiatric clinic in San Francisco. The "neurotic traits," such as phobias, obsessive-compulsive behaviors, and anxiety reactions, accounted for 23.8% of the problems reported. The psychiatric diagnoses of children referred to a clinic in Scotland were reported by Reid (1980). Out of 60 children, 13 (22%) were identified as exhibiting primarily a "neurotic disorder," including symptoms of depression, worry, and school phobia. Twelve were mildly retarded and one was severely mentally retarded. Finally, Benson (1985) surveyed 130 referrals to an outpatient mental health clinic in Illinois. Twenty-five percent of the sample were classified as "anxious-depressed withdrawal disorder" according to Quay's dimensional system (1979). Some of the presenting problems were depressed affect, low self-esteem, social withdrawal, and crying. There were more females than males placed in this group, more adults than children, and the clients tended to be in the mild to the moderate range of intellectual functioning.

The inpatient data on the frequency of occurrence of anxiety disorders and depression also hover around the 20% to 25% range. In an extensive study that tracked all births in a British city and reported follow-up data 22 years later, Richardson, Katz, Koller, McLaren, and Rubenstein (1979) found that 17% of the mentally retarded population could be described as "neurotic" and 26% as having a "neurotic disorder" in combination with another psychiatric disorder. By the term "neurotic disorder" the authors referred to "disturbance in emotions, nervous breakdowns, anxiety, need for tranquilizers, suicidal, self-destructive acts" (p. 280).

In a study conducted in an institution in the United States, teacher ratings of 252 residents on the Behavior Problem Checklist were factor analyzed and two anxiety-related factors were identified (Quay & Gredler, 1981). Items loading heavily on the "anxiety-withdrawal" factor were rated as present in 23% to 46% of the sample and included "self-conscious, feelings of inferiority, shyness, lack of self-confidence, easily flustered, hypersensitive, anxiety, passive, and suggestible." A second anxiety factor of three items was described as "unique to this analysis" and included "crying, tension, and nervous, jittery." These characteristics were rated as present in 25% to 30% of the residents.

When considered as a whole, significant numbers of mentally retarded children and adults are seen as anxious or depressed, regardless of the classification system used. Many surveys do not present sufficient data to determine how level of functioning, age, gender, or other variables may be associated with the diagnoses. Some reports do state that females are more likely to be identified as anxious or depressed than males, or that higher functioning individuals are more often diagnosed than lower functioning people. It is not clear whether the diagnostic disparity across levels of functioning represents a difference in the incidence of the disorders, or rather a reliance on verbal criteria in applying the labels.

ANXIETY DISORDERS

Assessment of Anxiety and Fear

Anxiety is an unpleasant emotional state with characteristic cognitive, behavioral, and physiological components. For example, anxiety may involve feelings of worry and apprehension and may be accompanied by increased pulse and respiration, sweaty palms, or dry mouth, and by avoiding situations in which anxiety occurs. Behaviorists view anxiety and fear as conditioned emotional responses. At one time, theorists distinguished fear from anxiety, because fear was said to have an identifiable source or object, whereas anxiety did not. The distinction between anxiety and fear is considered less useful presently when the focus is on overt behaviors.

The assessment of anxiety and fear in mentally retarded persons is similar to that with nonretarded persons in that the three response systems (motor or behavioral, cognitive or subjective, and physiological) may be evaluated. However, differences in verbal expression and cognitive development may alter both the observable indices of anxiety and the appropriate methods of assessment. Many assessment instruments have been adapted for mentally retarded persons from those developed for nonretarded children and adults.

Self-Report Measures of Anxiety and Fear

Many of the self-report measures of fear and anxiety were constructed from the perspective of a trait or dispositional view of personality. The individual is presumed to possess certain characteristics and to respond in a particular manner that is stable and consistent across situations. Thus, the self-report measures often do not provide the detailed descriptions of situational influences on responding that behaviorists require. In addition, many mentally retarded persons experience difficulty with self-report measures because of problems in labeling and/or reporting subjective experience. However, self-report measures offer the only method of assessing the subjective component of anxiety and fear.

Children's Manifest Anxiety Scale. The Children's Manifest Anxiety Scale (CMAS) (Castenada, McCandless, & Palermo, 1956) was developed for 4th, 5th, and 6th grade nonretarded children. It is a 42-item scale with an 11-item lie scale that addresses symptoms of anxiety. Some sample items are: "I get nervous when someone watches me work." "I worry about what other people think of me." "My hands feel sweaty." The respondent answers "Yes" or "No." The total score is the number of "Yes" answers to the anxiety items.

The CMAS has been characterized as vulnerable to acquiescence response set (Matthews & Levy, 1961). In addition, one study found that the factor structure of anxiety items differed greatly for mentally retarded and nonretarded individuals and that a high rate of "incorrect" responses to lie items was obtained from mentally retarded subjects (Flanigan, Peters, & Conry, 1969). It was concluded that the CMAS was not measuring the same construct in mentally retarded and in nonretarded children.

State-Trait Anxiety Inventory A-State Scale. The State-Trait Anxiety Inventory (STAI) A-State Scale was developed by Spielberger as a measure of a here-and-now mood state that may vary in response to perceived environmental threat, in contrast to trait anxiety, which is a relatively stable tendency of the individual to perceive events as threatening (Spielberger, 1973). The A-State scale is a 20-item questionnaire. The directions are to respond according to "how you feel right now, at this moment." The question stems are all "I feel. . . ." There are three response alternatives for each question. The choices for one item are: "very calm, calm, not calm." The scale is scored in the direction of high anxiety. In studies with mentally retarded persons, A-State anxiety scores were associated with levels of performance in athletic events (Levine & Langness, 1983) and varied predictably across stressful and nonstressful situations (Levine, 1985).

Fear Survey Schedule. The most commonly used self-report measure of fear is the Fear Survey Schedule (FSS) (Wolpe & Lang, 1964) and its variations. The questionnaire contains a list of many items that may arouse fear, such as lightning, insects, and blood. The respondent is asked to rate the intensity of fearfulness on a 5-point scale from "Not at all" to "Very much." The total score is used as an index of fearfulness.

Using a Fear Survey Scale designed for the study (89 items), mildly mentally retarded adults were compared to chronological age-and mental age-matched control groups (Duff *et al.*, 1981). Females reported greater fear than males. The mentally retarded subjects were intermediate between nonretarded children and nonretarded adults in the number of fears. There were some differences in the types of items reported as fear arousing by the mentally retarded subjects in comparison to the other two groups. For example, they were more fearful of doctors than nonmentally retarded children, and reported greater fear of thunder and lightning, hell, and germs than nonretarded adults. In general, the fears of mentally retarded subjects were more similar to the mental age-matched controls than to the chronological age-matched controls.

Psychopathology Instrument for Mentally Retarded Adults. The Psychopathology Instrument for Mentally Retarded Adults (PIMRA) was developed specifically for mentally retarded persons and was based on seven types of psychopathology as described in the third edition of the *Diagnostic and Statistical Manual of Mental Disorders* (DSM-III) (Matson, Kazdin, & Senatore, 1984). The seven subscales are schizophrenic disorder, affective disorder, psychosexual disorder, adjustment disorder, anxiety disorder, somatoform disorder, and personality disorder. Both a self-report and an informant version are available. On the self-report version, the respondent answers "Yes" or "No" to each question. Some of the questions on the anxiety subscale are: "Do you worry a lot?" "When things go bad for you do you feel OK?" "Do you feel relaxed most of the time?" In a factor-analytic study with 110 mentally retarded adults, the self-report version yielded two factors, anxiety (8 items) and social adjustment (5 items) (Matson *et al.*, 1984).

Fear Thermometer. The fear thermometer (Walk, 1956) offers a simple method of measuring self-reported fear. The subject is given a visual representation of a Likert-type scale and indicates the amount of fear experienced. A fear thermometer for children was devised by Kelley (1976), in which a different color was used for each level on the 5-point scale. The child may point to a number or manually move a marker to the appropriate fear level. The concrete presentation of the rating scale makes it a useful method of assessing situational anxiety with mentally retarded persons.

Interviews

Interviews may be conducted for a variety of purposes and may be structured or unstructured. In the assessment of anxiety and fear, mentally retarded persons may be interviewed to determine the circumstances in which they become anxious, the form that their anxiety response takes, and so forth. Structured interviews have been conducted with mentally retarded persons in a few studies to determine the stimuli that arouse fear.

In a study examining the fears of special education students aged 7 to 19 (Derevensky, 1979), students were chosen from educable mentally retarded (EMR), trainable mentally retarded (TMR), and learning disabled (LD) classes. During individual interviews, the students were asked, "What are things to be afraid of?" The responses were compared with those of nonretarded children. The mentally retarded children reported more fears and fears of many different types than nonretarded children.

A structured interview was also used to assess the fears of institutionalized, moderately mentally retarded adults aged 21 to 49 (Sternlicht, 1979). In two separate interviews, 22 subjects were asked what they were afraid of and what their friends were afraid of. Sternlicht categorized the fears as either preoperational (animals, supernatural/natural events) or concrete operational (physical injury, psychological stress) and reported that a developmental trend was present in the reports of fears. The criteria used for the categorization were not clearly stated, and there was no attempt to determine the reliability of the categorization.

Informant Reports

Parents, teachers, and staff may provide informant reports about mentally retarded persons. Generally, informant reports are obtained using global measures in which anxiety is one of several problem dimensions that are assessed.

The PIMRA informant scale contains the same 57 items that are included in the self-report version, worded as simple statements that are rated "Yes" or "No" for each subject. There are 7 items that pertain to anxiety disorders. The informant PIMRA factored into three factors: affective (14 items, including anxiety items), somatoform (5 items), and psychosis (5 items) (Matson *et al.*, 1984).

Behavioral Observation

One method of assessing the motor component of anxiety or fear is the Behavioral Avoidance Test (BAT) (Lang & Lazovik, 1963). The subject is asked to approach, touch, and handle the feared object during the test. In the event that a particular situation is feared, the person is asked to approach the situation, engage in the appropriate behaviors for the situation, and to generally stay in the situation as long as he or she can. Various measures of avoidance behavior are monitored, such as the distance covered, the time spent in the situation, response latency, and subject verbalizations. Some drawbacks have been noted in the use of BATs as an index of fear. There is no standard procedure that is used, the instructions vary from study to study, and little information has been gathered on the reliability and validity of the measure (Barrios, Hartmann, & Shigetomi, 1981).

Observer rating scales have been developed to assess nonretarded children's responses to specific anxiety-arousing situations, such as surgery and dental work (e.g., Melamed & Siegel, 1975). These scales are generally brief, objective, and tailored to the specific situation. One example of an observer rating scale for anxiety is the Preschool Observation Scale of Anxiety (POSA) by Glennon and Weisz (1978). A 30-item scale was constructed that was based on previously published literature on behavioral indices of anxiety. Some of the items are: "whines or whimpers," and "gratuitous hand movements." Nonretarded preschoolers gave self-reports of anxiety, were rated by teachers, and were observed by trained raters during 10-minute testing sessions. Some evidence for the validity and reliability of the POSA was obtained. Observer rating scales like the POSA may be useful to assess situational anxiety with mentally retarded persons.

Behavioral checklists may be used to assess the effects of interventions. For example, Luiselli (1980) developed a behavioral checklist to rate the effects of relaxation training. The scale contains nine items that are rated on a 5-point Likert scale, including forehead, neck, head, hands, and breathing. Each scale is anchored with behavioral descriptors. For example, the anchors for "forehead" are 1 = smooth and 5 = deeply furrowed or wrinkled. The interrater reliability of the checklist was .82.

Psychophysiological Assessment

Psychophysiological measures assess the third component of anxiety and fear. A number of different responses have been monitored for this purpose, including heart rate, pulse, respiration, blood pressure, muscle tension, and electrodermal activity. It has been widely reported that psychophysiological measures often do not correlate highly with self-report and/or behavioral measures, and that individuals exhibit patterns of responsivity that are reflected in some psychophysiological measures and not in others (e.g., Lang, 1971). In addition, psychophysiological measurement requires special equipment and technical expertise; the measurements may be affected by factors other than the ones of interest; and subjects may be frightened by the measurement process. For these reasons, there has been little psychophysiological measurement with fearful or anxious mentally retarded persons (Calamari, Geist, & Shahbazian, 1987; Peck, 1977). However, psychophysiological assessment offers a unique source of information for any comprehensive assessment, and is particularly useful when other methods of assessment are not feasible or are of questionable reliability.

Summary

The assessment of anxiety and fear in mentally retarded persons, as with other individuals, requires a comprehensive assessment with several sources of information and modes of response. The purpose of the assessment will affect the choice of measures used; for example, some self-report and informant measures are best suited for screening purposes, whereas others are appropriate for the assessment of an identified problem. The selection of assessment instruments is also guided by subject characteristics and situational factors. The subject's verbal/cognitive and motor abilities influence the selection of self-report and behavioral tests. Observer and informant ratings may be obtained, depending on the availability of reliable informants and of trained observers in accessible settings.

Few advances have been made in developing self-report, informant, and observer rating systems to assess anxiety in mentally retarded persons. The need for reliable observer and informant rating scales is especially acute in the assessment of nonverbal and severely mentally retarded individuals. Behavioral tests, including role-play tests, can be useful in assessing skill deficits and their contribution to the anxiety response.

Treatment of Anxiety and Fear

Respondent conditioning, operant conditioning, and observational learning principles have all been applied in the treatment of anxiety and fear. The most extensively researched behavioral intervention for the treatment of anxiety and fear is systematic desensitization, derived from respondent conditioning principles. As originally developed by Wolpe (1969), the procedure included an anxiety-inhibiting response, such as progressive muscle relaxation, paired with imaginal, hierarchical presentation of feared stimuli. Wolpe (1969) stated that other anxiety-inhibiting responses, such as eating, interpersonal relationships, and assertion, could be used instead of relaxation. In place of imaginal presentation of feared stimuli, *in vivo* presentation has frequently been used in the treatment of children's fears (Ollendick, 1979). The child makes approach responses to real-life stimuli, which are arranged from least to most anxiety arousing, while using relaxation skills.

Anxiety and fear have also been reduced via observational learning. The subject observes a model perform an approach response to the feared stimulus. Anxiety is presumably reduced, and responding is disinhibited through observing that the model's approach responses are not followed by aversive consequences and by the informational value of the model's responses (Bandura & Barab, 1973).

Finally, operant conditioning principles have been incorporated in behavioral treatment programs in which reinforcers are delivered contingent upon completion of hierarchy items. The research literature on the treatment of fear and anxiety with mentally retarded persons includes these techniques as well as combinations of interventions. The following section reviews some of this research.

Relaxation Training

Relaxation training has been used with mentally retarded children and adults for a variety of purposes. Harvey (1979) recommended relaxation training for mentally retarded clients with anxiety-related behavior problems. Specialized procedures have been developed that can make the training techniques appropriate for mentally retarded or multiply handicapped persons (Cautela & Grodin, 1978; Koeppen, 1974).

Following a review of studies in which relaxation training was used with developmentally disabled subjects, Luiselli (1980) concluded that most research failed to demonstrate that relaxation training was superior to other interventions and that, on the whole, the studies suffered from methodological shortcomings. A common problem was the failure to demonstrate that subjects became relaxed as a result of the training procedures.

A few recent studies have been concerned with the question of whether relaxation training can be effective with lower functioning individuals. Rickard, Thrasher, and Elkins (1984) worked with 20 adults from four IQ ranges, 85 to 100, 70 to 84, 55 to 69, and 40 to 54. The subjects were given three 30-minute relaxation training sessions, in which four types of verbal instructions were provided: to tense and relax muscle groups, to control breathing, to imagine pleasant scenes, and "to let go, relax and be at ease." Self-report ratings of relaxation on a 10-point scale were obtained pre- and postsession. The experimenter rated the subject's compliance with instructions, and an independent observer provided ratings for reliability checks. The lowest IQ group had some difficulty following instructions, and the two lowest groups had difficulty with the self-report ratings. But, individuals in the mildly mentally retarded and borderline ranges followed directions well. The authors stated that the self-report rating may have been too abstract for some subjects. Some researchers have handled this potential problem by devising a visual mode of presenting rating scales (e.g., Matson, 1981b).

In a second study to examine the influence of cognitive functioning levels on relaxation training effectiveness, auditory electromyograph (EMG) bio-feedback for frontalis muscle activity, modeling, and reinforcement were used in relaxation training sessions (Calamari *et al.*, 1987). Subjects were institutionalized adults in the profound to mild range of functioning. A control group listened to classical music. Tangible rewards were given to experimental subjects for EMG decreases, and the control subjects were rewarded on a yoked schedule. The experimental group exhibited significant reductions in muscle tension and in behavior ratings of relaxation following training. There were no effects attributed to the subject's level of functioning. The authors speculated that the auditory feedback may have assisted profoundly mentally retarded subjects in discriminating muscle tension and relaxation.

These studies have demonstrated that many mentally retarded persons can follow directions for a muscle tensing and relaxing procedure and that significant changes in tension can be obtained. The potential difficulty of some subjects in self-reporting muscle tension and relaxation could present an obstacle in effectively transferring the training to extratherapy situations. Greater flexibility and creativity in devising training procedures could increase the number of mentally retarded persons who could participate in relaxation training. Future research on relaxation training with mentally retarded persons could improve upon previous efforts by incorporating objective measures of relaxation effects and by evaluating the relative efficacy of the training in comparison to other interventions.

Respondent and Operant Conditioning

With few exceptions, the treatment of anxiety disorders in mentally retarded individuals has concentrated on the treatment of simple phobia. However, Benson (1985) noted that few phobia referrals were made to an outpatient clinic for developmentally disabled persons, and a survey of child clinicians found a low rate of referral for nonretarded children (Graziano & De-Giovanni, 1979). Although fears are common among mentally retarded individuals (Novosel, 1981), perhaps few are seen as so unusual in their object or intensity or to interfere significantly with the person's activities to warrant intervention.

The diagnostic criteria for simple phobia according to DSM-III-R (American Psychiatric Association, 1987) are: a persistent fear of a circumscribed stimulus; the stimulus provokes an anxiety response; the object or situation is avoided; the fear interferes with the person's functioning; and the person realizes that the fear is unreasonable (p. 245). Marks's (1969) definition of phobia adds the requirement that the fear is not age or stage specific. This permits the exclusion of fears that are considered normal for a particular developmental stage, such as separation anxiety in a 9-month-old.

Much of the anxiety treatment literature with mentally retarded persons consists of single case studies, with a few notable exceptions. Peck (1977) conducted one of the best experimental studies on the use of systematic desensitization as a treatment for fears in mentally retarded adults. Unfortunately, the results were somewhat equivocal because of a small sample size.

The study compared three types of desensitization—contact desensitization (therapist modeled and guided participation), vicarious symbolic (filmed model), and systematic desensitization (imaginal)—along with attention–control and no-treatment conditions. The subjects were adults with IQs ranging from 52 to 74. They were selected using a Fear Survey Schedule (FSS) and a Behavior Avoidance Test (BAT) for fear of rats or heights. In addition to the self-report and BAT measures, a fear thermometer, pulse rate, and observer ratings of fear and avoidance responses were obtained. The treatment groups ($n = 4$) received at most 15, 30-minute individual therapy sessions. A standard hierarchy, ordered for each subject, was used. There was a trend for the contact desensitization condition to be superior to the other conditions, although there were no significant differences between groups. Difficulties were reported in the ordering of the hierarchy items based on the subject's verbal descriptions, giving hand signals during relaxation training, and following practice procedures correctly.

There has been some concern that mentally retarded persons may have difficulty complying with the standard systematic desensitization procedures. In particular, there may be difficulty with the relaxation training or in imagining the feared stimuli. As a result, other approaches have been used in treating fears. A few studies used anxiety inhibitors other than relaxation in the treatment of a phobia. Jackson and King (1982) used reinforcement and laughter produced by tickling the subject to treat a phobic response to the sound of flushing toilets. The subject was a 4½-year-old autistic boy who attended a day school program. The phobic symptoms reported by the boy's teacher included "pupil dilation, trembling, increased muscle tonus, screaming, crying, tantrums, hyperventilation, and flight" (p. 365). *In vivo* desensitization with a 9-item anxiety hierarchy was used with tickling, verbal praise, and edible reinforcement (faded early in treatment). Generalization to other settings was incorporated into the response hierarchy. Three and six-month follow-up reports were obtained, and no fear symptoms were reported.

In a second study to use an alternate method of inhibiting anxiety, a phobia of physical examinations was treated with graded exposure and the presence of a nurse with whom the subject had a good relationship (Freeman, Roy, & Hemmick, 1976). The subject was a 7½-year-old boy with an IQ of 53. The phobic symptoms were to run screaming from the doctor, refuse to undress, temper tantrums, trembling, hyperactivity, and rapid breathing and pulse. The physical examination was divided into a number of steps that, at first, were performed by the nurse with the doctor present. While the physician performed more of the examination, the nurse was gradually faded from the examination room. No avoidance behavior was observed with the physician alone or in a generalization test with an unfamiliar doctor.

Playing checkers with the therapist was one component of the treatment program for a fear of mannequins that prevented a male with Down syndrome from going to stores and shopping malls (Waranch, Iwata, Wohl, & Nidiffer, 1981). The fear was a longstanding one, starting at age 5 and continuing to age 21. An FSS was administered pretreatment and did not identify other intense fears. A type of BAT was used in which the subject was asked to approach and touch three different sized mannequins while he was playing checkers with the therapist. During treatment, the subject played checkers while the smallest of three mannequins was gradually moved closer to him. Verbal prompts and reinforcement (unspecified type) were given for touching the mannequins. Later, the client was required to touch the mannequin between checker moves. In a generalization session at a shopping mall, the therapist reinforced the client with ice cream for touching four different mannequins. The parents continued to take their son to the mall for ice cream once a week for six months. During the 6-month follow-up, 40 trips were made to the shopping mall with no problems.

A combination of imaginal and *in vivo* presentation of stimuli was used in the treatment of an acrophobic adult with Down syndrome (IQ 33) (Guralnick, 1973). Over the course of 42 sessions, the subject was given brief relaxation training followed by imagining himself at successively greater heights. After imagining the scene without signaling anxiety, he engaged in the behavior in the session. Reinforcement with praise and edibles was given for remaining in the situation for longer time periods. Therapist observation and teacher reports were the outcome measures.

A different approach to the potential problem with imaginal presentation of feared stimuli is instead to present the stimuli visually. Rivenq (1974) treated a 13-year-old, borderline mentally retarded, institutionalized boy who exhibited an excessive fear of body hair. The subject was reinforced with candy and pastries for looking at pictures of hairy people. The pictures were brought closer to the subject, and the hair in the pictures became more noticeable as treatment progressed. The hair phobia was eliminated in four treatment sessions, according to therapist observations.

Visual presentation of stimuli and *in vivo* exposure were the treatment approaches given to neurologically impaired subjects, some of whom had IQs below 75, who were afraid of dogs or buses (Obler & Terwilliger, 1970). There were 15 treated subjects and 15 controls who were matched on several criteria. Treatment sessions lasted for 5 hours once a week. It was unclear if the controls were a no-treatment control or an attention placebo condition. The treatment group improved based on parent reports. Comparisons between high and low IQ groups, labeled "aware" and "unaware," showed no differences in response to treatment.

A critique of the Obler and Terwilliger (1970) study pointed out several methodological weaknesses, including the combination of treatment procedures, the use of both primary and secondary reinforcers, and a lack of clarity regarding the type of reinforcement schedule (Begelman & Hersen, 1971). The parent ratings were a poor measure and were not supplemented by more direct behavioral measures, and pretreatment ratings were incomplete. Further, the aware-unaware dimension was arbitrary and lacking foundation. Many of the criticisms leveled by Begelman and Hersen (1971) are valid for a number of the case study reports of phobia treatment with mentally retarded persons.

Because more mentally retarded individuals are living in community settings, the types of fears that are treated have shifted to those that interfere with community functioning. A few studies have focused on fears of riding in cars or buses, often a required means of transportation to community programs and activities. Mansdorf (1976) treated a mildly mentally retarded institutionalized woman (IQ 44) who was afraid of riding in a car to an off-grounds workshop. The subject was reinforced with tokens for *in vivo* exposure to hierarchy items. Initially, the therapist accompanied the patient. At follow-up 10 months later, the patient was traveling by car without signs of anxiety.

In another case study, an autistic boy who was afraid of riding a school bus was reinforced by his mother for graduated *in vivo* exposure to the bus (Luiselli, 1978). Prior to treatment, the 7-year-old cried, fell on the sidewalk, and tantrumed when asked to get on the bus. Crying continued during the ride. Treatment began with the mother and son sitting on the stationary bus. Brief stays were reinforced with praise and food. The mother was faded from the treatment while the amount of bus time was increased. Treatment for riding to school was completed in 7 days, and riding home from school was shaped in 2 days. A 1-year follow-up found no additional problems in bus riding.

A more extensive reinforcement program was administered by ward attendants to treat a severely mentally retarded male's toileting phobia (Luiselli, 1977). The 15-year-old resident had been toilet trained previously, but developed a fear of urinating in the toilet. Several procedures were used over the course of the treatment, making it difficult to determine what accounted for the treatment success. A time-out procedure for wet pants was used throughout treatment. Reinforcement for appropriate toilet use was a weekly trip with an attendant. At first, the trip was earned by obtaining stars given by staff for appropriate toilet use on a continuous schedule. The tokens were later discontinued and only praise was given. Next, a self-recording procedure was introduced, but it was discontinued when it was discovered that the subject was monitoring inaccurately. An intermittent token reinforcement program administered by staff with a daily, as well as a weekly, prize was the final intervention. Follow-ups at 4 months, 6 months, and 1 year were reported.

Modeling

The therapist, parents, and peers have all served as models in various treatment studies with mentally retarded individuals. Single or multiple models and mastery or coping models have been used. Tangible rewards and/or social reinforcement are typically provided following approach responses. In contact desensitization or participant modeling, the subject observes a live model approach the feared stimulus. Next, the model physically guides the subject through the approach response. Then, the subject performs the approach response alone. Participant modeling has been found to be more effective than live or filmed modeling in reducing fears in nonretarded children (Ollendick, 1979).

Contact desensitization was used with three mentally retarded adults who were afraid of escalators (Runyan, Stevens, & Reeves, 1985). The pretest consisted of a BAT of 25 items. During treatment, the therapist modeled the behavior and prompted or physically guided the subjects. Praise was given when a hierarchy item was successfully completed. At a 1-month follow-up, all three subjects were using escalators.

A peer mastery model was one element in the treatment of a toilet phobia in a 5-year-old, borderline mentally retarded boy at a day school (Wilson & Jackson, 1980). The child used a potty chair, but when encouraged to use the toilet, he screamed, cried, hyperventilated, and tried to escape. A 22-step hierarchy was developed in which the potty chair was gradually moved closer to the toilet, placed on it, and was eventually removed from the classroom bathroom. A peer model was used for Steps 4 to 8 only. Physical and verbal prompts were given at the beginning of each step, and verbal and social reinforcement were provided at the end. The child's mother replicated the procedure at home. In 33 school days, the program was completed and generalization tests were included. Three-week and 3-month follow-up tests were reported in which no further occurrence of the fear was noted.

Multiple-peer coping models were used in the treatment of a mildly mentally retarded woman's dog phobia (Jackson & Hooper, 1981). Self-report, BAT, parent, and observer ratings were obtained. Treatment sessions included presenting pictures of dogs. Treatment gains were maintained at a 2-month follow-up. The subject took less time to approach a dog and got closer to it. However, the self-report and parent report indicated fear of some dogs, specifically, those that barked or leaped. The authors concluded that it may be adaptive to fear these dogs and that it is difficult to teach the discriminations that would be necessary to determine when barking or leaping dogs should be avoided. According to the authors, the peer models were of most use in early stages, but later on, the exposure was more important. They also noted that the BAT is subject to demand characteristics and, in this case, variations in the dogs' behavior.

Participant modeling by the mothers of moderately mentally retarded girls aged 8 to 10 was studied by Matson (1981b) to treat a fear of talking to strange adults. The fear prevented parents from employing babysitters and restricted family social activities. The subjects were referrals to a mental health clinic. The pretreatment assessment included the Louisville Fear Survey Schedule (Miller, Barrett, Hampe, & Noble, 1972) that was completed by the parents, and a BAT in which the child was asked to introduce herself to a strange man at school. Self-ratings of fear were also obtained in this situation. The performance of the subject was compared to a matched "normal" control from the same classroom, selected on the basis of teacher ratings to be the least fearful of "safe" strangers. A multiple-baseline design across subjects was used. During the treatment phase, the mother gave a tangible reward for completing an approach response and greeting. The dependent measures were self-report fear ratings, the distance approached measured in feet, and the number of words spoken to the stranger. Generalization tests occurred in the child's home, with the father rating the child's behavior. The study was notable because of its use of "normal" child behavior as a comparison, the involvement of both parents in the treatment, and the use of multiple dependent measures that were collected at both pretest and posttest.

One of the few controlled group outcome studies in the anxiety treatment literature involved participant modeling by the therapist for fear of participating in community activities (Matson, 1981a). There were 12 subjects each in the treatment and no-treatment control groups, all mild or moderately mentally retarded adults. The study focused on fear of entering stores. The pretest measures included observer ratings of approach behavior, fearful statements, and shopping skill. Treatment, which was conducted in small groups over a 3-month period, began at the subject's workshop and involved a discussion of fears in general, an explanation of the treatment plan, and rehearsal with one subject when going to the grocery store and purchasing groceries. Subjects later went to a store and practiced grocery shopping, following a graduated hierarchy. The therapist and other subjects praised completion of the steps. The results indicated that the subjects who received participant modeling significantly improved in grocery shopping skills, and their level of fear was significantly decreased.

Summary

This brief review of the treatment of anxiety and fear in mentally retarded individuals has indicated that a variety of interventions are effective, with a number of different feared stimuli. The subjects successfully treated have included children and adults who ranged from severe to borderline in level of intellectual functioning. Several categories of phobic stimuli have been targeted, such as small animals, bodily injury, and interpersonal interactions.

Researchers have been creative in designing interventions to treat anxiety and fear. A variety of anxiety-inhibiting responses (relaxation, tickling, interpersonal relationship) and methods of presenting feared stimuli (imaginal, *in vivo*, visual) have been used. Modeling by peers or adults has also effectively increased approach responses. Several types of reinforcers, including food, tokens, and praise, have been given. In general, the maintenance of treatment effects has been good, with some studies reporting up to a 1-year follow-up. Generalization of treatment effects has been documented less frequently.

Many questions remain, however. One study reported difficulty constructing an anxiety hierarchy using subject report (Peck, 1977). Many studies did not explicitly state how the hierarchy was constructed, but it appears that many were generated by the therapist. Further, few studies have compared the effectiveness of different interventions, and the practice of combining interventions has meant that a "treatment of choice" has not been identified.

What are important subject variables in anxiety treatment with mentally retarded individuals? The individual's skills and developmental level must be considered in the design of interventions. The individual's imagery ability, ability to understand and follow directions, and potential to participate in hierarchy construction are all relevant factors. The degree to which the anxiety and fear are related to skill deficits also requires attention. Participant modeling may be recommended when *in vivo* exposure is feasible; the combination of anxiety reduction through exposure and information on appropriate behavior is especially appropriate for many mentally retarded individuals.

Treatment of Other Anxiety Disorders

Obsessive-compulsive disorder is the only anxiety disorder besides phobia that has been studied in any depth with mentally retarded persons. According to the definition of obsessive-compulsive disorder in the DSM-III-R (American Psychiatric Association, 1987), obsessions are persistent thoughts that are recognized as internally generated, whereas compulsive behaviors are repetitive, intentional behaviors that are performed "according to certain rules or in a stereotyped fashion" (p. 245). Compulsive behaviors may be performed to "neutralize" the obsessive thought. The person recognizes that the behavior is unreasonable, but resisting the compulsion leads to increased distress. Compulsive behavior types include "washers" and "checkers" (Foa & Steketee, 1979). Washers feel contaminated and excessively wash and clean, whereas checkers repeat actions to prevent unpleasant events. Depression, anxiety, and avoidance behaviors are commonly associated with obsessive-compulsive disorder.

The identification of obsessive-compulsive disorder among mentally retarded persons presents some difficulties. Limitations in verbal expression among lower functioning individuals prevent the determination of some of the diagnostic criteria for obsessive-compulsive disorder; for example, whether there are persistent ideas that the person tries to suppress, whether the behavior is designed to avoid future harm. These "motivational" qualities remain undetermined, and repetitive behaviors may be interpreted as purposeless, rather than anxiety-based. Behavioral interventions with mentally retarded persons have focused on the repetitive behaviors and have been less concerned with diagnostic criteria.

The repetitive behaviors of mentally retarded persons have been treated with overcorrection with considerable success (Foxx & Azrin, 1973; Matson & Stephens, 1981). In the Foxx and Azrin study, mouthing, head weaving, and hand clapping were reduced by overcorrection. In the case of hand mouthing, an overcorrection procedure was more effective than physical punishment, differential reinforcement of other behavior (DRO), and free reinforcement. Wall patting was reduced in the Matson and Stephens study (1981) by a hand overcorrection procedure, and face patting, hair flipping, and repetitive arm movements were treated in other subjects using similar interventions.

Repetitive behaviors have also been significantly reduced by a reinforcement program. An elderly, mildly mentally retarded woman living in an institution repeated a number of behaviors, including walking forward and back, turning corners and returning when enroute from one building to another (Cuvo, 1976). The woman was reinforced for reducing the amount of time she took to return to her unit from another building. Social and tangible reinforcement was given. Attendants administered the ABAB design program, and the woman reduced her travel time from 25 minutes to 10 minutes over the course of the program.

Repetitive behaviors can seriously interfere with work production as well as with interpersonal relationships. Overcorrection and a DRO procedure were combined in the treatment of three mildly mentally retarded men who engaged in clothes and body checking (Matson, 1982b). These behaviors are most similar to the compulsive behaviors that are treated in nonretarded individuals. The clients attended a sheltered workshop and lived in a community residence. DSM-III criteria were used to make the diagnosis of obsessive-compulsive disorder. During 30-minute training sessions, the clients were given work samples to complete and received tokens for not engaging in the target behavior for 1 minute. When the target behavior occurred, the clients performed an overcorrection procedure involving hand and arm movements. The therapist modeled appropriate work behavior. Treatment sessions were videotaped. Following each session, the subjects rated their anxiety level on a 1- to 7-point scale. The self-ratings of anxiety decreased with treatment as did the target behaviors. Ratings of randomly presented videotaped sessions by members of the community indicated that the clients' behavior was seen as more appropriate following treatment.

Conclusions

The assessment of anxiety disorders in mentally retarded individuals is complicated by the need to develop measures that are applicable to a wide range of functioning levels. The self-report measures of anxiety are most appropriate for mild to moderately mentally retarded persons. Informant reports of anxiety are a viable alternative or adjunct to self-report measures. The PIMRA informant measure (Matson et al., 1984) is promising and could be applied to a wide range of individuals, but the anxiety subscale has not yet been closely studied. Behavioral observation systems have not been well developed to assess anxiety in this population, and physiological measures seldom have been used.

Most of the treatment studies reviewed dealt with simple phobias. The behavioral interventions that were effective often involved combinations of treatment techniques, such as in vivo exposure, shaping, or modeling. Symbolic modeling has seldom been used with mentally retarded individuals (Peck, 1977), and no studies were found in which the treatment was flooding or implosion. Few group treatment studies have been completed, and few studies compared the relative effectiveness of interventions.

Many of the case studies were methodologically weak, relying on therapist or parent reports as the sole outcome measures. Little pretesting was done, and few attempts were made to determine a diagnosis using standard criteria. Tests of generalization of treatment effects and follow-up have been quite variable. The recent studies tend to be more complete in terms of assessment, generalization, and follow-up.

The relatively low rate of referral for treatment of anxiety disorders has previously been noted. Many mentally retarded individuals who could benefit from the interventions reported here have not been identified as needing treatment. The use of the PIMRA (Matson *et al.*, 1984) and other rating scales as screening instruments may lead to more complete assessment and treatment, when appropriate. It is possible that some behaviors that are labeled as noncompliance by caretakers, such as refusal to participate in community activities, may be anxiety-based and would respond to behavioral interventions. However, the distinction between fear and noncompliance may be difficult to make, particularly with less verbal individuals (Jackson, 1983).

DEPRESSION

As recently as 1983, an article was published with the title, "Do the Mentally Retarded Suffer from Affective Illness?" (Sovner & Hurley, 1983). The question was still considered a valid one, because there had been considerable debate about the matter for a number of years. Some writers proposed that mentally retarded individuals should be *more* susceptible to affective disorders because of their limited coping abilities and repeated failure experiences, whereas others doubted that "true" depressive disorders would occur among mentally retarded persons because of immature ego development. The evidence pro and con was debated in several articles (e.g., Gardner, 1967).

Part of the difficulty in answering the question has to do with the same issues that child clinicians have struggled with; that is, if children experience depression, is it presented in the same way, in different ways, or in both the same and different ways as in adults? Some researchers have proposed the concept of "masked depression" to refer to a type of depression in children in which the overt behavior may be aggressive, but the "underlying" disorder is that of depression (Cytryn & McKnew, 1972; Cytryn, McKnew, & Bunney, 1980). Not surprisingly, the debate over the legitimacy of masked depression as a diagnostic entity was lengthy and spirited (Carlson & Cantwell, 1980).

In regard to mentally retarded persons, Berman (1967) made an observation that was similar to the concept of masked depression. He noticed that a number of institutionalized individuals referred to him because of antisocial and aggressive behavior, upon interview, evidenced poor self-esteem and feelings of rejection. Berman labeled these individuals "depressed."

Although sufficient evidence has been gathered to indicate that mentally retarded individuals do, indeed, experience depressive disorders, the specific characteristics of the disorders and the ways in which they are manifested across a wide range of functioning levels have not been determined. The types of problem behaviors may vary as a function of developmental level, chronological age, or other factors. Thus, the identification, assessment, and treatment of depression in mentally retarded persons may require different methods for different subgroups of individuals (Matson, 1983).

The DSM-III-R divides the mood disorders (formerly affective disorders) into depressive and bipolar disorders. The depressive disorders include major depression and dysthymia (depressive neurosis). The primary characteristic of the depressive disorders is the presence of periods of depression without an occurrence of manic or hypomanic episodes. Some of the symptoms associated with depressed mood include sleep disturbances, low energy, low self-esteem, hopelessness, poor concentration, loss of interest in pleasurable activities, weight changes, and thoughts of death (American Psychiatric Association, 1987). The bipolar disorders include bipolar disorder and cyclothymia. The primary characteristic of the bipolar disorders is the presence of manic or hypomanic episodes. During manic or hypomanic episodes, the individual's mood is euphoric, self-esteem is high, there is a decreased need for sleep, the person speaks rapidly, is distractible, and makes many plans. The manic episode is differentiated from the hypomanic by a significant impairment in occupational functioning or interpersonal relationships (American Psychiatric Association, 1987). The following sections on the assessment and treatment of depression in mentally retarded individuals will deal primarily with the depressive disorders.

Assessment of Depression

The methods available for assessing depression in mentally retarded persons in varying degrees focus on the cognitive (poor concentration, worry), somatic or vegetative (sleep, eating, activity), or behavioral signs (slow speech, crying) of depressive disorders. The multidimensional nature of depression is reflected in the variety of approaches to assessment and treatment.

Self-Report Measures

There are several self-report measures of depression that have been used with mentally retarded individuals. In general, the adaptations that have been made to existing instruments developed for nonretarded children or adults have reduced the response alternatives and simplified the language.

Zung Depression Inventory. The Zung Self-Rating Depression Scale (Zung, 1965) is a 20-item scale developed on the basis of clinical diagnostic criteria. It contains 10 items phrased to be positively symptomatic of depression and 10 that are worded negatively. Some of the items are: "I still look forward to things as much as I used to"; "I would be better off dead"; and "I get tired for no good reason." The response alternatives are "Most of the time," "A good part of the time," "Some of the time," and "Never."

Beck Depression Inventory. The Beck Depression Inventory (Beck, Ward, Mendelson, Mock, & Erbaugh, 1961) includes 21 items, each focusing on a different symptom of depression. The respondent chooses from among four alternative statements for each item, for example: "I feel as though I am very bad or worthless"; "I feel quite guilty"; "I feel bad or unworthy a good part of the time"; "I don't feel particularly guilty."

The Children's Depression Inventory (CDI) (Kovacs, 1980/1981) is a downward extension of the Beck inventory for children aged 8 to 13. A 0 to 2 scoring system is used where "2" is scored for the most depressed of the three statements. One item offers the following statements to choose from: "I feel like crying everyday"; "I feel like crying many days"; and "I feel like crying once in awhile." The inventory has been widely used in studies of nonretarded children (e.g., Saylor, Finch, Spiroto, & Bennett, 1984).

Reynolds Adolescent Depression Scale. The Reynolds Adolescent Depression Scale (RADS) (Reynolds, 1987) was developed for nonretarded adolescents and covers the DSM-III symptoms of depression. It contains 30 items which the respondent rates on a 4-point scale from "almost always" to "hardly ever." Some items are: "I feel sad;" "I have trouble sleeping"; and "I feel like crying." The items are relatively simple, but the response alternatives may give some mentally retarded subjects difficulty.

PIMRA. This instrument for detecting psychopathology in mentally retarded adults (Matson *et al.*, 1984) has a 7-item depression subscale that has been studied fairly extensively. Some items are: "Do you have lots of energy?" "Do you have trouble sleeping?" "Do you feel sad?" The respondent answers "Yes" or "No." Individuals scoring high on the PIMRA depression subscale also scored high on the Beck and the Zung depression inventories (Senatore, Matson, & Kazdin, 1985).

Interviews

The most widely used index of depression based on a clinical interview is the Hamilton Rating Scale (Hamilton, 1960). The scale includes 17 dimensions that are rated on either a 0 to 2- or a 0 to 4-point scale. Some of the rated dimensions are depressed mood, guilt, insomnia, loss of weight, agitation, and somatic symptoms. The scale is recommended for use by skilled clinicians. In one study, the Hamilton scale was completed by outpatient clinicians or ward staff of mentally retarded adults and was found to correlate well with self-report Beck scores, the informant PIMRA total scores, and PIMRA depression subscale scores (Kazdin, Matson, & Senatore, 1983).

Informant Reports

The PIMRA has an informant version that includes a 7-item depression subscale (Matson *et al.*, 1984). The depression subscale score has been found to correlate highly with the Hamilton Rating Scale, but only low positive correlations were found between the subscale score and self-report measures of depression (Kazdin *et al.*, 1983). A cutoff score of 4 or greater was used to identify patients as depressed.

The psychometric properties of some informant scales may be superior to the corresponding self-report measures with mentally retarded adults. For example, Laman and Reiss (1987) found that the informant PIMRA depression subscale and a 4-item depression rating scale was a psychometrically sounder measure of depression in mentally retarded adults than any single self-report measure or combination of measures that included the RADS, Zung, and PIMRA self-report depression subscale.

Behavioral Observation

There has been greater development of observational measures of depressive disorders than of anxiety with mentally retarded individuals. Reid (1972) proposed that the diagnosis of depression in mentally retarded persons should take into account variations in behavior patterns. Working with inpatients 20 to 70 years of age, Reid (1972) diagnosed 21 patients as bipolar disorder based on observer ratings of activity, sleep patterns, and weight changes. In a second study, Reid and Naylor (1976) intensively studied four bipolar patients. Twice daily nursing ratings on activity level and withdrawal were kept as well as temperature, pulse, and sleep patterns. Clear patterns were identified that varied over a 4- to 9-week period. Reid's research has concentrated on the vegetative signs of depressive disorders, and many of the subjects were severely and profoundly mentally retarded.

Biochemical Measures

A considerable amount of research on depression has focused on physiological factors as concomitants or potential causes of depressive disorders. The Dexamethasone Suppression Test (DST) has been used in the diagnosis of depression in mentally retarded adults (Pirodsky et al., 1985). The procedure is to inject the subject with dexamethasone and examine blood cortisol levels; a high cortisol level is associated with depression. Pirodsky et al. (1985) tested 39 subjects and found that 5 had high cortisol readings. These subjects had been rated by staff as engaging in repetitive stereotyped movements, temper tantrums, and screaming/crying. It may be significant for defining the behavioral signs of depression in mentally retarded persons that the subjects with high cortisol readings in this study exhibited aggressive behaviors.

The Pirodsky et al. (1985) report was an initial study, and more research is needed on the validation of the test with mentally retarded individuals; nevertheless, the DST may offer an alternative assessment tool, particularly for severely/profoundly or nonverbal mentally retarded persons. However, a difficulty with the DST is that false positive results are associated with anticonvulsive drug use, thereby reducing the test's usefulness with a large number of mentally retarded persons (Pirodsky et al., 1985).

Characteristics and Correlates of Depression

Three psychosocial theories of the etiology of unipolar depression have guided research on the characteristics of depressive disorders and their treatment. Beck's cognitive theory of depression (1967) maintains that depressed individuals hold a negative cognitive schema that systematically distorts events and that they have negative cognitions about the self, the world, and the future. Lewinsohn's reinforcement theory of depression states that low levels of response contingent reinforcement, mediated by social skill deficits, cause depression (Lewinsohn, Hoberman, Teri, & Hautzinger, 1985). According to Seligman's learned helplessness theory (1975) and the reformulated attribution theory (Abramson, Seligman, & Teasdale, 1978), depression is due to faulty attributions about one's ability to control events and affect outcomes. Internal, stable, and global attributions for failure experiences contribute to pervasive, long-lasting depression.

Research with nonretarded adults, guided by these theories of depression, has identified some behavioral characteristics that are associated with depression. These include poor social skills (Libet & Lewinsohn, 1973; Youngren & Lewinsohn, 1980), weak social support (Paykel *et al.*, 1969), and learned helplessness (Seligman, 1975). Similar research has been conducted with mentally retarded adults, with greater emphasis given to the reinforcement and learned helplessness theories than to cognitive theory. Studies examining the behavioral characteristics or correlates of depression can provide information that may be useful in the prevention, assessment, and treatment of depressive disorders.

Social Skills and Social Support

Verbal interaction patterns have distinguished between depressed and nondepressed mentally retarded adults. Studying institutionalized subjects, Schloss (1982) found that depressed subjects exhibited negative affect in response to requests and to gain compliance, and that staff tended to interact with depressed patients more than peers did. In addition, people gave orders to depressed patients rather than make other kinds of statements and expressed negative affect to depressed patients more than to nondepressed patients. The results were seen as consistent with a reinforcement view of depression (Liberman & Raskin, 1974).

Verbal behavior patterns were also studied in an analog interview situation (Matson, Senatore, Kazdin, & Helsel, 1983). Two groups of mentally retarded adults, depressed and nondepressed, were identified based on their score on the Beck Depression Inventory. The subjects' responses to 10 Thematic Apperception Test (TAT) cards were rated on several dimensions, including the number of words spoken, negative self-statements, flat affect, crying, somatic complaints, latency and response time, and content of story. No difference between the two groups of subjects was found. The analog nature of the test situation was hypothesized to have affected the results.

The social skills and social support of depressed mentally retarded persons have also been studied. Reiss and Benson (1985) found that mentally retarded adults who were depressed, based on informant ratings and a self-report depression inventory, had lower levels of social support than disturbed/nondepressed and nondisturbed/nondepressed mentally retarded adults. Further, the depressed adults were rated poorer in social skills than the other two groups (Benson, Reiss, Smith, & Laman, 1985). To identify more specifically the social skill deficits of depressed mentally retarded adults, Laman and Reiss (1987) compared the supervisor ratings on the Social Performance Survey Schedule (SPSS) (Matson, Helsel, Bellack, & Senatore, 1983) of subjects who differed in level of depressed mood. Depressed mood was significantly negatively correlated with three of the four SPSS factors— Appropriate Social Skills, Assertiveness, and Sociopathic Behavior. When the subjects were divided into a High and a Low Depressed Mood group, 30 of the 57 SPSS items discriminated between the two groups, 15 were undesirable behaviors ("blames others for his/her problem," "complains"), and 15 were desirable behaviors ("shows enthusiasm for others' good fortunes," "asks if she or he can be of help"). In each case, depressed mood was associated with poorer social skills. The results indicate that the quality of interactions with depressed mentally retarded adults is negative, as Schloss (1982) found, and that the depressed adults are not necessarily withdrawn.

Learned Helplessness

Preliminary studies questioned whether mentally retarded individuals, in general, are more likely to be helpless than nonretarded persons. Two studies confirmed this hypothesis with chronological age-matched control subjects. Floor and Rosen (1975) compared the performance of mentally retarded adults and college students on questionnaire and behavioral tests of helplessness. The mentally retarded subjects were more helpless on all questionnaire measures (locus of control, coping, and passive dependency) and on some behavioral measures.

There is some evidence to suggest that mentally retarded people learn to be helpless during elementary school years. Weisz (1979) found that although mentally retarded children are not more helpless than nonretarded children in the early grades (ages $5\frac{1}{2}$, $7\frac{1}{2}$), by upper grade school (age $9\frac{1}{2}$) they are more helpless than nonretarded children. The finding was based on questionnaire and behavioral tests.

The finding that mentally retarded persons exhibited signs of helplessness did not necessarily indicate depression. The association between helplessness and depression in mentally retarded students was examined by Reynolds and Miller (1985). Adolescents in EMR classes were compared to regular class students on the Reynolds Adolescent Depression Scale and the Mastery Orientation Inventory (Reynolds & Miller, 1983), a questionnaire measure of academic helplessness. The EMR subjects were more depressed and more helpless than the control subjects.

Summary

Self-report and informant measures of depression have been used with mentally retarded children, adolescents, and adults. Generally, it has been found that mentally retarded persons can self-report mood states, but some care must be given to the wording of the questions and the response format.

However, at least one study found that informant ratings of depression were superior to self-ratings in terms of internal consistency (Laman & Reiss, 1987). Behavioral observation and biochemical tests have identified depressive disorders in some subjects and may provide critical information in the assessment of depression with nonverbal and severely/profoundly mentally retarded persons.

Poor social skills, weak social support, and helplessness have been identified as correlates of depression in mentally retarded individuals. The research results suggest some specific types of interventions, such as social skills training and family/social interventions would be appropriate in the prevention and treatment of depression. The finding that younger mentally retarded children were not helpless, but older children were (Weisz, 1979), suggests a possible course of the development of helplessness and perhaps depression.

Treatment of Depression

The treatment of depressed, mentally retarded individuals has been guided primarily by a reinforcement model of depression and has focused on specific social skills as the target behaviors. Three treatment studies have dealt with the behavioral characteristics of depression. In the first study, Matson, Dettling, and Senatore (1979) worked with a mildly retarded adult male subject who had a 10-year history of depression. He was prescribed imipramine during the course of behavioral treatment. In an AB design, three types of verbal statements, including negative self-statements, suicidal statements, and references to the past, were treated with "independence training." The training included live modeling, self-reinforcement, and self-monitoring. There were decreases in the targeted statements at posttest and 8-month follow-up. Ratings by professionals interacting with the subject in another setting also indicated improvement. Other positive effects of treatment were noted, such as greater participation in activities and self-reports of satisfaction.

In a second study to treat depression, social skills training was used in a multiple-baseline design across behaviors to alter the nonverbal speech patterns of a 10-year-old, borderline mentally retarded boy in an inpatient setting (Frame, Matson, Sonis, Fialkov, & Kazdin, 1982). The child's diagnosis of depression (major depression) was verified through psychiatric interview, mother's ratings on several questionnaire measures of depression, and ratings of a videotaped interview with the boy. The target behaviors were body posture, eye contact, poor speech quality (long latency, lack of clarity) and bland affect. The social skills training included instructions, modeling, role playing, feedback, and reward for participation in daily, individual training sessions. Improvements were noted in the targeted behaviors and were generally maintained at a 12-week follow-up. There was no test for generalization of treatment effects.

The best controlled study on the behavioral treatment of the symptoms of depression in mentally retarded adults was done by Matson (1982a). Four adults, two mildly and two moderately mentally retarded, participated in the multiple-baseline design across subjects. Assessment included a structured interview, which was videotaped, and three self-report depression inventories. Two "control" subjects who were not depressed were matched with each subject to provide a normative comparison on the target behaviors. The 40-minute individual treatment sessions consisted of information, modeling, role playing, feedback, and token reinforcement. A number of behaviors were targeted that had previously been identified as characteristic of depression, such as the number of words spoken, somatic complaints, irritability, grooming, negative self-statements, flat affect, eye contact, and speech latency. The target behaviors changed in the expected direction after treatment was initiated. The positive effects of treatment were maintained at 4- to 6-month follow-up. Also, significant improvements were obtained in the self-report depression inventories at posttest and follow-up.

Conclusions

The study of depression in mentally retarded persons has been quite limited. The identification and assessment of depression in this population can be a difficult process. Greater efforts to develop behavioral observation systems to monitor behavior patterns, such as activity level, eating, and sleep, may be fruitful in creating comprehensive assessment techniques that are applicable for a wide range of individuals. Biochemical tests may offer additional information that can be utilized in conjunction with other assessment methods. The self-report and informant methods that are currently in use require further evaluation to establish their reliability and validity with mentally retarded individuals and to outline their range of applicability. Standardized role-play tests and behavioral observation of specific verbal and nonverbal social skills are needed to identify social skills deficits and design appropriate training programs.

The three depression treatment studies have demonstrated that specific behaviors characteristic of depression can be changed with individual behavioral treatment and that the improvement is maintained for several months. The interventions were effective with both children and adults and with individuals who were moderate to borderline in intellectual functioning.

Depression encompasses several types of disorders with cognitive, physiological or somatic, and behavioral components. The treatment studies noted above have demonstrated changes in specific behaviors. Although the studies did not target the cognitive components of depression, some studies have noted "side effects" of treatment that suggest that these, too, may have been positively affected.

Some of the behavioral interventions that are used in the treatment of depression with mentally retarded individuals are described as social skills training. This approach is not a well-defined treatment package. Although the studies are explicit in detailing the behavioral techniques used (instructions, modeling, role playing, feedback, and reinforcement), the target behaviors and the practice situations varied from study to study. No standard treatment program for depression has been evaluated with mentally retarded subjects as has been done with nonretarded individuals (Bellack, Hersen, & Himmelhoch, 1981).

The treatment studies reviewed focused on remediating social skill deficiencies in depressed, mentally retarded individuals. However, the goals for effective social functioning for mentally retarded persons are not clear. Although there is evidence that depressed, mentally retarded people have greater social skill deficits than their nondepressed peers, there is little normative data on social skill development in mentally retarded children and adults. One treatment study (Matson, 1982a) included nondepressed subjects as controls to provide a performance standard for comparison with the depressed subjects. This method is excellent for gauging the clinical significance of treatment effects. Greater attention needs to be given to the goals of treatment with depressed, mentally retarded persons.

The three treatment studies comprise initial steps in the development of effective psychosocial interventions for depression with mentally retarded persons. Future studies may compare the effectiveness of individual treatments or systematically evaluate treatment combinations, such as pharmacological and psychosocial interventions (cf. Hersen & Bellack, 1984).

FUTURE DIRECTIONS

Anxiety disorders and depression occur in significant numbers among mentally retarded children and adults. It is only recently that screening instruments have been developed that could contribute to the early identification and referral of mentally retarded persons for psychological services (Matson et al., 1984). Further education efforts with teachers, counselors, and parents are needed to ensure that anxiety disorders and depression are recognized and receive appropriate attention.

The continued development of multimodal assessment tools is also required. Valuable preliminary work has been done with self-report, informant, observational methods, and physiological and biochemical measures. Norms are needed and validation studies are required on many of the instruments. Questions remain regarding the behavioral characteristics of anxiety disorders and depression for individuals of different levels of functioning. Future research will be concerned with developing new measures or adapting existing measures to better define anxiety disorders and depression in mentally retarded individuals of all ages and levels of functioning.

Research has indicated that there are effective behavioral interventions for the treatment of anxiety disorders and depression in mentally retarded persons, but the research that has been done could be improved methodologically. The anxiety treatment literature is more extensive than that of depression and has contributed a greater number of uncontrolled case studies. However, the recent research has begun to emulate behavioral treatment studies with other subject populations. There has been some improvement through the use of pretesting, follow-up, multiple outcome measures, and generalization tests.

The range of applicability of the effective interventions for anxiety disorder and depression in mentally retarded individuals is unclear. Future research will outline the boundaries for the selection or adaptation of interventions that are appropriate for individuals of various levels of functioning and skill level.

Future research on the treatment of anxiety disorders and depression may broaden the field by evaluating other treatments and by treating additional problems. The treatment of anxiety disorders has room to expand beyond interventions with simple phobias. Research on the treatment of depression may evaluate the efficacy of cognitive-behavioral interventions.

Research suggests that effective prevention programs could be developed for anxiety disorders and depression targeted at mentally retarded children and adolescents. Based on the association found between social skills and depression, it would seem that the systematic teaching of social/interpersonal skills in educational settings could be valuable in this regard. In the realm of anxiety disorders, individuals facing future anxiety-arousing situations could be targeted for prevention programs modeled on the preparation of nonretarded children for dental treatment (Melamed & Siegel, 1975).

REFERENCES

Abramson, L. Y., Seligman, M. E. P., & Teasdale, J. D. (1978). Learned helplessness in humans: Critique and reformulation. *Journal of Abnormal Psychology, 87,* 49–74.
American Psychiatric Association. (1987). *Diagnostic and statistical manual of mental disorders.* (3rd ed., rev.). Washington, DC: Author.
Bandura, A., & Barab, P. G. (1973). Processes governing disinhibitory effects through symbolic modeling. *Journal of Abnormal Psychology, 82,* 1–9.
Barrios, B. A., Hartmann, D. P., & Shigetomi, C. (1981). Fears and anxieties in children. In E. J. Mash & L. G. Terdal (Eds.), *Behavioral assessment of childhood disorders* (pp. 259–304). New York: Guilford Press.
Beck, A. T. (1967). *Depression: Causes and treatment.* Philadelphia: University of Pennsylvania Press.
Beck, A. T., Ward, C. H., Mendelson, M., Mock, J., & Erbaugh, J. (1961). An inventory for measuring depression. *Archives of General Psychiatry, 4,* 561–571.
Begelman, D. A., & Hersen, M. (1971). Critique of Obler and Terwilliger's "systematic desensitization with neurologically impaired children with phobic disorders." *Journal of Consulting and Clinical Psychology, 37,* 10–13.
Bellack, A. S., Hersen, M., & Himmelhoch, J. M. (1981). Social skills training for depression: A treatment manual. *JSAS Catalog of Selected Documents in Psychology, 10,* 92, (#2156).
Benson, B. A. (1985). Behavior disorders and mental retardation: Associations with age, sex, and level of functioning in an outpatient clinic sample. *Applied Research in Mental Retardation, 6,* 79–85.
Benson, B. A., Reiss, S., Smith, D. C., & Laman, D. S. (1985). Psychosocial correlates of depression in mentally retarded adults: II. Poor social skills. *American Journal of Mental Deficiency, 89,* 657–659.
Berman, M. I. (1967). Mental retardation and depression. *Mental Retardation, 5,* 19–21.

Calamari, J. E., Geist, G. O., & Shahbazian, M. J. (1987). Evaluation of multiple component relaxation training with developmentally disabled persons. *Research in Developmental Disabilities, 8,* 55–70.

Carlson, G. A., & Cantwell, D. P. (1980). Unmasking masked depression in children and adolescents. *American Journal of Psychiatry, 137,* 445–449.

Casteneda, A., McCandless, B. R., & Palermo, D. S. (1956). The children's form of the manifest anxiety scale. *Child Development, 27,* 317–326.

Cautela, J. R., & Groden, J. (1979). *Relaxation: A comprehensive manual for adults, children, and children with special needs.* Champaign, IL: Research Press.

Cuvo, A. J. (1976). Decreasing repetitive behavior in an institutionalized mentally retarded resident. *Mental Retardation, 14,* 22–25.

Cytryn, L., & McKnew, D. H. (1972). Proposed classification of childhood depression. *American Journal of Psychiatry, 129,* 149–154.

Cytryn, L., McKnew, D. H., & Bunney, W. E. (1980). Diagnosis of depression in children: A reassessment. *American Journal of Psychiatry, 137,* 22–25.

Derevensky, J. L. (1979). Children's fears: A developmental comparison of normal and exceptional children. *Journal of Genetic Psychology, 135,* 11–21.

Duff, R., LaRocca, J., Lizzet, A., Martin, P., Pearce, L., Williams, M., & Peck, C. (1981). A comparison of the fears of mildly retarded adults with children of their mental age and chronological age matched controls. *Journal of Behavior Therapy and Experimental Psychiatry, 12,* 121–124.

Flanigan, P. J., Peters, C. J., & Conry, J. L. (1969). Item analysis of the Children's Manifest Anxiety Scale with the retarded. *Journal of Educational Research, 62,* 472–477.

Floor, L., & Rosen, M. (1975). Investigating the phenomenon of helplessness in mentally retarded adults. *American Journal of Mental Deficiency, 79,* 565–572.

Foa, E. B., & Steketee, G. S. (1979). Obsessive-compulsives: Conceptual issues and treatment interventions. In M. Hersen, R. M. Eisler, & P. M. Miller (Eds.), *Progress in behavior modification* (Vol. 8, pp. 1–53). New York: Academic Press.

Foxx, R. M., & Azrin, N. H. (1973). The elimination of autistic self-stimulatory behavior by overcorrection. *Journal of Applied Behavior Analysis, 6,* 1–14.

Frame, C., Matson, J. L., Sonis, W. A., Fialkov, M. J., & Kazdin, A. E. (1982). Behavioral treatment of depression in a prepubertal child. *Journal of Behavior Therapy and Experimental Psychiatry, 13,* 239–243.

Freeman, B. J., Roy, R. R., & Hemmick, S. (1976). Extinction of a phobia of physical examination in a seven-year-old mentally retarded boy—A case study. *Behaviour Research and Therapy, 14,* 63–64.

Gardner, W. I. (1967). Occurrence of severe depressive reactions in the mentally retarded. *American Journal of Psychiatry, 124,* 386–388.

Glennon, B., & Weisz, J. R. (1978). An observational approach to the assessment of anxiety in young children. *Journal of Consulting and Clinical Psychology, 46,* 1246–1257.

Graziano, A. M., & DeGiovanni, I. S. (1979). The clinical significance of childhood phobias: A note on the proportion of child-clinical referrals for the treatment of children's fears. *Behaviour Research and Therapy, 17,* 161–162.

Guralnick, M. J. (1973). Behavior therapy with an acrophobic mentally retarded young adult. *Journal of Behaviour Therapy and Experimental Psychiatry, 4,* 263–265.

Hamilton, M. (1960). A rating scale for depression. *Journal of Neurology, Neurosurgery, and Psychiatry, 23,* 56–62.

Harvey, J. R. (1979). The potential of relaxation training for the mentally retarded. *Mental Retardation, 17,* 71–76.

Hersen, M., & Bellack, A. S. (1984). Effects of social skill training, amitriptylene, and psychotherapy in unipolar depressed women. *Behavior Therapy, 15,* 21–40.

Jackson, H. J. (1983). Current trends in the treatment of phobias in autistic and mentally retarded persons. *Australia and New Zealand Journal of Developmental Disabilities, 9,* 191–208.

Jackson, H. J., & Hooper, J. P. (1981). Some issues arising from the desensitization of a dog phobia in a mildly retarded female: Or should we take the bite out of the bark? *Australian Journal of Developmental Disabilities, 7,* 9–16.

Jackson, H. J., & King, N. J. (1982). The therapeutic management of an autistic child's phobia using laughter as the anxiety inhibitor. *Behavioural Psychotherapy, 10,* 364–369.

Kazdin, A. E., Matson, J. L., & Senatore, V. (1983). Assessment of depression in mentally retarded adults. *American Journal of Psychiatry, 140,* 1040–1043.

Kelley, C. K. (1976). Play desensitization of fear of darkness in preschool children. *Behaviour Research and Therapy, 14,* 79–81.

Koeppen, A. S. (1974). Relaxation training for children. *Elementary School Guidance and Counseling, 9,* 14–21.

Kovacs, M. (1980/1981). Rating scales to assess depression in school-aged children. *Acta Paedopsychiatrica, 46,* 305–315.

Laman, D. S., & Reiss, S. (1987). Social skills deficiencies associated with depressed mood in mentally retarded adults. *American Journal of Mental Deficiency, 92,* 224–229.

Lang, P. J. (1971). The application of psychophysiological methods to the study of psychotherapy and behavior change. In A. E. Bergin & S. L. Garfield (Eds.), *Handbook of psychotherapy and behavior change* (pp. 75–125). New York: Wiley.

Lang, P. J., & Lazovik, A. D. (1963). Experimental desensitization of a phobia. *Journal of Abnormal and Social Psychology, 66,* 519–525.

Levine, H. G. (1985). Situational anxiety and everyday life experiences of mildly mentally retarded adults. *American Journal of Mental Deficiency, 90,* 27–33.

Levine, H. G., & Langness, L. L. (1983). Context, ability and performance: Comparison of competitive athletics among mildly mentally retarded and nonretarded adults. *American Journal of Mental Deficiency, 87,* 528–538.

Lewinsohn, P. M., Hoberman, H., Teri, L., & Hautzinger, M. (1985). An integrative theory of depression. In S. Reiss & R. Bootzin (Eds.), *Theoretical issues in behavior therapy* (pp. 331–359). New York: Academic Press.

Liberman, R. P., & Raskin, D. E. (1974). Depression: A behavioral formulation. *Archives of General Psychiatry, 24,* 515–523.

Libet, J. M., & Lewinsohn, P. M. (1973). Concept of social skill with special reference to the behavior of depressed persons. *Journal of Consulting and Clinical Psychology, 40,* 304–312.

Luiselli, J. K. (1977). Case report: An attendant-administered contingency management programme for the treatment of a toileting phobia. *Journal of Mental Deficiency Research, 21,* 283–288.

Luiselli, J. K. (1978). Treatment of an autistic child's fear of riding a school bus through exposure and reinforcement. *Journal of Behaviour Therapy and Experimental Psychiatry, 9,* 169–172.

Luiselli, J. K. (1980). Relaxation training with the developmentally disabled: A reappraisal. *Behavior Research of Severe Developmental Disabilities, 1,* 191–213.

Mansdorf, I. J. (1976). Eliminating fear in a mentally retarded adult by behavioral hierarchies and operant techniques. *Journal of Behaviour Therapy and Experimental Psychiatry, 7,* 189–190.

Marks, I. M. (1969). *Fears and phobias.* New York: American Press.

Matson, J. L. (1981a). A controlled outcome study of phobias in mentally retarded adults. *Behaviour Research and Therapy, 19,* 101–107.

Matson, J. L. (1981b). Assessment and treatment of clinical fears in mentally retarded children. *Journal of Applied Behavior Analysis, 14,* 287–294.

Matson, J. L. (1982a). The treatment of behavioral characteristics of depression in the mentally retarded. *Behavior Therapy, 13,* 209–218.

Matson, J. L. (1982b). Treating obsessive-compulsive behavior in mentally retarded adults. *Behavior Modification, 6,* 551–567.

Matson, J. L. (1983). Depression in the mentally retarded: Toward a conceptual analysis of diagnosis. In M. Hersen, R. M. Eisler, & P. M. Miller (Eds.), *Progress in behavior modification* (Vol. 15, pp. 57–79). New York: Academic Press.

Matson, J. L., & Stephens, R. M. (1981). Overcorrection treatment of stereotyped behaviors. *Behavior Modification, 5,* 491–502.

Matson, J. L., Dettling, J., & Senatore, V. (1979). Treating depression of a mentally retarded adult. *British Journal of Mental Subnormality, 16,* 86–88.

Matson, J. L., Helsel, W. J., Bellack, A. S., & Senatore, V. (1983). Development of a rating scale to assess social skill deficits in mentally retarded adults. *Applied Research in Mental Retardation, 4,* 339–407.

Matson, J. L., Senatore, V., Kazdin, A. E., & Helsel, W. T. (1983). Verbal behaviors in depressed and nondepressed mentally retarded persons. *Applied Research in Mental Retardation, 4,* 79–83.

Matson, J. L., Kazdin, A. E., & Senatore, V. (1984). Psychometric properties of the psychopathology instrument for mentally retarded adults. *Applied Research in Mental Retardation, 5,* 81–89.

Matthews, C. G., & Levy, L. H. (1961). Response sets and manifest anxiety scores in a retarded population. *Child Development, 32,* 577–584.

Melamed, B. G., & Siegel, L. J. (1975). Reduction of anxiety in children facing hospitalization and surgery by use of filmed modeling. *Journal of Consulting and Clinical Psychology, 43,* 511–521.

Miller, L. C., Barrett, C. L., Hampe, E., & Noble, H. (1972). Factor structure of childhood fears. *Journal of Consulting and Clinical Psychology, 39,* 264–268.

Novosel, S. (1981). Psychiatric disorder in adults admitted to a hospital for the mentally handicapped. *British Journal of Mental Subnormality, 30,* 54–58.

Obler, M., & Terwilliger, R. F. (1970). Pilot study on the effectiveness of systematic desensitization with neurologically impaired children with phobic disorders. *Journal of Consulting and Clinical Psychology, 34,* 314–318.

Ollendick, T. H. (1979). Fear reduction techniques with children. In M. Hersen, R. M. Eisler, & P. M. Miller (Eds.), *Progress in behavior modification* (Vol. 8, pp. 127–168). New York: Academic Press.

Paykel, E. S., Myers, J. K., Dienelt, M. N., Klerman, G. L., Lindenthal, J. J., & Pepper, M. P. (1969). Life events and depression: A controlled study. *Archives of General Psychiatry, 21,* 753–760.

Peck, C. L. (1977). Desensitization for the treatment of fear in the high level adult retardate. *Behaviour Research and Therapy, 15,* 137–148.

Philips, I. (1967). Psychopathology and mental retardation. *American Journal of Psychiatry, 124,* 29–35.

Philips, I., & Williams, N. (1975). Psychopathology and mental retardation: A study of 100 mentally retarded children: I. Psychopathology. *American Journal of Psychiatry, 132* (12), 1265–1271.

Pirodsky, D. M., Gibbs, J. W., Hesse, R. A., Hsieh, M. C., Krause, R. B., & Rodriquez, W. H. (1985). Use of the dexamethasone suppression test to detect depressive disorders of mentally retarded individuals. *American Journal of Mental Deficiency, 90,* 245–252.

Quay, H. C. (1979). Classification. In H. C. Quay & J. Werry (Eds.), *Psychopathological disorders of childhood* (pp. 1–42). New York: Wiley.

Quay, H. C., & Gredler, Y. (1981). Dimensions of problem behavior in institutionalized retardates. *Journal of Abnormal Child Psychology, 9,* 523–528.

Reid, A. H. (1972). Psychoses in adult mental defectives: I. Manic depressive psychosis. *British Journal of Psychiatry, 120,* 205–212.

Reid, A. H. (1980). Psychiatric disorders in mentally handicapped children: A clinical and follow-up study. *Journal of Mental Deficiency Research, 24,* 287–298.

Reid, A. H., & Naylor, G. J. (1976). Short-cycle manic depressive psychosis in mental defectives: A clinical and physiological study. *Journal of Mental Deficiency Research, 20,* 67–76.

Reiss, S., & Benson, B. A. (1985). Psychosocial correlates of depression in mentally retarded adults: I. Minimal social support and stigmatization. *American Journal of Mental Deficiency, 89,* 331–337.

Reynolds, W. M. (1987). *Reynolds adolescent depression scale.* Odessa, FL: Psychological Assessment Resources.

Reynolds, W. M., & Miller, K. L. (1983). *Mastery orientation inventory.* Madison, WI: Department of Educational Psychology, University of Wisconsin-Madison.

Reynolds, W. M., & Miller, K. L. (1985). Depression and learned helplessness in mentally retarded and nonmentally retarded adolescents: An initial investigation. *Applied Research in Mental Retardation, 6,* 295–306.

Richardson, S. A., Katz, M., Koller, H., McLaren, J., & Rubenstein, B. (1979). Some characteristics of a population of mentally retarded young adults in a British city. A basis for estimating some service needs. *Journal of Mental Deficiency Research, 23,* 275–285.

Rickard, H. C., Thrasher, K. A., & Elkins, P. D. (1984). Responses of persons who are mentally retarded to four components of relaxation instruction. *Mental Retardation, 5,* 248–252.

Rivenq, B. (1974). Behavioral therapy of phobias: A case with gynecomastia and mental retardation. *Mental Retardation, 12,* 44–45.

Runyan, M. C., Stevens, D. H., & Reeves, R. (1985). Reduction of avoidance behavior of institutionalized mentally retarded adults through contact desensitization. *American Journal of Mental Deficiency, 90,* 222–225.

Saylor, C. F., Finch, A. J., Spiroto, A., & Bennett, B. (1984). The children's depression inventory: A systematic evaluation of psychometric properties. *Journal of Consulting and Clinical Psychology, 52,* 955–967.

Schloss, P. J. (1982). Verbal interaction patterns of depressed and nondepressed institutionalized mentally retarded adults. *Applied Research in Mental Retardation, 3,* 1–12.

Seligman, M. E. P. (1975). *Helplessness: On depression, development, and death.* San Francisco, CA: Freeman.

Senatore, V., Matson, J. L., & Kazdin, A. E. (1985). An inventory to assess psychopathology of mentally retarded adults. *American Journal of Mental Deficiency, 89,* 459–466.

Sovner, R., & Hurley, A. D. (1983). Do the mentally retarded suffer from affective illness? *Archives of General Psychiatry, 40,* 61–67.

Sovner, R., Hurley, A. D., & LaBrie, R. (1985). Is mania incompatible with Down's syndrome? *British Journal of Psychiatry, 146,* 319–320.

Spielberger, C. D. (1973). *State-trait anxiety inventory for children (STAIC) preliminary manual.* Palo Alto, CA: Consulting Psychologists Press.

Sternlicht, M. (1979). Fears of institutionalized mentally retarded adults. *Journal of Psychology, 101,* 67–71.

Walk, R. D. (1956). Self ratings of fear in a fear-invoking situation. *Journal of Abnormal and Social Psychology, 52,* 171–178.

Waranch, H. R., Iwata, B. A., Wohl, M. K., & Nidiffer, F. D. (1981). Treatment of a retarded adult's mannequin phobia through in vivo desensitization and shaping approach responses. *Journal of Behaviour Therapy and Experimental Psychiatry, 12,* 359–362.

Weisz, J. R. (1979). Perceived control and learned helplessness among mentally retarded and nonretarded children: A developmental analysis. *Developmental Psychology, 15,* 311–319.

Wilson, B., & Jackson, H. J. (1980). An in vivo approach to the desensitization of a retarded child's toilet phobia. *Australian Journal of Developmental Disabilities, 6,* 137–141.

Wolpe, J. (1969). *The practice of behavior therapy.* New York: Pergamon Press.

Wolpe, J., & Lang, P. J. (1964). A fear survey schedule for use in behavior therapy. *Behaviour Research and Therapy, 2,* 27–30.

Youngren, M. A., & Lewinsohn, P. M. (1980). The functional relationship between depression and problematic interpersonal behavior. *Journal of Abnormal Psychology, 9,* 333–341.

Zung, W. W. K. (1965). A self-rating depression scale. *Archives of General Psychiatry, 12,* 63–70.

15

Emotional Problems II

Autism

RON VAN HOUTEN

Autism was among the first developmental disorders to be treated utilizing a behavioral approach (Lovaas, Berberich, Perloff, & Schaeffer, 1966; Lovaas, Freitas, Nelson, & Whalen, 1967; Lovaas, Schaeffer, & Simmons, 1965; Risley & Wolf, 1967). The common behavioral characteristics of autism include social withdrawal and withdrawal from the physical environment; persistent, immediate echolalia; self-stimulation; occasional self-injurious behavior; a desire for the maintenance of sameness; and isolated areas of intelligence (Schreibman, 1975b). The prognosis for this disorder is poor, with only 1% to 2% obtaining normal functioning (Rutter, 1970) in the absence of aggressive therapy.

Many definitions of autism have been proposed (Churchill, Alpern, & DeMyer, 1971; Kanner, 1943; Ritvo & Freeman, 1978), and there is not complete agreement between these definitions (Schopler, 1978). A diagnosis of autism implies that a subset of symptoms is present from a larger set of symptoms. Hence, two children who are diagnosed autistic may exhibit different characteristics. Furthermore, because these "symptoms" are not functionally defined, their presence tells us little about controlling or causal factors in each individual case. Recent results reported by Lovaas (1987) provide some support for the hypothesis that autism may include several different disorders that have been grouped together because of the superficial features they have in common.

The purpose of this chapter is to examine the deficits and excesses observed in autistic children and to outline some specific treatment strategies.

CHARACTERISTICS OF THE AUTISTIC LEARNER

Behavior That Interferes with Learning

Lovaas (1987) reported the results of a well-controlled study on the recovery rates of young children who were diagnosed as autistic. This study com-

RON VAN HOUTEN • Department of Psychology, Mount Saint Vincent University, Halifax, Nova Scotia B3M 2J6, Canada.

pared the long-term results produced by a comprehensive and intensive behavioral treatment program with those produced by a minimum treatment plan administered to a control group. The results indicated that 47% of the experimental subjects achieved normal intellectual and educational functioning in contrast to only 2% of the control subjects. As part of the overall treatment plan, one treatment component involved making a loud reprimand and providing an occasional slap on the thigh contingent upon inappropriate self-stimulative, aggressive, and noncompliant behaviors. As a control procedure, some children in the treatment condition did not receive this portion of the treatment during a baseline period. This component was then introduced, removed, and reintroduced. During the baseline condition, when the contingent aversives produced a marked and sustained reduction in inappropriate behaviors as well as a large increase in appropriate behaviors. These play and language, were noted. These changes were judged to be inadequate to allow the children to be mainstreamed successfully. The introduction of contingent aversives produced a marked and sustained reduction in inappropriate behavior as well as a large increase in appropriate behaviors. These findings suggest that the presence of self-stimulation, aggression, and noncompliance can seriously interfere with learning in autistic children, thus clearly emphasizing the importance of bringing these behaviors under control. It is likely that a similar relationship exists with schizophrenic children.

The inverse relationship between aggression, noncompliance, self-stimulation, and learning reported by Lovaas has also been documented in a number of other studies. For example, Risley (1968) as well as Bucher and Lovaas (1968) found large improvements in imitative responding and eye contact in autistic children after punishment had been introduced to reduce either self-stimulation or noncompliance. In another study, Koegel and Covert (1972) demonstrated that autistic children did not acquire a discrimination while engaged in self-stimulation and that effective learning occurred only when self-stimulation was suppressed. It appears that self-stimulation interferes with attention to the task being taught. Punishment of self-stimulation eliminates this competing response and may also increase overall attention to environmental stimuli (Newsom, Favell, & Rincover, 1983). Lovaas, Newsom, and Hickman (1987) reviewed evidence that hallucinations may interfere with learning in schizophrenic children in much the same way as other forms of self-stimulation.

It has also been shown that the reduction of self-stimulation is associated with increases in appropriate toy play (Epstein, Doke, Sajwaj, Sorrell, & Rimmer, 1974; Harris & Wolchick, 1979; Koegel, Firestone, Kramme, & Dunlap, 1974). the results of these studies indicate that it is desirable to suppress self-stimulation once autistic children or adults have been taught more appropriate recreational activities.

Such behaviors as aggression, self-stimulation, extreme noncompliance and self-injury can interfere with learning in autistic children. These behaviors can also interfere with attempts to mainstream these children into natural settings, such as schools and recreational settings. Because most people find these behaviors bizarre, distasteful, or frightening, they will not tolerate their occurrence in community settings. For these reasons, it is essential that these inappropriate behaviors be brought under control early in the treatment process if a successful treatment outcome is to be obtained.

Overselectivity

It has been demonstrated that autistic children often respond only to one or two features of a multiple stimulus display. This phenomenon has been termed *stimulus overselectivity* (Lovaas, Schreibman, Koegel, & Rehm, 1971). The finding of overselectivity has been replicated within a number of stimulus modalities and is likely to be partially responsible for the difficulty autistic children and adults have in learning new behaviors (Koegel & Rincover, 1976; Koegel & Schreibman, 1977; Koegel & Wilhelm, 1973; Lovaas & Schreibman, 1971; Reynolds, Newsom, & Lovaas, 1974; Schreibman, 1975a; Schreibman & Lovaas, 1973). Overselectivity can occur between stimulus modalities, as in the case when a child responds to a teacher's idiosyncratic gesture or body movement rather than instructions, or it can be within the same modality, as in the case of a child intending to smudge marks on cards rather than color when a teacher attempts to teach a color discrimination using only one card for each color. The degree of stimulus overselectivity observed in autistic children has been shown to be related to mental age, being least pronounced in higher functioning autistic children (Wilhelm & Lovaas, 1976).

Because stimulus prompting procedures typically require responding to multiple cues, autistic children frequently become overly dependent upon the prompt (Koegel & Rincover, 1976). If autistic children are to benefit from prompting procedures, they need to attend more progressively to the relevant stimulus as the prompt is faded. A failure to do so will result in the child's behavior never coming under the control of the training stimulus.

Echolalia

Immediate echolalia is another characteristic of autistic and schizophrenic children that can interfere with language learning as well as with adaptive social functioning (Hingtgen & Bryson, 1972). Echolalia is most common in preschool and school-aged children, although it sometimes persists through adolescence into adulthood (Fay, 1969). Many autistic children also exhibit delayed echolalia, repeating words or phrases they have heard earlier (Fay, 1969). Echolalia is a normal phase of language development, peaking at about 30 months of age (Van Riper, 1963). Autistic children may persist at this behavior because they fail to progress to normal functional language. One possible explanation for echolalic speech (Carr, Schreibman, & Lovaas, 1975; Schreibman & Carr, 1978) is that it may function as a general strategy to verbal stimuli that the child has not learned to respond to appropriately. Once the child has learned to respond to a question or a request, echolalic responding tends to decline (Carr *et al.*, 1975; Risley & Wolf, 1967). Therefore, echolalic responding to a set of questions can be reduced by teaching the correct response to those questions. Nevertheless, little decline is noted in echolalic responding to novel questions.

Poor Generalization

Autistic children frequently show poor generalization to new situations as well as to stimuli that are close to the training stimulus. Stimulus overselectivity can contribute to this problem by restricting the aspects of a stimulus situation that acquire control over behavior.

In a carefully controlled study, Rincover and Koegel (1975) performed an assessment of stimulus control when autistic children failed to demonstrate generalization in a second setting. First, children were taught the response by a therapist working indoors. Next, a second therapist tested for generalization outdoors. Of those children who did not show generalization, each demonstrated control by some irrelevant feature, such as an inadvertent hand movement of the original therapist or the removal of hand restraint. Therapists who work with autistic persons must take care when they teach new behaviors that the correct stimuli acquire control.

ELIMINATING BEHAVIOR THAT COMPETES WITH EFFECTIVE TEACHING

Because the presence of high-frequency stereotypic behavior, noncompliance, and aggression are inversely related to treatment outcome (Lovaas, 1987), it is crucial that these behaviors be brought under control early in treatment. Although a variety of techniques are available to achieve this end, a good deal of clinical assessment as well as trial-and-error learning are often required in order to identify the best treatment approach for each child. With low functioning clients, it is important to perform a comprehensive assessment because seizure medication, ear infections, and other medical conditions may sometimes influence the frequency of tantrums, self-injury, aggression, or self-stimulation. In addition, it is important to perform a functional analysis to determine why the person engages in these behaviors. It has been demonstrated that inappropriate behavior can be maintained by social or material reinforcement, sensory reinforcement, or escape from work or teaching situations (Carr & Durand, 1985; Iwata, 1985; Iwata, Dorsey, Slifer, Bauman, & Richman, 1982). Knowledge of the function that the behavior serves can be helpful in designing an effective treatment plan.

Self-Stimulatory Behavior

Stereotypic behavior in autistic clients is frequently referred to as self-stimulatory behavior, reflecting the hypothesis that the inferred function of this behavior is to produce sensory or perceptual reinforcement. In a review of the literature on self-stimulatory behavior, Lovaas *et al.* (1987) cited a good deal of experimental evidence to support this hypothesis. Among the examples he included was evidence that access to sensory reinforcers can strengthen behaviors, the sensory extinction effect, the inverse relation between self-stimulation and other behaviors, the blocking effect of self-stimulation on the acquisition of new behaviors, and the response substitution effect.

Given the evidence that self-stimulatory behavior is most often maintained by sensory reinforcement, the most effective methods of treating it are sensory extinction or punishment in conjunction with the teaching of more acceptable ways of producing stimulation, such as toy play, looking at picture books, and the like.

Sensory extinction involves removing the sensory consequences of self-stimulation that maintain the behavior (Rincover, 1978a). For example, if twirling string is maintained by its visual consequence, it is possible to extinguish this behavior only by making available to the child string that has a rigid metal core that will not allow the production of the reinforcing consequence. Similarly, if twirling objects on a table is maintained by auditory consequences, then it should be possible to eliminate twirling by carpeting the table to dampen the sound. However, sensory extinction will prove effective only if the relevant perceptual reinforcer is isolated and removed following the behavior (Aiken & Salzberg, 1984; Maag, Rutherford, Wolchik, & Park, 1986; Rincover & Devany, 1982; Rincover, Cook, Peoples, & Packard, 1979; Rincover, Newsom, & Carr, 1979). Hence, it is necessary to identify experimentally whether a child spins an object to produce auditory or visual stimulation before sensory extinction can be employed effectively.

Although sensory reinforcement can be effective, it is not always practical or even possible to remove the reinforcing sensory consequences of a self-stimulatory behavior. In these instances, it is often necessary to employ punishment procedures to eliminate self-stimulatory behaviors.

One way to reduce or suppress self-stimulation is to follow it with a strong reprimand (Lovaas, 1987). If reprimands are to be effective, they must be firmly delivered and accompanied with strong nonverbal disapproval (Van Houten, Nau, MacKenzie-Keating, Sameoto, & Colavecchia, 1982). Studies have also shown that loud reprimands, which can sometimes produce a startle response, are more effective than soft reprimands in suppressing behavior (Doleys, Wells, Hobbs, Roberts, & Cartelli, 1976; McAllister, Stachowick, Baer, & Conderman, 1969; Risley, 1968). It is also important to interrupt or prevent the continuation or completion of the self-stimulatory behavior (Azrin & Wesolowski, 1980; Koegel *et al.*, 1974). This procedure is best accomplished by briskly stopping the behavior and quickly releasing the client, because any prolonged contact could prove reinforcing (Favell, McGimsey, & Jones, 1978). For example, if a young boy were to engage in self-stimulatory behavior using his hands, he should be reprimanded firmly while briskly placing his hands in his lap accompanied by the rapid release of his hands. The more rapidly this action can be completed, the better the success.

If a strong reprimand is not effective, it is possible to try another procedure, such as movement suppression time-out (Rolider & Van Houten,

1985b), overcorrection (Foxx & Bechtel, 1983), negative practice (Secan & Egel, 1986), or a spank (Lovaas, 1987). However, each of these procedures should only be administered under the close supervision of a qualified clinician.

Although in most instances self-stimulation is likely maintained by sensory reinforcement, there is evidence that it can serve as an escape response if it tends to postpone trials or shorten sessions (Durand & Carr, 1978). Rare instances when self-stimulation has been inadvertently shaped as an escape response should be easy to detect, because the behavior should not occur at a high frequency in situations in which demands do not occur, such as when the individual is alone. One way to treat self-stimulation, which functions as an escape response, is to provide rests on trials when self-stimulation does not occur. Another approach would be to punish instances of self-stimulation in the teaching situation. Finally, it may be possible to teach a somewhat more acceptable escape response, such as requests for help. However, if the task is at an appropriate level for the client and prompts are already being provided at an optimal level, this procedure should not be necessary. In this regard, it should be noted that making requests for help that is not really needed in order to avoid putting forth the effort required to learn a new task is a self-defeating escape response.

A final caution relating to the use of punishment should be noted. Lovaas (1987) has proposed the hypothesis that individuals who lack behaviors that could provide normal amounts of stimulation may develop self-stimulatory behaviors in order to provide the sensory stimulation needed to maintain the integrity of the central nervous system. Without self-stimulation, such clients may suffer some level of structural damage. For this reason, we should only punish self-stimulation in the context of an environment designed to teach functional skills that will replace the stimulation provided by these behaviors. As Lovaas (1987) stated,

> in certain situations, such as during periods when the individual is allowed privacy, or in severely understaffed wards with inadequately trained personnel, punishing self-stimulatory behavior without teaching and reinforcing alternatives would seem simply to constitute unnecessary and possibly harmful harassment, as well as probably being ineffective. (p. 59)

Furthermore, because response substitution commonly occurs when punishing self-stimulatory behavior, it is prudent to ensure that an alternative appropriate substitute be taught.

Tantrums, Aggression, and Severe Noncompliance

Most disruptive behaviors in autistic and psychotic children are negatively reinforced by their escaping academic, social, or vocational demands or by positive reinforcement in the form of attention or the presentation of material reinforcers, such as access to the opportunity to produce sensory reinforcement. In the teaching situation, disruptive behaviors, such as tantrums, aggression, and severe noncompliance, may serve to terminate or escape the teaching situation or to postpone or delay the presentation of the next trial or activity (Carr, 1977; Carr, Newsom, & Blinkoff, 1976, 1980; Iwata *et al.*, 1982; Romanczyk, Colletti, & Plotkin, 1980). If this type of behavior is successful, it can do a good deal of harm by preventing the child from receiving the most effective treatment possible and thereby prevent or delay recovery (Lovaas, 1987). Positive reinforcement in the form of attention or material gain can also maintain these behaviors (Carr & McDowell, 1980; Iwata *et al.*, 1982; Lovaas *et al.*, 1965; Patterson, 1980; Wahler, 1969).

Carr and Durrand (1985) presented data showing that aggression and tantrums could serve different functions for difficult children in a teaching situation. Two out of four of the children engaged in disruptive behavior when new material was introduced but not when material already mastered was employed. One child only engaged in disruptive behavior when the amount of teacher attention was reduced, and the last child engaged in disruptive behavior either when new work was introduced or when less attention was provided.

Several approaches can be helpful in treating behaviors that interfere with effective teaching. First, one should ensure that an adequate level of attention and other reinforcers are provided. Second, one can make certain that good teaching procedures are employed, which allow the child to have a high level of success. Third, disruptive behavior should not serve to produce positive attention or escape. Fourth, punishment can be introduced in order to suppress these disruptive behaviors.

Many punishment procedures have proven effective in eliminating tantrums and aggressive behaviors in handicapped and nonhandicapped children. These include reprimands (Lovaas, 1987), movement suppression timeout (Rolider & Van Houten, 1985a; Rolider & Van Houten, 1985b; Van Houten & Rolider, 1988), contingent exercise or effort (Luce, Delquadri, & Hall, 1980), overcorrection (Foxx & Bechtel, 1983), and spanks (Lovaas, 1987). Whenever any of these procedures are employed, one of the best early signs of whether they are going to be effective is whether you obtain good compliance following their application (Parrish, Cataldo, Kalko, Neef, & Egel, 1986). An easy way to test for compliance is to give the child several simple instructions in rapid succession following the application of punishment. If the inappropriate behavior occurs again at this point, punishment can be applied again until the child passes the compliance test. Increased compliance can also be observed in improved performance on academic tasks and in an increased level of eye contact with the therapist.

Generally, it is not as difficult to bring problem behavior under control in the home as it is to bring it under control in public places. Many parents encounter the same problem with their nonhandicapped children. One reason why it is more difficult to obtain control in public places is that it is difficult to apply most discipline procedures in a public place without disrupting ongoing activities. One way a parent may respond to this problem would be to avoid those social settings that are problematic. The major drawback associated with this "solution" is that it denies the child the opportunity to learn how to behave in these social situations and hence interferes with the child's more complete integration into the community.

Two methods that can be effective in treating this problem are tape-recorded mediated punishment (Rolider & Van Houten, 1985a) and recreating the scene (Van Houten & Rolider, 1988). When a tantrum or aggressive behavior in a public place involves an important auditory component, such as yelling or screaming, the parent can record the behavior in the public place on a small, tape recorder and then play back a segment at home, followed by the delivery of a reprimand and another form of punishment that has proven effective with the child. This procedure can then be repeated several times using different examples of the behavior.

In recreating the scene, the child can be guided manually through the behavior after recreating the setting variables as carefully as possible. Punishment can then be delivered in the same manner as described for the tape-recorded mediated procedures described above. Recreating the scene can also be employed when the major component of the behavior is motoric, as may be the case with some forms of aggressive behaviors, such as biting, hitting, or kicking. These two procedures can produce very rapid results. For example, the top half of Figure 1 shows the suppression of serious biting in an autistic child after one application of recreating the scene.

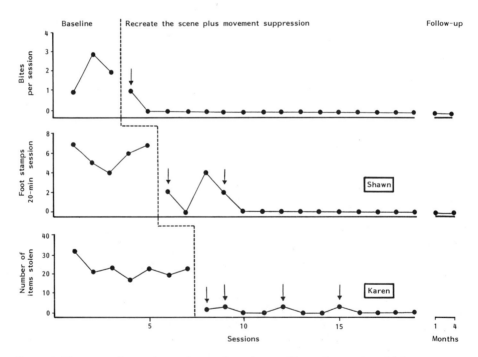

FIGURE 1. The upper frame shows the number of times Shawn bit another child per session during the baseline and the recreating the scene conditions. The arrow indicates the single session during which recreating the scene followed by movement suppression time-out procedures was applied three times after one incident of biting. From "Recreating the Scene: An Effective Way to Provide Delayed Punishment for Inappropriate Motor Behavior" by R. Van Houten and A. Rolider, 1988, *Journal of Applied Behavior Analysis, 21*, 191, Fig. 1. Copyright 1989 by the Society for the Experimental Analysis of Behavior, Inc. Reprinted by permission.

CHARACTERISTICS OF EFFECTIVE TEACHING

Researchers have identified a wide variety of procedures that have proven effective in teaching autistic and psychotic children. Many of these procedures are also effective with nonhandicapped children. The general sequence in the teaching situation should follow this pattern: A clear and simple instruction, often accompanied by prompts, should follow appropriate attending behavior; correct responses should be followed by reinforcement, and incorrect responses should be followed by punishment. Many small details can make a big difference in the type of results that are obtained. The variables described below are some of the factors that have proven to be important.

Seating Arrangement

The seating arrangement is a simple variable that can set the overall tone for the teaching session. Lovaas (1981) recommends a knee-to-knee teaching arrangement whereby the teacher sits facing the student with no desk or table between them and with the teacher's legs outside those of the student. A desk can then be positioned on the teacher's right or left, depending on whether he or she is right- or left-handed. This seating arrangement affords a high degree of control, because the teacher can easily provide physical contact with praise or reprimands, can stop or terminate a response, and can guide or otherwise manually prompt a behavior. Van Houten and Rolider (1989) have demonstrated that nonhandicapped children with small learning problems also reach criterion more rapidly in the knee-to-knee seating arrangement than with the standard desk in-between configuration.

Obtaining Compliance

If the child is going to learn, it is important that he or she learn to sit appropriately during the teaching situation. The knee-to-knee seating arrangement is ideally suited for teaching students to sit appropriately. Students should sit up straight, with their hands on their lap or on the teacher's knees, and should also be looking at either the teacher or the instructional materials. If a child engages in any inappropriate behaviors, such as throwing his or her arms up, this behavior should be followed by a strong clear reprimand, such as "hands down," while briskly placing the child's hands back on his or her lap. Further, it is very important to release the hands quickly in order to minimize the likelihood of reinforcing inappropriate behavior with prolonged physical contact. Appropriate sitting should be reinforced with lots of praise and other reinforcers early in the training until good control is established. In some cases, it may take very strong reprimands and lots of praise in order to teach appropriate sitting. However, the need to teach good sitting is unavoidable, because one cannot begin to teach until a reasonable degree of control and compliance has been attained.

Obtaining Eye Contact

It is difficult, if not impossible, to teach if the student does not attend to the teacher's face (a source of important stimuli) or to the instructional material. Eye contact can be prompted through the use of food or through other reinforcers that the child will visually follow. These prompts can be faded gradually, leaving control by the instruction "look at me," or by simply saying the child's name. It is important to adequately reinforce looking with a variety of reinforcers. Occasionally, even late in training, it is good to reinforce good eye contact with the use of a game, animal noises, or any other interpersonal stimulus that the child responds to as a reinforcer. Handicapped children are no different from other children in that they sometimes learn behaviors to escape work. One can take advantage of this by occasionally following good eye contact with a short break from work. Later in training, it is important to demand good eye contact. Negative reinforcement procedures, such as repeated demands, or holding the child's head until he or she looks, can also be very effective in establishing more dependable eye contact in autistic and psychotic children. A good description of these basic but important techniques can be found in Koegel and Schreibman (1982) or Lovaas (1981).

Use of Rapid Pacing

A good deal of data obtained with nonhandicapped, learning disabled, and educable mentally retarded individuals has demonstrated that rapid pacing, short time intervals, and short intertrial intervals lead to higher levels of performance (Allyon, Garber, & Pisor, 1976; Carnine, 1976; Van Houten & Little, 1982; Van Houten & Thompson, 1976). Koegel, Dunlap, and Dyer (1980) found that intertrial intervals as short as 5 seconds lead to poorer learning than shorter intertrial intervals of 1 or 2 seconds. Although one might explain these data in terms of a poor memory span in these children (Hingtgen & Bryson, 1972), this does not explain the presence of similar effects in nonhandicapped children (Carnine, 1976). Koegel and Schreibman (1982) also suggest that reinforcers should be selected in terms of how quickly they can be delivered and consumed in order to keep up a rapid pace.

Use of Effective Instructional Procedures

Because of the problems of overselectivity, it is crucial that one use clear instructions and prompts with autistic and psychotic children (Lovaas, 1981). Direct instructions like "say buh" or "touch horn" are preferable to instructions that contain a lot of chatter, such as "that's it Billy touch the horn, touch the horn now." Only the simple instructions are likely to acquire clear instructional control over the behavior.

Often it has been observed that autistic children respond before the instruction is completely delivered or prior to looking at the stimulus (Oppenheim, 1974). Examples include children reaching out to touch an object before the teacher has specified what to touch or beginning to repeat a word before the teacher has finished saying it. Dyer, Christian, and Luce (1982) demonstrated that autistic children showed better discrimination learning when they were required to wait several seconds before making a response. When presenting cards in labeling tasks, attention to the stimulus can be monitored by presenting the card in a different location on different trials, thus requiring the child to make an easily discriminable observing response. The instruction, for example, "what's this?" should not be presented until the child looks at the card. Dyer *et al.* (1982) increased performance by preventing a response by holding the child's hands for a period of time before letting him or her respond on a receptive labeling task or by delaying the instruction until after the stimulus had been present for several seconds in productive labeling tasks. One disadvantage of holding the child's hands is that performance will deteriorate once the procedure is discontinued. An alternative approach is to punish responses that occur before the instruction has been completely delivered with a reprimand. The advantage offered by this procedure is that the child learns to avoid responding until the stimulus has been delivered. A further delay can be introduced by teaching the child to withhold responding until he or she is instructed to respond, "touch it now."

Task Variation

Another factor that has been demonstrated to influence learning in autistic children and adults is task variation (Dunlap, 1984; Dunlap & Koegel, 1980; Winterling, Dunlap, & O'Neill, 1987). In the constant task condition, Dunlap and Koegel (1980) presented a single task, such as counting objects or color identification, throughout the entire session. In the varied task condition, the same task was interspersed with a variety of tasks from the child's curricula. In the varied task condition, no task was presented more than two times in succession. The results indicated that the children showed declining trends in correct responding during the constant task condition and improved performance during the varied task condition. In a follow-up study, Winterling *et al.* (1987) replicated these results and also showed that the varied task sequence produced much lower levels of disruptive and self-stimulatory behaviors than the constant task condition. The results of this research suggest that the repeated presentation of the same task may be aversive to the student and perhaps may produce escape-motivated behavior. The best way to avoid this problem is to ensure sufficient variety by rotating through the programs.

Use of Effective Prompts

A prompt is any stimulus added to a request, instruction, or question that usually will evoke the correct response. The correct use of prompts can increase the learning rate while maintaining a high level of success and reinforcement. Prompts are employed whenever new material is taught, unless the clinician suspects that they will not be needed because of increased generalization resulting from extended training on a variety of programs. Frequently, manual prompts are employed with autistic children by physically guiding their behavior. For example, a child who says "ah" when asked to say "oh" can be prompted to say "oh" by quickly rounding the child's lips by pressing in from both sides of the mouth while he or she is saying "ah." Manual prompts are easy to fade because children often find the physical manipulation mildly aversive and will attempt to avoid it by making the response on their own. Similarly, children can be prompted to clap by manually guiding their hands. It is important to remember that not all children will respond in the same way to a particular prompt. If a prompt fails to evoke the correct response, it should be modified until it is effective. Once a prompt is effective, it is necessary gradually to fade or drop the prompt. This can be done with the manual guidance by gradually reducing the amount of pressure applied, by gradually moving the locus of control further away, or by gradually prompting less of the behavior.

Another type of prompt is a stimulus prompt, such as modeling the correct response by holding up the picture of a dog and saying "dog" in order to get the child to say the correct label or by getting the child to imitate gargling water to prompt a hard c sound (unvoiced) or a g sound (voiced). This prompt can be dropped by reducing the volume of the prompt, by increasing the delay between presenting the picture card and the prompt (Lovaas, 1981), or by having the child take less of a sip of water.

Although the presence of immediate echolalia (i.e., repetition of one or more words in a temporally related sample of speech) is often utilized in teaching autistic and psychotic children to label pictures and objects, as well as to give correct answers to specific questions (Carr, Schreibman, & Lovaas, 1975; Ferrari, 1982; Risley & Wolf, 1967), these children will frequently persist on echoing questions to untrained stimuli. McMorrow and Foxx (1986) have speculated that it may be difficult to reduce echolalia to new stimuli by training correct responding to many stimuli, because the training programs all involve the reinforcement of echolalic responses early in training, since verbal prompts are frequently employed. One solution to this problem is to teach children with high levels of echolalia to respond with "I don't know" to novel questions (Schreibman & Carr, 1978).

Another solution is to use the point prompt procedure when teaching question answering (McMorrow & Foxx, 1986; McMorrow, Foxx, Faw, & Bittle, 1987). The point prompt procedure teaches correct verbal responding to questions without reinforcing echolalia by using a picture prompt (McMorrow et al., 1987). First, the person is taught to label items or picture cards when the teacher points to them. Second, these picture cards are used as a prompt in the following manner. The teacher holds up his index finger at eye level midway between himself and the student. If the student verbalizes while the question is being asked, or during the first second after the question was asked, a reprimand is delivered and the question is repeated. On trials, when the student does not echo the question, the teacher points to the picture card or item that prompts the answer to the question; that is, asking "what do you wear on your head," followed by pointing to a picture of a hat. A conditioned reinforcer, such as a nod or a smile, is then presented, and the picture card or object is covered by a piece of cardstock. The procedure is then repeated pointing at the cardstock. Correct responses are then reinforced. This nonverbal prompting procedure was effective in teaching correct responding to training stimuli and also reduced echolalia to untrained stimuli.

Another method frequently employed in teaching discriminations is to add a stimulus that is easy to discriminate and to fade it gradually. This procedure is most effective when the prompt involves exaggerating a critical feature of the relevant stimulus rather than adding an irrelevant stimulus that might prove difficult to drop (Rincover, 1978b; Schreibman, 1975a).

An alternative to fading prompts is to introduce a delay between the instruction or question and the prompt until the child responds before the prompt is delivered (Halle, Baer, & Spradlin, 1981; Halle, Marshall, & Spradlin, 1979; Lovaas, 1966). Charlop, Schreibman, and Thibodeau (1985) have also demonstrated that the time-delay procedure can be useful in increasing the spontaneous use of requests for reinforcers in autistic children. Their procedure involves having the teacher present an item, such as a cookie, and prompt a request by saying, "I want cookie." As the delay between the presentation of the item and the prompt was gradually increased, the children began to ask spontaneously for the item. Further, the results illustrated in Figure 2 show that requesting behavior generalized across people, settings, situations, and to objects that the children could label but had not learned to request. This type of generalization does not typically occur with autistic children (Lovaas, Koegel, Simmons, & Long, 1973; Rincover & Koegel, 1975). Similar results have been obtained using the delayed prompt procedure to teach autistic children to verbalize affection spontaneously (Charlop & Walsh, 1986). The incidental teaching procedures described by Hart and Risley (1975) also involve the use of delayed prompts and have been shown to promote generalization and spontaneity in autistic children (McGee, Krantz, & McClannahan, 1985). Thus, these procedures may prove very useful in promoting generalization. In addition, Touchette (1971) has argued that the time-delay procedure can be useful in avoiding the problem of overselectivity because the prompt and the training stimulus do not occur together and hence are not as likely to interfere with one another.

Use of Effective Consequences

It is very important to employ effective reinforcement and punishment procedures when teaching autistic and psychotic children. One way to enhance the efficacy of reinforcers and punishers with autistic children is to employ a variety of consequences (Egel, 1980, 1981; Charlop, Burgio, Iwata, & Ivanic, 1989). Egel (1980, 1981) found that a condition in which only one highly preferred reinforcer was available was not as effective as a condition in

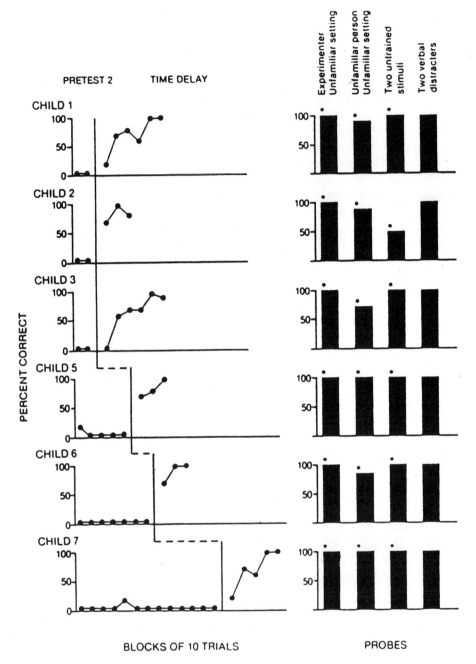

FIGURE 2. The percentage of spontaneous requests made per session during baseline and follow-ing the introduction of the time-delay procedure is shown on the left for each child and the percentage of probe trials in which spontaneous requests occur is shown on the right. All bars marked with an asterisk represent settings, stimuli, or distractor conditions during which there were no correct responses during baseline. From "Increasing Spontaneous Verbal Responding in Autistic Children Using a Time Delay Procedure" by C. Charlop, L. Schreibman, and M. G. Thibodeau, 1985, *Journal of Applied Behavior Analysis, 18,* 160, Fig. 1. Copyright 1985 by the Society for the Experimental Analysis of Behavior, Inc. Reprinted by permission.

which a variety of highly preferred reinforcers were available. Similarly Charlop *et al.* (in press) demonstrated that the use of a variety of relatively mild punishments was more effective in reducing the occurrence of inappropriate behavior than any of the consequences employed alone. These findings emphasize the importance of using a variety of reinforcing and punishing consequences in the teaching situation.

Another important factor is the use of functional reinforcers (Koegel & Williams, 1980; Neef, Walters, & Egel, 1984; Williams, Koegel, & Egel, 1981). Evidence points to a direct relationship between whether there is a functional relationship between the reinforcer and the response or antecedent stimulus. For example, Saunders and Sailor (1979) found that children acquired object labels for toys more rapidly when the toys were also used as reinforcers for the labeling response. In this instance, there is a direct relationship between the stimulus and the reinforcer. Koegel and Williams (1980) demonstrated a functional relationship between the response and the reinforcer. They found that autistic children learned to open a box faster when the reward was in the box than when it was handed to the child. This finding was replicated in a more closely controlled study in which the target behaviors and reinforcers were held constant. Williams *et al.* (1981) demonstrated that children learned to imitate a response, such as an outstretched hand, more rapidly when the reinforcer was placed in the child's hand rather than in the child's mouth, and that the same child learned to initiate opening the mouth more rapidly when the reinforcer was placed in the mouth rather in the outstretched hand. Neef *et al.* (1984) provided additional support to this finding by demonstrating that children learned to say "Yes" and "No" more rapidly when the response was related to the delivery of the reinforcer or a mild punisher than when the children were reinforced for a more abstract response, such as answering the question, "Is this a pencil?" The results of these studies highlight the importance of attempting to maintain a functional relationship between stimuli, responses, and reinforcers whenever possible with autistic children.

Maintaining a High Level of Alertness

Because many autistic and psychotic children have attentional deficits, it is desirable to maintain as high a level of arousal as possible in order to promote effective learning. In general, efforts to maintain compliance will also lead to high levels of alertness.

Employing Procedures That Promote Generalization and Maintenance

Many techniques have been developed to help promote generalization of treatment effects in autistic, schizophrenic, and nonhandicapped children (Baer, 1981; Shelton-Handleman, 1979; Stokes & Baer, 1977). One way to promote generalization is to have various persons teach the behavior in a variety of settings using a variety of slightly different teaching materials.

Stokes, Baer, and Jackson (1974) found that a greeting response did not generalize for some developmentally delayed children unless it had been taught by
several people. In general, the more people who teach a behavior, the greater
the likelihood of generalization. Having many people teach in a variety of
settings using a variety of materials also reduces the likelihood that an autistic
child will come under the control of extraneous cues as a result of stimulus
overselectivity.

Another method of promoting generalization and maintenance is to introduce delayed consequences following behavior (Dunlap & Johnson, 1985;
Dunlap, Koegel, Johnson, & O'Neill, 1987). Dunlap *et al.* (1987) were able to
maintain appropriate behavior in classroom and workshop settings through
the systematic thinning of reinforcement for appropriate behavior and then
gradually delaying the delivery of reprimands following inappropriate behavior. Delayed consequences have also been employed to extend treatment
gains to new settings in which control was absent (Rolider & Van Houten,
1985a; Van Houten & Rolider, 1988). The time-delay and point prompt procedures described earlier can also be employed in order to transfer control of
productive language from verbal stimuli to nonverbal environmental stimuli
(Charlop *et al.*, 1985; Charlop & Walsh, 1986; McMorrow & Foxx, 1986;
McMorrow *et al.*, 1987); so can the use of incidental teaching procedures,
because they involve both delayed prompting and teaching in a variety of
natural settings (McGee *et al.*, 1985).

Also, generalization can be promoted by teaching functional behavior
that makes contact with a natural contingency of reinforcement (Stokes &
Baer, 1977). Hence, it is better to teach behaviors that will serve to provide
positive reinforcers and terminate negative reinforcers in natural settings
rather than behaviors that have little utility outside of the teaching situation.
Further, it is also wise to ensure that the person is sensitive to the effects of
the reinforcers and punishers used in natural settings to control behavior.
Hence, it is crucial that approval be established as an effective reinforcer and
that reprimands be established as an effective punisher for each client.

Providing Training over a Large Portion of the Day

The results of a longitudinal study reported by Lovaas (1987) indicated
that it is essential for autistic children to receive many hours of effective
instruction each day if clinically significant treatment gains are to result.
Therefore, it is important that as many people as possible in the child's environment be taught how to teach appropriate behavior.

SUMMARY

Recent research on autism and childhood schizophrenia indicates that
there is a better chance of improvement and recovery provided these children
receive a sufficient amount of effective treatment. Effective treatment includes

the elimination of inappropriate behavior that can interfere with learning as well as integration of these children into community settings and the provision of many hours of behavioral treatment each day. New techniques show promise in eliminating problems, such as echolalia, and in promoting spontaneous and appropriate language.

References

Aiken, J. M., & Salzberg, C. L. (1984). The effects of sensory extinction procedure on stereotypic sounds of two autistic children. *Journal of Autism and Developmental Disorders, 14,* 291–299.

Allyon, T., Garber, S., & Pisor, K. (1976). Reducing time limits: A means to increase behavior of retardates. *Journal of Applied Behavior Analysis, 9,* 247–252.

Azrin, N. H., & Wesolowski, M. D. (1980). A reinforcement plus interruption method of eliminating behavior stereotypy of profoundly retarded persons. *Behaviour Research and Therapy, 18,* 113–119.

Baer, D. M. (1981). *How to plan for generalization.* Austin, TX: Pro Ed Publishers.

Bucher, B., & Lovaas, O. I. (1968). Use of aversive stimulation in behavior modification. In M. R. Jones (Ed.), *Miami Symposium on the prediction of behavior, 1967: Aversive stimulation.* Coral Gables, FL: University of Miami Press.

Carnine, D. W. (1976). Effect of two-teacher presentation rates on off-task behavior, answering correctly, and participation. *Journal of Applied Behavior Analysis, 9,* 199–206.

Carr, E. G. (1977). The motivation of self-injurious behavior: A review of some hypotheses. *Psychological Bulletin, 84,* 800–816.

Carr, E. G., & Durrand, V. M. (1985). Reducing behavior problems through functional communication training. *Journal of Applied Behavior Analysis, 18,* 111–126.

Carr, E. G., & McDowell, J. J. (1980). Social control of self-injurious behavior of organic etiology. *Behavior Therapy, 11,* 402–409.

Carr, E. G., Schreibman, L., & Lovaas, O. I. (1975). Control of echolalic speech in psychotic children. *Journal of Abnormal Child Psychology, 3,* 331–351.

Carr, E. G., Newsom, G. D., & Blinkoff, J. A. (1976). Stimulus control of self-destructive behavior in a psychotic child. *Journal of Abnormal Child Psychology, 4,* 139–153.

Carr, E. G., Newsom, G. D., & Blinkoff, J. A. (1980). Escape as a factor in the aggressive behavior of two retarded children. *Journal of Applied Behavior Analysis, 13,* 101–117.

Charlop, M. H., & Walsh, M. E. (1986). Increasing autistic children's spontaneous verbalizations of affection: An assessment of time delay and peer modeling procedures. *Journal of Applied Behavior Analysis, 19,* 307–314.

Charlop, M. H., Schreibman, L., & Thibodeau, M. G. (1985). Increasing spontaneous verbal responding in autistic children using a time delay procedure. *Journal of Applied Behavior Analysis, 18,* 155–166.

Charlop, M. H., Burgio, L. D., Iwata, B. A., & Ivanic, M. T. (in press). Stimulus variation as a means of enhancing punishment effects. *Journal of Applied Behavior Analysis.*

Churchill, D. W., Alpern, G. D., & DeMyer, M. K. (1971). *Infantile autism.* Springfield, IL: Charles C Thomas.

Doleys, D. M., Wells, K. C., Hobbs, S. A., Roberts, M. W., & Cartelli, L. M. (1976). The effects of social punishment on non-compliance: A comparison with timeout and positive practice. *Journal of Applied Behavior Analysis, 9,* 471–482.

Dunlap, G. (1984). The influence of task variation and maintenance tasks on the learning and affect of autistic children. *Journal of Experimental Psychology, 37,* 41–64.

Dunlap, G., & Johnson, J. (1985). Increasing the independent responding of autistic children with unpredictable supervision. *Journal of Applied Behavior Analysis, 18,* 227–236.

Dunlap, G., & Koegel, R. L. (1980). Motivating autistic children through stimulus variation. *Journal of Applied Behavior Analysis, 13,* 619–627.

Dunlap, G., Koegel, R. L., Johnson, J., & O'Neill, R. E. (1987). Maintaining performance of autistic clients in community settings with delayed contingencies. *Journal of Applied Behavior Analysis, 20,* 185–191.

Durand, V., & Carr, E. G. (1987). Social influences on "self-stimulatory" behavior: Analysis and treatment applications. *Journal of Applied Behavior Analysis, 20,* 119–132.

Dyer, K., Christian, W. P., & Luce, S. (1982). The role of response delay in improving the discrimination performance of autistic children. *Journal of Applied Behavior Analysis, 15,* 231–240.

Egel, A. L. (1980). The effects of constant vs. varied reinforcer presentation on responding by autistic children. *Journal of Experimental Child Psychology, 30,* 455–463.

Egel, A. L. (1981). Reinforcer variation: Implications for motivating developmentally disabled children. *Journal of Applied Behavior Analysis, 14,* 345–350.

Epstein, L. H., Doke, L. A., Sajwaj, T. E., Sorrell, S., & Rimmer, B. (1974). Generality and side effects of overcorrection. *Journal of Applied Behavior Analysis, 7,* 385–390.

Favell, J. E., McGimsey, J. F., & Jones, J. L. (1978). The use of physical restraint in the treatment of self-injury and as positive reinforcement. *Journal of Applied Behavior Analysis, 11,* 225–242.

Fay, W. H. (1969). On the basis of autistic echolalia. *Journal of Communication Disorders, 2,* 38–47.

Ferrari, M. (1982). Childhood autism: Deficits of communication and symbolic development. Distinctions from language disorders. *Journal of Communication Disorders, 15,* 191–208.

Foxx, R. M., & Bechtel, P. R. (1983). Overcorrection: A review and analysis. In S. Ayelrod & J. Apsche (Eds.), *The effects of punishment on human behavior* (pp. 133–220). New York: Academic Press.

Halle, J. W., Baer, D. M., & Spradlin, J. E. (1981). Teacher's generalized use of delay as a stimulus control procedure to increase language use in handicapped children. *Journal of Applied Behavior Analysis, 14,* 389–409.

Halle, J. W., Marshall, A. M., & Spradlin, J. E. (1979). Time delay: a technique to increase language use and facilitate generalization in retarded children. *Journal of Applied Behavior Analysis, 12,* 431–439.

Harris, S. L., & Wolchik, S. A. (1979). Suppression of self-stimulation: Three alternative strategies. *Journal of Applied Behavior Analysis, 12,* 185–198.

Hart, B., & Risley, T. R. (1975). Incidental teaching of language in the preschool. *Journal of Applied Behavior Analysis, 8,* 411–420.

Hingtgen, F. M., & Bryson, C. Q. (1972). Recent developments in the study of early childhood psychoses: Infantile autism, childhood schizophrenia, and related disorders. *Schizophrenia Bulletin, 5,* 8–54.

Iwata, B. A. (1985, August). *The experimental analysis of self-injurious behavior.* Paper presented at the 93rd annual convention of the American Psychological Association, Los Angeles.

Iwata, B. A., Dorsey, M. F., Slifer, K. F., Bauman, K. E., & Richman, G. S. (1982). Toward a functional analysis of self-injury. *Analysis and Intervention in Developmental Disabilities, 2,* 3–20.

Kanner, L. (1943). Autistic disturbances of affective contact. *Nervous Child, 2,* 217–250.

Koegel, R. L., & Covert, A. (1972). The relationship of self-stimulation to learning in autistic children. *Journal of Applied Behavior Analysis, 5,* 381–387.

Koegel, R. L., & Rincover, A. (1976). Some detrimental effects of using extra stimuli to guide learning in normal and autistic children. *Journal of Abnormal Child Psychology, 4,* 59–71.

Koegel, R. L., & Schreibman, L. (1977). Teaching autistic children to respond to simultaneous multiple cues. *Journal of Experimental Child Psychology, 24,* 299–311.

Koegel, R. L., & Schreibman, L. (1982). *How to teach autistic and other handicapped children.* Houston, TX: Pro Ed Publishers.

Koegel, R. L., & Wilhelm, H. (1973). Selective responding to the components of multiple visual cues by autistic children. *Journal of Experimental Child Psychology, 15,* 442–453.

Koegel, R. L., & Williams, J. A. (1980). Direct vs. indirect response reinforcer relationships in teaching autistic children. *Journal of Abnormal Child Psychology, 4,* 537–547.

Koegel, R. L., Firestone, P. B., Kramme, K. W., & Dunlap, G. (1974). Increasing spontaneous play by suppressing self-stimulation in autistic children. *Journal of Applied Behavior Analysis, 7,* 521–528.

Koegel, R. L., Dunlap, G., & Dyer, K. (1980). Intertrial interval duration and learning in autistic children. *Journal of Applied Behavior Analysis, 13*, 91–99.

Lovaas, O. I. (1966). A program for the establishment of speech in psychotic children. In J. K. Wing (Ed.), *Childhood autism*. Oxford: Pergamon Press.

Lovaas, O. I. (1981). *Teaching developmentally disabled children: The me book*. Baltimore: University Park Press.

Lovaas, O. I. (1987). Behavioral treatment and normal educational and intellectual functioning in young autistic children. *Journal of Consulting and Clinical Psychology, 55*, 3–9.

Lovaas, O. I., & Schreibman, L. (1971). Stimulus overselectivity of autistic children in a two stimulus situation. *Behaviour Research and Therapy, 9*, 305–310.

Lovaas, O. I., Schaeffer, B., & Simmons, J. Q. (1965). Building social behaviors in autistic children by use of electric shock. *Journal of Experimental Studies in Personality, 1*, 99–109.

Lovaas, O. I., Berberich, J. P., Perloff, B. F., & Schaeffer, B. (1966). Acquisition of imitative speech in schizophrenic children. *Science, 151*, 705–707.

Lovaas, O. I., Freitas, S., Nelson, K., & Whalen, C. (1967). Building social and preschool behaviors in schizophrenic and autistic children through non-verbal imitation training. *Behaviour Research and Therapy, 5*, 171–181.

Lovaas, O. I., Schreibman, L., Koegel, R., & Rehm, R. (1971). Selective responding by autistic children to multiple sensory input. *Journal of Abnormal Psychology, 77*, 211–222.

Lovaas, O. I., Koegel, R. L., Simmons, J. Q., & Long, J. S. (1973). Some generalization and follow-up measures on autistic children in behavior therapy. *Journal of Applied Behavior Analysis, 6*, 131–165.

Lovaas, O. I., Newsom, C., & Hickman, C. (1987). Self-stimulatory behavior and perceptual reinforcement. *Journal of Applied Behavior Analysis, 20*, 45–68.

Luce, S. C., Delquadri, J., & Hall, R. V. (1980). Contingent exercise: A mild but powerful procedure for suppressing inappropriate verbal and agressive behavior. *Journal of Applied Behavior Analysis, 13*, 583–594.

Maag, J. W., Rutherford, R. B., Jr., Wolchik, S. A., & Park, B. T. (1986). Sensory extinction and overcorrection in suppressing self-stimulation: A preliminary comparison of efficacy and generalization. *Education and Treatment of Children, 9*, 189–201.

McAllister, L. W., Stachowick, J. G., Baer, D. M., & Conderman, L. (1969). The application of operant conditioning techniques in a secondary school classroom. *Journal of Applied Behavior Analysis, 2*, 277–285.

McGee, G. G., Krantz, P. J., & McClannahan, L. E. (1985). The facilitative effects of incidental teaching on preposition use with autistic children. *Journal of Applied Behavior Analysis, 18*, 17–31.

McMorrow, M. J., & Foxx, R. M. (1986). Some direct and generalized effects of replacing an autistic man's echolalia with correct responses to questions. *Journal of Applied Behavior Analysis, 19*, 289–297.

McMorrow, M. J., Foxx, R. M., Faw, G. D., & Bittle, R. G. (1987). Cues-pause-point language training: Teaching echolalics functional use of their verbal labeling repertoires. *Journal of Applied Behavior Analysis, 20*, 11–22.

Neef, N., Walters, J., & Egel, A. L. (1984). Establishing generative yes/no responses in developmentally disabled children. *Journal of Applied Behavior Analysis, 17*, 453–460.

Newsom, C., Favell, J. E., & Rincover, A. (1983). The side effects of punishment. In S. Axelrod & J. Apsche (Eds.), *The effects of punishment on human behavior* (pp. 285–316). New York: Academic Press.

Oppenheim, R. C. (1974). *Effective teaching methods for autistic children*. Springfield, IL: Charles C Thomas.

Parrish, J. M., Cataldo, M. F., Kolko, D. J., Neef, N. A., & Egel, A. L. (1986). Experimental analysis of response covariation among compliant and inappropriate behaviors. *Journal of Applied Behavior Analysis, 19*, 241–254.

Patterson, G. R. (1980). Mothers: The unacknowledged victims. *Monographs of the Society for Research in Child Development, 45*, 5.

Reynolds, B. S., Newsom, C. D., & Lovaas, O. I. (1974). Auditory overselectivity in autistic children. *Journal of Abnormal Child Psychology, 2*, 253–263.

Rincover, A. (1978a). Sensory extinction: A procedure for eliminating self-stimulatory behavior in autistic and retarded children. *Journal of Abnormal Psychology, 6*, 299–310.

Rincover, A. (1978b). Variables affecting stimulus-fading and discriminative responding in psychotic children. *Journal of Abnormal Psychology, 87*, 541–553.

Rincover, A., & Devany, J. (1982). The application of sensory extinction procedures to self-injury. *Analysis and Intervention in Developmental Disabilities, 2*, 67–81.

Rincover, A., & Koegel, R. L. (1975). Setting generality and stimulus control in autistic children. *Journal of Applied Behavior Analysis, 8*, 235–246.

Rincover, A., Cook, R., Peoples, A., & Packard, C. (1979). Sensory extinction and sensory reinforcement principles for programming multiple adaptive behavior change. *Journal of Applied Behavior Analysis, 12*, 221–233.

Rincover, A., Newsom, C. D., & Carr, E. G. (1979). Using sensory extinction procedures in the treatment of compulsive-like behavior of developmentally disabled children. *Journal of Consulting and Clinical Psychology, 47*, 695–701.

Risley, T. (1968). The effects and side effects of the use of punishment with an autistic child. *Journal of Applied Behavior Analysis, 1*, 21–34.

Risley, T. R., & Wolf, M. M. (1967). Establishing functional speech in echolalic children. *Behaviour Research and Therapy, 5*, 73–78.

Ritvo, E. R., & Freeman, B. L. (1978). National Society for Autistic Children definitions of the syndrome of autism. *Journal of Autism and Childhood Schizophrenia, 8*, 162–167.

Rolider, A., & Van Houten, R. (1985a). Suppressing tantrum behavior in public places through the use of delayed punishment mediated by audio recordings. *Behavior Therapy, 16*, 181–194.

Rolider, A., & Van Houten, R. (1985b). Movement suppression time-out for undesirable behavior in psychotic and severely developmentally delayed children. *Journal of Applied Behavior Analysis, 18*, 275–288.

Romanczyk, R. G., Colletti, G., & Plotkin, R. (1980). Punishment of self-injurious behavior: Issues of behavior analysis, generalization and the right to treatment. *Child Behavior Therapy, 2*, 37–54.

Rutter, M. (1970). Autistic children: Infancy to adulthood. *Seminars in Psychiatry, 2*, 435–450.

Saunders, R., & Sailor, W. A. (1979). A comparison of three strategies of reinforcement on two-choice language problems with severely retarded children. *AAESPH Review, 4*, 323–333.

Schopler, E. (1978). On confusion in the diagnosis of autism. *Journal of Autism and Childhood Schizophrenia, 8*, 137–138.

Schreibman, L. (1975a). Effects of within-stimulus and extra-stimulus prompting on discrimination learning in autistic children. *Journal of Applied Behavior Analysis, 8*, 91–113.

Schreibman, L. (1975b). Attentional deficits in autistic children: Implications for teaching. *Clairemont Reading Conference, 39th Yearbook* (pp. 156–166), Clairemont, CA: Clairemont McKenna College.

Schreibman, L., & Carr, E. G. (1978). Elimination of echolalic responding to questions through the training of a generalized verbal response. *Journal of Applied Behavior Analysis, 11*, 453–463.

Schreibman, L., & Lovaas, O. I. (1973). Overselective response to social stimuli by autistic children. *Journal of Abnormal Child Psychology, 1*, 152–168.

Secan, K. E., & Egel, A. L. (1986). The effects of a negative practice procedure on the self-stimulation behavior of developmentally disabled students. *Education and Treatment of Children, 9*, 30–39.

Shelton-Handleman, J. (1979). Generalization by autistic-type children of verbal responses across settings. *Journal of Applied Behavior Analysis, 12*, 273–282.

Stokes, T. F., & Baer, D. M. (1977). An implicit technology of generalization. *Journal of Applied Behavior Analysis, 10*, 349–367.

Stokes, T. F., Baer, D. M., & Jackson, R. L. (1974). Programming the generalization of greeting responses in four retarded children. *Journal of Applied Behavior Analysis, 7*, 599–610.

Touchette, P. E. (1971). Transfer of stimulus control: Measuring the movement of transfer. *Journal of the Experimental Analysis of Behavior, 15*, 347–354.

Van Houten, R., & Little, G. (1982). Increasing response rate in special education children following on abrupt reduction in time limit in the absence of a token economy. *Education and Treatment of Children, 5*, 23–32.

Van Houten, R., & Rolider, A. (1988). Recreating the scene: An effective way to provide delayed punishment for inappropriate motor behavior. *Journal of Applied Behavior Analysis, 21,* 187–192.

Van Houten, R., & Rolider, A. (1989). An analysis of several variables influencing the efficacy of flashcard instruction. *Journal of Applied Behavior Analysis, 22,* 111–118.

Van Houten, R., & Thompson, C. (1976). The effects of explicit timing on math performance. *Journal of Applied Behavior Analysis, 9,* 227–230.

Van Houten, R., Nau, P., MacKenzie-Keating, S., Sameoto, D., & Colavecchia, B. (1982). An analysis of some variables influencing the effectiveness of reprimands. *Journal of Applied Behavior Analysis, 15,* 65–83.

Van Ripper, C. (1963). *Speech correction.* Englewood Cliffs, NJ: Prentice-Hall.

Wahler, R. G. (1969). Oppositional children: A quest for parental reinforcment control. *Journal of Applied Behavior Analysis, 2,* 159–170.

Wilhelm, H., & Lovaas, O. I. (1976). Stimulus overselectivity: A common feature in autism and mental retardation. *American Journal of Mental Deficiency, 81,* 26–31.

Williams, J. A., Koegel, R. L., & Egel, A. L. (1981). Response-reinforcer relationships and improved learning in autistic children. *Journal of Applied Behavior Analysis, 14,* 53–60.

Winterling, V., Dunlap, G., & O'Neill, R. E. (1987). The influence of task variation on the aberrant behaviors of autistic children. *Education and Treatment of Children, 10,* 105–119.

VI

Academic and Management Issues

16

Language Acquisition

JAMES F. McCOY AND JOSEPH A. BUCKHALT

INTRODUCTION

Most mentally retarded individuals have significant deficits in language. Many of the more severely impaired children exhibit little, if any, functional communicative skills. The development of a language acquisition training technology that allows the establishment of a functional communicative repertoire in mentally retarded children is critical if they are to learn how to exert effectively control over their environments. That is, for mentally retarded children to be able to obtain access to desired materials or activities, to obtain others' attention, to request information, and to make their needs and desires known to others, it is imperative that they be taught communicative language. This is not only the humane approach to take but also is in keeping with the normalization philosophy that we feel correctly guides the services for the mentally retarded individuals with whom we work.

The purpose of the present chapter is to review some of the major developments in language acquisition research with mentally retarded children. Because of the enormous amount of work in the area of language acquisition over the last few years, with numerous entire books devoted to the topic (e.g., Warren & Rogers-Warren, 1985) as well as chapters and research reports, our review has to be selective. First, a general chronology of the history of language acquisition training will be discussed. Next, we will describe some of the differences in didactic training and natural environment characteristics that seem important to consider in developing a technology of training communicative language. Then, a review of promising natural environment or milieu training procedures will be reviewed. Finally, a discussion of one promising future direction, increased parental involvement, will be provided.

JAMES F. McCOY • Department of Psychology, Auburn University, Auburn, Alabama 36849.   JOSEPH A. BUCKHALT • Department of Counseling and Counseling Psychology, Auburn University, Auburn, Alabama 36849.

HISTORICAL OVERVIEW

Few areas of applied research in mental retardation have received as much attention over the past three decades as language acquisition. Teaching mentally retarded persons to communicate as well as possible has been perceived by researchers as a very high priority. Techniques of language training are now routinely incorporated in prescriptive educational plans for mentally retarded persons of all ages and levels of impairment.

The evolution of research in language training seems to have progressed through three stages to this point. The first stage was initiated by the now classic theoretical "debate" regarding the nature of human language by Skinner (1957) and Chomsky (1959). Although neither Skinner's 1957 *Verbal Behavior* nor Chomsky's subsequent review (1959) contained any empirical data or even many suggestions as to how language might be practically facilitated, the works were important for at least two reasons. First, Skinner was perhaps the first researcher to suggest that although language was the most complex and sophisticated human behavior, it should nevertheless be amenable to explanation by principles that had been shown to govern other behaviors. This mere suggestion may have been incentive enough for some researchers to attempt to modify language when they might have otherwise been satisfied to study more elementary behaviors. However, the most important outcome seems to have been the enormous theoretical controversy generated by the two works that practically begged for empirical studies that might confirm one hypothesis or the other about how language is acquired. In the early 1960s, quite a number of studies were done primarily as demonstrations that language, like other behaviors, could indeed be modified with operant methods (e.g., Isaacs, Thomas, & Goldiamond, 1965; Sherman, 1963; Wolf, Risley, & Mees, 1964). Several of these first studies were done with psychotic adults or children who had previously used language but had become mute. Through the application of reinforcement procedures, effects that were termed "reinstatement" of language were obtained. Part of the rationale for selecting language-deficient populations for these first studies may have come from the realization of practical needs, although theoretical concerns probably also played a part. One might argue that if language can be initiated, shaped, and controlled via operant methods in the most severely impaired persons, then less severe impairments should pose less of a training problem.

Although behaviorists have typically chosen to attempt to remediate language in atypical individuals as a demonstration that language can be taught in a didactic fashion, psycholinguists have chosen to conduct more naturalistic, observational studies of nonhandicapped children. Their studies have been aimed at showing the structure and regularity of how children learn to speak in many different cultural contexts. And, of course, their intent has been to demonstrate that language develops in children without any explicit intentional efforts on the part of adults to teach it with the application of reinforcement or other behavioral principles. Of course, one might reasonably argue that, in addition to working with different strategies of research, the two groups of researchers were studying two essentially different problems. Although the psycholinguists were concerned with how language occurs naturally in average children, the behaviorists were more interested in how language would be taught to children who had failed to acquire it in the "normal" course of development. It seems that even though procedures may be developed to facilitate the acquisition of some language skills by a previously nonverbal mentally retarded child, those procedures may have nothing to do with the way a nonretarded child learns those same skills in his or her natural environment. Conversely, a comprehensive description of the structure and sequence of normal language development may or may not be particularly useful in teaching language to individuals for whom the normal environmental circumstances have been insufficient.

One of the first fairly comprehensive language programs that was based upon behavior modification principles was contained in Bereiter and Englemann's (1966) work, which addressed disadvantaged preschool children. By today's standards, the program was more explicit in the content of the curriculum to be taught than in the specific teaching methods to be used. Also, some degree of language usage (although assumed to be nonstandard) was expected of the children entering the program. Significant improvements in general training program models did not come about until the early to mid-1970s, and these models depended heavily upon a great number of limited individual studies that were done in the interim.

In a number of studies, the smallest definable unit of syntax, the *morpheme*, was chosen for training. Guess, Sailor, Rutherford, and Baer (1968), for example, trained a mentally retarded child in the use of plural morphemes. A subsequent series of studies showed moderate degrees of success in using reinforcement techniques to teach proper use of very limited grammatical rules, such as singular and plural endings, and present and past tenses of verbs (Baer & Guess, 1971, 1973; Guess, 1969; Sailor, 1971; Schumaker & Sherman, 1970). The theoretical rationale for choosing an area of training with such little apparent immediate relevance may have been two-fold. First, the choice of elementary morphemic usage derives from the propensity of operant researchers to subdivide complex tasks into their simplest discrete units for training in an analytic fashion. That logic would demand that the simplest grammatical element would be a starting place. A second reason, however, might have come from the previously mentioned controversy with the linguists. To demonstrate that true syntax could be taught directly through operant methods was to discredit much of what linguists were claiming about the way in which syntax is acquired.

As time progressed, more ambitious goals were accomplished by behavioral researchers. As early as 1970, Wheeler and Sulzer documented the training of complete sentences by a child whose speech had previously been telegraphic. Garcia, Guess, and Byrnes (1973) also showed that a severely mentally retarded girl who previously did not use sentences could be taught to do so through the use of modeling and reinforcement of imitation. Some degree of generalization to untrained sentences of similar form to those trained was also obtained. In 1972, Stremel presented the results of a training study in which three mentally retarded children were taught subject-verb-object constructions with shaping and reinforcement techniques.

During this period, some of the work was aimed not so much at building language skills in children who had none but rather at reducing the frequency of inappropriate language before appropriate patterns could be taught. One general program, which was pioneered by Lovaas (1968) with echolalic autistic children, has been to remove positive reinforcement for echoic responses, punish the responses in some instances, and bring the verbalizations under more appropriate environmental stimulus control through prompting and selective reinforcement. Several subsequent successful efforts at eliminating echolalia were reported by Risley and Wolf (1967), Johnston (1968), Tramontana and Shivers (1971), and others. Other inappropriate speech forms, such as diminished volume (Jackson & Wallace, 1974), perseverative speech (Butz & Hasazi, 1973), bizarre, schizophrenic-like speech (Barton, 1970), and elective mutism (Nolan & Pence, 1970), have been remediated successfully through operant procedures.

One purpose in referring to a small portion of the studies done during this period is to illustrate the piecemeal and somewhat haphazard progress, for some time, of behavioral studies of language training with language-deficient individuals. Since behavioral researchers tended to view the complexities of human language as an aggregation of discrete and simple individual skills, success at training the individual component skills was first necessary before comprehensive training could be accomplished. In retrospect, although behavioral researchers may have suffered somewhat from inadequate knowledge of the structure and sequence of language development in designing their first training studies, their early work did serve to demonstrate that certain aspects of language could indeed be modified via behavioral technology. Also, to be fair, the field of developmental psycholinguistics was relatively undeveloped when the behavioral studies began, so knowledge about how language develops in children was very limited initially, and has rather paralleled the growth of knowledge in behavioral training methods.

By the early to mid-1970s, a few researchers had become interested in piecing together information from the many individual training studies into comprehensive models of language training, and a second evolutionary stage was begun. By this time, not only were many individual demonstrations of the effectiveness of operant methodology available, but enough observational data had been gathered by developmental psycholinguists (e.g., Bloom, 1970; Brown, 1973) to give a clearer idea of how children's language is structured and how it changes. Not surprisingly, the training models which were initiated then and which now have continued to evolve, had some different orientations. The model prompted by Guess, Sailor, and Baer (1974, 1978) followed orthodox behavioral theory and method more closely than any others. Other models varied in the degree to which they incorporated psycholinguistic and cognitive-developmental theories. Miller and Yoder (1972, 1974), for example, were among the first researchers to suggest that the structure and sequence of material to be taught to mentally retarded children should be the same as that observed in normal children as reported, for example, by Bloom (1970), Brown (1973), and Schlesinger (1971). Bricker and Bricker (1974), in addition to agreeing that psycholinguistic studies might well dictate the content to be taught, believed that cognitive prerequisites, such as the sensorimotor skills discussed by Piaget, should also be entered into a language-training curriculum for mentally retarded children.

By the end of the 1970s, discrete language-training models had been developed and "field-tested" to a fairly complete degree. The models had been given adequate practical trials in the form of research and demonstration projects. Where research in the 1960s had been predominantly individual studies of relatively limited scope reported in professional journal articles, the 1970s saw the publication of chapters, monographs, and books that described the results of comprehensive, longitudinal applied research projects. Reviews of the area toward the end of the decade (e.g., Guess, Sailor, & Keogh, 1977; Mahoney, Crawley, & Pullis, 1979; McCoy & Buckhalt, 1981) often classified programs in terms of their theoretical orientation and intervention methods.

A "pure" behavioral model had been applied most fully by Guess, Sailor, and Baer (1974, 1976a,b, 1978), and models faithful to psycholinguistic theories had likewise been applied (Bloom & Lahey, 1978; Miller & Yoder, 1974). From a fairly early point, however, it began to be recognized that theoretical allegiance was less important than pragmatism in searching for what worked best. Among the first to recognize that an integrative approach was best were the Brickers (W. A. Bricker & D. D. Bricker, 1974; Lynch & W. A. Bricker, 1972). Their contention was that although operant techniques, such as reinforcement, shaping, prompting, and chaining, were the most effective teaching methods, knowledge from psycholinguistic research should form the content to be taught. Their views were the earliest indicators that an integrative approach would eventually prevail. If the views of Skinner and Chomsky were regarded initially as antithetical, they did provide the conflict for which a synthesis has now emerged and that characterizes the present era of research and application.

Even though individual research groups may continue to be categorized as more behavioral, more cognitive, or more psycholinguistic in orientation, recent textbooks and training curricula for the teachers of mentally retarded persons are noted for their eclecticism and integration. For example, McCormick and Goldman (1984), after describing psycholinguistic, behavioral, and developmental models, go on to state that

> it has become increasingly difficult to differentiate among program models in the eighties because of (a) considerably more dialogue among applied researchers, and (b) the gradual evolution toward a set of common tenets reflecting an almost universal concern for enhancing language use skills. (p. 202)

Although some areas of disagreement still exist (e.g., the production-comprehension issue), there is general agreement on many basic principles, such as the following:

1. The setting of language training should be as broad as possible, in-

cluding home, schoolroom, playground, and all settings where language is used.
2. All available significant persons—parents, teachers, peers—rather than a single language therapist should be involved.
3. The content of a program should come from our knowledge of how language normally develops in children.
4. Behavioral methods should form the core of instructional technology.
5. Generalization and maintenance are of great importance and must be planned from the beginning.
6. One cannot begin intervention too early. Language is built upon a foundation of social communication that precedes the emergence of language.

Didactic versus Natural Environment Characteristics

In the last few years, language acquisition research has shifted in focus from didactic approaches to milieu approaches that involve procedures in systematic language acquisition training in natural environmental contexts. Didactic approaches were extensively developed in the 1960s and 1970s and yielded a powerful technology based on behavior analysis, and are described by Guess *et al.* (1978) and McCoy and Buckhalt (1981). Milieu approaches have adapted many of the training procedures from didactic approaches, such as modeling, imitation, shaping, fading, and differential reinforcement, and have emphasized the development of the communicative function of language as opposed to vocabulary, form, syntax, and content of language. The major limitation of didactic approaches has been the difficulty in obtaining generalization of language from the training to the natural environment. The shift in emphasis to milieu approaches is an alternative strategy to solve the generalization problem, that is, the development of systematic language-training procedures that are applied in the everyday environments of mentally retarded children. Thus, generalization is assured because training takes place in the naturally occurring situations in which the language being trained is appropriate and normal for that context. Of course, other types of generalization become an issue, such as generalization of a language response from one natural context to another (e.g., classroom to playground, teacher to unfamiliar adult, across activities, etc.). (See Hart, 1985, for a detailed discussion of milieu approaches.)

It should be pointed out, however, that didactic approaches will probably need to be used to establish at least rudimentary language in many of the more severely mentally retarded children and then be supplemented with milieu approaches. The focus of the present section will be to review four promising milieu procedures. However, a contrast between the characteristics of didactic arrangements and the natural environment should highlight what a formidable task the development of highly effective milieu procedures is and will be.

Didactic	*Natural environment*
Training is conducted in a small (usually starkly furnished) room, with few materials, and with one-to-one instruction. Few distractions.	Training is conducted in a highly complex natural environment, such as structured and unstructured periods in a classroom full of other children and teachers, with many materials and activities concurrently available. Many distractions.
Reinforcement is artificial, salient, immediate, consistent, and delivered discretely.	Reinforcement is a natural consequence and is subtle, intermittent, and delivered in ongoing interactions.
Training procedures are precisely defined and systematically implemented for short periods out of the day.	Training is more informal, sporadic, and intuitive and can occur at any time and location.
There are adult-controlled sessions in which child's attention is directed. Brief utterances are modeled precisely at the child's level of functioning.	Any utterance is a potential model varied in topic length, amount, and quality with little control over child's attention.
Demand for the child to produce language is high, with many obvious opportunities to respond with language and resultant frequent responding.	Demand for the child to produce language is lower; also the child required to respond less frequently. Long periods of silence may be appropriate, and there are fewer opportunities to respond, which also may be more difficult for the child to discriminate.
The focus is on quality and quantity of phonemes, morphology, and syntax.	The focus is on the communicative function or the presumed intent of the utterance.

MILIEU APPROACHES

The contrast between the characteristics of the didactic environment and the natural environment are so obvious it should not be surprising, especially in retrospect, that generalization has been very disappointing. Milieu approaches have attracted the most interest in recent research because of their promise in solving the generalization problem. Milieu approaches that will be reviewed include interrupted behavior chain strategies, mand–model procedures, time-delay procedures, and incidental teaching.

Interrupted Behavior Chain Strategies

Interrupted behavior chain procedures involve identification of well-established chains, that is, ongoing, highly predictable sequences of purposeful behavior, and the consistent insertion of a language-training episode at the same point in the chain every time it occurs (Goetz, Gee, & Sailor, 1985; Goetz, Schuler, & Sailor, 1983; Hunt, Goetz, Alwell, & Sailor, 1986). Hunt *et al.* provided a good example of the potential of chain interruption procedures not only to train functional, communicative language in ongoing activities in the natural context but also to produce generalization of language to untrained chains. Three severely mentally retarded children, ages 6 and 7, participated in the study. Four chains were identified for each child that met the criterion of having at least three steps, each of which the children could at least initiate. In addition, each chain was evaluated for subjects' motivation for completion, by interrupting the chain and rating attempts to remove the obstacle and the amount of frustration. Chains, which were used, included both those that were performed spontaneously and independently as well as those that were not yet acquired and undergoing training. Examples of the chains and points of interruption included (1) just before putting a toothbrush in the mouth on a five-step toothbrushing chain, (2) when reaching for an item in the refrigerator in a five-step snack-obtaining chain, and (3) after throwing ball to partner in a six-step ballplaying chain. The language responses were different for each subject because of differing skill levels, but all consisted of responses to a pictorial communication system.

The interrupted chain procedure was evaluated with a multiple-baseline and a multiple probe design across subjects, which allowed determination of the efficacy of the interrupted chain procedure, the accelerated acquisition across experimental phases, and the generalization of language usage to untrained chains. Results showed that for all three subjects the interrupted chain procedure produced rapid acquisition of communicative language and, most importantly for each subject, communicative responses generalized to at least two untrained chains. In addition, data were collected on spontaneous occurrences of the target responses in numerous other activities. The highest functioning subject showed a remarkable spontaneous use of requesting items with the trained response on 51 occasions across 25 classroom and nonclassroom activities. Thus, the interrupted chain procedure may be a powerful milieu approach for producing acquisition, maintenance, and generalization of language. It should be a fruitful area of future research, and extension to vocal language for simple requests and elaborations of simple requests should be undertaken.

Mand–Model Procedures

The mand–model procedure was developed by Rogers-Warren and Warren (1980) and replicated by Warren, McQuarter, and Rogers-Warren (1984). The following sequence is used to provide a language-training opportunity in the child's ongoing activities in a natural environment, such as a classroom. First, a teacher displays several materials that are attractive and intrinsically reinforcing for the child. This action usually promotes the child's approach to the materials and the opportunity for both teacher and child to attend to the materials, at which time the teacher mands "Tell me what you want." If the child does not respond sufficiently, the teacher models an appropriate response. Finally, the teacher praises the child's appropriate response to the mand or for imitating the modeled language usage and gives the child access to the material. Rogers-Warren and Warren (1980) initially used mand–model procedures to facilitate generalization of language from a training setting to the classroom. Each of three language-delayed preschool children received 20 minutes of didactic language training each day. The mand–model procedure was introduced in the classroom during a free-play period and evaluated with a multiple-baseline design across subjects. Results showed that the mand–model procedure doubled and even tripled subjects' rates of verbalization. Also, increases in vocabulary and complexity of utterance also occurred. Warren *et al.* (1984) evaluated direct as opposed to generalization-enhancing effects of the mand–model procedure. Single and multiword utterances were trained in language-delayed preschool children in the classroom. Results showed that the mand–model procedure established the trained utterances and produced as well an increase in overall language complexity. In addition, increases in language occurred in a second classroom where training procedures were not in effect.

Thus, mand–model procedures hold considerable promise as a language-training procedure in the natural environment. Like the interrupted behavior chain strategy, more research is needed to establish the generality of the mand–model procedure across children with differing degrees of mental retardation and language delay, as well as an increased complexity of the language being trained.

Time-Delay Procedures

Several studies have examined time-delay procedures for language acquisition training in naturalistic settings. Time-delay was originally developed by Touchette (1971) as a transfer of the stimulus control procedure in visual discrimination learning research with mentally retarded subjects. A visual stimulus, which initially controlled correct responding, was used as a prompt to produce stimulus control by a new visual stimulus, which originally did not control correct responding. Initially, the prompt and the new stimulus were presented simultaneously; over trials, the new stimulus was presented at the start of each trial, and the prompt was presented after increasing increments of time. After several trials, the new stimulus would be presented, and several seconds would elapse before the prompt was presented. Eventually subjects learned to respond correctly to the new stimulus in the "time-delay" prior to the presentation of the prompt. Time-delay procedures have been used to establish a variety of skills in mentally retarded individuals, including following instructions (Striefel, Bryan, & Aikens, 1974), oral reading (McGee & McCoy, 1981) and bedmaking (Snell, 1982).

One of the first systematic investigations of the time-delay procedure for language acquisition training was conducted by Halle, Marshall, and Spradlin (1979). Six institutionalized mentally retarded children, who could vocally imitate, served as subjects. The goal of the study was to train subjects to request their meal when their food trays were presented. Initially, food trays were presented and "requesting" was modeled by staff, subjects then imitated the request and received their trays. Over meals, an increasing delay, up to 10 seconds, was introduced between tray presentation and staff modeling the request. A multiple-baseline design across subjects demonstrated that the time-delay procedure was effective in establishing the request response upon presentation of the tray and prior to staff modeling the response. In a second study, Halle, Baer, and Spradlin (1981) again used a multiple-baseline design across subjects to evaluate the time-delay procedure with six mentally retarded children in a special education classroom. Instead of increasing the delay interval, as in Halle *et al.* (1979), a fixed 5-second delay was used. Requesting (e.g., play materials, snack items, assignment materials) was established by presenting the materials and delaying modeling the request for 5 seconds. The item was given to the children after they imitated the request or made the request prior to the prompt. When items were presented prior to the prompt, the time-delay procedure produced consistently large increases in requests for all subjects. In other words, stimulus control of requesting transferred from the imitative stimuli that were modeled by teachers to the items or the activities. Noteworthy were some generalization results. After training with the time-delay procedure on several requests, children started making requests for additional items and for assistance, such as help in zipping a coat prior to recess, asking for a pencil, or asking for permission to leave an activity. Apparently, the teachers began using the time-delay procedure in these other situations in which they previously preempted speech by anticipating a child's desire, or the teachers were previously responding to the children's nonverbal cues. This finding attests to the relative ease of implementing the time-delay procedure as well as its high degree of flexibility.

The time-delay procedure has been used successfully by Charlop, Schreibman, and Thibodeau (1985) to increase the spontaneous speech of seven developmentally delayed children who were also diagnosed as autistic. Four highly preferred reinforcers (food and drinks) were selected for each subject. Two reinforcers were used in each session and were alternated randomly across trials. When subjects were attending, the experimenter presented one of the items and immediately modeled the request "I want (reinforcer's label)." If the child imitated, the reinforcer was delivered. Incorrect responding resulted in the teacher saying "No" and removing the item. Contingent upon correct responding, the delay interval was increased in 2-second increments up to a total of 10 seconds. Training continued until a child correctly responded in the presence of the object, prior to modeling the request for 18 out of 20 consecutive trials. Results showed the time-delay procedure was effective in producing requests when objects were presented (prior to the prompt) in all subjects. In addition, generalization data showed requests occurred when the reinforcer was presented by unfamiliar persons in non-training environments.

As mentioned previously, time-delay procedures are flexible and easy to use as a milieu training procedure in language acquisition. If children vocally imitate, then modeling the language response can be used as a prompt, which initially controls the child's response. Time-delay training may be used to transfer stimulus control over language from the prompt to the naturally occurring appropriate stimuli within the child's everyday environment.

Incidental Teaching

Incidental teaching was initially developed by Hart and Risley (1968, 1975) as a procedure to enhance and elaborate the language of economically disadvantaged preschool children. Recently, researchers have modified and extended incidental teaching procedures that hold considerable promise as a milieu training strategy for mentally retarded children with severe language deficits. Incidental teaching involves the following steps (Hart & Risley, 1982). The child initiates an interaction with an adult (teacher) concerning a topic of momentary, presumably high interest to the child. The teacher focuses full attention on the child and the child-chosen topic. The teacher requests a language response from the child, which may consist of asking "What do you want?" thus prompting the language response by modeling, or asking for an elaboration of the child's language. Finally, the teacher reinforces the child's language response by stating "That's right," repeating what the child said, and giving the child whatever it was that he or she initiated. For example, a child might approach a toy cabinet that a teacher is close to and stare intently at a toy car on an upper shelf. The teacher then takes the opportunity for a brief incidental teaching episode by focusing attention on the child, which signals the child to emit the request of "car." If the child does not respond, the teacher can prompt the response of "car" or, if the teacher knows that the child is capable of a more elaborate response than the single-word utterance, can wait for an elaboration or prompt one by saying, "Oh, do you want the blue car?" and requiring the child to say "I want the blue car" before giving the car to the child. A critical aspect of the systematic use of incidental teaching is for teachers to be intimately aware of the child's language repertoire so that the child's language responses are challenging but within the child's ability to perform. In addition, incidental teaching episodes should be initiated by the child, should occur in the natural ongoing flow of behavior, and should be kept brief. An excellent recent review of incidental teaching procedures for language acquisition training by Warren and Kaiser (1986) covers many issues beyond the scope of this chapter.

McGee, Krantz, Mason, and McClannahan (1983) conducted one of the first investigations of incidental teaching with two severely developmentally delayed children. Receptive-labeling skills were taught during a routine daily activity of lunch preparation in a group home setting, and generalization was assessed later in the day in a one-to-one, discrete-trials session. A multiple baseline across four sets of lunch materials (sandwiches, vegetables, snacks, and packing materials) was used to evaluate the incidental teaching procedures. Incidental teaching consisted of making a request for the subject to "Give me _____," and then having the subject select from three target objects and two distractor objects from the kitchen counter. If the child selected the correct object, the teacher said, "Good, you gave me the _____," and if an incorrect selection occurred, the teacher repeated the request while simultaneously prompting the correct object by pointing. Results showed rapid acquisition of receptive labeling and generalization of that skill across settings. Subsequent studies have shown incidental teaching to be effective in establishing a wide variety of language skills, including preposition use (McGee, Krantz, & McClannahan, 1985), answering yes or no questions (Neef, Walters, & Egel, 1984), and requesting with sign language (Carr & Kologinsky, 1983).

In an interesting recent extension of the incidental teaching research, Haring, Neetz, Lovinger, Peck, and Semmel (1987) evaluated training special education teachers to use four different incidental teaching strategies. A multiple-baseline design across three classrooms was used to evaluate the effectiveness of self-instructional manuals and daily preplanning of activities in increasing teachers' use of incidental teaching procedures. The self-instructional manuals included material on four procedures: giving students choices, blocking access to materials or activities, placing objects out-of-reach, and giving students objects that were not in the context of an event (e.g., giving them a book at lunchtime). Sessions took place during all activity transitions during the school day. Results showed strong effects for the intervention package in increasing incidental teaching episodes. During baseline, an average of only one episode per teacher per day occurred, whereas, after intervention, an average of 5.9 episodes per teacher per day occurred. This study clearly demonstrates that teachers often do not provide naturalistic language-training opportunities, but that they may be easily trained to do so.

Integration of Approaches

A comprehensive model of language acquisition training can be constructed by combining didactic and milieu approaches. Many mentally retarded children, particularly the more severely impaired, will need the intensive training afforded by the one-to-one, massed practice, distraction-free training provided by the didactic approach. Selection of language targets, though, should emphasize functional communicative responses that the child will have many opportunities to use in the natural environment. Milieu approaches should then be used to increase the language acquired in didactic training in the natural environment as well as to produce language elaboration and generalization within natural environmental contexts. The four milieu approaches that have been reviewed seem to represent a hierarchy of procedures in terms of the degree of adult control that is exerted over training opportunities in the natural environment. Halle (1987) suggested a similar integration of approaches, based upon an elegant conceptual analysis of the source of stimulus control over spontaneous language usage in the natural environment.

Chain interruption procedures (Hunt *et al.*, 1986) appear to represent the greatest degree of adult control over training. Chains are selected that occur throughout the day in many contexts and are interrupted at a step just prior to receiving the natural reinforcer inherent in the task. The language response is required to continue the chain. Thus, there are very clearly defined opportunities for potentially numerous training episodes each day.

Mand–model procedures appear to represent the next degree of adult control over training opportunities. The procedure starts with a teacher providing the child with several attractive, presumably reinforcing materials. A clear opportunity for a training trial is provided; however, the child may not attend to and approach the materials, thus negating the training opportunity. If too much additional prompting is used to obtain child approach and attention, this might be counterproductive by inadvertently reinforcing lack of attention or oppositional behavior. So, a critical step in the mand–model procedure appears to be dependent upon the child being momentarily more interested in the materials than any other competing stimuli in the environment. If the child approaches and attends when offered the materials, it is likely that a successful training episode will occur with teacher manding, "Tell me what you want," and so forth.

Time-delay procedures appear to contain slightly less adult control over training opportunities than mand–model procedures. The purpose of time-delay training is to transfer stimulus control over the child's language responses from adult-modeled language to nonverbal stimuli (in the environment, such as objects, activities, etc.). For example, rather than manding a verbal response, the teacher displays an object and then briefly delays modeling the appropriate response. The child's response has to come under the more remote stimulus properties of the object rather than the more salient stimulus properties of an adult mand for language.

Incidental teaching represents the greatest degree of child control and the least degree of adult control of the four milieu procedures under discussion. The first step in incidental teaching episodes involves an initiation by the child of an interaction with an adult, often for assistance. For example, a teacher might be drinking from a water fountain that is too high for the child to reach. The child approaches and says "water" or looks at the waterspout while licking his or her lips. The teacher then has the opportunity for an incidental teaching episode by requiring an elaboration, "I want water," or prompting a verbal response to the nonverbal cues. Once the child initiates, the adult has an opportunity for language training. However, the entire process obviously depends upon the child's initiation and the immediate responsiveness on the part of the teacher. Many severely mentally retarded children may exhibit extremely low rates of initiations, thus preventing opportunities for this powerful procedure for teaching language.

In summary, an integrated model of language intervention training could consist of didactic training of communicative responses and concurrent use of interrupted chain procedures in the natural environment. As language is learned in the chains, use of the mand–model procedure could be implemented and then the time-delay procedures. Finally, incidental teaching could be employed. This sequence of more intensive, adult-controlled to increasingly more natural, child-controlled learning could be employed concurrently and sequentially to many communicative responses.

Parent–Child Interaction as a Basis for Language Acquisition

Only in the last 10 years have serious attempts been made to involve parents directly in the training of language skills in their mentally retarded children. In the earlier years, researchers trained language skills in the laboratory and clinic and then checked for generalization of that training to the home environment. Garcia and DeHaven's (1974) review, for example, catalogued the mixed results that were obtained with such a research strategy. Rather than summarize all the studies that have included generalization to the home, perhaps one example may be used in illustration. Garcia, Bullet, and Rust (1977) conducted a study specifically aimed at fostering generalization of training across settings, from classroom to home. After training mentally retarded children through the use of imitation and reinforcement procedures to label pictures with complex sentences in a classroom, the use of these sentences at home was measured. It was discovered that the children did not begin to use the trained sentences at home until some of the sentences were actually trained in the home setting.

Some of the shortcomings of early behavioral language intervention programs may have been because of an overreliance upon highly skilled intervention "experts" as primary trainers, and attempts to teach language out of its natural physical and social context. Current research in language training is characterized by greater attention to parent–child interaction and to the social function aspects of language acquisition.

With such a firm historical foundation of concern for the functional aspects of behavior, it is surprising that early behavioral intervention models appear to have lost sight of the natural functions of language. The production and reception of language serve primarily social functions. Although it is undeniable that language also serves some individual, private functions, as in the case of self-guided behavior, most of its functions occur in interactions among two or more persons in reciprocal communication. Recognition of this fact led to the suggestion that programs in language training be located within their natural social context. Mahoney, for example, has advocated an "ecological" mode of training (Mahoney, 1975; Mahoney & Seely, 1976; Mahoney *et al.*, 1979), and MacDonald has termed his approach "environmental" language intervention (e.g., MacDonald, 1976).

An assumption of the ecological (or environmental) model is that language training can best be accomplished within the context of the child's daily activities and interactions with its caregiver, usually the mother. For example, if a goal of language training is to get the child to express the utterance "go out" when he or she wishes to do so, the best time to teach it is when the child actually wishes to go outside, the best place to teach it is the context of his or her familiar surroundings, and the best person to teach it is probably the most frequent caregiver. It would be difficult to envision a clinical teaching situation more desirable than that just described. Many training programs have been overly "trainer-oriented," with the trainer initiating all teaching exercises and disregarding what the child may actually be intending or interested in at any particular moment. One effect of such training is the high degree of stimulus control over language exerted by the trainer and the structured training environment.

Almost all current programs have begun to focus on pragmatic communication in an interactive setting. As McCormick and Schiefelbusch (1984) state:

> In addition to psycholinguistic, behavioral, and/or developmental assumptions, these newer programs place heavy emphasis on intentions (what communicative function the utterance or nonverbal behavior serves) and social appropriateness. The concern is less with what the child can say and how he says it than with what he can accomplish with language. (pp. 209–210)

An additional example of the current emphasis on social interaction is the work of Bricker, who argues that the alternating "turn-taking" interaction between parent and infant is of critical importance (D. Bricker & Carlson, 1981; D. Bricker & Schiefelbusch, 1984).

> Mutual stimulation should be arranged for the caregiver and infant in recurring daily contacts (usually caregiving or play), where each partner can stimulate the responses of the other. Stimulation should be frequent and sustained, with the adult responding sensitively and directly to the infant's initiations. The adult should model and prompt responses to sustain and accelerate the infant's social-communication activities. The initial goal of intervention should not be to teach the infant specific words or other speech events, but to enhance the infant's reciprocal social-communication acts that are fundamental to the development of referential language. (D. Bricker & Schiefelbusch, 1984, p. 245)

The way in which parents and their young children communicate both verbally and nonverbally must be understood more fully. If one assumes with MacNamara (1972) that language communication is preceded by, and dependent upon, much social dialogue between parent and infant that is nonverbal, understanding all aspects of this process seems critical. A great deal of evidence exists already supporting the notion that very early parent–child communication occurs. Kagan's (1967) research with infants and facial schemata suggests that infants have the ability to discriminate human faces from the first few months of life. Research also suggests that infants can process differentially speech sounds at a very early age (Morse, 1974). Although these two areas document the infant's receptive communicative potential, more evidence suggests that infants' capacity for productive communication is also present at a very early age. Among the behaviors that are capable of acquiring early communicative function are crying, smiling and other facial gestures, babbling, eye contact, and numerous motor behaviors. Shaffer's (1971) early investigations into infants' so-called signaling ability, including smiling, have been of particular benefit, as have Bell's (1968, 1974) summaries of the numerous ways in which the active participation of the infant can affect the infant–caregiver interaction.

It has been suggested that one source of delayed or deficient communicative competence is that mentally retarded infants' behaviors are difficult to interpret and "read" (Dunst, 1983; McCoy & Buckhalt, 1981). Recently, Yoder (1987) has provided evidence that even trained observers have difficulty agreeing on the presence or absence and interpretation of mentally retarded infants' communicative cues. It is also the case that individual differences in parental abilities to discriminate cues may affect social interactions upon which language is built. It has long been contended that some parents could differentiate varying infant states by listening to cries independent of contextual cues (Wolff, 1969), and several writers (Lamb & Easterbrooks, 1981; McCoy & Buckhalt, 1981) have suggested that parents differ in their discriminative sensitivity.

The work of Fraiberg (1974, 1977) with blind infants and their mothers may provide a model that is useful to the design of facilitative language interventions for mentally retarded infants. Fraiberg first observed that the communication system between mother and child was not optimal because of the blind infants' deficiencies in the normal ways in which infants signal various messages. For example, she found that the absence of eye contact and the delayed smiling responses of blind infants tended to cause mothers to misinterpret the infants' emotional states and to feel rebuffed by the infants. One result was the provision of fewer verbal interactions, and this state of affairs may have contributed to later delays in language development. When mothers were trained to be more aware of the blind infants' motoric patterns, which often were responsive to maternal stimulation when smiling and eye contact were absent, mothers reported more positive feelings and, more importantly, changed their styles of interacting with the infants. If the ecological model is correct in assuming that a healthy communication system is critical to language development, perhaps parents of mentally retarded infants could be sensitized to their child's communication signals, which may be less pronounced, slower in development, or more idiosyncratic than those of a similar-aged nonretarded infant. In behavioral parlance, such a procedure would consist of sensitizing parents to the discriminative stimuli that govern their interactive behaviors with the infant.

One research issue that has been given considerable recent attention is whether parents of mentally retarded children are more "directive" than parents of nonretarded children. In this sense, directiveness refers to a greater frequency of commands and questions as well as a tendency not to be responsive to the child's ongoing activity or attempts to initiate interactions. Mahoney and Powell (1984) have argued that parents of mentally retarded children who are learning language should be taught to allow the child to select and direct social interactions. By allowing the child's interests and initiations to guide interactions, the child may discover that language affords some degree of control over the environment (of which the parent is a critical part) and may develop intrinsic motivation for using language. Mahoney (1987) has presented some evidence that his Transactional Intervention Program can result in mentally retarded children's developing greater communication skills when parents are taught to focus on child-oriented topics and to respond to the child's attempts to communicate.

Although the majority of studies have found parents of mentally retarded children to be more directive than parents of similar-aged nonretarded children (Cardoso-Martin & Mervis, 1981; Eheart, 1982; Stoneman, Brody, & Abbott, 1983; Terdal, Jackson, & Garner, 1976), a recent 2-year longitudinal study with six Down syndrome and four nonretarded children, which began when the children were 12 months old, revealed that differences in directiveness disappeared when children were matched for mental age. All parents showed similar decreases in directiveness over time, but the changes began later for the mentally retarded children (Maurer & Sherrod, 1987). Apparently, parents adjust many aspects of their language according to the perceived competence of the child rather than to the child's chronological age.

The conclusions of Maurer and Sherrod (1987) regarding directiveness parallel those made earlier concerning complexity of parental language. Working from the assumption that parents of mentally retarded children may infer lower receptive understanding and reduce the complexity of their speech, several researchers (e.g., Buckhalt, Rutherford, & Goldberg, 1978; Buium, Rynders, & Turnure, 1974; Marshall, Hegrenes, & Goldstein, 1973) found that language complexity was indeed lower. Subsequent studies, which matched mentally retarded and nonretarded children for mental age or "language-age," suggested that parents of all children adjusted the complexity of their language according to the capabilities of the child (e.g., Rondal, 1977, 1980).

It is now generally recognized that an important consideration for optional language development is the presence of a good "interactional match," in which parents are aware of the child's level of development and are attuned to the child's immediate needs and interests. Mahoney and Powell (1984), for example, suggested that parents regulate their own interactive behaviors by matching them with their child's developmental level, interaction style, and the activities in which the child shows interest through self-initiated activities.

SUMMARY

Research on language acquisition with mentally retarded and other seriously developmentally delayed children (e.g., autistic and pervasive developmental disorder) has a short but remarkable history. There are few areas in the behavioral sciences that have witnessed such tremendous growth and progress in the last quarter of a century. If the next 25 years are as progressive as the last 25 years, severely language deficient children, regardless of their diagnostic label and degree of handicap, will most likely receive training that will provide them with a communicative language repertoire far greater than we can imagine today. As we noted in the introduction to this chapter, our review had to be limited and focused because of the proliferation of knowledge concerning language acquisition.

First, we reviewed the relatively short history in terms of major trends. Next, there was treatment of the emerging trend within behavioral circles to concentrate more upon the development of sound, systematic, and replicable procedures to move training into the natural environment with milieu training procedures. Finally, a discussion of potentially fruitful issues concerning the primary caregivers—parents—was presented with an emphasis on developmental research. We feel behavioral clinicians and researchers might be less aware of this work, and it may be important to consider in the future evolution of devising increasingly more effective language intervention strategies.

ACKNOWLEDGMENTS. The clerical and editorial assistance of Patricia C. Watson made the writing of this chapter much more enjoyable. We thank her for many hours of extra work.

REFERENCES

Baer, D. M., & Guess, D. (1971). Receptive training of adjectival inflections in mental retardates. *Journal of Applied Behavior Analysis, 4*, 129–139.

Baer, D. M., & Guess, D. (1973). Teaching productive noun suffixes to severely retarded children. *American Journal of Mental Deficiency, 77*, 498–505.

Barton, E. S. (1970). Inappropriate speech in a severely retarded child: A case study in language conditioning and generalization. *Journal of Applied Behavior Analysis, 3*, 209–217.

Bell, R. Q. (1968). A reinterpretation of the direction of effects in studies of socialization. *Psychological Review, 75*, 81–95.

Bell, R. Q. (1974). Contributions of human infants to caregiving and social interaction. In M. Lewis & L. A. Rosenblum (Eds.), *The effect of the infant on its caregiver* (pp. 1–19). New York: Wiley.

Bereiter, C., & Engelmann, S. (1966). *Teaching disadvantaged children in the preschool.* Englewood Cliffs, NJ: Prentice-Hall.

Bloom, L. (1970). *Language development: Form and function in emerging grammars.* Cambridge, MA: MIT Press.

Bloom, L., & Lahey, M. (1978). *Language development and language disorders.* New York: Wiley.

Bricker, D., & Carlson, L. (1981). Issues in early language intervention. In R. L. Schiefelbusch & D. Bricker (Eds.), *Early language: Acquisition and intervention* (pp. 477–515). Baltimore: University Park Press.

Bricker, D., & Schiefelbusch, R. (1984). Infants at risk. In L. McCormick & R. Schiefelbusch (Eds.), *Early language intervention* (pp. 243–265). Columbus, OH: Charles E. Merrill.

Bricker, W. A., & Bricker, D. D. (1974). An early language training strategy. In R. L. Schiefelbusch & L. L. Lloyd (Eds.), *Language perspectives: Acquisition, retardation, and intervention* (pp. 431–468). Baltimore: University Park Press.

Brown, R. (1973). *A first language: The early stages.* Cambridge: Harvard University Press.

Buckhalt, J., Rutherford, R., & Goldberg, K. (1978). Verbal and nonverbal interactions with mothers with their Down's syndrome and nonretarded infants. *American Journal of Mental Deficiency, 82*, 337–343.

Buium, N., Rynders, J., & Turnure, J. (1974). Early maternal linguistic environment of normal and Down's syndrome language-learning children. *American Journal of Mental Deficiency, 79,* 52–58.

Butz, R. A., & Hasazi, J. E. (1973). The effects of reinforcement on perseverative speech in a mildly retarded boy. *Journal of Behavior Therapy and Experimental Psychiatry, 4,* 167–170.

Cardoso-Martin, C., & Mervis, C. B. (1981, March). *Maternal speech to prelinguistic Down syndrome children.* Paper presented at Gatlinburg Conference for Research on Mental Retardation/Developmental Disabilities, Gatlinburg, TN.

Carr, E. G., & Kologinsky, E. (1983). Acquisition of sign language by autistic children: II Spontaneity and generalization effects. *Journal of Applied Behavior Analysis, 16,* 297–314.

Charlop, M. H., Schreibman, L., & Thibodeau, M. G. (1985). Increasing spontaneous verbal responding in autistic children using a time delay procedure. *Journal of Applied Behavior Analysis, 18,* 155–166.

Chomsky, N. (1959). Review of B. F. Skinner, *Verbal behavior. Language, 35,* 26–58.

Dunst, C. (1983). Communicative competence and deficits: Effects on early social interactions. In E. McDonald & D. Gallagher (Eds.), *Facilitating social-emotional development in the young multiply handicapped child.* Philadelphia: Home of Merciful Saviour Press.

Eheart, B. K. (1982). Mother-child interactions with retarded and nonretarded preschoolers. *American Journal of Mental Deficiency, 87,* 20–25.

Fraiberg, S. (1974). Blind infants and their mothers: An examination of the sign system. In M. Lewis & L. A. Rosenblum (Eds.), *The effect of the infant on its caregiver.* New York: Wiley.

Fraiberg, S. (1977). *Insights from the blind: Comparative studies of blind and sighted infants.* New York: New American Library.

Garcia, E. E., & DeHaven, E. (1974). Use of operant techniques in the establishment and generalization of language: A review and analysis. *American Journal of Mental Deficiency, 79,* 169–178.

Garcia, E. E., Guess, D., & Byrnes, J. (1973). Development of syntax through imitation of a model. *Journal of Applied Behavior Analysis, 6,* 299–310.

Garcia, E. E., Bullet, J., & Rust, F. P. (1977). An experimental analysis of language training generalization across classroom and home. *Behavior Modification, 1,* 531–550.

Goetz, L., Schuler, A., & Sailor, W. (1983). Motivational considerations in teaching language to students with severe handicaps. In M. Hersen, V. Van Hasselt, & J. Matson (Eds.), *Behavior therapy for the developmentally and physically disabled* (pp. 57–77). New York: Academic Press.

Goetz, L., Gee, K., & Sailor, W. (1985). Using a behavior chain interruption strategy to teach communication skills to students with severe disabilities. *Journal of the Association for the Severely Handicapped, 10*(1), 21–30.

Guess, D. (1969). A functional analysis of receptive language and productive speech: Acquisition of the plural morpheme. *Journal of Applied Behavior Analysis, 2,* 55–64.

Guess, D., Sailor, W., Rutherford, G., & Baer, D. (1968). An experimental analysis of linguistic development: The productive use of the plural morpheme. *Journal of Applied Behavior Analysis, 1,* 225–235.

Guess, D., Sailor, W., & Baer, D. M. (1974). To teach language to retarded children. In R. L. Schiefelbusch & L. L. Lloyd (Eds.), *Language perspectives: Acquisition, retardation, and intervention* (pp. 529–563). Baltimore: University Park Press.

Guess, D., Sailor, W., & Baer, D. M. (1976a). *Functional speech and language training for the severely handicapped: Part I. Persons and things.* Lawrence, KS: H & H Enterprises.

Guess, D., Sailor, W., & Baer, D. M. (1976b). *Functional speech and language training for the severely handicapped: Part II. Action with persons and things.* Lawrence, KS: H & H Enterprises.

Guess, D., Sailor, W., & Keogh, W. (1977). *Language intervention programs and procedures for handicapped children: A review of the literature.* Final Project Report, U. S. Office of Education, Division of Mental Health and Mental Retardation of the Social and Rehabilitation Services Department of the State of Kansas.

Guess, D., Sailor, W., & Baer, D. M. (1978). Children with limited language. In R. L. Schiefelbusch (Ed.), *Language intervention strategies* (pp. 101–143). Baltimore: University Park Press.

Halle, J. (1987). Teaching language in the natural environment to individuals with severe handicaps: An analysis of spontaneity. *Journal of the Association for Persons with Severe Handicaps, 12,* 28–37.

Halle, J. W., Marshall, A., & Spradlin, J. (1979). Time delay: A technique to increase language use and facilitate generalization in retarded children. *Journal of Applied Behavior Analysis, 12*, 431–439.

Halle, J. W., Baer, D. M., & Spradlin, J. E. (1981). An analysis of teachers' generalized use of delay in helping children: A stimulus control procedure to increase language use in handicapped children. *Journal of Applied Behavior Analysis, 14*, 389–409.

Haring, T. G., Neetz, J. A., Lovinger, L., Peck, C., & Semmel, M. I. (1987). Effects of four modified incidental teaching procedures to create opportunities for communication. *Journal of the Association for Persons with Severe Handicaps, 12*, 218–226.

Hart, B. (1985). Naturalistic language training strategies. In S. F. Warren & A. Rogers-Warren (Eds.), *Teaching functional language* (pp. 63–88). Austin, TX: Pro-Ed.

Hart, B., & Risley, T. (1968). Establishing use of descriptive adjectives in the spontaneous speech of disadvantaged preschool children. *Journal of Applied Behavior Analysis, 1*, 109–120.

Hart, B., & Risley, T. (1974). Using preschool materials to modify the language of disadvantaged children. *Journal of Applied Behavior Analysis, 7*, 243–256.

Hart, B., & Risley, T. (1975). Incidental teaching of language in the preschool. *Journal of Applied Behavior Analysis, 8*, 411–420.

Hart, B., & Risley, T. (1982). *How to use incidental teaching for elaborating language*. Lawrence, KS: H & H Enterprises.

Hunt, P., Goetz, L., Alwell, M., & Sailor, W. (1986). Using an interrupted behavior chain strategy to teach generalized communication responses. *Journal of the Association of the Severely Handicapped, 11*, 196–204.

Isaacs, W., Thomas, J., & Goldiamond, I. (1965). Application of operant conditioning to reinstate verbal behavior in mute psychotics. *Journal of Abnormal Psychology, 70*, 155–164.

Jackson, D. A., & Wallace, R. F. (1974). The modification and generalization of voice loudness in a fifteen-year-old retarded girl. *Journal of Applied Behavior Analysis, 7*, 461–471.

Johnston, M. K. (1968). Echolalia and automatism in speech: A case report. In H. N. Sloane, Jr., & B. D. MacAulay (Eds.), *Operant procedures in remedial speech and language training* (pp. 185–194). Boston: Houghton Mifflin.

Kagan, J. (1967). The growth of the "face" schema: Theoretical significance and methodological issues. In J. Hellmuth (Ed.), *Exceptional infant* (Vol. 1, pp. 335–348). New York: Brunner/Mazel.

Lamb, M. E., & Easterbrooks, M. A. (1981). Individual differences in parental sensitivity, origins, components, and consequences. In M. E. Lamb & L. R. Sherrod (Eds.), *Infant social cognition: Empirical and theoretical considerations* (pp. 127–150). Hillsdale, NJ: Lawrence Erlbaum.

Lovaas, O. I. (1968). A program for the establishment of speech in psychotic children. In H. N. Sloane, Jr., & B. D. MacAulay (Eds.), *Operant procedures in remedial speech and language training* (pp. 125–154). Boston: Houghton-Mifflin.

Lynch, J., & Bricker, W. A. (1972). Linguistic theory and operant procedures: Toward an integrated approach to language training for the mentally retarded. *Mental Retardation, 10*, 12–17.

MacDonald, J. D. (1976). Environmental language intervention. In F. B. Withrow & C. J. Nygren (Eds.), *Language, materials, and curriculum management for the handicapped learner*. Columbus, OH: Charles E. Merrill.

MacNamara, J. (1972). Cognitive basis of language learning in infants. *Psychological Review, 77*, 282–293.

Mahoney, G. (1975). An ethological approach to delayed language acquisition. *American Journal of Mental Deficiency, 80*, 139–148.

Mahoney, G., & Seely, P. (1976). The role of the social agent in language acquisition: Implications for language intervention. In N. R. Ellis (Eds.), *International review of research in mental retardation* (Vol. 8. pp. 57–103). New York: Academic Press.

Mahoney, G. J. (1987, April). *Maternal communication style with mentally retarded children*. Paper presented at the Society for Research in Child Development, Baltimore.

Mahoney, G. J., & Powell, A. (1984). *Transactional intervention program: A demonstration early intervention project for birth through three-year-old handicapped infants*. Ann Arbor: University of Michigan.

Mahoney, G. J., Crawley, S., & Pullis, M. (1979). Language intervention: Models and issues. In B. K. Keogh (Ed.), *Advances in special education* (Vol. 1, pp. 39–57). Greenwich, CT: JAI Press.

Marshall, N. R., Hegrenes, J., & Goldstein, S. (1973). Verbal interactions: Mothers with their retarded children versus mothers and their nonretarded children. *American Journal of Mental Deficiency, 77*, 415–419.

Maurer, H., & Sherrod, K. B. (1987). Context of directives given to young children with Down syndrome and nonretarded children: Development over two years. *American Journal of Mental Deficiency, 91*, 579–590.

McCormick, L., & Goldman, R. (1984). Designing an optimal learning program. In L. McCormick & R. Schiefelbusch (Eds.), *Early language intervention* (pp. 201–241). Columbus, OH: Charles E. Merrill.

McCormick, L., & Schiefelbusch, R. (1984). *Early language intervention.* Columbus, OH: Charles E. Merrill.

McCoy, J. F., & Buckhalt, J. A. (1981). Language acquisition. In J. L. Matson & J. R. McCartney (Eds.), *Handbook of behavior modification with the mentally retarded* (pp. 281–330). New York: Plenum Press.

McGee, G. G., & McCoy, J. F. (1981). Training procedures for acquisition and retention of reading in retarded youth. *Applied Research in Mental retardation, 2*, 263–276.

McGee, G. G., Krantz, P. J., Mason, D., & McClannahan, L. E. (1983). A modified incidental-teaching procedure for autistic youth: Acquisition and generalization of receptive object labels. *Journal of Applied Behavior Analysis, 16*, 329–338.

McGee, G. G., Krantz, P. J., & McClannahan, L. E. (1985). The facilitative effects of incidental teaching on preposition use by autistic children. *Journal of Applied Behavior Analysis, 18*, 17–31.

Miller, J. F., & Yoder, D. E. (1972). A syntax teaching program. In J. E. McLean, D. E. Yoder, & R. L. Schiefelbusch (Eds.), *Language intervention with the retarded: Developing strategies* (pp. 191–211). Baltimore: University Park Press.

Miller, J. F., & Yoder, D. E. (1974). An ontogenetic language teaching strategy for retarded children. In R. L. Schiefelbusch & L. L. Lloyd (Eds.), *Language perspectives: Acquisition, retardation, and intervention* (pp. 505–528). Baltimore: University Park Press.

Morse, P. A. (1974). Infant speech perception: A preliminary model and review of the literature. In R. L. Schiefelbusch & L. L. Lloyd (Eds.), *Language perspectives: Acquisition, retardation, and intervention* (pp. 19–53). Baltimore: University Park Press.

Neef, N. A., Walters, J., & Egel, A. L. (1984). Establishing generative yes/no responses in developmentally disabled children. *Journal of Applied Behavior Analysis, 17*, 453–460.

Nolan, J. D., & Pence, C. (1970). Operant conditioning principles in the treatment of a selectively mute child. *Journal of Consulting and Clinical Psychology, 35*, 265–268.

Risley, T. R., & Wolf, M. M. (1967). Establishing functional speech in echolalic children. *Behavior Research and Therapy, 5*, 73–88.

Rogers-Warren, A., & Warren, S. (1980). Mands for verbalization: Facilitating the display of newly trained language in children. *Behavior Modification, 4*, 361–382.

Rondal, J. (1980). Fathers' and mothers' speech in early language development. *Journal of Child Language, 7*, 353–369.

Rondal, J. A. (1977). Maternal speech in normal and Down's syndrome children. In P. Miller (Ed.), *Research to practice in mental retardation* (pp. 239–243). Baltimore: University Park Press.

Sailor, W. (1971). Reinforcement and generalization of productive plural allomorphs in two retarded children. *Journal of Applied Behavior Analysis, 4*, 305–310.

Schlesinger, I. M. (1971). Production of utterances and language acquisition. In D. I. Slobin (Ed.), *The ontogenesis of grammar.* New York: Academic Press.

Schumaker, J., & Sherman, J. A. (1970). Training generative verb usage by imitation and reinforcement procedures. *Journal of Applied Behavior Analysis, 3*, 273–287.

Shaffer, H. R. (1971). *The growth of sociability.* Baltimore: Penguin.

Sherman, J. A. (1963). Reinstatement of verbal behavior in a psychotic by reinforcement methods. *Journal of Speech and Hearing Disorders, 28*, 398–400.

Skinner, B. F. (1957). *Verbal behavior.* New York: Appleton-Century-Crofts.

Snell, M. E. (1982). Analysis of time delay procedures in teaching daily living skills to retarded adults. *Analysis and Intervention in Developmental Disabilities, 2,* 3–14.

Stoneman, Z., Brody, G. H., & Abbott, D. (1983). In-home observations of young Down syndrome children with their mothers and fathers. *American Journal of Mental Deficiency, 87,* 591–600.

Stremel, K. (1972). Language training: A problem for retarded children. *Mental Retardation, 10,* 47–79.

Striefel, S., Bryan, K. S., & Aikens, D. A. (1974). Transfer of stimulus control from motor to verbal stimuli. *Journal of Applied Behavior Analysis, 7,* 123–135.

Terdal, L., Jackson, R. H., & Garner, A. M. (1976). Mother-child interactions: A comparison between normal and developmentally delayed groups. In E. J. Marsh, L. A. Hamerlynck, & L. C. Handy (Eds.), *Behavior modification and families.* New York: Brunner/Mazel.

Touchette, P. E. (1971). Transfer of stimulus control: Measuring the moment of transfer. *Journal of the Experimental Analysis of Behavior, 15,* 347–354.

Tramontana, J., & Shivers, O. (1971). Behavior modification with an echolalic child: A case note. *Psychological Reports, 29,* 1034.

Warren, S. F., & Kaiser, A. P. (1986). Incidental language teaching: A critical review. *Journal of Speech and Hearing Disorders, 51,* 291–299.

Warren, S. F., & Rogers-Warren, A. K. (Eds.). (1985). *Teaching functional language.* Austin, TX: Pro-Ed.

Warren, S. F., McQuarter, R. J., & Rogers-Warren, A. K. (1984). The effects of mands and models on the speech of unresponsive socially isolate children. *Journal of Speech and Hearing Disorders, 47,* 42–52.

Wheeler, A. J., & Sulzer, B. (1970). Operant training and generalization of a verbal response form in a speech-deficient child. *Journal of Applied Behavior Analysis, 3,* 139–147.

Wolf, M. M., Risley, T. R., & Mees, H. (1964). Application of operant conditioning procedures to the behavior problems of an autistic child. *Behaviour Research and Therapy, 2,* 305–312.

Wolff, P. H. (1969). The natural history of crying and other vocalizations in early infancy. In B. M. Foss (Ed.), *Determinants of infant behavior* (Vol. 4, pp. 87–109). London: Methuen.

Yoder, P. J. (1987). Relationship between degree of infant handicap and clarity of infant cues. *American Journal of Mental Deficiency, 91,* 639–641.

17

Academic Training

PAUL WEISBERG

INTRODUCTION

Diagnosticians who evaluate individuals having trouble with certain academic content areas often look for basic flaws within the individual as the source of the difficulty. This approach leads to classifying the individual according to some presumed or real disability, and the information that is provided to the teacher centers on that deficiency; for instance, poor auditory sequencing, inability to generalize, or sporadic attention. Sometimes, nothing is gained because the teacher already knows about the deficit, having encountered frequent samples of it from the learner in the classroom. If a remedy is suggested, it is in a form that does not mention or find fault with the current academic program or with the teaching procedures (Engelmann, Granzin, & Severson, 1979). Indeed, the person providing the remedy probably has not looked at the program or set foot in the classroom.

Given such a one-sided approach to evaluation, few professionals ever consider that the failure is due to instructional flaws. Engelmann (1980) suggested that we critically examine academic programs and tasks to see if, on logical grounds, they are free from introducing misconceptions and if they have the teaching examples organized so that a generalized and efficient form of learning is predictable. Thus, an early and essential step in judging academic performance is to "diagnose the program." Should a learner make no progress when presented with a well-designed program, we can more appropriately rule out an instructional variable and ascribe the failure to a learner flaw. An underlying theme of this chapter is to identify, evaluate, and explicate aspects of academic programs for mentally retarded individuals, a group that is highly in need of special consideration in classroom and daily living settings (Browder & Snell, 1987; Etzel & Le Blanc, 1979).

THE LANGUAGE OF INSTRUCTION

If told to "touch the letter under the second truck" or "write your name in the lower right-hand corner," many handicapped individuals would not

PAUL WEISBERG • Department of Psychology, University of Alabama, Tuscaloosa, Alabama 35487.

understand the meaning of such work as *under, second, lower,* and *corner* if presented separately or in sentences. To master the language of academic concepts and operations, students need to be directly taught and tested on the essential academic vocabulary and how to deal with increasingly more complex terms and relationships. A description of some of these teaching methods together with relevant research follows.

Teaching Object Characteristics by Modeling

When teaching any naive learner to attend to the critical attribute or feature of basic concepts, such as *truck, red, over,* or *larger than,* it would be pointless to use dictionary definitions because they refer to additional concepts with features that are also foreign to the learner. Moreover, we cannot use words to describe the attributes of these concepts in ways that permit the learner to discriminate reliably between examples and nonexamples of the concepts. Instead, we must model and present concrete examples and nonexamples in a sequence that permits the learner to reach a correct interpretation of the concept feature. Figure 1 presents a prototypic sequence for teaching *over* according to Engelmann and Carnine's (1982) programming logic.

Before showing the examples, the teacher says, "Watch the ball. I'll tell if it's over or not-over the table." The first six examples are modeled. The teacher says, "it's not over," for the negative examples (S−) in Steps 1, 2, and 6. She says, "it's over," for the positive examples (S+) in Steps 3, 4, and 5. During the test segment in Steps 7 to 12, the learner answers "yes" or "no" to the question, "Is it over?" Having the same object (ball held in hand) used for both S+ and S− rules out the maximum number of irrelevant stimuli and thus reduces the number of teaching examples. The teacher's wording is similarly restricted in order to place primary emphasis on the features of the examples. Modeling a range of S+ and S− examples enhances correct identification of the novel examples presented during the test segment.

The examples are always in view. After the ball is positioned into the location shown and the concept is labeled as "over" or "not-over," the ball is quickly moved and repositioned to form the next example. This means that examples are continuously converted to create the next S+ or S−. A minimum-difference change occurs between the examples in Steps 2 and 3; the

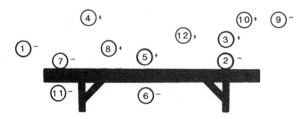

FIGURE 1. Sequence of positive (+) and negative (−) examples for teaching the concept *over.*

ball is moved upward a bit, but no other stimulus changes are made. Although the movement is meager, it should be noticeable because of the ball's previous stationary position in Step 2. That the change is important is signaled through the new wording at Step 3—"it's over." Other minimum-difference changes, which equally teach a discrimination between important object characteristics, occur at Steps 5 and 6 and at 9 and 10.

The same sequence used in teaching *over* can be used for all prepositional concepts as well as for adjectives (e.g., *green, big, smooth*) and action verbs. Only the teaching material and wording would need to be altered (and sometimes the sequence would start with modeled S+ examples). For these concepts, S+ examples can also be easily converted into S− examples (or vice versa) in one operation by changing the relevant concept feature. Other concepts that are also single dimensional, but whose concept feature is based upon relative changes, are comparative concepts (e.g., *getting greener, bigger than, smoother than*). They, too, can be taught in essentially the same way as *over* and lend themselves to continuous S+/S− conversions. Finally, there are noun concepts in which many attributes serve to distinguish between the S+ and S− examples. Such concepts have vocabulary labels that stand for a number of features in simple objects (car, dogs, chair, quarters), object classes (vehicles, animals, furniture, coins), and symbols (letters, numbers, shapes). Because most nouns possess multidimensional concept features, one noun cannot be transformed into another noun within a single operation. Thus, continuous conversions are not possible. Nonetheless, their concept feature can be taught by modeling positive examples ("this is a truck") and negative examples ("this is not a truck") and by appropriate testing.

It is best to teach a new concept in a restrictive setting. However, once a criterion performance is attained, programming for generalization is imperative. The concept feature must be extended systematically to new objects, and variations must be made in teacher wording and questioning procedures (e.g., asking "where" questions), in mode of stimulus presentation (e.g., presenting pairs of S+ and S− examples as pictures), and in the nature of the response convention (e.g., asking the learner to label the concept or to produce a concept example). The details for programming these variations are given in Engelmann and Carnine (1982).

There is a growing body of research to support the efficacy of Engelmann and Carnine's (1982) teaching procedures with instructionally naive and handicapped individuals. Williams and Carnine (1981) found that variation in the teacher's wording during the testing of preschoolers for their understanding of *diagonal* had a deleterious effect. Keeping to the same wording during testing results in a 50% better performance. Concerning whether the initial teaching stimuli should be constant or varied across trials, Carnine (1980b) found that consistency worked best in teaching preschoolers to discriminate angles of 90 degrees or more. Variations in the teaching stimuli required three times as many trials for learning than nonvaried stimuli. If pairs of S+ and S− examples are used in training, they should contain the same irrelevant stimuli and differ only on the relevant concept feature. Carnine (1980a) found that minimal-pair differences produced the best transfer in preschoolers who were taught *on* (called "flot"); the greater the number of irrelevant stimuli contained within S+ and S− pairs, the worse the transfer.

Stimulus conversion procedures offer great promise for teaching the basic vocabulary of single-dimensional concepts found in many language, academic, and vocational programs because they focus the learner's attention immediately on the relevant concept feature. Taking the lead from Carnine's (1980b) findings that dynamic presentations (of movable stimuli) were more effective than static presentations (nonmovable pairs of stimuli on cards), Gersten, White, Falco, and Carnine (1982) extended the efficacy of dynamic presentations for teaching *diagonal* to mildly and moderately handicapped young children in special education classes. These presentations were also successful for teaching *slanted* to severely handicapped adults in a work-activity center. Using TV displays for presenting the concepts *parallel* and *diameter*, Weinheimer and Weisberg (1987) found that educably mentally retarded (EMR) third graders trained by continuous conversion procedures did as well as chronological age-matched nonhandicapped students trained by noncontinuous procedures (stimuli removed from view between trials), and they reached criterion in half as many trials as handicapped peers trained by noncontinuous conversions. Sims (1984) taught the concept *longer than* (called "protraction") and found that 100% of nonhandicapped kindergartners learned through continuous conversions, whereas only 10% learned through noncontinuous stimulus conversions.

Handicapped learners will often form an interpretation of an object characteristic that is different from the one intended by the teacher. Although these misconceptions show up during tests of generalization, when novel S+ and S− examples are presented, they can be traced to faulty stimulus programming practices that are present during training (Engelmann & Carnine, 1982; Horner, Bellamy, & Colvin, 1984). One kind of generalization error, called a "misrule" (Engelmann & Carnine, 1982), occurs when irrelevant stimuli are always or sometimes associated with S+ but not with S−. Under these conditions, generalization stimuli containing the irrelevant features will often be selected incorrectly as instances of the concept features (Carnine, 1980a). For instance, by inadvertently training handicapped individuals to cross a street "independently" after another person begins to cross (whose actions serve as irrelevant stimuli), these individuals could easily learn a misrule about crossing and ignore relevant traffic signs (Horner *et al.*, 1984). Misrules can be minimized or eliminated if the same irrelevant stimuli are programmed in both S+ and S− presentations, either when they appear together or sequentially.

A second error appears when a novel S− is readily accepted as an instance of the positive concept feature. The phenomenon is called *overgeneralization*, and it is due to the absence of S− examples during discrimination training or the selection of the wrong kind. Overgeneralizing is likely when no S− examples are used in training (Carnine, 1980b; Williams & Carnine, 1981); or when S− examples are used, they result in easy discriminations that leave the learner unprepared for the difficult discriminations during the generalization tests. The latter circumstance prevailed when handicapped adults were taught to select and reject target grocery items (Horner, Albin, & Ralph, 1986). Training with S+ required the selection of grocery items that matched a photograph of that item. Training with S− required the rejection of an item that was not in the photo. Use of S− as the training stimuli that were maximally different from S+ (bottle of Heinz Ketchup vs. can of Star Kist Tuna) led to incorrect acceptance of novel S− items: for example, Carnation Tuna was selected as a purchasable item when and S+ picture of Star Kist Tuna was shown. However, use of minimally different S− items in training (can of Nine-Lives Cat Food vs. Star Kist Tuna) resulted in appropriate rejection of novel S− items. Although training with minimally different pairs can result in more errors during early acquisition, the increased precision during generalization is well worth the effort (Horner *et al.*, 1986).

A third error occurs when a novel S+ is rejected as an instance of the positive concept feature. The phenomenon, known as *undergeneralization*, occurs when the range of S+ values is not sufficiently sampled. Selecting an S+ training set limited to land vehicles (truck, bus, motorcycle) in order to teach the concept *vehicles* will likely result in the rejection of some novel S+ objects (airplane, boat) during a generalization test. Restricting the S+ range during academic training often occurs when practice is given on a limited range of problems (e.g., using only fractions with numerators consisting of two digits and denominators of 100 as the basis for training decimal conversions), and students are then expected to generalize to new, but related conversion problems (e.g., doing conversions with untrained single- and triple-digit numerators) (Carnine, 1980a). Selecting a representative set of positive examples is critical for teaching the general case. According to Becker (1986), a general case has been taught when after teaching some members of a set, the student responds correctly to any member.

TEACHING VOCABULARY WITH SYNONYMS AND DEFINITIONS

If one word is known, it can be used as a synonym to describe the meaning of a new, unknown word. According to Carnine and Silbert (1979), the major instructional steps are: (1) presenting the synonym ("another word for *over* is *above*"); (2) testing for understanding by presenting positive and negative examples (positioning a stimulus in various spatial locations and asking questions about *above*); and (3) reviewing the new word in a context of familiar and related concept words (asking questions about *above*, *over*, and *under*). The same sequence can be applied to teaching terms related to subtraction. First, if *minus* was previously learned through presentations of minus equations, then *subtraction* could be taught as a synonym ("subtraction means minus"). Second, several equations could be presented ($4 - 2, 5 + 3, 5 - 3, 6 + 1$) and the same question asked of each ("Do we subtract in this problem?"). Third, the new word would be reviewed within a related set. If *add* was previously taught as a synonym for *plus*, then questions about both terms would be asked, "What does subtract (add) tell us to do?" In a similar vein, the words *sell, lose,* and *give away* could be taught as synonyms for *minus* or *subtract.*

Definitions can be used to build vocabulary when learners know the words in the definition and when the concept is too complicated to be explained by a synonym. There are usually three steps to follow. First, the teacher constructs a definition, preferably by specifying a small class to which the word belongs and by telling how the word differs from other class members as in, "An exit is a door that leads out of a building." Second, positive and negative examples are presented to test understanding. Pictures of doors of a closet, movie theater, restaurant, and restroom are shown, and the learner is asked if each door is an exit, followed by a request for justification ("How do you know?"). Third, the new word is reviewed along with other previously taught definitions. The definition should be constructed in a way that is understandable to students rather than being technically correct. Defining a parallelogram as, "a rectangle that has two slanted sides" is a functional and adequate description for the instructionally naive even if it might meet with some disapproval on technical aspects.

Given that the teaching of comprehension in classrooms is done infrequently (Durkin, 1978–1979), there is an urgent need for a compendium of core vocabulary terms whose meanings are stated as synonyms or definitions and whose supportive positive and negative examples are communicated in a precise and useful manner for the instructionally naive.

TEACHING RELATIONSHIPS AND OTHER FORMS

Basic concepts can be combined by relating one empirical fact to another one so that the learner, when given one fact, can make an inference about the other one. Consider this two-part empirical relationship, "the heavier the car, the more gas it will use." Taught this relationship and presented two cars of different weights, the learner can predict that the heavier one will use more gas without the need to observe or measure the gas consumption. There are innumerable scientific facts and logical-based principles that have this same two-part structure and thus imply the same teaching sequence (Engelmann & Carnine, 1982). Many such facts are inherent in daily living and need to be taught. The food-pricing relationship of "heavier chicken costs more money" is one, as are the scores of facts dealing with the health and well-being of the individual (e.g., "smoking more cigarettes makes it harder to breathe"). Woodward, Carnine, and Gersten (1988) developed a computer simulation of the health profiles of real-life characters. Their program separately presented and integrated many facts dealing with nutrition, exercise, smoking, drinking, and stress management. Mildly handicapped high school students who were taught the simulation program recalled more facts than control students taught by reading about the facts (78% vs. 56% correct recall).

Another way to develop relationships is through transformations, as in the conversions of decimals into percentages, singular nouns into plural forms, standard time into digital time, and in the hundreds of other ways symbolic material is manipulated. Baer and Guess (1973) taught severely mentally retarded children how to convert a verbal description of an action shown in a picture into a noun suffix as in, "This man writes": "He is _____." Noun suffixes learned during training generalized to nontrained descriptions of verbs. H. B. Clark and Sherman (1975) presented examples of pronoun-verb-noun statements ("He is a baker") to EMRs who were taught to convert them into the past tense by saying, "Yesterday, he baked," in response to the generative transformational question, "What did he do yesterday?" On other occasions, the training examples were converted into the future tense or into the past tense. Not only did verb-transformation training substantially improve statements made during training, but generative answers to questions about nontrained examples also occurred. These findings imply that if a system for relating changes in one set of examples to changes in a corresponding set of responses is provided, generalizations are possible because all examples come under the control of the same transformation principle.

Major Instructional Variables

The three instructional variables that are essential for a successful program are: (1) organization of instruction and allotment of teaching time; (2) program design; and (3) teacher presentation procedures. All three must be present. A well-designed program and an effective teacher will not produce appreciable gains if instructional time is limited. Similarly, that same program with adequate instructional time will not be successful if the teacher is unskilled. Finally, a skilled teacher with adequate time will have limited success if the program is poorly designed.

Organization of Instruction

A hallmark of the mastery learning approach (Bloom, 1976) is that complex learning units can be mastered by 90% of learners if they are given adequate time and instruction to master the basic subskills. The difference in learning rate between the fastest and slowest learners is likely to be greatest on the first unit of a series of related tasks, but that difference shrinks over the remaining learning units if extra time and help are given to those who need it.

More recently, investigators (Englert & Thomas, 1982; Stevens & Rosenshine, 1981) have found a pattern of classroom practices that can lead to better academic outcomes with handicapped students. These classroom management procedures involve frequent testing, placing students in appropriate instructional groups, and organizing instruction in the classroom and throughout the school to ensure effective use of resources and time. Making more effective use of classroom time should translate into increased learner opportunity to make more active and appropriate academic responses.

Weisberg, Sims, and Weinheimer (1983) identified 14 areas for enhancing overall classroom efficiency. Some of these included reducing the number of interfering nonacademic routines (such as transitional activities), using instructionally "dead time" for oral speed-drills on the components of academic routines, grouping students by performance levels rather than by diagnostic labels, coordinating efforts between regular and remedial teachers so that the same instructional strategies and skills are emphasized, providing academically relevant seatwork during homeroom time, and having parents and responsible volunteers assist in academic endeavors, such as listening to students read, evaluating spelling performance, and firming up counting activities. Detailed examples for maximizing instructional time and minimizing extraneous activities can be found in Paine, Radicchi, Rosellini, Deutchman, and Darch (1983). Orelove (1982) has provided general guidelines for developing classroom schedules for severely handicapped students.

Aspects of Program Design

Inappropriate selection and organization of the teaching examples within a program, coupled with a complicated instructional vocabulary, can contribute a sizable amount to the confusion and ultimate struggles that low-performing students exhibit. Given the current state of knowledge and technological advances in the principles of programming, it is alarming that so many commercial programs and curricular materials are designed in a way to induce learning failures (see Beck & McCaslin, 1978; Engelmann, 1982). Described below are several principles that on the surface, make good sense and yet are poorly utilized by many professionals who have the responsibility to design academic programs.

Continuous Teaching of Explicit Strategies

When possible, students should be taught to work a broad set of related tasks or problems using a consistent multistep procedure instead of requiring them to memorize each discrete task. Often, students see the operations for one kind of problem demonstrated but are rarely provided step-by-step instruction in how to apply the steps to other related problems. In beginning addition, when symbols like $4 + 2 = \square$ are provided, pictures of objects or counters are written under the 4 and 2. The teacher counts and "joins" the two groups and then asks, "How many in all?" Note that the students can do the problem without ever attending to the number symbols; they need only count the objects. The difficulty occurs when problems consisting only of numbers are given. It is the experience of Silbert, Carnine, and Stein (1981) that, unless taught, low-performing students will not draw objects for symbols and count them. Similarly, students are commonly taught the main idea of a written passage and given examples in which the main idea is always expressed by the first sentence. When given another passage that contains no sentence that expresses the main idea, many students will continue to choose the first sentence (Engelmann, 1982).

Frequently, strategies are developed out of well-formulated academic objectives that apply to many situations. However, arbitrarily defined objectives can often prevent or interfere with the use of highly useful strategic approaches to teaching. The familiar but restricted first-grade objective, "shall identify and name the 12-hour positions of a clock, such as 1 o'clock, 2 o'clock, and so forth," often translates into a series of rote-memory operations that will have little application to learning other time positions. There is a program (Hofmeister, Atkinson, & Hofmeister, 1975) that takes a generalizable time-telling approach and does not begin with the o'clock positions. Instead, counting minutes (in multiples of five) for the big hand and determining the hour for the little hand are initially taught, making it possible to learn a large range of times. If the o'clock times are an imposed beginning objective, teachers might inadvertently opt for nonstrategic teaching and rote learning instead of a more generalizable strategy.

A perfectly adequate strategy will never get off the ground if it is first applied to a large mix of irregular examples. About 80% of English words are phonetically regular (in which the most common sounds for letters are pronounced) or approach regularity. Initially, a strategy of sounding out words should be applied to a sequence of regular words followed by intermittent presentation of irregular words. When this is done, children with IQs of 70 can be taught generalizable word-attack skills (Gersten, Becker, Heiry, & White, 1984). However, the strategy will fail if the introductory words come from popular basal-reader series or the first 40 words of the well-known Dolch (1936) sight wordlist because half the words from these sources are irregular (Carnine & Silbert, 1979; Weisberg *et al.*, 1983).

Sequencing of Skills

Sequencing involves determining the order for introducing new information and strategies. Three sequencing guidelines are to (1) teach preskills prior to the introduction of strategies that require their application; (2) teach easier skills before more difficult ones; and (3) separate over time strategies and information that are easily confused with each other (Carnine & Silbert, 1979; Engelmann & Carnine, 1982). Within any content area, the problem types causing the most difficulty are generally those with lots of steps in the strategy and those with many similar to other strategies (Silbert *et al.*, 1981).

The chances of a multistep instructional routine being run smoothly and with accuracy are probably greater if each of the component steps or preskills is introduced separately, is reviewed, and then is integrated with other skills before the entire strategy is presented (Engelmann & Carnine, 1982). Moreover, the wording used in teaching the preskills should be as close as possible to that used in the consolidated routine. By not preteaching the preskills and not using consistent wording, the routine can become unduly long, require many difficult discriminations, and thus result in a high error rate and learner resistance (Engelmann & Carnine, 1982).

The more difficult items are those that look alike (*b-d*, 6-9, then-them, a square and rectangle, similar looking labels for cans of green vegetables) and/or those whose names sound alike, such as similar sounding short vowel sounds (*e-i*), consonants (*f-v*), and words (four-five, triangle-rectangle). Sometimes, the difficulty is caused because arbitrarily arranged sequences, like the alphabet, govern the sequencing of information. The first four lowercase letters have high visual similarity (*a, b, c, d*), and two letters (*b-d*) contain both visual and auditory similarity. Concepts can be made easier if subtypes of academic content (like uppercase and lowercase letters) are first identified, and examples from regular subtypes (*Oo, Pp, Ss*) are taught before irregular subtypes (*Aa, Gg, Dd*). The same can be done for sequencing the teen numerals, with regularity based on how the second digit is read; thus, 14, 16, 17, 18, 19 before 11, 12, 13, and 15 (Engelmann & Carnine, 1982). Note that students can still learn to rote count and say the alphabet even though the sequence for identifying printed numerals and letters is changed.

One way to lessen difficulty is to separate in time items that are similar in sound and/or appearance. In some programs, many lessons are appropriately interposed between similar items like *b* and *d* and *m* and *n*. In others, highly similar and very difficult items appear inappropriately one after another, such as teaching the sounds for the five short vowel sounds followed by the five long vowel sounds. At least two or more nonsimilar members should come between the similar ones. Carnine (1976b) contrasted two separation orders for teaching the difficult *e-i* sound discrimination: Preschoolers learned a similar separated order (*e c m u s i*) in 178 trials and a similar together order (*e i u c m s*) in 293 trials.

An easy-to-hard progression can contribute to learner success during the easy discrimination and may lead to the gradual development of attention to important stimulus features that are necessary for the hard discrimination (Carnine, 1980c). The benefits of this progression are most apparent when there is some logical or empirical basis for ordering difficulty level and there is a programmed sequence for teaching the difficult discriminations. However, when a reliable basis for responding is not taught, providing only easy discriminations of a concept early may be deleterious and, as explained earlier, can lead to concept overgeneralizations.

Providing Discrimination Practice and Cumulative Review

Adequate time must be spent reviewing concepts and operations so low-performing students can master and retain them. Engelmann's (1982) analysis of how basal readers teach the main idea revealed that an average of 62 days intervened between two teaching examples of that concept. Serious delays in reviewing material have been identified in programs that teach spelling (Collins, 1983), vocabulary (Carnine & Silbert, 1979), and fractions (Kelly, Carnine, Gersten, & Grossen, 1986).

It is impossible to specify an exact number of practice trials appropriate to all students and for all tasks. Carnine's (1977) data on word-recognition training suggest that it is best to give massed practice until some performance standard is reached rather than to give a fixed number of trials to all students. In general, the more stringent the performance criterion, the better the retention of material (Carlson & Minke, 1975). Criterion performance should be set higher for low performers, especially if the new material is to be integrated with other information or skills. The information provided in the answer and the number of steps in a task will qualify the criteria for mastery and the amount of practice needed; tasks that involve labeling (where guessing is less likely) or a few steps will require less rigorous criteria than "yes or no" answers or tasks with many steps.

Only tasks that can be done through application of previously taught strategies should be practiced. If a variety of problem types have been taught, they should be presented together in a mixed set to teach students to discriminate the application of previously taught strategies (Engelmann & Carnine, 1982; Vargas, 1984). Given words of a particular type to read on a given day (short *a* vowel words on one day, short *i* words on another day, and short *e* on another), reading during that day may be perfectly adequate. This does not prove that the short *e* and short *i* words can be discriminated, and, in all likelihood, performance will suffer when words with different vowel sounds appear together.

An effective review process is to introduce and practice new items in a context of previously taught, related materials. Once the new item is mastered, additional items are added to the set one at a time, and both the new and the old are reviewed cumulatively (Becker, Engelmann, & Thomas, 1975). When moderately and severely mentally retarded preschoolers were taught functional words, Fink and Brice-Gray (1979) found that reviewing the words cumulatively produced faster acquisition than reviewing then pairwise (173 vs. 244 trials for mastery) and better recall (90% vs. 48%). Cumulative review procedures have been successfully applied to teaching letter–sound correspondences (Carnine, 1976b), alphabet letters and colors (Kincaid, Weisberg, & Sims, 1981), and spelling (Neef, Iwata, & Page, 1980). Recall is strong after cumulative review, probably because the interfering effects of other interpolated material are minimized, which is otherwise not possible when items are separately reviewed. Cumulative review further allows multifeature concepts to be learned incrementally while new members, containing some but not all of these features, are added to the set of related concepts (Becker, 1986). Students may also prefer this review process because of the opportunity to receive reinforcement for redoing familiar items while learning new and, perhaps, difficult items (Neef *et al.*, 1980).

As set size gets larger, it is time consuming and logistically difficult to review all members together. Engelmann and Carnine (1982) suggested selective review, using six to eight items. The reviewed items should (1) tend to have high error rates, (2) be those recently introduced, (3) be those not recently reviewed, and (4) be highly similar to the newest member. Although a new item should be presented initially with previously trained items that are maximally dissimilar to it, once mastered, the new item should be reviewed increasingly among items similar to it. Thus, there should be two formats in an instructional program: (1) introductory tasks in which item discrimination is relatively easy, and (2) review tasks in which harder discriminations can be expected.

Teacher Presentation Procedures

In general, early primary-grade teachers must be proficient in a variety of teacher-directed presentation procedures that maintain student participation in oral question and answer exchanges during small group or individualized instruction. Intermediate- and secondary-grade teachers must be more skilled in managing students who are working independently by monitoring written answers to worksheet exercises. In both cases, teachers must convey warmth and support, yet demand high-quality academic work (Rosenshine, 1983).

Teaching procedures may be divided into two major areas (Silbert et al., 1981). The first considers those teacher behaviors that maintain a high level of student attentiveness and participation during group instruction. The second considers those behaviors that ensure student mastery of the skills being taught. These include monitoring, correcting, and diagnosing student errors.

Securing and Maintaining Attention

Students are more attentive to a lively, fast-paced presentation that evokes a great deal of active and frequent responding. Asking lots of questions that are brief, concise, and at a low cognitive level provides more opportunities for success and is related to achievement in basic skills (Rosenshine, 1983). Carnine (1976a) found that a faster-paced presentation (12 questions per minute) for teaching decoding skills was associated with a higher percentage of correct answers (80%) and more on-task behavior (90%) than a slower-paced presentation (5 questions per minute), in which the corresponding values were 10% and 30%, respectively. Suggesting that the teaching pace be picked up, whenever possible, may appear illogical when applied to low-IQ individuals. These individuals are slower in thinking, so the pacing, it is claimed, should match that slowness. However, part of the problem is that distractibility is higher in slower-paced tasks, perhaps resulting in the teacher nagging at the nonattentive learner to get on-task. Of course, some tasks demand slower pacing, such as those that require the application of rules and the covert processing of information.

Teaching the learner to respond to clear-cut signals that indicate where to look and when to answer can improve student attention and the rate of group responding (Cowart, Carnine, & Becker, 1973). Signals also provide the extra time instructionally naive students need for framing an answer (Becker & Carnine, 1980). Attention to salient concept features is also facilitated through dynamic presentations (Gersten, White, Falco, & Carnine, 1982), through specific questions that prompt an answer about a feature (Koegel, Dunlap, Richman, & Dyer, 1981), and through shadowing techniques, such as circling part of a configuration while talking about that part.

Task-related attentional behaviors can be promoted further through a variety of consequent events. Prescriptions for establishing individual and group reinforcement contingencies that can promote time-on-task abound, and the interested reader is referred to Becker (1986) and to Paine et al. (1983). Worth noting is that although time-on-task appears to be a necessary condition for improvements in academic abilities, it is not a sufficient condition. For example, Carnine (1976a) reported that math-computation skills in primary-grade children did not get any better despite improved rates of attention to teacher-directed activities.

Monitoring, Correcting, and Diagnosing Errors

Monitoring student performance for accuracy and correcting errors appropriately were two practices that distinguished most a teacher's effectiveness in elevating student achievement (Gersten, Carnine, & Williams, 1982). In group situations, teachers need to watch the students' eyes to see if they are attending and watch their mouths and listen during oral responding. Often, errors can be anticipated and prevented. For example, during decoding, the vowel sound of CVC words is frequently misidentified by low performers. Having them identify the vowel before they sound out words can improve performance substantially (Fink, 1976). Precorrection procedures have further reduced errors in object identification tasks (Ausman & Gaddy, 1974), spelling (Greenwood, Delquadri, & Hall, 1984), and math problems (Lovitt & Curtiss, 1968).

Fink and Carnine (1975) showed the value of immediately correcting mistakes whenever they occur. The accuracy of answering math facts both in training and in posttests by preschoolers was about 50% higher during correction phases than during noncorrection phases. Moreover, students should attend to the feedback they receive. When students graphed worksheet errors, the number declined significantly compared to when they were simply told the number of errors (Fink & Carnine, 1975).

Not all mistakes are corrected the same way. Concept discrimination errors require the teacher to model the missed positive and/or negative example, test for the missed example, back up several examples, and then retest on all preceding examples including the missed one. Labeling errors requires a three-step procedure of (1) modeling the correct response, (2) providing practice with other examples using an alternation pattern, and (3) testing after some delay. For example, if a student misidentifies 5 as 3, the teacher would first model the correct answer ("this is 5"). Then, if other familiar numerals in the task were 4, 2, and 7, the teacher would alternate between them and 5, making sure to increase the number of familiar items between any two occasions of the mislabeled item. Thus, 5, 7, 5, 2, 4, 5, 2, 7, 4, 5, is an acceptable alternation pattern. Delayed testing is done later, possibly after another task. Alternation and delayed testing are excellent procedures for building long-term recall. Factural errors (e.g., "What does the big hand of the clock tell about?") require a model-test procedure and, if necessary, a delayed test.

In correcting errors during a multistep problem-solving task or for a complex application, process feedback is necessary. Whenever possible, the teacher should prompt the learner to use the previously taught strategy or rule that generates the answer or solution rather than to furnish those answers directly. Carnine (1980d) found that an effective sounding-out strategy for decoding words was abandoned by beginning readers when the teacher provided whole-word (nonstrategic) answers to incorrect answers. The long-er nonstrategic correction procedures were in force, the greater were the number of errors, and the harder it was to reinstate the original sounding-out routine.

To correct errors that arise from an improper or poorly coordinated string of responses, as might occur during statement repetition, counting, or hand-writing, the teacher should model the sequence, lead or run through the sequence with the student (or physically guide them) until they can make all responses independently, and then test them. Much practice is necessary during the leading phase, and it may e necessary to use shaping and chaining procedures during which only a few steps are firmed at a time.

Diagnosis of errors involves the determination of their source, and re-mediation involves the reteaching of the skill based on the diagnosis (Arter & Jenkins, 1979). Remediation is a more long-term affair than correcting be-cause, in the latter condition, the teacher knows exactly what question or request the student missed and thus can rectify the error immediately. Errors diagnosed because of poor motivation can be remediated through a change in reinforcement contingencies. Skill-deficit errors can be diagnosed by examin-ing worksheets and by observing and asking students how they worked a problem (Vargas, 1984). Elaborations of these remedies are reported in En-gelmann and Carnine (1982) and in Haring and Bateman (1977).

READING

According to Browder and Snell (1987), one of four tactics can be taken when handicapped individuals need to read printed materials in various set-tings. The first approach has a teacher read for the individual; thus, no train-ing is given. The second approach also bypasses reading instruction but has a designed prosthesis that substitutes for reading words. For example, instead of teaching recipe reading, pictures show the sequence for meal preparation and cooking (Robinson-Wilson, 1977). The third approach teaches a limited set of words for a special activity, as when the words on road signs or those on a laundry machine form the core. The fourth approach attempts to teach generative reading, enabling a very large set of words to be acquired that cuts across different activities. This procedure requires a large investment of in-structional time, but the individual ends up with greater self-sufficiency.

The second approach, using instructional booklets of pictures and log-ographic symbols to communicate meaning otherwise denoted by words, is fast becoming an accepted way of enabling prereading, nonverbal, and illite-rate individuals to function in community settings (e.g., Horner et al., 1986) and participate in home-living activities like cooking and meal preparation (Johnson & Cuvo, 1981; Robinson-Wilson, 1977). This approach has its roots in graphic communication systems (Clark, 1984), and the various forms will not be reviewed here. Worth mentioning, however, is that the recognition of pictographic symbols was found to be more readily acquired, maintained, and generalized to daily situations by severely handicapped, nonverbal adolescents than the more noniconic, concept-based Blissymbols (Hurlburt, Iwata, & Green, 1982).

Teaching Word Recognition

The meaning–emphasis approach, which seeks to develop instant whole-word recognition, is the one most often used for nonhandicapped school children (Carnine & Silbert, 1979) and, judging from the research literature, it is probably the dominant method for teaching reading to handicapped individuals of all ages. Code emphasis or phonic programs constitute another approach. Here, reading is seen as learning a printed code to match the words in the spoken language. The DISTAR (Direct Instruction Systems for Teaching and Remediation) program (Engelmann & Bruner, 1983) is a synthetic phonics program frequently used with handicapped individuals (Gersten & Maggs, 1982), though it is appropriate for all beginning readers (Becker, 1986; Weisberg, 1988). The differences between meaning- and code-emphasis programs are most pronounced in the beginning stages of reading. It is at this time when a decision must be made whether to begin with smaller units consisting of sounds from which words are derived, or to begin with the larger, whole-word unit followed, perhaps, by learning the sound elements within the word (Chall, 1983).

Reading Procedures

Figure 2 shows the two-part sequence used in the DISTAR program for teaching beginning word recognition. The teacher initially models each of the steps for segmenting and blending words, but the goal is to have the students do by themselves all the steps for decoding words. Eventually, they learn to

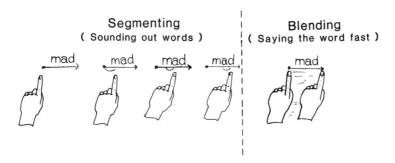

FIGURE 2. Segmenting and blending words in the DISTAR reading program. During segmenting, the individual (teacher or student) begins by touching the ball to the left and then loops from letter to letter, saying each sound without pausing between them. The continuous sounds (*m* and *a*) are said for 2 seconds early in training and later for 1 second. The stop sounds (*d*) are said for an instant. During blending, the individual touches the ball and slashes under the entire word, saying the word at its spoken rate—mad!

sound out words subvocally, and, with much practice, they also learn formats that teach sight reading (Carnine & Silbert, 1979).

Bracey, Maggs, and Morath (1975) found that children with IQs of 30 to 40, within 41 hours of intensive DISTAR instruction, could learn 22 sounds, decode 200 words, and had the requisite skills to decode many nontrained words containing the taught sounds. Nonreading moderately mentally retarded preadolescents receiving 30-minute lessons daily of DISTAR for $3\frac{1}{2}$ years, which was preceded and accompanied by language training, came to read at an entering third-grade level (Booth, Hewitt, Jenkins, & Maggs, 1979). The DISTAR approach has also engendered solid decoding skills in large numbers of poverty-level children both in preschool (Engelmann, 1970; Weisberg, 1988) and in the elementary grades (Becker, Engelmann, Carnine, & Maggs, 1982) as well as in learning-disabled children (Lloyd, Epstein, & Cullinan, 1981) and in middle-class, advantaged children (Becker, 1986).

Whole-word teaching procedures for mentally handicapped individuals have taken several forms. In time-delay training, a word is initially modeled or prompted, then the teacher gradually increases the time between successive re-presentations of the word until the student can identify it without any help (Browder, Hines, McCarthy, & Fees, 1984). In picture fading, a word is associated with a picture that is graphically faded, either by making it lighter or by removing its components until only the word remains (Dorry & Zeaman, 1973). In matching-to-sample tasks, as in the Edmark reading program (1984), students point to a target word initially in the presence of dissimilar distractor stimuli, and later in a context in which the distractors increasingly resemble the target configuration. In Sidman's (1971) cross-modality matching, individuals learn whole words through an indirect route that is based on equivalence training: One of several pictures and printed words are separately matched to a common dictated word, and, as a result of these trained equivalences, the word is correctly matched to its picture referent even though the word-picture equivalence was never trained (Sidman, Cresson, & Wilson-Morris, 1974). Sometimes, untrained oral reading has also emerged (Sidman et al., 1974). Finally, there are look-say or sight methods in which words are placed on flash cards for handicapped students to read (Feinberg, 1975; Goldberg & Rooke, 1967).

Picture-Prompting Procedures

The picture-prompting/picture-fading technique deserves special consideration because of its questionable value for building durable reading skills, despite its frequent use with low performers (Samuels, 1970; Weisberg, Packer, & Weisberg, 1981). Given a picture–word pair, the picture will dominate in securing instant attention because it requires lower cognitive effort and is a more compelling and familiar stimulus than a printed word (Samuels, 1970). Research shows that kindergarten children have overwhelmingly chosen the picture over the word as the "reading" response (Duell, 1968), suggesting that when the word is presented alone, students will fail to identify it from among other words. Duell and Anderson (cited in Duell, 1968) attempted to teach color words to nonhandicapped kindergarteners by having the actual colors appear on the letters within each word. Eventually, the color prompts were removed, and all the words came to be printed in black. "Reading" was perfect as long as the color referent remained, but upon its removal, the words were inconsistently identified. Not surprisingly, many words were called "black."

To get around the fact that, normally, the controlling structural features of referents and words are different, Miller and Miller (1968) modified conventional words to make them resemble the referent or concept (e.g., the word *candy* appeared in striped, peppermint-type lettering or the word *jump* appeared to make jumping movements). Through contiguous pairings of iconic accentuated words with their conventional printing, teenagers (mean IQ of 55) subsequently read the conventional word better than in a nonaccentuated training condition. However, in an independent word-discrimination task in which the learner had to point to the target word from among others, accentuated training was not superior to nonaccentuated training.

Aside from the limited transfer from picture to word recognition, there are concerns about the absolute levels of reading performance once the picture is removed. During immediate tests of recall, word identification has been close to 100% after the last picture–word trial (Dorry & Zeaman, 1973; Walsh & Lamberts, 1979). Unfortunately, during delayed recall tests as short as one day, performance plummeted to 50% for children with IQs between 23 and 55 (Dorry & Zeaman, 1973) and to less than 1% for teenagers with a mean IQ of 44 (Walsh & Lamberts, 1979). These results are particularly discouraging because the words trained have been highly dissimilar, easy to discriminate nouns (e.g., *apple, bell, horse, dog, elephant*), and the participants received ample practice during the picture-fading phase. It is also the case that since only nouns, some adjectives, and some verbs can be represented pictorially, these restrictions will leave the reader with a limited vocabulary. Those words not easily represented include noncontent words (prepositions, adverbs, conjunctions, nominatives, auxiliary verbs) as well as those that refer to tense (*run, ran, running*) and number (*none, some, all*). Without being able to read the noncontent words, most reading becomes meaningless. Finally, based on the story-reading tendencies of nonhandicapped children (Samuels, 1970), it is the poorer readers who become dependent upon looking at the illustration. These "picture readers" continually shift their gaze from the text to the picture, and are thus most distracted by them.

The upshot is that a spurious kind of reading can be established through picture prompting, but it will be limited to a rebuslike system having only specialized use. To expect that reading printed words will automatically ensue when the prompts are removed ignores the research literature and, worse yet, it fails to consider the development of erroneous reading habits and the personal hardships encountered by the beginning student. If anything, the literature suggests that word recognition is better when no pictures are used than when they are (Harzem, Lee, & Miles, 1976; Samuels, 1970; Walsh & Lamberts, 1979).

Word Selection

In code programs, words containing the most common sound for a letter or letter combination should be taught earlier than words containing the minor sound. For example, the sound for *c* is pronounced "k" in about 80% of the words and in the remaining as "s." Other things being equal, words such as *cot, lock, corn, can,* and *cake* should occur earlier than *cent, cereal,* and *city.* Not to do so could discourage a naive reader from learning about phonetic regularity. Other word-selection considerations for phonic programs like DISTAR are word type (e.g., CVC words before CCVC words), whether the initial sound is a continuous versus a stop sound (e.g., *mit, fan, sit* are easier to decode than *kit, tan,* and *bid*), location of a consonant blend—with blends at the end of words presented before blends at the beginning (*milk* and *nest* are generally easier than *frog* and *stop*)—word length (shorter words are easier to sound out than longer ones), and word familiarity (*mud, jump* before *mid* and *lump*). Elaboration of these and other variables related to word sequence can be found in Carnine and Silbert (1979).

Popular appeal and utility are usually the chief concerns for initial word selection in whole-word, meaning-emphasis programs. Thus, should circumstances dictate mastery of a related set of words, say those for colors, numerals, tools (in a vocational setting), or foods (for shopping), they would probably be taught together as whole words without regard to the phonic programming guidelines mentioned above. As long as the related word set is kept small and used in a restricted setting, whole-word teaching is an acceptable approach, though, at times, certain word pairs (*blue-brown, four-five, beans-beets*) will likely be confused. However, should the goal be broader based, such as mastering the most frequently occurring words from Grades 1 to 3 (Dolch, 1936) or the 200 most essential survival words (Wilson, 1963), then problems are likely to result because whole-word training does not lead to generative reading.

Generative Reading

By first teaching the common sounds for letters, together with a strategy for segmenting and blending sounds, generalized decoding can be developed in mentally retarded populations (Booth *et al.*, 1979). Again, this is possible only if the order of sound and word introduction is controlled in the beginning stages of reading. By the time 10 sounds have been mastered, there is the potential for reading 720 three-sound words, 4,320 four-sound words, and 21,600 five-sound words (Becker *et al.*, 1975). Not all will be real words, but the reader is nevertheless furnished with consistent word-attack skills. After 40 sounds, a basis for reading a large percentage of the English language has been established. Irregularities still have to be taught, but the reader is at least afforded the skills to attack any new word.

Whole-word teaching is unlikely to produce generative reading (Becker, 1986; Carnine, 1977). Being able to sight-read *yellow* and *man* is not helpful in decoding words, such as *yesterday, red, mad,* and *look.* One means to help naive readers sight-read and memorize new words is to program highly dissimiliar words. Such programming, however, can give the false impression that reading is progressing smoothly until new words similar to the old ones are increasingly presented, as they must be fore the development of a reading vocabulary. It is then that whole-word reading breaks down for the low performer. Weisberg (1988) reported that it is the "little" words that are particularly troublesome: *in-on, then-them, not-no, stop-spot, and-any, ran-run.* Analyzing the word errors of EMR teenagers (mean IQ of 63) trained by whole-word procedure, Mason (1978) found that they guessed at words, discounted letter–sound relationships, and chose, instead, short and common word patterns. Specifically, they turned unfamiliar words into familiar words (*skimp* into *ship, coax* into *coat*), read only a common shorter word embedded within an uncommon word (*bus* for *bush, yes* for *yeast*), made more errors on the end than on the beginning of a word (*seem* for *seep*), and frequently misread consonant clusters (*much* for *mush*).

Meaning-emphasis approaches use a combination of instructional procedures for drawing attention to the word: word length, word configuration, initial and ending letters, and context and picture cues. Such a multifaceted cue approach can lead to rather complex teacher explanations that leave the naive reader utterly confused (Carnine & Silbert, 1979). In addition, when they fail to read a word, a picture or context clue might be given. If that fails, they are simply told the word. This correction is often inappropriate because it may foster the attitude that, "if you don't get the word, the teacher will tell it to you." Thus, students are guaranteed to get the word through guessing which, after a while, becomes the predominant reading strategy (Weisberg, 1988). Obviously, what these beginning students need is a simpler, more dependable word-attack strategy that applies to all words.

Rate of Learning

The rate at which new words are introduced into such code programs as DISTAR is low at first, because the early lessons are spent in teaching and integrating the component skills for a decoding strategy. With continued training, the rate should accelerate positively as more sounds are presented and decoding performances are firmed. By Lesson 40 of DISTAR Reading, only 8 new words are taught, but by Lessons 80, 120, and 160, the numbers are, respectively, 49, 62, and 118. Meaning-emphasis programs can present a higher rate in the beginning, particularly if word dissimilarity is high, but the rate is not likely to accelerate and may even falter because word similarity is being increased and decoding strategies are not being taught. This means that program impact is best evaluated after long-term instruction. That program directors and decision makers need to know both the kind of behaviors promoted by a program as well as the time frame necessary for their development cannot be overemphasized, because one might be tempted to discontinue DISTAR reading instruction if it is observed in its early stages (Weisberg, 1988).

Comparative Studies

Studies on the effects of different reading approaches with handicapped populations have been extremely limited. In a fairly comprehensive review of reading studies, Chall (1983) concluded that the benefits of a beginning code program held for all the IQ ranges she studied. By the end of Grade 3, slow learners taught explicit (or synthetic) phonics began to outperform those students who were taught by a meaning-emphasis program or by an indirect-phonics program, wherein students are expected to induce phonic generalizations. In the nationwide Follow-Through project evaluating poverty-level children from kindergarten to third grade, the program producing the best reading outcomes, with reading scores reaching the 41st percentile, was DISTAR, a direct synthetic-phonics program. Sponsors of other models generally used meaning-emphasis programs, and, on the average, the children read at the 20th percentile or lower (Becker *et al.*, 1982). Working with poverty-level preschoolers, Weisberg (1988) found a strong correlation between decoding and number of reading lessons completed that was independent of entry IQ. Although still in preschool, those who had two years of DISTAR read and comprehended text that was intended for a beginning second grade.

In one of the few comparative studies with mentally retarded persons, Apffel, Kelleher, Lilly, and Richardson (1975) used teacher-collected, criterion-referenced data to judge the reading progress of moderately mentally retarded preadolescents. About 65% of those in the DISTAR reading program were considered to have made good progress. Those taught by the Rebus program (Woodcock, 1967), in which words are paired with pictures, produced a good progress rate of only 26%. In a large-scale project by Vandever, Maggart, and Nasser (1976), over 100 EMR primary-grade children (mean IQ of 65) received word recognition training in either the Edmark, the Merrill (a psycholinguistic), or the Sullivan (code-emphasis) programs. On the first 150 words in each program, 50 were correctly read by the Edmark-trained students, and about 35 by those in the other programs after one school year. There were no differences on 15 words common to each program. The reading of 35 nontrained words was never higher than 10% for any program. Taken together, these findings led Vandever *et al.* (1976) to wonder whether the Edmark program was fostering relatively rapid initial word recognition at the expense of teaching generalized reading skills.

Teaching Reading Comprehension

The design of instruction for reading comprehension is exceedingly more difficult in scope and preparation than that involved in decoding. The programmer must consider three variables that affect comprehension: (1) the size of the content unit (phrases, sentences, paragraphs), (2) the sheer number and complexity of different skills involved, and (3) the knowledge base against which the reader evaluates a comprehension message. Learning deficiencies in any of these areas will lead to misunderstandings of textual material. The problem is compounded if decoding is poor and, consequently, words are not identified reliably or read fast enough. Slow decoding results in pauses that prevent recall of previously read material, and, ultimately, comprehension suffers (Gough, 1976). Increasing the reading rate can lead to gains in comprehension (Perfetti, 1977), but initial emphasis should be given to word accuracy rather than fluency (Carnine & Silbert, 1979).

Size of the Content Unit

Comprehension training should begin as soon as possible, even if it is initially limited to picture–word matching exercises. As passages get longer, matching phrases and, later, sentences to pictures and dictated descriptions should be added as comprehension exercises. In addition, literal questions should be orally asked throughout the reading lesson. To help students who, while reading, do not group words into phrases, organizational prompts could be employed, such as leaving extra space between the phrases within the sentence (Oaken, Weiner, & Cromer, 1971). To facilitate passage reading, advanced organizers that summarize upcoming content could be employed, and the low performer should be pretaught the meaning of special words. A number of deficits could interfere with the comprehension of larger units (e.g., phrasing errors, lack of expression, over- or underreliance on context). Although there are procedures to correct these deficiencies (Carnine & Silbert, 1979), they have not been fully implemented with the mentally retarded.

Skills for Comprehension

The type and number of comprehension skills required by the primary grades can become sizeable if they are based upon a listing of the separate skills that are needed for specific reading materials (Levin, 1971–1972). The current trend in comprehension training, however, is to teach multipurpose skills that can be applied from training with selected reading sources to a wide range of untrained sources (Jenkins, Stein, & Osborn, 1981). Some factors that qualify what skills are needed are the size and complexity of the reading unit, whether literal or inferential questions are asked, whether questions are asked before, during, and/or after each passage reading, whether the comprehension items are in oral or written form, and whether the passage calls for simplifying complex constructions. Sample formats for teaching beginning and more sophisticated skills are provided in Carnine and Silbert (1979).

There are two lines of research for studying comprehension skills in the mentally retarded. One evaluates whether the skills for functional reading, usually of a limited kind, can be created. Students are taught the words for concepts, such as size, color, and shape. They are then given passages that, when correctly read, result in verifiable environmental changes: "Put the little, blue square in the big box." Brown and Perlmutter (1971) taught direction-following at the sentence level to trainable mentally retarded (TMR) teenagers. Nine sentences, "The penny is _____ the box," were constructed and varied in meaning by the insertion of one of nine prepositions; for example, "on top of," "to the left of," "under," and so forth. The student had to re-position a penny in a nearby box so its location conformed to the meaning of the target sentence. That it took 60 hours to learn to read and understand the directions of all nine sentences is somewhat disconcerting, but it is probably due to the weak reading skills established through prior whole-word memo-rization training.

The second line of research seeks to establish multipurpose comprehen-sion skills through strategy training. For instance, Kameenui, Carnine, and Maggs (1980) attempted to directly teach mildly handicapped third to fifth graders two skills that were related to simplifying complex constructions. To teach the ability to understand passive-voice constructions ("Bill was teased by Jane"), a modeling procedure was used along with lots of "who" ques-tions ("Who did the teasing?" "Who got teased?"). The other skills involved learning how to break down a sentence containing a clause into two simple sentences. Thus, "Henry, who kissed Joan, ran home crying," was converted into "Henry kissed Joan" and "Henry ran home crying." These two com-prehension skills were successfully trained using both oral and written sen-tences and resulted in the gradual development of the ability to simplify sentences in untrained passages.

Language and Comprehension

Comprehension tasks frequently require verbal competencies and infor-mation about the world that many mentally retarded individuals lack. With-out having language skills for sequencing, summarizing, and making inferen-ces about content, these individuals will be at a loss in answering more complex comprehension questions. Thus, it is essential that a good language program accompany a reading program. Better yet, the two should be coordi-nated with the prerequisite skills that are important for reading, such as answering "who" questions or identifying pronoun antecedents, taught dur-ing language instruction.

Understanding concepts represented by words pervades every com-prehension task. Carroll (1971) estimated that vocabulary-concept knowledge constitutes 80% of comprehension. Currently, teachers do not provide sys-tematically the necessary vocabulary skills that students need; Durkin (1978–1979) found that fourth-grade teachers spend 1% of their reading time in comprehension instruction. In addition, many basal tests have serious design flaws that prevent clear understanding of concepts, and they often presume background knowledge beyond the experience of most children (Beck, McKeown, McCaslin, & Burkes, 1979). Although vocabulary can be taught through the methods cited earlier (e.g., modeling concepts, providing syn-onyms and definitions), one problem with vocabulary training is that it is not generative. Instead, each vocabulary word needs to be taught separately. To lessen the load, Becker (1977) has proposed that if core words are first identi-fied and taught, they can serve as the basis for defining other unknown but related words. If the basic and related vocabularies were taught prior to their appearance in reading material, teachers and students would benefit im-mensely.

MATHEMATICS AND RELATED INSTRUCTION

The four domains common to most mathematics curricula are: math concepts, math computations, math facts, and math problem-solving applications. Although these areas may appear initially as separate strands in a program, they will become increasingly interwoven as math sophistication and application are acquired. The interrelationships can be illustrated by discussing the component skills for money usage. Learning about coin value entails mastery of simple facts, such as "a nickel is worth 5 cents," and an understanding of the concepts of "worth" or "equal to." Learning to classify different coins according to their monetary value and to make comparative statements involves knowledge of concepts, such as most, least, and seriation. Counting coins of the same denomination requires use of multiplication computations as in skip counting by five for nickels. Problem-solving tasks, like coin summation problems, require bringing into play all of the previous concepts, facts, and computation skills as well as the integration of other math components. The same applies for more complex applications, as when one needs to learn to compute change during grocery shopping.

Math Concepts

Although there are a multitude of concepts that have found their way into math curricula, not all are necessary or relevant for many handicapped individuals. Browder and Snell (1987) doubted whether common elementary school concepts dealing with geometric shapes, set theory, and Roman numerals are essential to the mastery of computation skills and are significantly related to the daily living of these individuals. Some concepts are best taught through a well-formulated and logically sequenced language program. Teaching the understanding of various kinds of classification and class-inclusion concepts, which are essential for certain kinds of math-story problems, is one such language-reasoning domain. Other language-related concepts include learning about spatial relationships (e.g., *over*, *between*) directionality, movement, and opposites (like *open* vs. *closed* figures, *straight* vs. *curved* lines), all of which can be taught as basic language concepts. Typically, when math concepts appear in a math program, the expectation is that students already know them or will develop an immediate understanding. Because explicit procedures for teaching language-based concepts are not normally provided within math programs, instructionally naive students will lose out because of their deficiencies in the language of instruction.

Piaget (1953) has long argued that children should have intuitive understanding of several mathematical concepts before they are placed in a formal program. McClennen and Harrington (1982) claim that certain stage-based tendencies, such as the inability to take the viewpoint of another (namely, the teacher), can prevent egocentric children from being taught teacher-generated logical explanations. Similarly, given two rows of objects equal in number but not of the same length, preoperational children who can count will center on the most outstanding perceptual feature of one row, such as its length, rather than on the number of objects in each row. Although these tendencies are widespread, mildly retarded individuals can succeed at number and other conservation tasks when trained through rule-governed procedures (Hendler & Weisberg, 1988).

Frequently, attempts to develop conceptual foundations for mathematical skills introduce alternative problem-solving strategies for the same skill, and often the strategies are taught concurrently (Silbert et al., 1981). This situation is particularly true for many basal math programs. The assumption that students will better understand an algorithm by being exposed to multiple strategies is prevalent. According to Silbert et al. (1981), multiple strategies often confuse the instructionally naive and fragment the teaching time so that no strategy is mastered.

Computations

The procedures for teaching the computations for addition, subtraction, multiplication, and division are inventions; there is no right way to construct them. The powerful routines are those that are serviceable for a large range of problems. Based on the program-design principles of Engelmann and Carnine (1982), the following guidelines are offered for the development of computational skills: (1) the steps in a computation should consist of only those critical behaviors for problem solution; (2) every functional behavior must be overt, especially during the early stages of instruction; (3) corrective feedback should be provided at each step; (4) covert behaviors should systematically replace the overt behaviors until the entire sequence can be done independently; (5) the component preskills at each step should be pretaught before training is begun on the entire routine; and (6) the mathematical "language" that is used to teach each step should be communicated in a direct and immediate way using a simplified language.

In many cases, conventional ways of doing computations will need to be modified to make each step more teachable. For example, algebraic addition calculations of the form $4 + \square = 6$ are troublesome. Many students treat the unknown (or box) as a place to write the sum, probably as a result of experience with unknowns being sums in regular addition problems and the failure to understand what equality means. Thus, they add 4 and 6 and end up with 10. To give a specific illustration of how to prevent this misrule and to demonstrate generally the kind of detail found in a multistep strategy, Table 1 shows a format, adapted from Silbert et al. (1981), for teaching a missing-addend strategy.

Before doing this problem, the students would have been taught the necessary component skills of symbol identification (for +, =, and $\square$) numeral identification (1 through 6), understanding the equality rule, which side of an equation to start counting on, drawing lines for numbers, counting from a lower number to a higher target number, drawing lines under a box for each number counted, counting the lines under a box, and writing numerals in a box for the number of lines counted. Worth noting is that many of these

TABLE 1
Sample Format for Teaching a Missing-Addend Strategy[a]

Teacher	Learner
(Write on board:) 4 + ☐ = 6	
1. Read this problem.	"Four plus how many equals six"
2. This is a new kind of problem. It doesn't tell us how many to plus. We have to figure out how many to plus. What must we figure out?	"How many to plus."
3. We use the equal rule to help us. The equal rule says we must end up with the same number on this side (point to 4 + ☐) and the other side of the equal (point to 6). First, we figure the side we start counting on. (Point to 4 + ☐.) Do I start counting on this side? Why not?	"No" "The box does not tell how many lines to make."
(Point to 6.) Do I start counting on this side? Yes. The six tells me to make six lines. (Draw six lines under the 6.)	"Yes"
4. We want to end up with the same number on both sides. (Point to 4 + ☐.) How many on this side now?	"Four"
I'll draw four lines. (Draw four lines under 4.) Think. How many do we need to end up with on this side?	"Six"
To correct: We want to end up with the same number on this side as on the other side. What number do we end up with on the other side? (Repeat Step 4.)	"Six"
5. We have four. We want to end up with six. Count as I make the lines. Tell me when to stop. (Point to 4.) How many in this group? Get it going. (Draw lines under box as students count.)	"Four" "fffooouuurrr . . . five, six, stop!"
To correct: If students do not say stop after saying 6, tell them, "We ended up with 6 on the other side. We must end up with 6 on this side." (Then repeat from Step 5.)	
6. What number did we end up with? We made the sides equal. Are we going to write 6 in the box?	"Six" "No"
To correct: If students say yes, "We must count the lines under the box to see what number goes in the box."	
7. The number of lines under the box tells us what numeral to write in the box. How many lines do we have under the box? So, what numeral should I write in the box?	"Two" "Two"
(Write 2 in the box.)	
8. Four plus how many equals six? Say the whole statement.	"Two" "Four plus two equals six"

[a]From *Direct Instruction Mathematics* (pp. 116–117) by J. Silbert, D. Carnine, and M. Stein, 1981, Columbus, OH: Charles E. Merrill. Copyright 1981 by Bell & Howell Company. Adapted by permission.

concepts and skills will be useful for subsequent computations, such as regular and algebraic subtraction tasks.

The format in Table 1 is an introductory one and contains many steps, each performed at the overt level. Later formats of this problem type would attempt to shorten the number of steps and "covertize" the process. This can be done by dropping steps, merging several steps together and teaching the learner to regroup them into a shorter form, and/or giving the learner an inclusive direction ("work the rest of the problem yourself and write the answer"). The sample problems for the introductory format would be done on the blackboard by the teacher. This presentation is therefore highly structural and represents Step A of the progression toward the development of independent seatwork activities, as outlined by Silbert *et al.* (1981). Step B presents structured worksheets during which the teacher guides the students through the steps in applying the Step A strategy to problems on their worksheets. Step C contains less-structured worksheet problems in which the number of steps and prompts are reduced, and the students are required to do larger task segments under systematically decreasing teacher guidance. In Step D, low-structure worksheets are given, and the teacher monitors the students closely during worksheet activities until they develop accuracy rates of 85% or better and can complete problems within preset time restrictions. In Step E, teacher support is withdrawn, and the students work all problems independently under the Step D accuracy and fluency criteria.

There has been scant research on how to develop independent seatwork activity through programmed sequencing of tasks, and there is almost none with handicapped individuals. One study (Paine, Carnine, White, & Walters, 1982) assessed the effect of the pattern of structure on column multiplication problems by three low-achieving students. One finding was that the presentation of Steps A and B had a negligible impact on improving correct performance during independent seatwork beyond the baseline level of 19%. Instatement of Step C, however, elevated independent performance to 80% correct, and it is likely that instatement of Step D, stressing problem accuracy and fluency, would have generated even higher levels of mastery.

Problem Solving

Unless pretaught that the verbs *buy*, *find*, and *gets more* usually denote addition operations and that *loses*, *spends*, and *gives away* denote subtraction, low-performing students will have trouble with simple oral and written story problems containing these words. Even when taught, they may fail to notice a change in verb usage and then may work a problem incorrectly. Thus, they may subtract upon hearing the word *spends* in this problem: "Bill has many nickels. He spends 8 nickels on Monday and spends 4 nickels on Tuesday. How many nickels does he spend together?" Because the larger number also appears first, that may further signal subtraction, especially if previous subtraction problems began with the large number.

Problem difficulty is substantially increased when the story problem contains irrelevant quantities, requires two or more different operations, and involves large numbers. The use of unfamiliar words and syntax further compounds the difficulty level. To do addition or subtraction problems involving classification, students will need to distinguish between the number for the larger group (superordinate class), which when given requires subtraction, and the numbers for the smaller groups (subordinate classes), which when given requires addition. Then, there are complex action problems that do not lend themselves to a phrase-by-phrase translation into an equation, as in "Susan needs 15 plates to set a table. She has 5 plates so far. How many more plates does she need?" Finally, there are comparison problems that give two quantities, and the wording determines whether the differences between them are added or subtracted.

Silbert *et al.* (1981) identified the dimensions of these story problems and outlined the order to teach them. They also developed specialized formats for converting each problem type into an appropriate equation and provided strategies for teaching the kind of arithmetic operation to employ. Along these lines, Darch, Carnine, and Gersten (1984) taught skill-deficient fourth graders to discriminate story problems involving multiplication versus division operations. In one treatment, the students were first taught whether the quantities identified the "big number" (larger group) or two "little numbers" (smaller group). Subsequently, they were taught essentially that if the problem tells about the "big number" and it uses the same number again and again (as conveyed by the words *each* or *every*), then it is a division problem. Conversely, if it does not tell about the big number and it uses the same number again, it is a multiplication problem. Students taught an explicit translation strategy were able to write the correct computation statement 85% of the time. Those who were taught by basal methods that stressed open-ended discussions bringing into play everyday experiences got 63% correct. Moreover, significantly more students taught by explicit strategies reported liking the way the stories were taught and tended to use the rules more often than the basal students.

Kameenui, Carnine, Darch, and Stein (1986) found that explicit strategies were more effective than basal methods in teaching single-digit subtraction, fraction skills, and beginning division skills to regular education students possessing different math abilities. That sorely needed research with handicapped individuals may be forthcoming is indicated by the research of Kelley *et al.* (1986) with these students in high school. When taught by strategic approaches employing videodisk technology, complex fraction problems were more successfully solved and retained than when taught by basal approaches.

SOME MATHEMATICAL APPLICATIONS

As with reading, one of four approaches can be taken to help handicapped individuals meet the demands of daily living involving math skills (Browder & Snell, 1987). The first approach bypasses math instruction altogether, as when a trainer gives someone exact change for a bus or a vending machine. The second approach involves teaching the use of a prosthesis as a substitute for math-related activities, as when the individual carries a coin-matching card showing the kind and number of coins to use for a bus or a vending machine. The third approach teaches skills that are specific to one activity, as when coin-summation calculations are taught just for vending machines. The fourth approach teaches generalized skills that enable the handicapped individual to perform math operations for a variety of daily activities.

Monetary Usage

There has been a fair amount of studies devoted to teaching moderately handicapped adolescents specific money skills that deal with counting coins to match prices from one cent to a dollar (Bellamy & Buttars, 1975; Borakove & Cuvo, 1976), choosing different combinations of coins to equal values from five cents to fifty cents (Trace, Cuvo, & Criswell, 1977), and computing coin change of given purchase prices less than a dollar and change requirements of less than forty-nine cents (Cuvo, Veitch, Trace, & Konke, 1978). In these studies, a model-lead-test sequence has been the primary instructional procedure. Initially, the instructor demonstrates the sequence of computations to be taken, helps the students perform these steps when necessary, and then allows for independent practice and review. Silbert et al. (1981) have outlined more strategic approaches toward monetary calculations, wherein students are taught certain rules to follow during coin-summation and change-counting tasks. However, the effectiveness of these rule-governed procedures need to be validated with handicapped individuals and compared to other training procedures.

Browder and Snell (1987) have noted that group-home living and shopping routines require far more use of dollar bills than coins. One approach is to teach the classification and use of bills by the usual prices required for certain goods. For example, one-dollar bills are used for small, over-the-counter purchases but ten-dollar bills for major purchases like groceries and clothes. Another approach is to teach more refined skills for a variety of contexts. This procedure will entail learning about bill summations, equivalences, and change computations, and the more difficult operation of expressing total prices in dollars and cents (e.g., $2.32) from which other prices are to be added or subtracted. One possibility to circumvent time-consuming pencil and paper operations is to teach various computations with a calculator. Horton (1985) found that EMR adolescents using calculators generally exceeded the computational performances of nonhandicapped peers using paper and pencil.

Time Telling and Calendar Operations

Learning to tell time nowadays can begin with standard face or digital clocks, after which the conversion of one form of time into the other can be taught. Using a standard clock, time can be estimated roughly by attending only to the smaller hour hand and saying, "The time is between 2 and 3 o'clock," or, when it is directly at some number, "The time is 8 o'clock." Partington, Sundberg, Iwata, and Mountjoy (1979) taught EMR adolescents with a time-telling program that required minimal skills. Initially, the face of a standard clock was covered with a "before" or an "after" cover that was shown on the left and on the right side in order to teach, respectively, the identification of specific numbers as being before or after the hour. With the covers removed, the minute hand was then positioned progressively between 1 to 29 minutes on the before and after sides, and this procedure was integrated with that of saying the hours. Identification of half-hour times was taught last. The result was a complete description of the time. In contrast, the Hofmeister *et al.* (1975) clock program requires the preskill of counting by 5 to 55 and teaches expression of all times in terms of minutes (in multiples of 5) *after* the hour. Such expressions should make conversion to digital time easier than programs that teach before the hour.

Teaching generalized time telling with standard clocks can pose problems especially when critical stimuli, like the numerals, are deleted or modified by typeset. Digital clocks provide greater consistency and perhaps allow more easily acquired subskills for time telling than standard clocks. Evaluation of digital time telling procedures is needed.

Finding the dates on a calendar and locating the days on which they fall is probably the individual's first encounter with tabular information. Traditional methods of teaching calendar operations usually wait until the students know all the ordinal numbers from first to thirty-first before any date is taught. The procedure then requires the introduction of the months one at a time but does not provide an opportunity for locating dates from among several months presented simultaneously. Weisberg's (1986) program teaches date statements ("The date is July third") immediately after the first five ordinal numbers and the names of three months can be identified. Upon program completion, preschoolers can locate targeted dates and days from sets of four simultaneously presented months in which all the words are abbreviated.

Being able to carry out the steps in telling time or in "reading" a calendar does not mean that the individual will know what time lunch is served, how many seconds there are in a minute, or when his mother's birthday occurs. Conversely, knowing these facts does not imply anything about the ability to do the steps. If different variables control multistep operations and the understanding of facts, we should not expect automatic generalization from one kind of controlling dimension to the other. Too often, behavioral inventories treat the two as the same and encourage unfair assessment.

CONCLUDING REMARKS

The concepts and routines of a full academic program consist of an enormous amount of tasks. Obviously, not all of the tasks can be taught at the same time, so special consideration must be given to the appropriate selection and sequencing of relevant teaching examples. In the past, the selection and ordering of tasks have more or less been guided by tradition and, sometimes, by invented developmental "principles." For example, despite research to the contrary (Carnine & Silbert, 1979), many educators still teach alphabet letter names on the premise that they are prerequisites for decoding words. (Even without familiarity with the research, our own experience of learning to read a foreign language should alert us to the nonsignificance of letter names.) Similarly, many educators still believe that children should begin to write using wide-diameter pencils, even though there are no hard data for this developmental supposition and the existing data argue against this practice (Sims & Weisberg, 1982).

The barrage of dead-end skills and wasted effort found in many educational settings needs to be replaced by a logical analysis of the structure of academic content and skill repertoires of the kind formulated by Engelmann and Carnine (1982). Their proposal stipulates that, through a search for common structures across academic content areas, we will be in a better position to design programs that will lead the student to make generalizations across these content areas. Guidelines for the selection, sequencing, and integration of the teaching examples that lead to logically consistent strategies is another goal, and one that is often neglected in many programs (Beck *et al.*, 1979; Engelmann, 1982). Finally, there is the whole area of developing and of continuing with those classroom organizations and teacher-delivery systems that allow the mentally retarded and any individual to learn more in less time and to process previously taught material automatically and with confidence.

ACKNOWLEDGMENTS. Support was furnished in part by the Office of Sponsored Programs of the University of Alabama under the direction of Dr. Robert L. Wells. The author is especially grateful to Bruno Andracchio and Roberta Weisberg for their critical comments and to Connie Sulentic and Mary Al-Akhdar for their careful preparation of this chapter.

References

Apffel, J. A., Kelleher, J., Lilly, M. S., & Richardson, R. (1975). Developmental reading for moderately retarded children. *Education and Training of the Mentally Retarded, 10,* 229–235.
Arter, J. A., & Jenkins, J. R. (1979). Differential diagnostic-prescriptive teaching: A critical appraisal. *Review of Educational Research, 49,* 517–555.
Ausman, J. O., & Gaddy, M. R. (1974). Reinforcement training for echolalia: Developing a repertoire of appropriate verbal responses in an echolalic girl. *Mental Retardation, 12,* 20–21.
Baer, D., & Guess, D. (1973). Teaching productive noun phrases to severely retarded children. *American Journal of Mental Deficiency, 77,* 489–505.
Beck, I. L., & McCaslin, E. S. (1978). *An analysis of dimensions that affect the development of code-breaking ability in eight beginning reading programs.* Pittsburgh: University of Pittsburgh, Learning Research and Development Center.
Beck, I. L., McKeown, M. G., McCaslin, E. S., & Burkes, A. (1979). *Instructional dimensions that may affect reading comprehension: Examples from two commercial reading programs.* (LRDC Publication 1979 No. 20). Pittsburgh: University of Pittsburgh, Learning Research and Development Center.

Becker, W. C. (1977). Teaching reading and language to the disadvantaged—What we have learned from field research. *Harvard Educational Review, 47*, 518–543.

Becker, W. C. (1986). *Applied psychology for teachers: A behavioral-cognitive approach.* Chicago: Science Research Associates.

Becker, W. C., & Carnine, D. W. (1980). Direct instruction: An effective approach to educational intervention with the disadvantaged and low performers. In B. B. Lahey & A. K. Kazdin (Eds.), *Advances in clinical and child psychology* (Vol. 3, pp. 429–473). New York: Plenum Press.

Becker, W. C., Engelmann, S., & Thomas, D. R. (1975). *Teaching 2: Cognitive learning and instruction.* Chicago: Science Research Associates.

Becker, W. C., Engelmann, S., Carnine, D. W., & Maggs, A. (1982). Direct instruction technology: Making learning happen. In P. Karoly & J. J. Steffen (Eds.), *Improving children's competence: Advances in child behavioral analysis and therapy* (pp. 151–204). Lexington, MA: D. C. Heath.

Bellamy, T., & Buttars, K. L. (1975). Teaching trainable level retarded students to count money: Toward personal independence through academic instruction. *Education and Training of the Mentally Retarded, 10*, 18–26.

Bloom, B. S. (1976). *Human characteristics and school learning.* New York: McGraw-Hill.

Booth, A., Hewitt, D., Jenkins, W., & Maggs, A. (1979). Making retarded children literate: A five-year study. *Australian Journal of Mental Retardation, 5*, 257–260.

Borakove, L. S., & Cuvo, A. J. (1976). Facilitative effects of coin displacement on teaching coin summation to mentally retarded adolescents. *American Journal of Mental Deficiency, 81*, 350–356.

Bracey, S., Maggs, A., & Morath, P. (1975). The effects of a direct phonic approach in teaching reading with six moderately retarded children. *The Slow Learning Child, 22*, 83–90.

Browder, D., Hines, C., McCarthy, L. J., & Fees, J. (1984). Sight word instruction to facilitate acquisition and generalization of daily living skills for the moderately and severely retarded. *Education and Training of the Mentally Retarded, 19*, 191–200.

Browder, D. M., & Snell, M. E. (1987). Functional academics. In M. E. Snell (Ed.), *Systematic instruction of persons with severe handicaps* (pp. 436–468). Columbus, OH: Charles E. Merrill.

Brown, L., & Perlmutter, L. (1971). Teaching functional reading to young trainable students. *Education and Training of the Mentally Retarded, 6*, 74–84.

Carlson, J. G., & Minke, K. A. (1975). Fixed and ascending criteria for unit mastery learning. *Journal of Educational Psychology, 67*, 96–101.

Carnine, D. W., & Silbert, J. (1979). *Direct instruction reading.* Columbus, OH: Charles E. Merrill.

Carnine, D. W. (1976a). Effects of two teacher presentation rates on off-task behavior, answering correctly, and participation. *Journal of Applied Behavior Analysis, 9*, 199–206.

Carnine, D. W. (1976b). Similar sound separation and cumulative introduction in learning sound correspondences. *Journal of Educational Research, 69*, 368–372.

Carnine, D. W. (1977). Phonic versus look-say: Transfer to new words. *The Reading Teacher, 30*, 636–640.

Carnine, D. W. (1980a). Three procedures for presenting minimally different positive and negative instances. *Journal of Educational Psychology, 72*, 452–456.

Carnine, D. W. (1980b). Relationships between stimulus variations and the formation of misconceptions. *Journal of Educational Research, 74*, 106–110.

Carnine, D. W. (1980c). Two letter discrimination sequences: High-confusion-alternatives first versus low-confusion-alternatives first. *Journal of Reading Behavior, 12*, 41–47.

Carnine, D. W. (1980d). Phonic versus whole-word correction procedures following phonic instruction. *Education and Treatment of Children, 3*, 323–330.

Carnine, D. W. (1980e). Preteaching versus concurrent teaching of the component skills of a multiplication algorithm. *Journal for Research in Mathematics Education, 11*, 375–379.

Carroll, J. B. (1971). *Learning from verbal discussion in educational media: A review of the literature.* Princeton, NJ: Educational Testing Service.

Chall, J. A. (1983). *Learning to read: The great debate* (updated edition). New York: McGraw-Hill.

Clark, C. R. (1984). A close look at the standard rebus system and blissymbolics. *Journal of the Association for Persons with Severe Handicaps, 9*, 37–48.

Clark, H. B., & Sherman, J. A. (1975). Teaching generative use of sentence answers to three forms of questions. *Journal of Applied Behavior Analysis, 8*, 321–330.

Collins, M. (1983). Teaching spelling: Current practices and effective instruction. *Direct Instruction News, 3*(1), 14–15.

Cowart, J., Carnine, D. W., & Becker, W. C. (1976). The effects of signals on attending, responding, and following directions in direct instruction. In W. C. Becker & S. Engelmann (Eds.), *Analysis of achievement data on six cohorts of low-income children from 20 school districts in the University of Oregon Direct Instruction Follow Through Model* (Technical Report 76-1) (pp. 67–98). Eugene, OR: University of Oregon.

Cuvo, A. J., Veitch, V. D., Trace, M. W., & Konke, J. L. (1978). Teaching change computation to the mentally retarded. *Behavior Modification, 2,* 531–548.

Darch, C., Carnine, D., & Gersten, R. (1984). Explicit instruction in mathematics problem-solving. *Journal of Educational Research, 77,* 351–359.

Dolch, E. W. (1936). A basic sight vocabulary. *Elementary School Journal, 36,* 456–460.

Dorry, G., & Zeaman, D. (1973). The use of a fading technique in paired-associate teaching of a reading vocabulary with retardates. *Mental Retardation, 11,* 3–6.

Duell, O. K. (1968). An analysis of prompting procedures for teaching a sight vocabulary. *American Educational Research Journal, 5,* 675–686.

Durkin, D. (1978–1979). What classroom observation reveals about reading comprehension instruction. *Reading Research Quarterly, 14,* 481–533.

Edmark reading program. (1984). Seattle: Edmark Associates.

Engelmann, S. (1970). The effectiveness of direct verbal instruction on IQ performance and achievement in reading and arithmetic. In J. Hellmuth (Ed.), *Disadvantaged child* (Vol. 3. pp. 339–361). New York: Brunner/Mazel.

Engelmann, S. (1980). Toward the design of faultless instruction: The theoretical basis of concept analysis. *Educational Technology, 2,* 28–36.

Engelmann, S. (1982). A study of 4th–6th grade basal reading series. *Direct Instruction News, 1, 1,* 4–5, 19.

Engelmann, S., & Bruner, E. (1983). *Reading Mastery I and II: DISTAR Reading.* Chicago: Science Research Associates.

Engelmann, S., & Carnine, D. (1982). *Theory of instruction: Principles and applications.* New York: Irvington Publishers.

Engelmann, S., Granzin, A., & Severson, H. (1979). Diagnosing instruction. *Journal of Special Education, 13,* 355–363.

Englert, G. S., & Thomas, C. C. (1982). Management of task involvement in special education classrooms: Implications for teacher preparation. *Teacher Education and Special Education, 5,* 3–10.

Etzel, B. C., & LeBlanc, J. M. (1979). The simplest treatment alternative: The law of parsimony applied to choosing appropriate instructional control and errorless-learning procedures for the difficult-to-teach child. *Journal of Autism and Developmental Disabilities, 9,* 361–382.

Feinberg, P. (1975). Sight vocabulary for the TMR child and adult: Rationale, development and application. *Education and Training of the Mentally Retarded, 10,* 246–252.

Fink, W. T. (1976). Effects of a pre-correction procedure on the decoding errors of two low-performing first-grade girls. In W. C. Becker & S. Engelmann (Eds.), *Analysis of achievement data on six cohorts of low-income children from 20 school districts in the University of Oregon Direct Instruction Follow Through Model* (Technical Report 76-1) (pp. 33–39). Eugene, OR: University of Oregon.

Fink, W. T., & Brice-Gray, K., (1979). The effects of two teaching strategies on the acquisition and recall on an academic task by moderately and severely retarded preschool children. *Mental Retardation, 17,* 8–12.

Fink, W. T., & Carnine, D. W. (1975). Control of arithmetic errors using informational feedback and graphing. *Journal of Applied Behavioral Analysis, 8,* 461.

Gersten, R. M., & Maggs, A. (1982). Five year longitudinal study of cognitive development of moderately retarded children in a direct instruction program. *Analysis and Intervention in Developmental Disabilities, 2,* 239–243.

Gersten, R. M., Carnine, D. W., & Williams, P. B. (1982). Measuring implementation of a structured educational model in an urban school district: An observational approach. *Educational Evaluation and Policy Analysis, 4,* 67–69.

Gersten, R. M., White, W. A. T., Falco, R., & Carnine, D. (1982). Teaching basic discriminations to handicapped and non-handicapped individuals through a dynamic presentation of instructional stimuli. *Analysis and Intervention in Developmental Disabilities, 2*, 305–317.

Gersten, R. M., Becker, W. C., Heiry, T. J., & White, W. A. T. (1984). Entry IQ and yearly academic growth of children in direct instruction programs: A longitudinal study of low SES children. *Educational Evaluation and Policy Analysis, 6*, 109–121.

Goldberg, I., & Rooke, M. (1967). Research and educational practices with mentally deficient children. In N. Haring & R. Schiefelbusch (Eds.), *Methods of special education* (pp. 112–136). New York: McGraw-Hill.

Gough, P. B. (1976). One second of reading. In H. H. Singer & R. B. Ruddell (Eds.), *Theoretical models and processes of reading* (pp. 34–50). Newark, DL: International Reading Association.

Greenwood, C. R., Delquadri, J. C., & Hall, R. V. (1984). The opportunity to respond and student academic performance. In W. L. Heward, T. E. Heron, D. S. Hill, & J. Trap-Porter (Eds.), *Focus on behavior analysis in education* (pp. 58–88). Columbus, OH: Charles E. Merrill.

Haring, N. G., & Bateman, G. (1977). *Teaching the learning disabled child.* Englewood Cliffs, NJ: Prentice-Hall.

Harzem, P., Lee, I., & Miles, T. R. (1976). The effects of pictures and learning to read. *British Journal of Educational Psychology, 46*, 323–327.

Hendler, M., & Weisberg, P. (1988). *Conservation acquisition, maintenance, and generalization by mentally retarded children using equality-rule training.* Manuscript submitted for publication.

Hofmeister, A. M., Atkinson, C. M., & Hofmeister, J. B. (1975). *Programmed time telling.* Eugene, OR: Engelmann-Becker Press.

Horner, R. H., Bellamy, G. T., & Colvin, G. T. (1984). Responding in the presence of nontrained stimuli: Implications of generalization error patterns. *Journal of the Association for Persons with Severe Handicaps, 9*, 287–296.

Horner, R. H., Albin, R. W., & Ralph, G. (1986). Generalization with precision: The role of negative teaching examples in the instruction of generalized grocery item selection. *Journal of the Association for Persons with Severe Handicaps, 11*, 300–308.

Horton, S. (1985). Computational rates of educable mentally retarded adolescents with and without calculators in comparison to normals. *Education and Training of the Mentally Retarded, 20*, 14–24.

Hurlburt, B. I., Iwata, B. A., & Green, J. D. (1982). Nonvocal language acquisition in adolescents with severe physical disabilities: Blissymbol versus iconic stimulus formats. *Journal of Applied Behavior Analysis, 15*, 241–258.

Hurley, O. L. (1975). Reading comprehension skills vis-à-vis the mentally retarded. *Education and Training of the Mentally Retarded, 10*, 10–14.

Jenkins, J. R., Stein, M. L., & Osborn, J. R. (1981). What next after decoding? Instruction and research in reading comprehension. *Exceptional Education Quarterly, 2*, 27–39.

Johnson, B. F., & Cuvo, A. J. (1981). Teaching cooking skills to mentally retarded persons. *Behavior Modification, 5*, 187–202.

Kameenui, E., Carnine, D., & Maggs, A. (1980). Instructional procedures for teaching reversible passive voice and clause constructions to three mildly handicapped children. *The Exceptional Child, 27*, 29–40.

Kameenui, E., Carnine, D., Darch, C., & Stein, M. (1986). Two approaches to the development of mathematics instruction. *Elementary School Journal, 86*, 633–650.

Kelly, B., Carnine, D., Gersten, R., & Grossen, B. (1986). The effectiveness of videodisc instruction in teaching fractions to learning handicapped and remedial high school students. *Journal of Special Education Technology, 8*(2), 5–17.

Kincaid, M. S., Weisberg, P., & Sims, Jr., E. V. (1981). Using tokens as instructional stimuli to teach academic skills to children during a token-exchange period. *Perceptual and Motor Skills, 52*, 223–233.

Koegel, R. L., Dunlap, G., Richman, G. S., & Dyer, K. (1981). The use of specific orienting cues for teaching discrimination tasks. *Analysis and Intervention in Developmental Disabilities, 1*, 187–198.

Levin, J. R. (1971–1972). Comprehending what we read: An outsider looks in. *Journal of Reading Behavior, 4*, 18–29.

Lloyd, J., Epstein, M. H., & Cullinan, D. (1981). Direct teaching for learning disabilities. In J. Gottlieb & S. Strichart (Eds.), *Developmental theory and research in learning disabilities* (pp. 278–309). Baltimore: University Park Press.

Lovitt, T. C., & Curtiss, K. (1968). Effect of manipulating an antecedent event on mathematics response rate. *Journal of Applied behavior Analysis, 1,* 329–333.

Mason, J. M. (1978). Role of strategy in reading by mentally retarded persons. *American Journal of Mental Deficiency, 85,* 467–473.

McClennen, S., & Harrington, L. (1982). A developmentally-based functional mathematics program for retarded and autistic persons. *Journal of Special Education Technology, 5,* 23–30.

Miller, A., & Miller, E. E. (1968). Symbol accentuation: The perceptual transfer of meaning from spoken to printed word. *American Journal of Mental Deficiency, 73,* 200–208.

Neef, N. A., Iwata, B. A., & Page, T. J. (1980). The effects of interspersal training versus high-density reinforcement on spelling acquisition and retention. *Journal of Applied Behavior Analysis, 13,* 153–158.

Oaken, R., Weiner, M., & Cromer, W. (1971). Identification, organization and reading comprehension for good and poor readers. *Journal of Educational Psychology, 62,* 71–78.

Orelove, F. P. (1982). Developing daily schedules for classrooms of severely handicapped students. *Education and Treatment of Children, 5,* 59–68.

Paine, S. C., Carnine, D. W., White, W. A. T., & Walters, G. (1982). Effects of fading teacher presentation structure (covertization) on acquisition and maintenance of arithmetic problem-solving skills. *Education and Treatment of Children, 5,* 93–107.

Paine, S. C., Radicchi, J., Rosellini, L., Deutchman, L., & Darch, C. (1983). *Structuring your classroom for academic success.* Champaign, IL: Research Press.

Partington, J. W., Sundberg, M., Iwata, B. A., & Mountjoy, P. T. (1979). A task-analysis approach to time-telling instruction for normal and educable mentally impaired children. *Education and Treatment of Children, 2,* 17–29.

Perfetti, C. A. (1977). Language comprehension and fast decoding: Some psycholinguistic prerequisites for skilled reading comprehension. In J. T. Guthrie (Ed.), *Cognition, curriculum, and comprehension.* Newark, DL: International Reading Association.

Piaget, J. (1953). How children form mathematical concepts. *Scientific American, 189*(5), 74–79.

Robinson-Wilson, M. A. (1977). Picture recipe cards as an approach to teaching severely and profoundly retarded adults to cook. *Education and Training of the Mentally Retarded, 12,* 69–73.

Rosenshine, B. (1983). Teaching functions in instructional programs. *Elementary School Journal, 83,* 335–351.

Samuels, J. S. (1970). Effects of pictures on learning to read, comprehension and attitudes. *Review of Education Research, 40,* 397–407.

Sidman, M. (1971). Reading and audio-visual equivalents. *Journal of Speech and Hearing Research, 14,* 5–13.

Sidman, M., Cresson, Jr., O., & Wilson-Morris, M. (1974). Acquisition of matching to sample via mediated transfer. *Journal of the Experimental Analysis of Behavior, 22,* 261–273.

Silbert, J., Carnine, D., & Stein, M. (1981). *Direct instruction mathematics.* Columbus, OH: Charles E. Merrill.

Sims, E. V. (1984). *Effects of continuous versus noncontinuous presentations and magnitude of difference between examples and nonexamples on acquisition and transfer of a comparative concept.* Unpublished doctoral dissertation, University of Alabama.

Sims, E. V., & Weisberg, P. (1982, September). *Behavioral analysis of handwriting.* Paper presented at the Conference of Behavior Analysis in Education, Ohio State University, Columbus.

Stevens, R., & Rosenshine, B. V. (1981). Advances in research on teaching. *Exceptional Education Quarterly, 2,* 1–10.

Trace, M. W., Cuvo, A. J., & Criswell, J. L. (1977). Teaching coin equivalence to the mentally retarded. *Journal of Applied Behavior Analysis, 10,* 18–92.

Vandever, T. R., Maggart, W. T., & Nasser, S. (1976). Three approaches to beginning reading instruction for educable mentally retarded children. *Mental Retardation, 14,* 29–32.

Vargas, J. S. (1984). What are your exercises teaching? An analysis of stimulus control in instructional materials. In W. L. Heward, T. E. Heron, T. E. Hill, & J. Trap-Porter (Eds.), *Focus on behavior analysis in education* (pp. 126–141). Columbus, OH: Charles E. Merrill.

Walsh, B. F., & Lamberts F. (1979). Errorless discrimination and picture fading as techniques for teaching words to TMR students. *American Journal of Mental Deficiency, 83,* 473–479.

Weinheimer, B., & Weisberg, P. (1987). Acquisition of basic concepts by mentally retarded and nonretarded children through video-presented, stimulus conversion procedures. *Journal of Special Education Technology, 9,* 45–53.

Weisberg, P. (1986, May). Developing and evaluating calendar formats for instructionally naive students. In R. S. Weisberg (Chair), *Field testing of recent direct instruction programs.* Symposium conducted at the meeting of Association for Behavior Analysis, Milwaukee.

Weisberg, P. (1988). Direct instruction in the preschool. *Education and Treatment of Children, 11,* 349–363.

Weisberg, P., Packer, R. A., & Weisberg, R. S. (1981). Academic training. In J. L. Matson & J. R. McCartney (Eds.), *Handbook of behavior modification with the mentally retarded* (pp. 331–411). New York: Plenum Press.

Weisberg, P., Sims, E. V., & Weinheimer, B. A. (1983). Academic skills. In J. L. Matson & S. E. Breuning (Eds.), *Assessing the mentally retarded* (pp. 335–396). New York: Grune & Stratton.

Williams, P., & Carnine, D. W. (1981). Relationship between range of examples and of instructions and attention in concept attainment. *Journal of Educational Research, 74,* 144–148.

Wilson, C. T. (1963). An essential vocabulary. *The Reading Teacher, 17,* 94–96.

Woodcock, R. W. (1967). Peabody rebus reading program. Circle Pines, MN: American Guidance Service.

Woodward, J., Carnine, D., & Gersten, R. (1988). Teaching problem solving through a computer simulation. *American Educational Research Journal, 25,* 72–86.

18

Sexual Behavior

Ramasamy Manikam and Dinah S. Hensarling

Increased knowledge about the causes of mental retardation, though still incomplete, has given impetus to a movement toward normalization of lifestyles of mentally retarded persons. With this growing emphasis on normalization, issues regarding sexuality and the sexual rights of mentally retarded persons have come to the forefront. Immediately, two issues arise when discussing sexual behavior as it relates to persons who are classified as mentally retarded. First, the classification "mentally retarded" encompasses a group of individuals with a very wide range of behaviors, of levels of functioning, of physical capabilities, and of social competencies. For example, behaviors that are expected from persons who are classified as profoundly mentally retarded differ greatly from behaviors that are expected from those who are classified as moderately mentally retarded. It is therefore meaningless to speak in generalizations about traits, capabilities, and behavior of mentally retarded persons as a homogeneous group. The second issue is the notion of appropriate versus inappropriate sexual behavior. What is meant by appropriate sexual expression, and do the same values hold for mentally retarded persons? In general, society's goals remain unclear regarding what constitutes normal sexual behavior for persons functioning within a normal range of intelligence; the issue becomes muddier still with regard to mentally retarded persons. Regrettably, among some professionals and staff members working with mentally retarded people, the question of appropriate versus inappropriate sexual behavior continues not only to remain unanswered but unasked. Strides in conceptualizing what healthy sexual behavior is regarding mentally retarded persons will do much to ease the tensions that are felt by all who work closely with these persons.

Normalization

In an attempt to identify appropriate sexual behavior, it is helpful to understand the concept of normalization. Kempton (1977a) has delineated the various rights of normalization in reference to mentally retarded persons as

Ramasamy Manikam and Dinah S. Hensarling • Department of Psychology, Louisiana State University, Baton Rouge, Louisiana 70803.

follows: (1) the right to receive training in social-sexual behavior that will open more doors for social contact with people in the community; (2) the right to all the knowledge about sexuality that they can comprehend; (3) the right to enjoy love and to be loved by the opposite sex, including sexual fulfillment; (4) the right of the opportunity to express sexual impulses in the same form that are socially acceptable for others; (5) the right to birth control services, which are specialized to meet their needs; (6) the right to marry; (7) the right to have a voice in whether or not they should have children; and (8) the right for supportive services that involve those rights as they are needed and are feasible. Using the concept of normalization, restrictions on sexual behavior should originate from physical and/or mental limitations only.

Among the individuals who are classified as mentally retarded, most fall into the mild and moderate range and, within this range, most develop normal reproductive capabilities (Salerno, Park, & Giannini, 1975). Typically, there is a lag between physical maturation and social maturation among mentally retarded persons. This lag is lengthened by an array of societal attitudes and by environmental constrictions creating sexual difficulties that might otherwise be avoided. There are many variables that potentially impact the social/sexual development of mentally retarded persons. Among these factors are (1) parental attitudes; (2) attitudes held by professionals as well as direct caregivers; (3) the quantity and quality of sex education provided to mentally retarded persons, their parents, and staff personnel; and (4) social interaction opportunities and access to models.

This chapter will open with a review of the variables impacting on the development of sexual behavior of mentally retarded persons. Following this, there will be a discussion of curriculum and resources, knowledge, attitudes, and behavior about sexuality held by mentally retarded persons. Finally, a discussion on behavioral programming to develop appropriate social and sexual behaviors and on the treatment of inappropriate behaviors will close the chapter.

PARENTAL ATTITUDES

Parents of mentally retarded persons represent a major source of sexual information about mentally retarded persons. Consequently, parents' attitudes about sex in general and the sexuality of their children in particular can profoundly impact the mentally retarded person's sexual development. Parental attitudes toward the sexuality of their mentally retarded children is best described as ambivalent. Although the parents of normal children often have difficulties facing the sexuality of their offspring, the parents of mentally retarded individuals often feel anxious and uncomfortable when faced with the sexuality of their children. Frequently, these parents lack a general knowledge about sex, which will only exacerbate the discomfort and the anxiety that they feel. Several studies have been implemented that explore the attitudes held by parents regarding sex education for their mentally retarded children, as well as parental knowledge about sex. Ambivalency of parents regarding sex education for their children has been reported by many researchers (Alcorn, 1974; Dupras & Tremblay, 1976; Hall, Morris, & Barker, 1973). Often, parents lack knowledge about sex, feel anxious about discussing sexuality, and frequently have sexual difficulties themselves (Goodman, 1976). Among parents, major sexual concerns pertain to the limited judgment, vulnerability, promiscuity, homosexuality, and masturbation, if these are demonstrated by their mentally retarded children. As indicated from these parental concerns, sexuality is a topic many parents feel inept to address competently.

Some interesting attitudes have become apparent. For example, Turchin (1974) found that mothers of mentally retarded offspring felt that masturbation was more appropriate for their mentally retarded sons than for their mentally retarded daughters. Furthermore, many parents may adopt the attitude that their mentally retarded children are incapable of demonstrating control over sexual behavior; whereas other parents may adopt the view that their children are innocent (a sort of asexual being) and thus may oppose sex education, which would destroy that innocence (Alcorn, 1974). Watson and Rogers (1980) found that parents of moderate mentally retarded children anticipated that the sexual events in the lives of their children would occur later than similar events in the lives of children without handicaps. Although many parents have expressed discomfort with sex education, others have voiced a need for it; 88% of the parents in the Watson and Rogers (1980) study approved of sex education for their children, specifically requesting that it be focused on methods of contraception. Because parents' knowledge and attitudes about sexuality potentially influence the sexual behavior of their mentally retarded offspring, the aforementioned studies suggest that a beneficial path toward normalizing mentally retarded persons would be the provision of sex education for parents of mentally retarded persons.

PROFESSIONAL ATTITUDES

Direct caregivers of mentally retarded persons often feel the underpinnings of pressure to avoid any event that would damage the reputation of their facility (Greengross, 1976). Often, these caregivers not only feel responsible for general care and education, but also that it is their "duty" to constrict manifestations of sexual behavior among the residents under their care. This feeling of responsibility tends to be reinforced by the system, the supervisors, and the parents. Frequently, the authoritative stance that professionals and staff take results in systems that tend to produce residents who are acquiescent and who respond best to authoritative injunctions. This type of learning can be in direct conflict when assertion and personal decision making are required (Craft & Craft, 1983). Thus, for example, a sexual relationship represents an equal relationship, that is, an adult to an adult (as opposed to a slanted relationship of a parent to a child) and inherently requires competencies in assertion and in decision making in the mentally retarded person.

Mulhern (1975) surveyed residential staff regarding sexual behavior of mentally retarded persons. Sixty-seven percent believed that the adjustment problems of their residents were due to sexual frustration. On the other hand, the only forms of sexual expression that received majority approval were private masturbation, brief kissing, and private petting. Responses to the survey indicated that the majority of staff are confronted with sexual behavior which they feel should not be permitted, and that many staff members are faced with prohibitions of sexual behavior in residents which they feel should be permitted. Also, respondents evinced a greater tolerance for private sex-related activities as opposed to public activities. Mitchell, Doctor, and Butler (1978) found that 72% of residential staff approved of limited heterosexual contact, for example, handholding. Only 33.6% deemed "kissing standing up" acceptable, and 9.25% approved of intercourse anywhere within the facility. Overall, less approval for homosexual behavior was found when compared to heterosexual behavior. Also, sexual behavior while couples were alone was significantly more acceptable. An apt commentary on prevalent attitudes regarding sexuality and mentally retarded persons is the finding of the Mitchell *et al.* (1978) study: a large number of caregivers felt that no sexual behavior on the part of residents was acceptable. Coleman and Murphy (1980) found that masturbation received a high percentage (88%) of approval among staff, but there was a rapid decline in approval when sexual activity involved others. A majority of respondents believed that mentally retarded persons should be permitted to marry and have children; many added qualifying addenda, such as if they have a sense of responsibility, have good jobs, and so forth. Researchers have noted more restrictive attitudes by caretakers when compared to the general public (McEwen, 1977; Mitchell *et al.*, 1978).

Problems can occur using attitudinal surveys in that they are sometimes insensitive to certain operative nuances. For example, administrators and staff of mental retardation facilities have voiced difficulty in making statements about appropriate or inappropriate sexual behavior among their mental retardation population, especially in light of the dramatic differences in behavioral competencies among mentally retarded individuals (Coleman & Murphy, 1980; Mulhern, 1975). Many respondents feel that consideration of maturity level and social abilities in concert with IQ should be the determining factors when delineating appropriate sexual behavior. Surveys sensitive to these variables need to be employed when attitudes are being measured.

STAFF BURNOUT

A relevant issue when discussing professional/staff attitudes about sex and mentally retarded persons pertains to problems that are due to staff burnout. Such burnout and physical and emotional exhaustion can occur among staff as a result of their intense and intimate work with mentally and/or physically handicapped people over time. Shanley (1986) noted that staff burnout becomes manifest in behaviors that demonstrate distancing and avoiding of residents. Distancing behaviors might include escaping to the staff room to avoid contact with residents, ridiculing the residents, feeding the residents in a hurried and noninteractive fashion, or bathing residents in a similar fashion. Typically, direct caregivers are underpaid and often feel that they are at odds with the professional staff of the institution. Through feeding, toileting, bathing, and grooming mentally retarded persons under their care, caregivers profoundly impact the attitudes and sexual identity of these individuals. Messages given to mentally retarded residents about their sexuality or their physical body are potentially strongly negative when they receive regular physical contact from burned-out and frustrated direct caregivers. Ways to minimize the negative effects of burnout should be implemented when working conditions are such that staff are at risk.

SYSTEM POLICIES

Directly affecting the attitudes of professionals toward sexual behavior are the system policies (or lack thereof) about appropriate sexual expression of persons under their care. Several researchers have explored the impact of these system policies. Direct caregivers often receive little direction from the system for which they work concerning appropriate sexual expression for mentally retarded persons under their care. Policies regarding sexual behavior of mentally retarded persons are often vague or nonexistent (Deisher, 1973; Mitchell et al., 1978). When policies have been established, facility staff are often unaware of their contents. Mulhern (1975) reported that only 23% of the mental retardation units responding to his survey had policies governing sexual behavior. Saunders (1979) reported that staff were unclear and inconsistent in their understanding of sexual behavior policies adopted by their facilities. Findings such as these suggest that questions about appropriate sexual behavior as it relates to mentally retarded persons are not being asked at the systems level.

SEX EDUCATION

Sex education is another variable affecting sexual behavior of mentally retarded persons. The lack of sexual knowledge by parents and staff can impede appropriate sexual maturity among mentally retarded persons, as was noted in the previous discussion of attitudes. Whatever comprises normative sexual behavior for mentally retarded persons begs further clarification in the literature and in applied settings. Facility staff have difficulty allowing mentally retarded persons under their care the freedom of interaction with others in ways suggesting sexual underpinnings. Because of the pressure felt by professional staff, any overtly sexual behavior among residents tends to be labeled problematic, and is dealt with accordingly. A system for evaluating and facilitating appropriate sexual conduct of mentally retarded individuals is needed, which takes into account variability in IQ, adaptive behavior, and social skills. Monat (1982) provided guidelines about the different behaviors to expect from mildly, moderately, severely, and profoundly mentally retarded persons in terms of sexual behavior and comprehension of sex education training. Examples elucidating problems and educational needs of these specific groups are also given. These guidelines illustrate how difficult it is to speak of the mentally retarded population in general terms. Hall and Sawyer (1978) proposed a workshop that was designed to develop sexual behavior standards within a facility. A primary purpose of the workshop format is to facilitate, as opposed to hinder, appropriate sexual expression among mentally retarded persons.

The human condition includes the need for human companionship, love, and sexual relationships—mentally retarded persons notwithstanding (Gordon, 1973). Mentally disabled persons have difficulty learning about these needs and acquiring sufficient social skills that would make them obtainable (Franzblau, Green, & Rothenberger, 1979). (See also Chapter 12, "Social Skills," in this volume, regarding specific treatment procedures.) A paucity of effective sex education programming has plagued institutions and schools for the mentally retarded, which has led to undue ignorance as well as vulnerability among this special population. This lack of sex education often leads to sexual difficulties among mentally retarded persons (Gordon, 1973).

Coleman and Murphy (1980) found a high percentage (87%) of sex education programs among facilities for mentally retarded persons. Although the majority of the programs provided sex education, few allowed the residents the freedom within the facility to express sexuality, except through private masturbation. They pointed out that we should not be overly critical of administrators and staff who appear to be projecting a double message; they are responsible to and are pressured by the community and the guardians of the persons under their care. Brantlinger (1985) failed to find the high percentage rates found by Coleman and Murphy (1980); only 42% of the special education teachers that were surveyed had ever programmed sex education. Respondents also acknowledged awareness of frequent sexual activity and misinformation among persons under their care. This situation may be partially explained by the results of Abramson, Parker, and Weisberg (1988), who found that a low percentage of special education teachers were receiving training in sex education instruction.

Haight and Fachting (1986) as well as others noted that sex education for disabled persons has focused on physiological aspects of sexuality, thus relegating love, maturity, and relational stress to peripheral issues. They contended that these peripheral issues are equally important for effective sex education programming, especially for disabled persons who often live in isolation and encounter little exposure to appropriate social modeling and correct information. Reviewing curriculum materials in human sexuality instruction with learning disabled persons, Haight and Fachting (1986) reported that topics covered by these texts included emotional development, physical development, venereal disease, and contraception. A minority of the texts addressed communication, responsibility for pregnancy, self-concept, normalcy, and decision making. Topics inadequately addressed or ignored were: love, marriage, intimacy, romance, privacy, sexual deviance, sexual abuse, consequences of early pregnancy, maturity, sexual roles, and relational stress. The neglect of sexual abuse is particularly disturbing because sexual abuse of people with disabilities is a major problem facing health professionals (Berkman, 1986; Corin, 1986). Given the problem, it seems apparent that mentally retarded persons require instruction in recognizing and reporting sexual abuse.

Johnson (1981, reported in Haight & Fachting, 1986) suggested that sex education should include instruction in sex roles and responsibilities, sexual feelings, self-concept, love, intimacy, romance, marriage, privacy, respect, incest, sexual abuse, decision-making strategies, as well as other traditional physiologically oriented topics. Eastman (1985, cited in Haight & Fachting, 1986) included touching, communication, and limitations to sexual involvement faced by disabled persons as important issues to be addressed.

McCary and McCary (1982) delineated guidelines for instruction in human sexuality, and two of them deserve emphasis here: (1) addressing the emotional aspects may be as important as the biological aspects; and (2) children should be taught that sexual exploitation and manipulation of others is as reprehensible as any other form of manipulation. These issues obviously need to be addressed in a formal structured manner, such as in sex education programs.

Implementing Sex Education Programs

Sex education training programs that are geared to staff and parents of mentally retarded persons can not only increase their awareness of the sexuality of mentally retarded persons but also sensitize them to the specific sexual problems that these persons face. The more comfortable professionals and parents become in discussing sexual issues, the more capable they become in developing healthy sexual attitudes among people under their care. The need for staff and parent sex education to include ways to increase awareness of their own sexuality has been stressed (Monat, 1982). Successful sex education programming for mentally retarded persons seems to include effective education for parents, staff, and the clients, with a major goal being to develop a comfort level that allows for appropriate sexual exploration and expression (Kempton, 1977b; Monat, 1982).

When implementing sex education programming, a needs assessment is advisable, which would include assessing individuals' knowledge about sex and areas in which knowledge is lacking. Once accomplished, need-specific programming can be implemented. The integrity of programming can be enhanced by adequately training the staff. Monat (1982) advocated sex education training in the classroom and the natural environment by as many staff members as possible. Wilson and Baldwin (1976) demonstrated that staff members who volunteer for sex education training improved their knowledge and attitudes about sexuality and the mentally retarded. They warned that a selection bias may occur when sex education training is provided on a voluntary basis; that is, staff members who already hold open-minded attitudes toward sexuality and the mentally retarded may be more likely to volunteer for training. Therefore, all staff members should undergo sex education training to maximize effective programming and consistency across staff.

Sex education strategies for mentally retarded persons must be specific and clear, because this special population learns best with concrete communications rather than subtle messages. Their opportunities for exposure to accurate direct knowledge are small when compared to the normal population. This situation is particularly true for residents in mental retardation centers, where exposure to meaningful models is often lacking.

Training for all staff should be provided, and the material presented should be composed of consistent and clear terminology in order to avoid confusion and strengthen the learning process. As is the case with most teaching strategies regarding mentally retarded persons, sex education teaching strategies should be concrete, repetitive, and geared to meet the specific needs of these individuals. Effective sex education may well occur in the context of an individual's natural environment as opposed to formal classroom instruction. Because classroom instruction runs into generalization difficulties, steps should be taken to overcome this limitation (Monat, 1982).

OPPORTUNITIES FOR SOCIAL INTERACTION

Among variables potentially affecting sexual expression of mentally retarded people are opportunities for varied social contact. Mentally retarded persons living within an institutional setting are often inordinately limited in types of social interaction. The following are four typical characteristics of these settings: (1) All residents are treated alike and are required to do the same thing. (2) A split exists between system staff and persons under their care (residents/students) (Shanley, 1986). (3) Residents are isolated from society over time to the degree that the institution affects/controls every aspect of their lives (Goffman, 1961). (4) In what Goffman refers to as "role dispossession," the mentally retarded person can no longer present different concepts of self to different individuals and groups; that is, he or she develops one role identity because of the interaction with the same people in the same setting day after day.

ATTITUDES OF MENTALLY RETARDED PERSONS

Knowledge about sex and attitudes held by mentally retarded persons could potentially affect the appropriateness of the sexual expression they exhibit. Several studies have explored attitudes and the knowledge base of mentally retarded persons about sexual topics (Brantlinger, 1985; Edmonson & Wish, 1975; Fischer & Krajicek, 1974; Hall & Morris, 1976). Fischer and Krajicek (1974) used pictures to determine mentally retarded adolescents' information about sex-role identification, body parts, menstruation, pregnancy, masturbation, intimate interpersonal behavior, and childbirth. Results indicated that approximately one half had acquired adequate terminology, but few conceptually understood sexual situations, such as intercourse, pregnancy, and childbirth. Through the use of semistructured interviews, Edmonson and Wish (1975) assessed the level of understanding of 18 moderately retarded men on homosexuality, masturbation, dating, marriage, intercourse, pregnancy, childbirth, and anatomical terminology. The median rate of correct responses was a low 28%, and only one respondent answered as many as one half of the items correctly. Brantlinger (1985) explored the attitudes and knowledge about sexual topics of 13 mildly mentally retarded students. Although there was great variation, all respondents were inadequately informed about sex and sexuality. Brantlinger noted that all but three students implied that sex was dirty and nasty. This finding is not surprising because attitudes that are held are based on erroneous information or only partial information.

As can be gleaned from the aforementioned studies, the mentally retarded population suffers from severe deficits with regard to their level of understanding of sexual functioning and their own sexuality in general. These studies indicate a definite need for the provision of effective sex educational programming for this special population. Healthy attitudes toward sexuality cannot be acquired in the face of erroneous information, and appropriate sexual behavior cannot be expected in the face of unhealthy attitudes about sexuality.

STERILIZATION

The practice of sterilization arose as a convenient and effective method to counter unwanted pregnancies among mentally retarded women. A request for sterilization may originate from concerned parents, concerned professionals, a mentally retarded woman's efforts to avoid pregnancy, or a mentally retarded couple's choosing to remain childless. Regardless of who makes the request, sterilization as a means of contraception for mentally retarded persons is a controversial procedure, one that raises ethical and legal questions for parents and guardians of mentally retarded persons, for professionals, and for society as well. When others (e.g., guardians or parents) request sterilization, the question quickly arises as to who will be the beneficiary. And the answers to this are sometimes the parents, the caregivers, or the good of society. Concern for hereditary transmission of mental retardation to offspring, and the child-rearing abilities of potential mentally retarded parents have motivated some to advocate sterilization.

Advocates argue that (1) the mentally retarded reproduce at a higher rate than the nonretarded population, and that (2) mentally retarded persons are more likely to bear children with mental deficits than nonretarded persons (Murphy, Coleman, & Abel, 1981). A majority of studies show a lower reproduction rate among the mentally retarded when compared to the nonretarded population (Floor, Baxter, Rosen, & Zisfein, 1975; Reed & Anderson, 1973). Less opportunity for heterosexual relationships (e.g., marriage) may be a mediating variable operating in these findings. Murphy *et al.* (1981) suggested that as normalization experiences increase, this trend may change.

Research indicates a higher rate of mental retardation among the offspring of mentally retarded persons. Bass (1963) reported that among 25 studies measuring mental retardation rates among the offspring of mentally retarded persons, great variability was present; rates varied from 2.5% to 83%. He noted that some of the variability in rates may be due to variability in the criteria that were used for mental retardation classification. Murphy *et al.* (1981) suggested that sampling bias (the means by which samples were obtained) represents another probable cause of varied rates in these studies. Reed and Anderson (1973) found a mean IQ of 74 for offspring in which both parents were mentally retarded, an IQ of 90 when only one parent was mentally retarded, and an IQ of 107 when neither parent was mentally retarded. The findings of Scally (1973) approximate these results.

The transmission of hereditary defects is usually evident among individuals in the severe range of mental retardation and usually includes physical defects as well (MacLean, 1983). But the etiology of few cases of mental retardation is clearly genetically linked, and 83% of the mentally retarded population were born to nonretarded parents.

Debate and unresolved issues surrounding sterilization of mentally retarded persons suggest that great caution should be taken when considering this option. Evans (1980) reviewed the legal issues involved in sterilization of mentally retarded persons in Canada. In light of legislative action and case law, medical doctors should refuse a request for sterilization (1) when requested on nonmedical grounds, for example, as a contraceptive measure, and (2) when the request is made for a mentally retarded person under the age of 16 (unless physical well-being is at stake). Current regulations of the United States Department of Health and Human Services prohibit persons under 21, people residing in institutions, or persons who are ruled mentally incompetent from sterilization procedures at their own or another's consent (Andron, 1983).

A more popular solution to the misfortunes of sexuality and the handicapped has been proposed through education, and thus, curricula and resource materials have become a major area of emphasis.

CURRICULA AND RESOURCES

The goal of sex education should be to enable clients to acquire adequate knowledge, appropriate attitudes, and values in order to be able to deal with their own sexuality, to relate appropriately to others, and to initiate and sustain pleasurable sexual experiences (Abramson, Parker, & Weisberg, 1988). Unfortunately, many programs are geared to discourage and intimidate, and even to stop individuals from participating in sexual activities. This solution appears to be due to society's inability to come to grips with the fact that mentally handicapped individuals deserve the same rights as others to fully experience their own sexuality. A serious question more difficult to resolve than teaching prerequisite skills is the development and implementation of a curriculum to provide education in sexuality. The issue of what to teach has social, cultural, and religious implications. The authors would argue that behavioral technology can be helpful in problem resolution only when agreement to instruct has occurred, and those who are given the privilege to teach are adequately trained in behavioral technology and are accountable for change. Nevertheless, some general guidelines can be formed. The curricula should tackle three domains, knowledge, attitude, and behavior.

Mentally handicapped individuals generally have little accurate knowledge about sexuality, with most of their information coming from peers (Gebhardt, 1973). Kempton (1977a) reported that many mentally retarded couples did not know about sexual intercourse, and many mentally handicapped women believe that intercourse should not be pleasurable. Brantlinger (1985) found that his subjects varied greatly regarding knowledge about sexual topics, but that none could be described as being "well informed." Reading a portion of the transcript from an interview presented by Brantlinger, it was amazing how little, as well as how wrong, the information generally was. Brantlinger rightfully pointed out the deleterious consequences that could result if these individuals were left to be sexually active while having major distortions in their views.

For mentally handicapped individuals, knowledge on sexuality is important for many reasons and has been argued for by many authorities (Craft & Craft, 1983; Gordon, 1973; Johnson, 1975; Kempton, 1977b). Lack of such knowledge all too often can lead to exploitation (Shindell, 1975). Gordon (1973) noted that for the victims of these unknowing individuals unwanted pregnancy, because of lack of safeguards, is often the result. Incestous behavior, too, can occur when they are ignorant of morals and ethics. Hall and Morris (1976) found that many of their subjects could not accurately describe or identify venereal disease, family planning, and birth control. Through interviews, Fischer and Krajicek (1974) found that their sample of 16 moderately mentally retarded children (aged 10 to 17 years) varied greatly in their knowledge of sex in such areas as interest, sexual identification, and bodily parts and functioning. Many youngsters who are both mentally handicapped and mentally average often see sex and love as synonymous (Renshaw, 1982). Because of their limited exposure to normal individuals, mentally handicapped individuals would be more prone to this behavior and would do almost anything to keep the friendship of others. In studying sexual knowledge of mentally retarded adolescents living at home, Backer (1973) found that few had more than passing knowledge on concrete aspects of sexual behaviors, and even less on such topics as conception, contraception, and venereal disease. Parents and caretakers would prefer that the mentally handicapped person know less about sex (Craft & Craft, 1983), for fear that knowing too much would make the individuals practice indiscriminately what they know (Szymanski, 1977). In general, professionals believe that such a fear is largely unwarranted and has been proven false from the observations carried out by Edgerton and Dingman (1964), who found that mentally retarded individuals were able to control their impulses and obey societal rules. This finding supports the fact that given proper and sufficient education and knowledge, mentally handicapped individuals have the potential to control, decide upon, choose, and reject sexual activity in a far better fashion than generally believed.

Programs to provide sex education for the mentally handicapped are much talked about, but there is little evidence that much teaching on sexuality is being provided in schools in special education classes (Brantlinger, 1985). There are not many systematic programs in sex education for mentally retarded persons, and what little there is largely confined to basic anatomy and physiology, which is inadequate. The curriculum should go beyond this to include such topics as sexual techniques, contraception, pregnancy, venereal diseases, masturbation, homosexuality, and planned parenthood. Furthermore, even when children have received sex education, frequently a misunderstanding of the information has been found, even among normal individuals (Brantingler, 1985). This situation cannot be any better among mentally retarded individuals who are intellectually weak. This situation was the case in the study carried out by Edmonson and Wish (1975), who found that although subjects obtained understanding on anatomy and sexual activity, misinformation was rampant.

Melone and Lettick (1983) outlined a well thought-out program on sex education at Benhaven (in New Haven, Connecticut) that was designed primarily for autistic individuals. It should be borne in mind, however, that most autistic individuals are mentally retarded. Their program contains six units, each having specific behavioral objectives and goals. The units comprise (1) identification of body parts, (2) menstruation, (3) masturbation, (4) physical examination, (5) personal hygiene, and (6) social behavior, with a built-in pre- and posttest. Teachers are given material on what to teach, how to teach, how to structure the group, and what is the duration of each lesson. Specific guidelines are also provided with regard to the vocabulary to be used and the prerequisite skills needed by the students prior to the introduction of each new unit. These researchers reported that the program was highly successful, though they did point to aspects that were weak and needed modifications and adaptations.

Penny and Chataway (1982) reported a sex education program for mentally retarded persons by the Family Planning Association of South Australia. This program constituted six teaching sessions focusing on six topics: (1) development of the adolescent body, (2) reproduction and fetal development, (3) personal relationships and sexual responsibility, (4) male and female roles, (5) planning for parenthood, and (6) contraception and venereal disease. Although the program was individually focused, the researchers did conduct group sessions as the situation warranted and they reported that the program was successful. However, methodological flaws prevented them from arguing any stronger on the efficacy of the program. Patullo and Barnard (1968) developed a successful program to teach menstrual hygiene to a 14-year-old female. In another program, Foxx and McMorrow (1984) demonstrated the effectiveness of an innovative sex education program that they had carried out with institutionalized mentally handicapped adults who were mild and moderately mentally handicapped. They used a commercially available table game to develop social sexual skills. Their posttraining evaluation showed improvement in all skill areas; in addition, generalization was also noted. It should not be concluded that the sex education program can only be successful with the mild mentally handicapped individuals because the case for teaching the moderately handicapped has also been convincing (Bass, 1975; Fujita, 1970; Kempton, 1977). Curriculum content for mentally retarded persons should take into consideration the individual characteristics of these different levels of mental retardation.

Monat (1982) reviewed the sexual characteristics of mentally retarded populations and found that there is not much difference in sexual behavior between the mildly mentally retarded and the nonretarded populations. Whereas the moderately retarded groups tend to function more at a primary reinforcement level, severely mentally retarded individuals, on the other hand, exhibit weak control of sexual impulses and commonly lack development of psychosocial sexual behavior. They have limited ability to predict or forsee the consequences of sexual behavior and are unable to comprehend societal rules. However, profoundly mentally retarded persons deal with only the most basic level of sexual behavior, and this, in most cases, is limited to masturbation. This behavior may result in physical harm because of lack of knowledge and skill, and information on masturbation would be helpful in the programming.

There is no shortage of resources to teach sex education to mentally retarded persons. Any and all material developed for individuals with average intelligence, of which there is an abundance, can be modified and utilized. Even though adaptations and modifications are generally necessary when this material is presented, nevertheless, there is still an impressive array of material available, as, for example, slides on "Sexuality in the Mentally Handicapped" (Kempton, 1978). In fact, such materials as *A Resource Guide in Sex Education for the Mentally Retarded* (1971, which was published jointly by the American Association for Health, Physical Education and Recreation, and the Sex Information Council of the United States, would be helpful for those who are interested in setting up programs and gaining resources. A list of relevant sex education sources and curriculum materials is provided in the Appendix of this chapter. It has to be emphasized, however, that some commercial materials are based on research and knowledge. Many educational programs have a kind of obvious logic to their use and will differ in their degree of effectiveness. Furthermore, the books and visual aids that are available largely depict middle-class values of systems that are foreign to the mentally retarded individual (Meyers, 1971). However, any limitations to the acquisition of knowledge of sexuality and the practice of sexual behavior are often imposed by parents and caretakers rather than the resources or the mental capacity of handicapped individuals.

Little research on sexual behavior of mentally retarded persons has occurred, and scant attention has been paid to developing specific teaching programs and developing appropriate sexual skills for them. The available literature is long on measuring the attitudes of others and knowledge of sexuality among mentally handicapped individuals, but short on programs, treatment procedures, and improvement in residential environments.

Sexuality is one of the most difficult and disturbing issues faced by institutional administrators and staff. Consequently, many have opted to avoid the issue, as evinced by the lack of policies guiding sexual behavior. Most likely, part of the difficulty stems from the fact that there are no quick and easy answers. Even though institutional staff members may sometimes have the knowledge about the sexual needs of mentally retarded persons, all too often they avoid the issue because of legal implications and opposition from the community or parents. A more direct path should be taken with caretakers and parents to help them deal with their attitudes and lack of knowledge about the sexuality of mentally retarded persons. This goal can be accomplished only through training and education. The problems with the status of mentally retarded individuals, both in their knowledge base and behavioral repertoire, seem to be in large part a consequence of the attitudes of parents and caretakers. All caretakers should be provided with mandatory instruction on behavior management and training before they are allowed to work with mentally retarded persons. Also, school personnel should be trained to deal with the issues of the sexuality of mentally handicapped persons with confidentiality, respect, and appropriate strategies.

Curricula to educate mentally handicapped persons about sexuality should go beyond piecemeal activities, and each school should have a full program dealing with all aspects of health, hygiene, and sexual behaviors. Empirically validated techniques and methods should be employed in the teaching and training of sexual behaviors to mentally retarded persons. Commercial programs and guides should be adapted and modified so that they are appropriate to the level of retardation and the language ability of the handicapped person.

It is very important and morally desirable that mentally retarded persons be provided with the education and skills necessary for full functioning in the area of human sexuality. The present trend of ignoring their needs and punishing their inappropriate behavior, with the sole aim of eliminating that behavior, is largely unnecessary and inappropriate.

Behavioral strategies have been shown to be effective in treating inappropriate behaviors related to the sexuality of mentally retarded persons. However, large-scale studies are few, and there is a lack of follow-up data for long-term effect, maintenance, and generalization. Implementors of behavioral strategies, especially parents and caretakers, do not seem to have sufficient knowledge and skills to be effective. For behavioral strategies to work in practice, service providers must assess, monitor, and periodically employ booster sessions at the conclusions of treatment. Poorly designed treatment plans that are inappropriately implemented do more harm than good.

APPENDIX: RESOURCE MATERIAL FOR PLANNING AND TEACHING SEXUALITY PROGRAMS

Printed Materials

American Association for Health, Physical Education and Recreation, and Sex Information and Education Council of the United States. *A Resource Guide in Sex Education for the Mentally Retarded* (Washington, DC: American Association for Health, Physical Education and Recreation, 1971).

American Foundation for the Blind, Inc. *Sex Education for the Visually Handicapped in Schools and Agencies: Selected Papers* (American Foundation for the Blind, 15 West 16th Street, New York, NY 10011).

This material includes programs on beginning sex education programs. Also contains behavioral objectives and learning activities.

Bass, M. S. (1976). *Developing Community Acceptance of Sex Education for the Mentally Retarded.* New York: Human Sciences Press.

Kempton, W., & Forman, R. (1976). *Guidelines for Training on Sexuality and the Mentally Handicapped.* Philadelphia: Planned Parenthood Association of Southeastern Pennsylvania.

McKray, B., Young, C., & Bigley, L. (1979). *Sex Education for Individuals with Developmental Disabilities: An Annotated Bibliography.* Iowa City: University of Iowa.

A Selected Bibliography on Sexuality, Sex Education and Family Planning for Use in Mental Retardation Programs (1976). Minneapolis: Planned Parenthood of Minnesota.

Sex Information and Education Council of the United States: A Bibliography of Resources in Sex Education for the Mentally Retarded (1973). New York: Human Sciences Press.

Films and Filmstrips

All Women Have Periods. 11-minute, 16mm, or an 8mm cassette, color film. Perennial Education, Inc., 477 Roger Williams, P.O. Box 855, Ravinia, Highland Park, IL 60035.

This is a film which deals with menstrual hygiene for developmentally disabled persons.

Birth Control Methods: A Simplified Presentation for the Mentally Retarded. Perennial Education, Inc., 1825 Willow Road, P.O. Box 236, Northfield, IL 60093.

Sex and the Handicapped. 18-minute, 16mm color film. Focus International, Inc., 1 East 53rd Street, New York, NY 10022.

The ABC's of Sex Education for Trainable Persons. 20-minute, 16mm color film. Educational Division, Hallmark Film and Recordings, Inc., 51 New-Plant Court, Owing Mills, MD 21117.

Prepared as an inservice program dealing with how to teach bodily functions, reproduction and social behavior, and responsibilities. Discusses such topics as masturbation, homosexuality, social acceptability, and protection from exploitation.

"Sexuality and the Mentally Handicapped." Winnifred Kempton Slide Series, Omega Films, 133 Manville Road, Unit No. 19, Scarborough, Ontario M1L 4J7.

For teaching the mentally handicapped. Comes with slides, teacher's guide, and scripts. Topics are: parts of the body, male puberty, social behavior, human reproduction, birth control, venereal disease, marriage, and parenting.

"Fertility Regulation for the Mentally Retarded." SIECCAN, 423 Castlefield Avenue, Toronto, Ontario M3J 1P3.

Methods of fertility regulation, their advantages and disadvantages are discussed. Topics include the pills, IUDs, anatomy and physiology of the reproductive cycle.

"The EASE Curriculum." Omega Films, 133 Manville Road, Unit No. 19, Scarborough, Ontario M1L 4J7.

Curriculum for the developmentally handicapped and the retarded adult. Acromym stands for Essential Adult Sex Education. Consists of curriculum guide, pretest and posttest, teaching picture cards, filmstrip, audiocassettes, birth-control and menstrual kit, pupil profile sheet. Deals with four instructional units: biological, sexual behavior, health, and relationships. Companion to the slide series "Sexuality and the Mentally Handicapped."

"Sex Education Slides." Edvick Communications, P.O. Box 3612, Portland, OR 97208.

Slides to aid sex education curriculum for the trainable and moderate level mentally handicapped individuals.

"Like Other People." City Films Distribution, 376 Wellington Street, West, Toronto, Ontario M5V 1E3.

Deals with the sexual, emotional, and social needs of the physically and mentally handicapped persons.

"Your Body during Adolescence." McGraw-Hill Text Films, 330 West 42nd Street, New York, NY 10036.

Provides an outline and discussion of 18 teenagers of different body types, the various stages of development, the structure and function of male and female reproductive organs, puberty, and the roles of the glands.

"The Human Body: The Reproductive System." Coronet Institutional Films, 65 East South Water Street, Chicago, IL 60601.

Graphic presentation of the male and female reproductive systems.

"As Boys Grow." Medical Arts Production, 414 Mason Street, San Francisco, CA 94102.

Deals with developmental behaviors of males, ejaculation, masturbation, and fertilization.

"Story of Menstruation." Kotex Corporation, Kimberly-Clark Corp., North Lake Street, Neenah, WI 54956.

Animated (10-minute) film with diagrams by Walt Disney. Explains the physiology of menstruation.

"Teaching Personal Hygiene and Good Conduct to Teenagers." Harris County Center for the Retarded, Inc., P.O. Box 13403, Houston, TX 77019.

Focuses on hygiene and behavior problems. Includes 6 filmstrips for girls and 5 filmstrips for boys.

REFERENCES

Abramson, P. R., Parker, T., & Weisberg, S. R. (1988). Sexual expression of mentally retarded people: Educational and legal implications. *American Journal of Mental Retardation, 93*(3), 328–334.

Alcorn, D. E. (1974). Parental views on sexual development and education of the trainable mentally retarded. *Journal of Special Education, 8,* 119–130.

Andron, L. (1983). Sexuality counseling with developmentally disabled couples. In A. Craft & M. Craft (Eds.), *Sex education and counselling for mentally handicapped people* (pp. 254–286). Tunbridge Wells: Costello Press.

Backer, H. (1973). Sexual knowledge and attitudes of mentally retarded adolescents. *American Journal of Mental Deficiency, 77,* 706–709.

Bass, M. S. (1963). Marriage, parenthood, and prevention of pregnancy. *American Journal of Mental Deficiency, 68,* 318–333.

Bass, M. S. (1975). Sex education for the handicapped. *Family Coordinator, 23*(1), 27–33.

Berkman, A. (1986). Professional responsibility: Confronting sexual abuse in people with disabilities. *Sexuality and Disability, 7,* 89–95.

Brantingler, E. A. (1985). Mildly mentally retarded secondary students' information about and attitudes toward sexuality and sexuality education. *Education and Training of the Mentally Retarded, 21*(1), 99–108.

Coleman, E. M., & Murphy, W. D. (1980). A survey of sexual attitudes and sex education programs among facilities for the mentally retarded. *Applied Research in Mental Retardation, 1,* 269–276.

Corin, L. (1986). Sexual assault of the disabled: A survey of human service providers. *Sexuality and Disability, 7,* 110–116.

Craft, A., & Craft, M. (1983). *Sex education and counseling for mentally handicapped people,* Baltimore: University Park Press.

Craft, A., & Craft, M. (1985). Sexuality and personal relationship. In M. Craft, J. Bicknell, & S. Hollins (Eds.), *Mental handicap: A multi-disciplinary approach* (pp. 177–196). Philadelphia: Baillière Tindall.

Deisher, R. W. (1973). Sexual behavior of retarded in institutions. In F. F. de la Cruz & G. D. LaVeck (Eds.), *Human sexuality and the mentally retarded* (pp. 51–56). New York: Brunner/Mazel.

Dupras, A., & Tremblay, R. (1976). Path analysis of parents' conservatism toward sex education of their mentally retarded children. *American Journal of Mental Deficiency, 81,* 162–211.

Edgerton, R. B., & Dingman, H. F. (1964). Good reasons for bad supervision: Dating in a hospital for mentally retarded. *Psychiatric Quarterly Supplement, 38,* 221–223.

Edmonson, B., & Wish, J. (1975). Sex knowledge and attitudes of moderately retarded males. *American Journal of Mental Deficiency, 80,* 172–179.

Evans, K. G. (1980). Sterilization of the mentally retarded—A review. *Canadian Medical Association Journal, 123,* 1066–1070.

Fischer, H. L., & Krajicek, M. J. (1974). Sexual development in the moderately retarded child: Level of information and parental attitudes, *Mental Retardation, 12,* 351–354.

Floor, L., Baxter, D., Rosen, M., & Zisfein, L. (1975). A survey of marriages among previously institutionalized retardates. *Mental Retardation, 13,* 33–37.

Foxx, R. M., & McMorrow, M. J. (1984). Teaching social/sexual skills to mentally retarded adults. *American Journal of Mental Deficiency, 89*(1), 9–15.

Franzblau, S. H., Green, J. H., & Rothenberger, G. S. (1979). Educating the learning disabled adolescent about sexuality. *Journal of Learning Disabilities, 12,* 576–580.

Fujita, B. (1970). Sexuality, contraception and the mentally retarded. *Social Medicine, 18*(2), 58–65.

Gebhardt, P. (1973). Sexual behavior of the mentally retarded. In F. F. de La Cruz & G. D. LaVeck (Eds.), *Human sexuality and the mentally handicapped.* New York: Brunner/Mazel.

Goffman, E. (1961). *Asylums: Essays on the social situation of mental patients and other inmates:* Harmondsworth, England: Penguin.

Goodman, R. (1976). Family planning programs for the mentally retarded in institutions and community. *Family Coordinator, 24*(1), 29–35.

Gordon, S. (1973). Sex education for neglected youth: Retarded, handicapped, emotionally disturbed and learning disabled. In S. Gordon (Ed.), *The sexual adolescent* (pp. 62–98). Boston: Duxbury Press.

Greengross, W. (1976). *Entitled to love.* London: Mallaby Press.

Haight, S. L., & Fachting, D. D. (1986). Materials for teaching sexuality, love, and maturity to high school students with learning disabilities. *Journal of Learning Disabilities, 19*, 344–350.

Hall, J. E., & Morris, H. L. (1976). Sexual knowledge and attitudes of institutionalized adolescents. *American Journal of Mental Deficiency, 80*(4), 382–387.

Hall, J. E., & Sawyer, H. W. (1978). Sexual policies for the mentally retarded. *Sexuality and Disability, 1*(1), 34–43.

Hall, J. E., Morris, H. L., & Barker, H. R. (1973). Sexual knowledge and attitude of mentally retarded adolescents. *American Journal of Mental Deficiency, 77*, 706–709.

Johnson, W. R. (1975). *Sex education and counseling of special groups.* Springfield, IL: Charles C Thomas.

Kempton, W. (1977a). Sex education for the mentally handicapped. *Sexuality and Disability, 1*, 137–146.

Kempton, W. (1977b). The sexual adolescent who is mentally retarded. *Journal of Pediatric Psychology, 2*(3), 104–107.

Kempton, W. (1978). Sex education for the mentally handicapped. *Sexuality and Disability, 1*, 137–146.

MacLean, R. (1983). Birth control techniques and counselling for a mentally handicapped population. In A. Craft & M. J. Craft (Eds.), *Sex education and counselling for mentally handicapped people* (pp. 24–112). Turnbridge Wells: Costello Press.

McCary, J. L., & McCary, S. P. (1982). *McCary's human sexuality.* Belmont, CA: Wadsworth.

McEwen, J. L. (1977). Survey of attitudes toward sexual behavior of institutionalized mental retardates. *Psychological Republic, 41*, 874.

Melone, M. B., & Lettick, A. L. (1983). Sex education at Benhaven. In E. Schopler & G. B. Mesibov (Eds.), *Autism in adolescents and adults* (pp. 169–186). New York: Plenum Press.

Meyers, J. H. (1971). Sex and the mentally retarded. *Medical Aspects of Human Sexuality, 5*, 94–118.

Mitchell, L., Doctor, R. M., & Butler, D. C. (1978). Attitudes of caretakers toward the sexual behavior of mentally retarded persons. *American Journal of Mental Deficiency, 83*, 289–296.

Monat, R. K. (1982). *Sexuality and the mentally retarded.* San Diego: College Hill Press.

Mulhern, T. J. (1975). Survey of reported sexual behavior and policies characterizing residential facilities for retarded citizens. *American Journal of Mental Deficiency, 79*, 670.

Murphy, W. D., Coleman, E. M., & Abel, G. G. (1981). Human sexuality in the mentally retarded. In J. L. Matson & F. Andrasik (Eds.), *Treatment issues and innovations in mental retardation* (pp. 581–643). New York: Plenum Press.

Patullo, A. W., & Barnard, K. E. (1986). Teaching menstrual hygiene to the mentally retarded. *American Journal of Nursing, 68*(12), 2572–2575.

Penny, R. C., & Chataway, J. G. (1982). Sexual education for mentally retarded persons. *Australia and New Zealand Journal of Developmental Disabilities, 8*(4), 204–212.

Reed, S. C., & Anderson, B. E. (1973). Effects of changing sexuality on the gene pool. In F. F. de la Cruz & G. D. LaVeck (Eds.), *Human sexuality and the mentally retarded* (pp. 111–125). London: Butterworth.

Renshaw, D. C. (1982). Helping patients with sex problems in the 1980's. *Psychosomatics, 23*(3), 291–294.

Salerno, L. J., Park, J. L., & Giannini, M. J. (1975). Reproductive capacity of the mentally retarded. *Journal of Reproductive Medicine, 14*, 123–129.

Saunders, J. (1979). Staff members' attitudes towards the sexual behavior of mentally retarded residents. *American Journal of Mental Deficiency, 84*, 206–208.

Scally, B. G. (1973). Marriage and mental handicap: Some observations in Northern Ireland. In F. F. de la Cruz & G. D. LaVeck (Eds.), *Human sexuality and the mentally retarded.* London: Butterworth.

Schulman, E. D. (1980). What about sexual activities and marriage for the retarded adults. In E. D. Schulman (Ed.), *Focus on the retarded adults: Programs and services* (pp. 284–312). St. Louis: C. V. Mosby.

Shanley, E. (1986). *Mental handicap: A handbook of care.* London: Churchill Livingstone.

Shindell, P. E. (1975). Sex education program and the mentally handicapped. *Journal of School Health, 45*(2), 88–90.

Szymanski, L. S. (1977). Psychiatric diagnostic evaluation of mentally retarded individuals. *Journal of the American Academy of Child Psychiatry, 16*, 67–87.

Turchin, G. (1974). Sex attitudes of mothers of retarded children. *Journal of School Health, 44*(9), 490–492.

Watson, G., & Rogers, R. S. (1980). Sexual instructions for the mildly retarded and normal adolescent: A comparison of educational approaches, parental expectations and pupil knowledge and attitude. *Health Education Journal, 39*(3), 88–95.

Wilson, R. R., & Baldwin, B. A. (1976). A pilot sexuality training workshop for staff at an institution for the mentally retarded. *American Journal of Public Health, 66,* 77–78.

Index

DATE DUE
